Applied Pharmaceutics

Applied Pharmaceutics

Edited by **Erica Helmer**

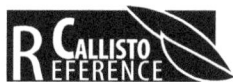

R **C**ALLISTO
REFERENCE

New York

Published by Callisto Reference,
106 Park Avenue, Suite 200,
New York, NY 10016, USA
www.callistoreference.com

Applied Pharmaceutics
Edited by Erica Helmer

International Standard Book Number: 978-1-63239-748-5 (Hardback)

The publisher's policy is to use permanent paper from mills that operate a sustainable forestry policy. Furthermore, the publisher ensures that the text paper and cover boards used have met acceptable environmental accreditation standards.

Trademark Notice: Registered trademark of products or corporate names are used only for explanation and identification without intent to infringe.

Printed in the United States of America.

Contents

Preface

This book outlines the processes and applications of applied pharmaceutics in detail. It will unravel the recent studies in this field. The field of pharmaceutics refers to the practice of forming new medicines from existing drugs, which are useful, harmless and efficient for the human body. Some of the key components of this field include molecular drug design, novel drug delivery, conventional dosage forms, nanotechnology, etc. This book includes topics that are of utmost significance to this field and are bound to provide incredible insights to the readers. It is a collective contribution of a renowned group of international experts. Students, researchers, pharmacists, doctors, and all associated with the discipline of pharmaceutics will find this book full of crucial and unexplored concepts.

This book has been the outcome of endless efforts put in by authors and researchers on various issues and topics within the field. The book is a comprehensive collection of significant researches that are addressed in a variety of chapters. It will surely enhance the knowledge of the field among readers across the globe.

It gives us an immense pleasure to thank our researchers and authors for their efforts to submit their piece of writing before the deadlines. Finally in the end, I would like to thank my family and colleagues who have been a great source of inspiration and support.

Editor

An Overview of the CNS-Pharmacodynamic Profiles of Nonselective and Selective GABA Agonists

Xia Chen,[1] Sanne de Haas,[2] Marieke de Kam,[2] and Joop van Gerven[2]

[1] *Phase I Unit of Clinical Pharmacological Research Center, Peking Union Medical College Hospital, 100032 Beijing, China*
[2] *Centre for Human Drug Research, 2333 CL Leiden, The Netherlands*

Correspondence should be addressed to Xia Chen, connie1976@vip.sina.com

Academic Editor: Keith Wafford

Various $\alpha_{2,3}$ subtype selective partial GABA-A agonists are in development to treat anxiety disorders. These compounds are expected to be anxiolytic with fewer undesirable side effects, compared to nonselective GABA-A agonists like benzodiazepines. Several $\alpha_{2,3}$ subtype selective and nonselective GABA-A agonists have been examined in healthy volunteers, using a battery addressing different brain domains. Data from five placebo-controlled double-blind studies were pooled. Lorazepam 2 mg was the comparator in three studies. Three $\alpha_{2,3}$-selective GABAA agonists (i.e., TPA023, TPACMP2, SL65.1498), one α_1-selective GABAA agonists (zolpidem), and another full agonist (alprazolam) were examined. Pharmacological selectivity was assessed by determination of regression lines for the change from baseline of saccadic-peak-velocity- (ΔSPV-) relative effect, relative to changes in different pharmacodynamic endpoints (ΔPD). SPV was chosen for its sensitivity to the anxiolysis of benzodiazepines. Slopes of the ΔSPV-ΔPD relations were consistently lower with the $\alpha_{2,3}$ selective GABA-A agonists than with lorazepam, indicating that their PD effects are less than their SPV-effects. The ΔSPV-ΔPD relations of lorazepam were comparable to alprazolam. Zolpidem showed relatively higher impairments in ΔPD relative to ΔSPV, but did not significantly differ from lorazepam. These PD results support the pharmacological selectivity of the $\alpha_{2,3}$-selective GABA-A agonists, implying an improved therapeutic window.

1. Introduction

Anxiety is a psychological and physiological state with somatic, emotional, cognitive, and behavioral components [1], which dominates thinking and leads to disturbance of daily functioning. Serotonergic antidepressants, either selective serotonin reuptake inhibitors (SSRIs) or serotonin-norepinephrine reuptake inhibitors (SNRIs), are currently prescribed as the 1st-line treatment for several anxiety disorders. However, the slow onset of therapeutic effect and the presence of sexual side effects prevent these drugs from more extensive use and lead to lack of treatment compliance [2]. Moreover, SSRIs/SNRIs cause transient increase of anxiety during the first few weeks of administration. All these clinical experiences provide space for the use of benzodiazepines (BZDs) in acute anxiety episodes.

Benzodiazepines are the most commonly prescribed anxiolytic drugs, although treatment guidelines generally limit their use to several weeks to prevent the occurrence of tolerance and dependence. Benzodiazepines are allosteric modulators of the $GABA_A$ receptors that affect the central nervous system (CNS) as full GABAergic agonists [3]. As a consequence, these drugs have detrimental effects on alertness, memory, postural stability, and muscle tone. In loss-of-function studies conducted in point-mutated mice [4], different subtypes of $GABA_A$ receptors have been found responsible for the specific aspects of benzodiazepine pharmacology: (1) α_1-containing receptors are associated with sedative effects of benzodiazepines [5, 6]; (2) α_2/α_3-containing receptors are related to anxiolysis and analgesia [7, 8]; (3) α_5-receptors are associated with cognition [9, 10]. BZDs exert their CNS actions in a concentration-related manner [11]. The anxiolytic, hypnotic, muscle relaxant, and amnesic effects of BZDs generally appear concomitantly, and the onset and duration of action of the compounds correlate closely with their pharmacokinetic properties. The effect profile of BZDs has been attributed to their non-selective agonism at the α_1, α_2, α_3, and α_5 subunit-containing $GABA_A$ receptors. To improve the pharmacological and functional selectivity, novel GABAergic anxioselective compounds are

TABLE 1: *In vitro* pharmacological property of the GABAergic compounds.

Compound	α_1		α_2		α_3		α_5		α_1/α_2-ratio
	K_i (nM)	Efficacy° (%)	K_i (nM)	Efficacy°(%)	K_i (nM)	Efficacy°(%)	K_i (nM)	Efficacy° (%)	
TPA023* [26]	0.27	0[#]	0.31	11	0.19	21	0.41	5	0
TPACMP2* [13]	0.22	18	0.40	23	0.21	45	0.23	18	0.78
SL65.1498[#] [28]	17	45	73	115	80	83	215	48	0.39
Zolpidem	20 [29]	75[§] [30]	400 [29]	78[§] [30]	400 [29]	80[§]	5000 [29]	9[§] [30]	0.96

° Relative efficacy is defined as the extent of the potentiation of GABA-A EC20-equivalent current produced by the compound compared to that produced by a nonselective full agonist (chlordiazepoxide/diazepam).
* Mean values of 3 experiments in Xenopus oocytes with human recombinant $\alpha\beta3\gamma2$ receptors; efficacy relative to chlordiazepoxide.
[#] Mean values of 3 experiments in hek293 cells with recombinant rat receptors $\alpha\beta2\gamma2$; efficacy relative to chlordiazepoxide.
[§] Mean values of 3 experiments in Xenopus oocytes with human recombinant $\alpha\beta2\gamma2$ receptor; efficacy relative to diazepam.

TABLE 2: Component tests of the Neurocart battery and the related CNS domains.

Neurocart test	Targeted function	Related CNS areas
Saccadic eye movement	Neurophysiologic function	Superior colliculus, substantia nigra, amygdala
Smooth pursuit	Neurophysiologic function	Midbrain
Adaptive tracking	Visuomotor coordination	Neocortex, basal nuclei, brain stem, cerebellum
Body sway	Balance	Cerebellum, brain stem
Visual verbal learning test (VVLT)	Memory	Hippocampus
VAS Bond and Lader	Alertness, mood, calmness	Cortex, prefrontal cortex
VAS Bowdle	Feeling high, internal and external perception	Cortex, prefrontal cortex, amygdala

evaluated using recombinant human GABA$_A$ receptors during preclinical development. The GABAergic effect profile of a compound is characterized by the affinity of the ligand for the receptor and by the *in vitro* efficacy of the compound at each GABA$_A$ receptor subtype. In the past years, several partial GABA$_A$ agonists have been developed, which have a relatively high *in vitro* efficacy at α_2/α_3 subtypes compared with α_1 or α_5 subtypes. Such α_2/α_3 subtype-selective partial GABA agonists are anticipated to have favorable therapeutic effect and to be less sedating or cognition impairing (Table 1).

Based on nonclinical investigations with *in vitro* assays and animal models of anxiety, the human pharmacology of novel GABAergic agents is approached through sequential clinical studies regarding pharmacokinetics, receptor occupancy, and pharmacodynamics (PD) in healthy volunteers. Direct links have been proposed between plasma drug concentration and receptor occupancy [4], as well as between plasma drug concentration and pharmacodynamic parameters [12–15]. Such pharmacokinetic/pharmacodynamic (PK/PD) relationships warrant the assessment of surrogate biomarkers in healthy volunteers treated with single doses of selective novel GABAergic compound(s).

More than 170 pharmacodynamic tests or test variants have been developed to assess the CNS effects of benzodiazepines [11]. De Visser et al. analyzed the interstudy consistence, sensitivity, and pharmacological specificity of the frequently used biomarkers. Saccadic peak velocity (SPV) and visual analogue scale of alertness (VAS$_{alertness}$) were identified as the most sensitive parameters for benzodiazepines. Both tests showed consistent effects to a variety of benzodiazepines at different doses.

During the past fifteen years, the Centre for Human Drug Research (CHDR) has established a selection of computerized neuropsycho-pharmacodynamic tests called the Neurocart battery. The components of this battery target a variety of neurophysiological and/or neuropsychological domains (Table 2). Of this battery, adaptive tracking, saccadic eye movements, and body sway were proved sensitive to the sedating effects of sleep deprivation [16], as well as benzodiazepines and other GABAergic drugs. In the recent years, the Neurocart battery was used in a series of phase I studies to assess CNS pharmacodynamics of partial $\alpha_{2,3}$ subtype selective GABA$_A$ agonists. Both nonselective and/or selective GABA$_A$ agonists were administered as single oral dose to healthy volunteers. Clear distinctions of effect profile were observed in these trials [12–14]. The objective of this paper was to characterize the pharmacodynamic effect profiles of novel anxioselective GABA$_A$ agonists and identify suitable biomarkers to distinguish $\alpha_{2,3}$ subtype-specific GABA$_A$ agonists from full GABA$_A$ agonists like benzodiazepines.

2. Methods

Five clinical studies, all of which are published [12–15, 17], were conducted at the CHDR in healthy volunteers after approval from the Ethics Review Board of Leiden University Medical Centre. All subjects provided written inform consent for study participation. Each trial was designed as single-dose, cross-over or parallel-armed, randomized, double-blind, placebo- and/or positive-controlled study. The subjects took single oral doses of a selective GABAergic compound, placebo-, and/or a nonselective benzodiazepine. Three studies used lorazepam 2 mg as a positive control, whereas in the studies with zolpidem 10 mg and alprazolam 1 mg, these drugs were the only GABAergic study medications. Data of all studies came from the same research center and were pooled from the studies-specific electronic databases kept by the center. *In vitro* pharmacological parameters of novel compounds were extracted from the Investigator's Brochures and published articles. These parameters provide reliable information about the subtype selectivity of each compound, but it is more difficult to compare the pharmacological properties between the drugs. Due to the diversity of cell types and $GABA_A$ receptor homologies used in the whole-cell patch clamping assays, the links between *in vitro* pharmacology and human *in vivo* effects are considered less quantitative and semiquantitative comparisons are preferred.

2.1. Treatments. Three novel drugs designed to be $\alpha_{2,3}$ subtype selective were dosed in three of the above-mentioned studies (for each dose group, the number of study participants is provided in parentheses): TPA023 0.5 mg, 1.5 mg ($n = 12$) [12]; TPACPM2 (MK0343) 0.25 mg, 0.75 mg ($n = 12$) [13]; SL65.1498 2.5 mg, 7.5 mg, and 25 mg ($n = 20$) [14]. Zolpidem is a hypnotic with a high affinity for α_1-subtypes, and alprazolam is a nonselective GABAergic anx-anxiolyticiolytic. Zolpidem 10 mg ($N = 14$) [15] and alprazolam 1 mg ($N = 20$) were administered in another two studies, respectively.

2.2. Pharmacodynamic Assessments

2.2.1. Saccadic Eye Movement. Saccadic eye movements are very sensitive to a variety of mostly CNS-depressant drugs [18, 19]. Saccadic peak velocity has been shown to be closely related to the anxiolytic properties of benzodiazepines [4]. Since partial $\alpha_{2,3}$-subtype-selective $GABA_A$ agonists are developed to be anxiolytic, it was expected that these compounds would reduce saccadic peak velocity, similar to what is typically observed with benzodiazepines. Therefore, saccadic peak velocity was used as a biomarker for the anxiolytic properties of the $GABA_A$ agonists, to which all other pharmacodynamics effects were compared in this meta-analysis. Recording and analysis of saccadic eye movements was conducted with a microcomputer-based system for sampling and analysis of eye movements. The program for signal collection and the AD converter were from Cambridge Electronic Design (CED Ltd., Cambridge, UK), the amplifiers were supplied by either Nihon Kohden (Nihon Kohden, Life Scope EC, Tokyo, Japan) or Grass (Grass-Telefactor, An Astro-Med, Inc. Product Group, Braintree, USA), and the sampling and analysis scripts were developed at CHDR (Leiden, The Netherlands).

2.2.2. Smooth Pursuit. The same systems as used for saccadic eye movements were also used for measuring smooth pursuit. For smooth pursuit eye movements, the target moves sinusoidally at frequencies ranging from 0.3 to 1.1 Hz, in steps of 0.1 Hz. The amplitude of target displacement corresponds to 22.5 degrees eyeball rotation to both sides. Four cycles were recorded for each stimulus frequency. The method has been validated at CHDR by Van Steveninck based on the work of Bittencourt et al. [20] and the original description of Baloh et al. [21].

2.2.3. Visual Analogue Scales (VASs). Visual analogue scales as originally described by Norris [22] were used previously to quantify subjective effects of benzodiazepines [19]. From the set of sixteen scales, three composite factors were derived as described by Bond and Lader [23], corresponding to alertness, mood, and calmness. These factors were used to quantify subjective drug effects.

2.2.4. Body Sway. The body sway meter measures body movements in a single plane, providing a measure of postural stability. Body sway was measured with an apparatus similar to the Wright ataxiameter, which integrates the amplitude of unidirectional body movement transferred through a string attached to the subject's waist. Two-minute measurements were made in the anteroposterior direction with eyes open and closed, with the subject standing comfortably on a firm surface with their feet slightly apart. The method has been used before to demonstrate postural instability due to benzodiazepines [24, 25].

2.2.5. Adaptive Tracking. The adaptive tracking test as developed by Hobbs and Strutt was used, according to specifications of Atack et al. [26]. The adaptive tracking test is a pursuit-tracking task. A circle of known dimensions moves randomly across a screen. The test subject must try to keep a dot inside the moving circle by operating a joystick. If this effort was successful, the speed of the moving circle increases. Conversely, the velocity was reduced if the test subject cannot maintain the dot inside the circle. The adaptive tracking test is a measure of visuomotor coordination that has proved to be very sensitive of various psychoactive drugs [27].

Table 3 summarizes the pharmacodynamic tests used in the different studies.

2.3. Statistical Analysis. Individual graphs are generated for each pharmacodynamic variable (*y*-axis) versus SPV change from baseline (*x*-axis). Summary graphs are generated with lorazepam and one other treatment per graph, for all GABAergic treatments.

A regression analysis of change from baseline of body sway (ΔSway), tracking (ΔTrack), VAS alertness ($\Delta VAS_{alertness}$), or VAS calmness ($\Delta VAS_{calmness}$) against the change from baseline of SPV (ΔSPV) was performed with a mixed effect model on the available individual data. The fixed factor was the GABAergic treatment and treatment by saccadic peak velocity, while the random factors were subject slope and intercept. The values of body sway were analyzed after log-transformation, while the other parameters were taken without transformation. The estimates of the slopes of the linear relations of these ΔSPV-relative effect profiles were compared between each dose of subtype-selective $GABA_A$ agonists and lorazepam. The estimates of slopes, their estimated difference, and the *P* values were tabulated. Thereafter, summary plots were generated, combined with the population regression line as calculated in the regression.

All statistical analyses were carried out with SAS for Windows v9.1.3 (SAS institute, inc., Cary, NC, USA).

TABLE 3: Use of pharmacodynamic tests in each study.

Study	CHDR99112	CHDR0102	CHDR0105	CHDR0614	CHDR0407
compound	TPA023	TPACMP2	SL65.1498	Alprazolam	Zolpidem
comparator	Lorazepam	Lorazepam	Lorazepam	NA	NA
SEM	Done	Done	Done	Done	Done
Sway	Done	Done	Done	Done	Done
VAS BL	Done	Done	Done	Done	Done
Smooth	ND	ND	Done	Done	Done
Track	ND	ND	ND	Done	Done

ND: not done; NA: not applicable; SEM: saccadic eye movement; Smooth: smooth pursuit; Sway: body sway; VAS BL: VAS Bond and Lader; Track: adaptive tracking.

TABLE 4: Results of the linear model for saccadic peak velocity change from baseline and log body sway change from baseline by treatment with treatment by SPV change from baseline as interaction.

Treatment	ΔSPV-relative relation	Item	Estimate of treatment	Estimate of lorazepam	P value
TPA023 1.5 mg	ΔSway-ΔSPV	Slope	−0.00048	−0.00305	<0.0001
		Intercept	−0.01316	0.1292	<0.0001
	ΔVAS$_{alertness}$-ΔSPV	Slope	0.03312	0.126	0.0001
		Intercept	0.4551	−4.4739	0.0021
TPACMP2 0.75 mg	ΔSway-ΔSPV	Slope	−0.00027	−0.00305	<0.0001
		Intercept	0.03784	0.1292	0.0009
	ΔVAS$_{alertness}$-ΔSPV	Slope	0.09884	0.126	0.2525
		Intercept	−1.4465	−4.4739	0.0397
SL65.1498 25 mg	ΔSway-ΔSPV	Slope	−0.00128	−0.00305	0.0003
		Intercept	0.0222	0.1292	<0.0001
	ΔVAS$_{alertness}$-ΔSPV	Slope	0.04193	0.126	0.0009
		Intercept	0.2453	−4.4739	<0.0001
	ΔSmooth-ΔSPV	Slope	0.01554	0.1099	<0.0001
		Intercept	−1.4483	−6.2553	<0.0001
Alprazolam 1 mg	ΔSway-ΔSPV	Slope	−0.00204	−0.00305	0.0667
		Intercept	0.001788	0.1292	<0.0001
	ΔVAS$_{alertness}$-ΔSPV	Slope	0.0734	0.126	0.0763
		Intercept	−0.628	−4.4739	0.0254
	ΔTrack-ΔSPV	Slope	0.0747	0.0572	0.1545
		Intercept	0.3023	−4.0742	<0.0001
	ΔSmooth-ΔSPV	Slope	0.08077	0.1099	0.2808
		Intercept	−1.4025	−6.2553	0.0002
Zolpidem 10 mg	ΔSway-ΔSPV	Slope	−0.0033	−0.00305	0.7336
		Intercept	0.06014	0.1292	0.0127
	ΔVAS$_{alertness}$-ΔSPV	Slope	0.1526	0.126	0.5231
		Intercept	−3.2697	−4.4739	0.5219
	ΔTrack-ΔSPV	Slope	0.0489	0.0572	0.6240
		Intercept	−0.9123	−4.0742	<0.0001
	ΔSmooth-ΔSPV	Slope	0.09771	0.1099	0.7412
		Intercept	−3.8439	−6.2553	0.0815

3. Results

3.1. ΔSPV-ΔSway Relation (Δ = Change from Baseline). Average changes from baseline of body sway against SPV within the investigational time course (i.e., 6 hours after dose) were plotted by study. Figure 1 demonstrates clear distinctions between the ΔSPV-relative effect profile of lorazepam 2 mg

and most doses of the $\alpha_{2,3}$-subtype selective compounds (i.e., TPA023 1.5 mg, TPACMP2 0.75 mg). The full GABA$_A$ agonist alprazolam is similar to lorazepam. The slope of the ΔSPV-ΔSway plots for zolpidem is slightly steeper than for lorazepam.

As was revealed by the statistical analysis using the mixed linear model (Table 4), the estimated differences

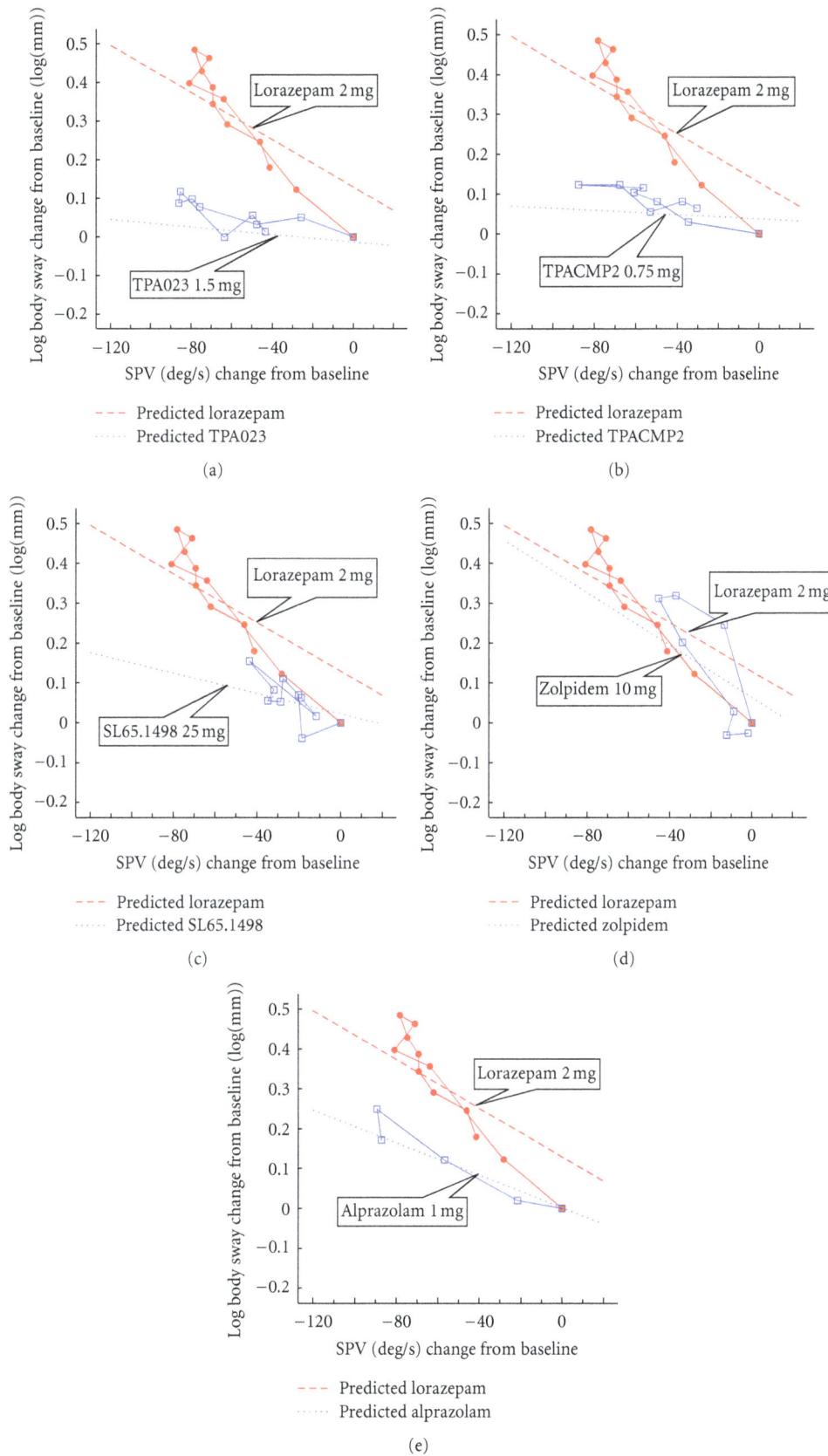

FIGURE 1: ΔLogSway (log mm)-ΔSPV (deg/sec) relative effect profile of TPA023 1.5 mg, TPACMP2 0.75 mg, SL65.1498 25 mg, zolpidem 10 mg, and alprazolam 1 mg versus lorazepam 2 mg, respectively. (Blue open square: investigational compound; red closed circle: lorazepam 2 mg; blue dot line: the comparator drug; red dash line: lorazepam 2 mg.)

of the slope of regression lines are statistically significant between lorazepam and the $\alpha_{2,3}$ subtype selective partial GABAergic treatment of TPA023 1.5 mg, TPACMP2 0.75 mg, and SL65.1498 25 mg. There is no statistically significant difference between the slopes for lorazepam and alprazolam, and the difference with zolpidem suggested by the average plots (Figure 1) is not confirmed by the model (Table 4).

3.2. ΔSPV-$\Delta VAS_{alertness}$ Relation. Figure 2 plots the average values of $\Delta VAS_{alertness}$ versus ΔSPV obtained from individual subjects per study. As was found for the ΔSPV-$\Delta Sway$ relations, a similar difference to lorazepam was observed with novel subtype selective GABAergic compounds. The slopes of the regression line of the ΔSPV-$\Delta Sway$ relation for TPA023 1.5 mg and SL65.1498 25 mg are statistically shallower than the slope for lorazepam, respectively. No statistical differences can be demonstrated for TPACMP2 0.75 mg, alprazolam 1 mg, or zolpidem 10 mg.

3.3. ΔSPV-$\Delta Smooth$ Relation. Figure 3 and Table 4 provide the ΔSPV-relative effect profiles and the slopes and intercept for smooth pursuit after alprazolam, zolpidem, and SL65.1498. Smooth pursuit was not determined with the other partial agonists. Statistically significant differences are found in the slope of regression lines with SL65.2498 25 mg. Zolpidem and alprazolam show comparable slopes to lorazepam.

3.4. ΔSPV-ΔPD Relations versus In Vitro Pharmacological Properties. This analysis surmises that comparisons of ΔSPV-ΔPD profiles represent the underlying pharmacological characteristics of subtype selective and nonselective GABA$_A$ agonists. A further corroboration of this approach could be provided by a comparison of ΔSPV-ΔPD profiles with the underlying pharmacological properties. This should be possible in principle, but the quantitative preclinical information provided in Table 1 was derived from different sources which in themselves were incomparable, despite the fact that all programs used oocyte-clamp assays to characterize the different GABAergic compounds. Some of these differences could be diminished by calculation of the ratio of relative efficacy on the α_1 GABA$_A$ subunit to that on the α_2 subunit, as a benchmark of α_2-specificity of the GABAergic compounds. This calculated ratio is provided in Table 1. Although the number of compounds in this overview is too small for any meaningful statistical evaluation, it is interesting that the four compounds for which this could be calculated showed a close relationship between α_1/α_2-efficacy ratios and ΔSPV-ΔVAS alertness ratios with borderline statistical significance ($r^2 = 0.86$, two-sided $P = 0.0727$). Due to the absence of *in vitro* pharmacological data and the difference of experimental settings of the trail with alprazolam, alprazolam was not included into the present analysis.

4. Discussion

This analysis was performed to explore the central nervous system (CNS) effects of various GABAergic agents and characterize the pharmacodynamic effect profiles of these compounds in healthy volunteers and correlate such profiles to their pharmacological properties.

A battery of CNS pharmacodynamic tests was administered to healthy volunteers who were dosed with GABAergic compound(s). The composition of the CNS battery was based on the sensitivity of the measurements to nonselective GABAergic treatments, and on the coverage of a wide range of different CNS domains (Table 2). This approach enabled us to identify unique effect profiles for pharmacologically distinct GABAergic treatments, including (1) traditional, pharmacologically nonselective, full GABAergic compounds at their clinical dose(s) (i.e., lorazepam 2 mg and alprazolam 1 mg), (2) a marketed GABAergic compound with high α_1-subtype affinity (i.e., zolpidem 10 mg), and (3) several novel, $\alpha_{2,3}$-subtype selective GABAergic compounds at different investigational doses.

The new class of partial subtype selective GABA agonists was expected to be anxiolytic but less sedating and cognition impairing, as indicated by the preclinical *in vitro* and *in vivo* data. The anxiolytic effects of nonselective GABAergic agonists are accompanied by somnolence, impaired locomotion, and cognitive disturbance. These clinical side effects are reflected by the pharmacodynamics effects of lorazepam or alprazolam on VAS$_{alertness}$ (measure of subjective sedation), body sway (measure of postural instability), and adaptive tracking (measure of visuomotor coordination). Memory testing was not performed frequently and consistently enough to allow a comparative analysis among the different compounds. However, the original publication of the TPA023-study provides indications that the partial subtype selective GABA agonist has fewer cognitive effects than the partial subtype selective GABA agonist. In this study, lorazepam 2 mg showed clear memory reductions, which did not occur with a dose of TPA023 1.5 mg that caused comparable SPV reductions [12].

Saccadic peak velocity (SPV) has previously been shown to be closely related to the anxiolytic doses of benzodiazepines [11], and SPV was therefore used as a reference parameter. As expected, SPV showed significant responses to almost every GABAergic compound investigated in these six studies [12–14]. In contrast to lorazepam or alprazolam, which influenced each output parameter of the saccadic eye movement test (i.e., SPV, saccadic reaction time, and inaccuracy), the α_1-(zolpidem) or $\alpha_{2,3}$-subtype selective GABAergic compounds (TPA023, TPACMP2, SL65.1498) only affected SPV.

At their highest investigational dose, the effect size of TPA023 and TPACMP2 on SPV was comparable to the effects observed with lorazepam or alprazolam, whereas the effect of SL65.1498 was only marginally significant on SPV. In almost all these cases, the impact on other CNS effects was lower. This by itself is an indication of pharmacological selectivity, but a comparison based merely on overall or maximum effects could obscure some of the more subtle pharmacological differences (like the findings of SL65.1498 study) when the pharmacodynamic biomarker is less sensitive to the drug or if the dose of a drug

(a)

(b)

(c)

(d)

(e)

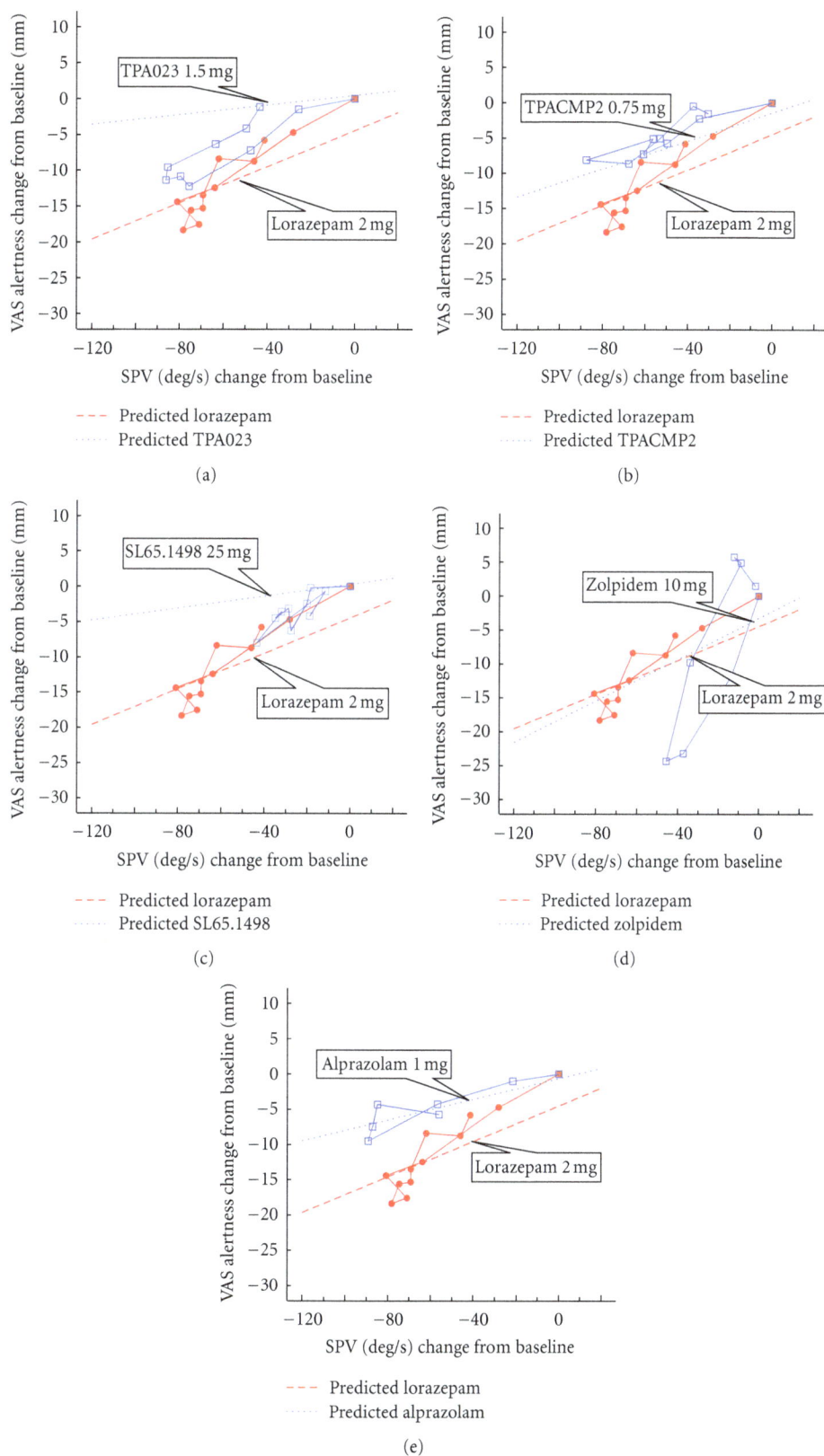

FIGURE 2: $\Delta VAS_{alertness}$-ΔSPV relative effect profile of TPA023 1.5 mg, TPACMP2 0.75 mg, SL65.1498 25 mg, zolpidem 10 mg, and alprazolam 1 mg versus lorazepam 2 mg, respectively. (Blue open square: investigational compound; red closed circle: lorazepam 2 mg; blue dot line: the comparator drug, red dash line; lorazepam 2 mg.)

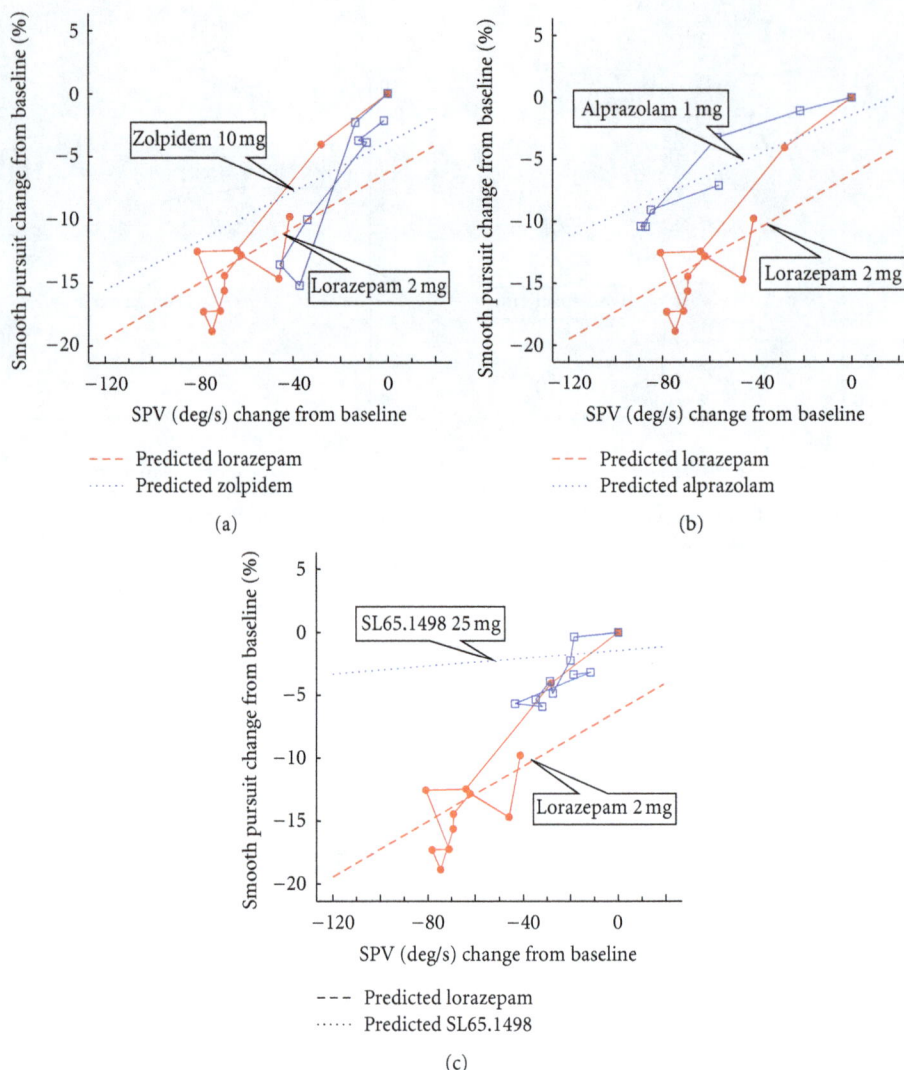

FIGURE 3: ΔSmooth-ΔSPV relative effect profile of SL65.1498 25 mg, zolpidem 10 mg, and alprazolam 1 mg versus lorazepam 2 mg, respectively. (Blue open square: investigational compound; red closed circle: lorazepam 2 mg; blue dot line: the comparator drug, red dash line; lorazepam 2 mg.)

is subtherapeutic. The relationships between the ΔSPV-effects and other pharmacodynamic (ΔPD) effects provide a complete profile of the differential effects, at each time point after drug administration. These outputs reflect the degree of $\alpha_{2,3}$ selectivity and may therefore also be indicators for anxioselectivity. Based on these perceptions, a GABAergic compound with "flat" regression lines in the ΔSPV-relative plotting graphs would show anxiolysis with reduced off-target effects in clinical settings. For most of the novel compounds described in this overview, there are no clinical reports of anxiolytic effects or improved tolerability. However, a recent article on TPA023, the oldest compound in this meta-analysis, reported reduced anxiety in a preliminary clinical trial at doses that were also used in our pharmacodynamic studies [4]. No detailed comparative information is available on the therapeutic window in these clinical trials.

We found that the ΔSPV-relative effect profiles of $\alpha_{2,3}$ subtype-specific GABAergic compounds are similar among

each other but different from lorazepam 2 mg. The absolute slopes of the regression lines for the ΔSPV-ΔPD relations are generally lower with the selective GABA$_A$ agonists than with the benzodiazepines. The results of alprazolam were comparable to lorazepam, which provides additional confidence that the analyses reflect pharmacological differences as well as similarities. Zolpidem seemed to be the only major exception, since this α_1 subtype-selective GABAergic compound produced considerably steeper average slopes for certain ΔSPV-relative profiles than lorazepam or alprazolam, whereas the statistical population model did not reveal statistically significant differences between zolpidem and the benzodiazepines. This could reflect a limitation of the population model for ΔSPV-ΔPD relationships, which was chosen to be simple and unbiased, but necessarily had to ignore some rather complex individual response relationships. The analyses were based on linear slope estimates without a fixed intercept. In reality, however, all individual data points started at a fixed intercept (at $T = 0$, when ΔSPV and

ΔPD were both zero), and, in many cases, the ΔSPV-ΔPD relationships were not linear, and zolpidem even formed loops when the SPV effect displayed a different time course than the PD effect. In almost all other cases, however, the statistical analyses and the graphical representations of the average relationships provide accurate representations of the individual plots.

This meta-analysis indicates that comparisons of ΔSPV-ΔPD profiles are able to identify pharmacological differences between subtype selective and nonselective GABA$_A$ agonists. A comparison of ΔSPV-ΔPD profiles with the underlying pharmacological properties was refuted by the very small number of compounds for which this could be compared. Nonetheless, strong relationships (with an R-value of 0.93) between the α_1/α_2-ratios of the four compounds for which this could be determined and their ΔSPV-ΔVAS$_{alertness}$ ratios. Clearly this remains to be confirmed with larger numbers of compounds. Still, the consistent ΔSPV-relative profiles of the selective GABAergic compounds suggest potential links between the preclinical profiles and the ΔSPV-relative pharmacodynamics profiles of these compounds. Moreover, TPACMP2 showed a distinct ΔSPV-ΔVAS$_{alertness}$ relation but shared a similar ΔSPV-ΔSway relation with the other $\alpha_{2,3}$-subtype-selective GABAergic agonists. The relatively large amount of sedation with TPACMP2 could reflect the relatively high ratio of α_1/α_2-efficacy of TPMCMP2 compared to the other compounds. Similarly, the large efficacy of zolpidem is compatible with its steep ΔSPV-ΔVAS$_{alertness}$ ratio and the strong hypnosedative effect of this z-hypnotic in the clinic.

5. Conclusion

TPA023, TPACMP2, and SL65.1498 are members of the novel experimental drug family of $\alpha_{2,3}$-subtype selective receptor agonists. *In vitro* pharmacological properties of these compounds indicate higher binding affinity and relative efficacy at the $\alpha_{2,3}$-subunits. *In vivo* preclinical studies with animal models translated such pharmacological properties into potential of anxiolysis and relatively reduced off-target effects in comparison with nonselective full GABAergic agonists like benzodiazepines.

The Neurocart battery is a collection of validated tests amenable to the effects of various CNS-acting drugs. Components of this battery were shown to be sensitive to different rapid-onset CNS effects of the benzodiazepines, in which reduction of saccadic peak velocity displays features of a GABAergic anxiolytic biomarker, whereas impairments of body sway, adaptive tracking, and memory are translated to effects that are less desirable for an anxiolytic drug. Most novel GABAergic compounds showed dose-dependent responses to saccadic peak velocity but did not affect the other CNS effects to the same extent, indicative of the pharmacoselectivity of these new compounds. Moreover, the ΔSPV-relative effect profiles provide information about dose potency and effect specificity. This battery is suitable to not only present the general depressive effects of benzodiazepines but also demonstrate the pharmacological selectivity and specificity of the novel GABAergic compounds. Comparative

effect profiling as used in these studies can provide clear indications for the pharmacological selectivity and specificity of novel GABAergic compounds in healthy volunteers. This is a valuable approach for the early drug development of this new drug class, which will hopefully contribute novel anxiolytics with an improved therapeutic window to patients with anxiety disorders.

References

[1] M. E. P. Seligman, E. F. Walker, and D. L. Rosenhan, *Abnormal Psychology*, W.W. Norton & Company, New York, NY, USA, 4th edition, 2000.

[2] A. S. Eison and U. L. Mullins, "Regulation of central 5-HT$_{2A}$ receptors: a review of in vivo studies," *Behavioural Brain Research*, vol. 73, no. 1-2, pp. 177–181, 1995.

[3] G. Wong and P. Skolnick, "High affinity ligands for "diazepam-insensitive" benzodiazepines receptors," *European Journal of Pharmacology—Molecular Pharmacology Section*, vol. 225, no. 1, pp. 63–68, 1992.

[4] J. R. Atack, "Subtype-selective GABA$_A$ receptor modulation yields a novel pharmacological profile: the design and development of TPA023," *Advances in Pharmacology*, vol. 57, pp. 137–185, 2009.

[5] R. M. McKernan, T. W. Rosahl, D. S. Reynolds et al., "Sedative but not anxiolytic properties of benzodiazepines are mediated by the GABA$_A$ receptor α1 subtype," *Nature Neuroscience*, vol. 3, no. 6, pp. 587–592, 2000.

[6] J. K. Rowlett, D. M. Platt, S. Lelas, J. R. Atack, and G. R. Dawson, "Different GABA$_A$ receptor subtypes mediate the anxiolytic, abuse-related, and motor effects of benzodiazepine-like drugs in primates," *Proceedings of the National Academy of Sciences of the United States of America*, vol. 102, no. 3, pp. 915–920, 2005.

[7] J. Knabl, R. Witschi, K. Hösl et al., "Reversal of pathological pain through specific spinal GABA$_A$ receptor subtypes," *Nature*, vol. 451, no. 7176, pp. 330–334, 2008.

[8] J. Knabl, U. B. Zeilhofer, F. Crestani, U. Rudolph, and H. U. Zeilhofer, "Genuine antihyperalgesia by systemic diazepam revealed by experiments in GABA$_A$ receptor point-mutated mice," *Pain*, vol. 141, no. 3, pp. 233–238, 2009.

[9] J. R. Atack, P. J. Bayley, G. R. Seabrook, K. A. Wafford, R. M. McKernan, and G. R. Dawson, "L-655,708 enhances cognition in rats but is not proconvulsant at a dose selective for α_5-containing GABA$_A$ receptors," *Neuropharmacology*, vol. 51, no. 6, pp. 1023–1029, 2006.

[10] T. M. Ballard, F. Knoflach, E. Prinssen et al., "RO4938581, a novel cognitive enhancer acting at GABAA α_5 subunit-containing receptors," *Psychopharmacology*, vol. 202, no. 1–3, pp. 207–223, 2009.

[11] S. J. De Visser, J. P. Van Der Post, P. P. De Waal, F. Cornet, A. F. Cohen, and J. M. A. Van Gerven, "Biomarkers for the effects of benzodiazepines in healthy volunteers," *British Journal of Clinical Pharmacology*, vol. 55, no. 1, pp. 39–50, 2003.

[12] S. L. De Haas, S. J. De Visser, J. P. Van Der Post et al., "Pharmacodynamic and pharmacokinetic effects of TPA023, a GABA$_A$ $\alpha_{2,3}$ subtype-selective agonist, compared to lorazepam and placebo in healthy volunteers," *Journal of Psychopharmacology*, vol. 21, no. 4, pp. 374–383, 2007.

[13] S. L. De Haas, S. J. De Visser, J. P. Van Der Post et al., "Pharmacodynamic and pharmacokinetic effects of MK-0343, a GABA$_A$ $\alpha_{2,3}$ subtype selective agonist, compared to lorazepam

and placebo in healthy male volunteers," *Journal of Psychopharmacology*, vol. 22, no. 1, pp. 24–32, 2008.

[14] S. L. De Haas, K. L. Franson, J. A. J. Schmitt et al., "The pharmacokinetic and pharmacodynamic effects of SL65.1498, a GABA$_A$ 2,3 selective agonist, in comparison with lorazepam in healthy volunteers," *Journal of Psychopharmacology*, vol. 23, no. 6, pp. 625–632, 2009.

[15] S. L. De Haas, R. C. Schoemaker, J. M. A. Van Gerven, P. Hoever, A. F. Cohen, and J. Dingemanse, "Pharmacokinetics, pharmacodynamics and the pharmacokinetic/ pharmacodynamic relationship of zolpidem in healthy subjects," *Journal of Psychopharmacology*, vol. 24, no. 11, pp. 1619–1629, 2010.

[16] A. L. Van Steveninck, B. N. M. Van Berckel, R. C. Schoemaker, D. D. Breimer, J. M. A. Van Gerven, and A. F. Cohen, "The sensitivity of pharmacodynamic tests for the central nervous system effects of drugs on the effects of sleep deprivation," *Journal of Psychopharmacology*, vol. 13, no. 1, pp. 10–17, 1999.

[17] J. M. P. Baas, N. Mol, J. L. Kenemans et al., "Validating a human model for anxiety using startle potentiated by cue and context: the effects of alprazolam, pregabalin, and diphenhydramine," *Psychopharmacology*, vol. 205, no. 1, pp. 73–84, 2009.

[18] A. L. Van Steveninck, S. Verver, H. C. Schoemaker et al., "Effects of temazepam on saccadic eye movements: concentration-effect relationships in individual volunteers," *Clinical Pharmacology and Therapeutics*, vol. 52, no. 4, pp. 402–408, 1992.

[19] A. L. Van Steveninck, H. C. Schoemaker, M. S. M. Pieters, R. Kroon, D. D. Breimer, and A. F. Cohen, "A comparison of the sensitivities of adaptive tracking, eye movement analysis, and visual analog lines to the effects of incremental doses of temazepam in healthy volunteers," *Clinical Pharmacology and Therapeutics*, vol. 50, no. 2, pp. 172–180, 1991.

[20] P. R. M. Bittencourt, P. Wade, A. T. Smith, and A. Richens, "The relationship between peak velocity of saccadic eye movements and serum benzodiazepine concentration," *British Journal of Clinical Pharmacology*, vol. 12, no. 4, pp. 523–533, 1981.

[21] R. W. Baloh, A. W. Sills, W. E. Kumley, and V. Honrubia, "Quantitative measurement of saccade amplitude duration, and velocity," *Neurology*, vol. 25, no. 11, pp. 1065–1070, 1975.

[22] H. Norris, "The action of sedatives on brain stem oculomotor systems in man," *Neuropharmacology*, vol. 10, no. 2, pp. 181–191, 1971.

[23] A. Bond and M. Lader, "The use of analogue scales in rating subjective feelings," *British Journal of Medical Psychology*, vol. 47, pp. 211–218, 1974.

[24] A. L. Van Steveninck, R. Gieschke, H. C. Schoemaker et al., "Pharmacodynamic interactions of diazepam and intravenous alcohol at pseudo steady state," *Psychopharmacology*, vol. 110, no. 4, pp. 471–478, 1993.

[25] A. L. Van Steveninck, A. E. Wallnöfer, R. C. Schoemaker et al., "A study of the effects of long-term use on individual sensitivity to temazepam and lorazepam in a clinical population," *British Journal of Clinical Pharmacology*, vol. 44, no. 3, pp. 267–275, 1997.

[26] J. R. Atack, K. A. Wafford, S. J. Tye et al., "TPA023 [7-(1,1-dimethylethyl)-6-(2-ethyl-2H-1,2,4-triazol-3-ylmethoxy)-3-(2-fluorophenyl)-1,2,4-triazolo[4,3-b]pyridazine], an agonist selective for α2- and 3-containing GABA$_A$ receptors, is a nonsedating anxiolytic in rodents and primates," *Journal of Pharmacology and Experimental Therapeutics*, vol. 316, no. 1, pp. 410–422, 2006.

[27] R. G. Borland and A. N. Nicholson, "Visual motor coordination and dynamic visual acuity," *British Journal of Clinical Pharmacology*, vol. 18, no. 1, pp. 69S–72S, 1984.

[28] G. Griebel, G. Perrault, J. Simiand et al., "SL651498: an anxioselective compound with functional selectivity for α_2- and α_3-containing γ-aminobutyric acid$_A$ (GABA$_A$) receptors," *Journal of Pharmacology and Experimental Therapeutics*, vol. 298, no. 2, pp. 753–768, 2001.

[29] F. Crestani, J. R. Martin, H. Möhler, and U. Rudolph, "Mechanism of action of the hypnotic zolpidem in vivo," *British Journal of Pharmacology*, vol. 131, no. 7, pp. 1251–1254, 2000.

[30] E. Sanna, F. Busonero, G. Talani et al., "Comparison of the effects of zaleplon, zolpidem, and triazolam at various GABA$_A$ receptor subtypes," *European Journal of Pharmacology*, vol. 451, no. 2, pp. 103–110, 2002.

Analgesic and Anti-Inflammatory Activity of *Pinus roxburghii* Sarg.

Dhirender Kaushik,[1] Ajay Kumar,[1] Pawan Kaushik,[1] and A. C. Rana[2]

[1] *Institute of Pharmaceutical Sciences, Kurukshetra University, Kurukshetra 136 119, India*
[2] *Rayat College of Pharmacy, Ropar, Punjab 144 533, India*

Correspondence should be addressed to Dhirender Kaushik, dkaushik.apti@gmail.com

Academic Editor: Abdelwahab Omri

The Chir Pine, *Pinus roxburghii*, named after William Roxburgh, is a pine native to the Himalaya. *Pinus roxburghii* Sarg. (Pinaceae) is traditionally used for several medicinal purposes in India. As the oil of the plant is extensively used in number of herbal preparation for curing inflammatory disorders, the present study was undertaken to assess analgesic and anti-inflammatory activities of its bark extract. Dried and crushed leaves of *Pinus roxburghii* Sarg. were defatted with petroleum ether and then extracted with alcohol. The alcoholic extract at the doses of 100 mg/kg, 300 mg/kg, and 500 mg/kg body weight was subjected to evaluation of analgesic and anti-inflammatory activities in experimental animal models. Analgesic activity was evaluated by acetic acid-induced writhing and tail immersion tests in Swiss albino mice; acute and chronic anti-inflammatory activity was evaluated by carrageenan-induced paw oedema and cotton pellet granuloma in Wistar albino rats. Diclofenac sodium and indomethacin were employed as reference drugs for analgesic and anti-inflammatory studies, respectively. In the present study, the alcoholic bark extract of *Pinus roxburghii* Sarg. demonstrated significant analgesic and anti-inflammatory activities in the tested models.

1. Introduction

Inflammation is the response to injury of cells and body tissues through different factors such as infections, chemicals, and thermal and mechanical injuries [1]. Most of the anti-inflammatory drugs now available are potential inhibitors of cyclooxygenase (COX) pathway of arachidonic acid metabolism which produces prostaglandins. Prostaglandins are hyperalgesic, potent vasodilators and also contribute to erythema, edema, and pain. Hence, for treating inflammatory diseases, analgesic and anti-inflammatory agents are required [2]. Nonsteroidal anti-inflammatory drugs (NSAIDs) are the most clinically important medicine used for the treatment of inflammation-related diseases like arthritis, asthma, and cardiovascular disease [3]. Nonsteroidal anti-inflammatory drugs (NSAIDs) are among the most widely used medications due to their efficacy for a wide range of pain and inflammatory conditions [4]. However, the long-term administration of NSAID may induce gastro-intestinal ulcers, bleeding, and renal disorders due to their nonselective inhibition of both constitutive (COX-1) and inducible (COX-2) isoforms of the cyclooxygenases enzymes [5–7]. Therefore, new anti-inflammatory and analgesic drugs lacking those effects are being searched all over the world as alternatives to NSAIDs and opiates [8, 9]. Medicinal plants are believed to be an important source of new chemical substances with potential therapeutic effects. The research into plants with alleged folkloric use as pain relievers, anti-inflammatory agents, should therefore be viewed as a fruitful and logical research strategy in the search for new analgesic and anti-inflammatory drugs [10].

Pinus roxburghii Sarg. is the only tree with an ornamental specimen and having different medicinal values found in the Himalayan region of Bhutan, Nepal, Kashmir, Sikkim, Tibet and other parts of North India [11]. The plant is belonging to family Pinaceae commonly known as Chir Pine [12]. It consists of 110–120 species distributed throughout temperate regions of the Northern Hemisphere, and more than 40 taxonomic treatments have been recognized of several major divisions within the genus [13].

Pinus roxburghii Sarg. has many medicinal uses, the wood is aromatic, deodorant, haemostatic, stimulant, anthelmintic, digestive, liver tonic, diaphoretic, and diuretic. It is useful in eye, ear, and pharynx diseases, foul ulcers, haemorrhages, haemoptysis, worn infections, flatulence, liver diseases, bronchitis, inflammations, skin diseases, pruritus, and giddiness [11].

The chief chemical constituents of turpentine oil from *Pinus roxburghii* Sarg. are α-pinene, β-pinene, car-3-ene and longifolene [14, 15] hydrocarbons (d- and l-pinene), resin acids, camphene, fenchene, dipentene, and polymeric terpenes [16, 17].

Based on the above findings, *Pinus roxburghii* Sarg. bark extract was evaluated for its analgesic and anti-inflammatory effects on experimental induced pain and inflammation.

2. Material and Methods

2.1. Plant Material.
The stems bark of *Pinus roxburghii* Sarg. were collected from the hilly region of Morni, District Panchkula, Haryana, in the month of December 2008 and was authenticated by FRI, Dehradun, Uttarakhand, India, where a voucher specimen no. 129 FHH was deposited for future reference.

2.2. Preparation of Extract.
Shade dried coarse powdered bark of *Pinus roxburghii* Sarg. in a quantity sufficient as per the volume of extractor was packed in thimble (made of filter paper sheet). A sufficient volume of alcohol was added to the reservoir, and hot continuous extraction process in a Soxhlet extractor was started. This extraction process was continued for about 48 hours or until alcohol coming down the siphoning tube became colourless. The excess of alcohol was distilled under reduced pressure using rotatory vacuum evaporator. (Heidolph Laborota 4011, digital). A brown residue was recovered from flask with 12% yield.

2.3. HPLC Analysis.
Samples of alcoholic bark extract of *Pinus roxburghii* Sarg. were analysed without any treatment.

The HPLC system (Shimadzu, Japan) consisted of a diode array detector (SPDM10AVP), solvent delivery module (LC-10ATVP), online degasser (DGU-14A), an autoinjector (SIL-10ADVP), flow channel system (FCV-14AH), system controller (SCL-10AVP), and a reversed-phase HPLC column (RP-18, 250 mm × 4.6 mm, 5 μm particle size, Sigma, USA). The flow rate of the HPLC was 1 ML/min, and the mobile phase 0.05% TFA in ACN: 0.05% TFA in water (gradient) for 70 min. Standards of chlorogenic acid, rutin and querctin were injected separately (10 ML). Chemical compounds in the samples were identified by comparison of their retention times (Rt) with the standards. Data analysis was carried out using Class VP V6.12 SP2 software (Shimadzu, Japan).

2.4. Animals.
Wistar rats (150–250 gm) and Swiss albino mice (20–25 gm) of either sex, brought from National Institute of Pharmaceutical Education and Research, Mohali, were kept in the Animal House of Institute of Pharmaceutical Sciences, Kurukshetra University, Kurukshetra. Animals were housed at standard conditions of temperature (22 ± 1°C) and 12/12 h light/dark cycle. They were fed with standard pellet diet (Ashirwad Industries, Ropar, Punjab) and had free access to water. Five animals are used in each group. Permission for conduct of these experiments were obtained from, Institutional Animal Ethics Committee (IAEC).

2.5. Acute Toxicity Study.
Toxicity studies conducted as per internationally accepted protocol drawn under OECD guidelines 425 in Swiss albino mice.

3. Pharmacological Activity

3.1. Anti-Inflammatory Activity

3.1.1. Carrageenan Induced Paw Edema Method.
Carrageenan-induced paw inflammation was produced according to the method described by Winter et al. [18]. One hour after oral administration of the alcoholic extract of *Pinus roxburghii* Sarg. (100, 300, and 500 mg/kg), reference drug (indomethacin, 10 mg/kg) or vehicle (tween 80 (5%)), an injection of 0.1 ML of carrageenan (1% carrageenan suspended in 0.9% NaCl) was made into the right hind limb of each rat under the subplantar aponeurosis.

Measurement of paw volume was done by means of volume displacement technique using plethysmometer (Ugo Basile no. 7140) immediately after carrageenan injection and after 1, 2, 3, and 4 hr.

Percetages of inhibition were obtained using the following ratio:

$$\frac{(V_t - V_o) \text{ control} - (V_t - V_o) \text{ treated}}{(V_t - V_o) \text{ control}} \times 100. \quad (1)$$

V_t is the average volume for each group after treatment, and V_o is the average volume for each group before any treatment.

3.1.2. Cotton Pellet Granuloma Method.
Cotton pellet granulomas produced according to the method described by Winter and Porter [19]. Sterile cotton pellets (20 ± 0.5 mg) were implanted subcutaneously in the abdomen region of the rats. The animals received alcoholic bark extract of *Pinus roxburghii* Sarg. (100, 300 and 500 mg/kg), reference drug (diclofenac sodium, 50 mg/kg) or vehicle (tween 80 (5%)), orally, once a day through an oral cannula over seven consecutive days. On the 8th day, the rats were sacrificed, the cotton pellets removed, pellets dried up to constant weight at 60°C and the net dry weight, that is, after subtracting the weight of the cotton pellets, was determined.

3.2. Analgesic Activity

3.2.1. Acetic Acid Induced Writhing Test Method.
The method used in this test has been described by Koster et al. [20]. The total number of writhings following intraperitoneal administration of acetic acid solution (1%, 10 mL/kg) was recorded over a period of 10 min, starting 5 min after acetic acid injection. The mice were treated with the alcoholic bark extract of *Pinus roxburghii* Sarg. (100, 300, and 500 mg/kg),

TABLE 1: Protective efeect of *Pinus roxburghii* Sarg. on paw edema induced by carrageenan in rat.

Groups	Drug (dose), route	Change in paw volume (mL) Mean ± SEM Time (hr)			
		1 hr	2 hr	3 hr	4 hr
Control	Tween 80 (5%) p.o	0.71 ± 0.12	0.93 ± 0.01	1.8 ± 0.03	1.9 ± 0.02
Standard	Indomethacin (10 mg/kg), p.o	0.21 ± 0.06(70.4)	0.23 ± 0.02**(75.26)	0.41 ± 0.01**(77.22)	0.35 ± 0.09(81.56)
AB	100 mg/kg, p.o	0.61 ± 0.17(14.08)	0.92 ± 0.17(1.07)	0.89 ± 0.13**(50.55)	1.07 ± 0.19(43.68)
AB	300 mg/kg, p.o	0.63 ± 0.14(11.21)	0.78 ± 0.19(16.12)	0.79 ± 0.20**(56.11)	1.87 ± 0.14(1.57)
AB	500 mg/kg, p.o	0.39 ± 0.12(45.07)	0.52 ± 0.13(44.08)	0.68 ± 0.11**(62.22)	0.68 ± 0.11(64.21)

$n = 5$. Results are expressed as mean ± SEM. Percentage inhibition are in brackets.
$*P > 0.05$, $**P < 0.01$ as compared to control, AB = alcoholic bark extract.

or vehicle (tween 80 (5%)) or standard drug (diclofenac sodium, 50 mg/kg), 30 min before administration of acetic acid. The number of writhings and stretching was recorded and permitted to express the percentage of protection.

3.2.2. Tail Immersion Test in Rats. The procedure described by Aydin et al. [21] was used to conduct this test. 3 cm of the tail was introduced in hot water at a temperature of $55 \pm 0.5°C$. Within a few minutes, the rats reacted by withdrawing the tail. The reaction time was recorded with a stopwatch. The animals were treated by alcoholic extract of *Pinus roxburghii* Sarg. (100, 300 and 500 mg/kg), or water (vehicle) or standard drug (diclofenac sodium, 50 mg/kg), 30 min before the immersion of the tail. The time reaction is taken at 1, 2, 3, and 4 after administration of different preparations.

3.2.3. Statstical Analysis. All values were expressed as mean ± SEM, and data was analyzed by one way analysis of variance (ANOVA) followed by Dunnett's *t*-test using GraphPad InStat.

4. Results

4.1. Acute Toxicity Test of Plant Extract. Alcoholic extract of the plant *Pinus roxburghii* Sarg. was found safe at the dose of 5000 mg/kg according to OECD guidelines 425.

4.2. HPLC Analysis. A correct assignment to the various compounds was not possible. From UV spectra and retention times of the main peaks, some compound classes contained in the extract have been determined. High-performance liquid chromatography (HPLC) revealed the presence of bioflavonoids, quercetin, chlorogenic acid, and rutin (Figure 1).

4.3. Anti-Inflammatory Activity

4.3.1. Carrageenan-Induced Paw Edema in Rats. In the carrageenan-induced oedema test, the paw volumes and percentages of ages of inhibition by the alcoholic extract of *Pinus roxburghii* Sarg. and standard drugs are shown in Table 1. Injection of carrageenan was done 1 h after oral administration of the extract (100, 300, and 500 mg/kg), indomethacin (reference drug) and water. Measurement of paw size was

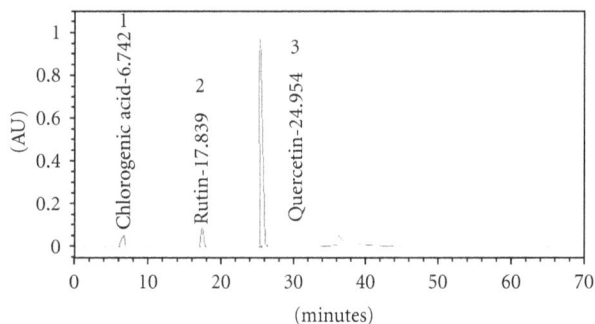

FIGURE 1: HPLC analysis of *Pinus roxburghii* Sarg. (Pinaceae) showing presence of chlorogenic acid (1), rutin (2) and quercetin (3).

taken before carrageenan injection and then 1, 2, 3, and 4 h after carrageenan injection. The alcoholic extract of *Pinus roxburghii* Sarg. at all doses showed a significant inhibition of paw oedema at third hour as compared to reference drug (Table 1).

4.3.2. Cotton Pellet Granuloma. Table 2 shows that the alcoholic bark extract of *Pinus roxburghii* Sarg. exhibited a significant and dose-related inhibition of the dried weight of the cotton pellet granuloma. The inhibitory values for 100, 300, and 500 mg/kg of the extract were 31.11%, 36.13% and 56.93% ($P > 0.01$), respectively. Diclofenac sodium (reference drug) and water inhibited granuloma tissue formation with a value of 92.87 ($P > 0.01$) %, a slightly higher value than that observed with the 80 mg/kg dose of the *Pinus roxburghii* Sarg. extract.

4.4. Analgesic Activity

4.4.1. Acetic Acid Induced Writhing Test in Mice. The alcoholic extract of *Pinus roxburghii* Sarg. (100, 300, and 500 mg/kg) dose significantly and dependently reduced the number of abdominal constriction induced in mice by a solution of acetic acid 1%. This dose-dependent protective effect reached a maximum inhibition of 80.95% at the dose of 500 mg/kg. Diclofenac sodium (reference drug) exerted a significant protective effect, with percentage of protection of 90 (Table 3).

TABLE 2: Protective efeect of *Pinus roxburghii* Sarg. on cotton pellet induced granuloma.

Groups	Drug (dose), route	Weight of dry Cotton Pellet Granuloma (mg)	% protection
Control	Tween 80 (5%) p.o	202 ± 0.23	0
Standard	Indomethacin (10 mg/kg), p.o	14.4 ± 3.3**	92.87
AB	100 mg/kg, p.o	139 ± 3.2	31.11
AB	300 mg/kg, p.o	129 ± 1.1	36.13
AB	500 mg/kg, p.o	87 ± 9.1**	56.93

$n = 5$. Results are expressed as mean ± SEM. $*P > 0.05$, $**P < 0.01$ as compared to control, AB = alcoholic bark extract.

TABLE 3: Protective efeect of *Pinus roxburghii* Sarg. on writhing induced by acetic acid.

Groups	Drug (dose), route	No of wriths (Mean ± SEM)	% Protection
Control	Acetic acid (0.6% V/V), i.p	42 ± 11.6	0
Standard	Diclofenac Sodium (50 mg/kg), p.o	4.2 ± 1.0**	90
AB	100 mg/kg, p.o	25.4 ± 4.8	39.52
AB	300 mg/kg, p.o	17.4 ± 1.9**	58.57
AB	500 mg/kg, p.o	8.0 ± 2.0**	80.95

$n = 5$. Results are expressed as mean ± SEM. $*P > 0.05$, $**P < 0.01$ as compared to control, AB = alcoholic bark extract.

4.4.2. Tail Immersion Test in Rats. As presented in Table 4, alcoholic extract of *Pinus roxburghii* Sarg. in doses of 500 mg/kg ($P < 0.01$) body weight showed a significant elongation of reaction time, 30 minutes after oral administration of the extract. After 60 minutes, the alcoholic extract of *Pinus roxburghii* Sarg. in doses of 300 mg/kg ($P < 0.05$) and 500 mg/kg ($P < 0.05$) body weight showed a significant elongation. After 90 minutes alcoholic extract of *Pinus roxburghii* Sarg. in doses of 300 mg/kg ($P < 0.05$) and 500 mg/kg body weight showed a significant ($P < 0.05$) elongation of reaction time. After 120 minutes alcoholic extract of *Pinus roxburghii* Sarg. in doses of 100 mg, 300 mg, and 500 mg/kg body weight showed no significant elongation of reaction time.

5. Discussions

Carrageenan-induced edema has been commonly used as an experimental animal model for acute inflammation and is believed to be biphasic. The early phase (1-2 h) of the carrageenan model is mainly mediated by histamine, serotonin, and increased synthesis of prostaglandins in the damaged tissue surroundings. The late phase is sustained by prostaglandin release and mediated by bradykinin, leukotrienes, polymorphonuclear cells, and prostaglandins produced by tissue macrophages [10, 22]. Since the extract/fractions significantly inhibited paw edema induced by carrageenan in the second phase, this finding suggests a possible inhibition of cyclooxygenase synthesis by the extract and this effect is similar to that produced by nonsteroidal anti-inflammatory drugs such as indomethacin, whose mechanism of action is inhibition of the cyclooxygenase enzyme.

The inflammatory granuloma is a typical feature of an established chronic inflammatory process [23, 24]. The cotton pellet granuloma method has been widely employed to evaluate the transudative, exudative, and proliferative components of chronic inflammation, because the dried weight of the pellets correlates well with the amount of granulomatous tissue [25]. We found a dose-dependent inhibition of granuloma formation in mice, suggesting that the aqueous stem bark extract of *Pinus roxburghii* Sarg. inhibits chronic inflammation processes during the late phases of acute inflammation.

The brain and spinal cord play a major role in central pain mechanisms. The dorsal horn of the spinal cord is endowed with several neurotransmitters and receptors including substance P, somatostatin, neuropeptide Y, inhibitory amino acid, nitric oxide, endogenous opioids, and the monoamines which are the major targets for pain and inflammation [26]. The tail immersion test was considered to be selective to examine compounds acting through opioid receptor; all the extract/fractions increased pain threshold which means basal latency, which indicates that it may act *via* centrally mediated analgesic mechanism. Narcotic analgesics inhibit both peripheral and central mechanism of pain, while nonsteroidal anti-inflammatory drugs inhibit only peripheral pain [27]. The extract inhibits pain with both mechanisms, suggesting that the plant extract may act as a narcotic analgesic. On the other hand, acetic acid-induced writhing model represents pain sensation by triggering localized inflammatory response. Such pain stimulus leads to the release of free arachidonic acid from the tissue phospholipid [28]. The acetic acid induced writhing response is a sensitive procedure to evaluate peripherally acting analgesics. The response is thought to be mediated by peritoneal mast cells [29], acid sensing ion channels [30], and the prostaglandin pathways [31]. Flavonoids may increase the amount of endogenous serotonin or may interact with 5-HT$_2$A and 5-HT$_3$ receptors which may be involved in the mechanism of central analgesic activity [32]. Moreover, EtOAc extract showed highest analgesic activity in all the experimental modelo which may be due to its high flavonsid contents which are responsible for free radical scavenging activity, as

TABLE 4: Protective efeect of *Pinus roxburghii* Sarg. on tail withdrawal reflex induced by tail immersion.

Groups	Drug (dose), route	Reaction time (min) Mean ± SEM			
		30 min	60 min	90 min	120 min
Control	Tween 80 (5%), p.o	1.0 ± 0.1	1.4 ± 0.2	1.5 ± 0.2	2.8 ± 0.2
Standard	Diclofenac sodium (50 mg/kg), p.o	$5.8 \pm 0.2^{**}$	$8.2 \pm 0.2^{**}$	$8.4 \pm 0.2^{**}$	$8.8 \pm 0.2^{**}$
AB	100 mg/kg, p.o	1.4 ± 0.2	2.4 ± 0.3	2.8 ± 0.2	3.4 ± 0.2
AB	300 mg/kg, p.o	1.8 ± 0.2	$3.2 \pm 0.2^*$	$4.4 \pm 0.4^*$	$6.2 \pm 1.5^*$
AB	500 mg/kg, p.o	$2.8 \pm 0.4^{**}$	$3.2 \pm 0.4^*$	$4.6 \pm 0.2^*$	5.4 ± 1.9

$n = 5$. Results are expressed as mean ± SEM. $^*P > 0.05$, $^{**}P < 0.01$ as compared to control, AB = alcoholic bark extract.

these free radicals are involved during pain stimulation, and antioxidants showed reduction in such pain [33].

The results of the present study have shown that the crude extract of the investigated plant exhibited very high anti-inflammatory and analgesic activities. These activities may be linked with the presence of polyphenolic compounds present in the extract. The HPLC analysis of AB extract shows the presence of bioflavonoids, quercetin, and rutin, which are reported to be anti-inflammatory, antiasthmatic, analgesic anti-inflammatory, and antioxidant, and these findings are in concordance with our results. Many plants containing flavonoids have been shown to have diuretic, laxative, antispasmodic, anti-hypertensive, and anti-inflammatory actions [34]. Flavonoids and saponins are well known for their ability to inhibit pain perception as well as anti-inflammatory properties due to their inhibitory effects on enzymes involved in the production of the chemical mediator of inflammation [35].

The ability of flavonoids to inhibit eicosanoid biosynthesis has been documented. Eicosanoids, such as prostaglandins, are involved in various immunological responses and are the end products of the cyclooxygenase and lipoxygenase pathways [36]. Further, flavonoids are able to inhibit neutrophils degranulation and thereby decrease the release of arachidonic acid [37]. Thus, the presence of flavonoids in the extract/fractions of *Pinus roxburghii* Sarg. might be responsible for the anti-inflammatory and analgesic activity in Swiss albino mice and rats.

References

[1] O. A. Oyedapo, C. O. Adewunmi, E. O. Iwalewa, and V. O. Makanju, "Analgesic, antioxidant and anti-inflammatory related activities of 2^1-hydroxy-2,4^1-dimethoxychalcone and 4-hydroxychalcone in mice," *Journal of Biological Sciences*, vol. 8, no. 1, pp. 131–136, 2008.

[2] M. Anilkumar, "Ethnomedicinal plants as anti-inflammatory and analgesic agents," in *Ethnomedicine: A Source of Complementary Therapeutics*, pp. 267–293, Research Signpost, India, 2010.

[3] F. Conforti, S. Sosa, M. Marrelli et al., "The protective ability of Mediterranean dietary plants against the oxidative damage: the role of radical oxygen species in inflammation and the polyphenol, flavonoid and sterol contents," *Food Chemistry*, vol. 112, no. 3, pp. 587–594, 2009.

[4] IMS Health, IMS National Sales Perspectives TM, 2005.

[5] A. Robert, "Antisecretory, antiulcer, cytoprotective and diarrheogenic properties of prostaglandins," *Advances in Prostaglandin and Thromboxane Research*, vol. 2, pp. 507–520, 1976.

[6] B. M. Peskar, "On the synthesis of prostaglandins by human gastric mucosa and its modification by drugs," *Biochimica et Biophysica Acta*, vol. 487, no. 2, pp. 307–314, 1977.

[7] H. Tapiero, G. Nguyen Ba, P. Couvreur, and K. D. Tew, "Polyunsaturated fatty acids (PUFA) and eicosanoids in human health and pathologies," *Biomedicine and Pharmacotherapy*, vol. 56, no. 5, pp. 215–222, 2002.

[8] M. G. Dharmasiri, J. R. A. C. Jayakody, G. Galhena, S. S. P. Liyanage, and W. D. Ratnasooriya, "Anti-inflammatory and analgesic activities of mature fresh leaves of *Vitex negundo*," *Journal of Ethnopharmacology*, vol. 87, no. 2-3, pp. 199–206, 2003.

[9] N. Kumara, "Identification of strategies to improve research on medicinal plants used in Sri Lanka," in *Proceedings of the WHO Symposium*, pp. 12–14, University of Ruhuna, Galle, Sri Lanka, 2001.

[10] M. Gupta, U. K. Mazumder, P. Gomathi, and V. T. Selvan, "Antiinflammatory evaluation of leaves of *Plumeria acuminata*," *BMC Complementary and Alternative Medicine*, vol. 6, article 36, 2006.

[11] C. J. Earle, "Pinus roxburghii Sargent 1897," http://www.conifers.org/pi/pin/roxburghii.htm.

[12] B. Sharad and A. Bohra, "Antibacterial potential of three naked-seeded (Gymnosperm) plants," *Natural Product Radiance*, vol. 7, no. 5, pp. 420–425, 2008.

[13] A. J. Eckert and B. D. Hall, "Phylogeny, historical biogeography, and patterns of diversification for Pinus (Pinaceae): phylogenetic tests of fossil-based hypotheses," *Molecular Phylogenetics and Evolution*, vol. 40, no. 1, pp. 166–182, 2006.

[14] V. P. S. Verma and R. K. Suri, "Geographic variation in the chemical composition of turpentine oil of chirpine (PrS)," *Indian Perfumer*, vol. 22, pp. 179–181, 1978.

[15] M. Smaleh, O. P. Sharma, and N. P. Dobhal, "Chemical composition of turpentine oil from pleoresin (Pinus roxburghii Sargent) Indian oerfumer," *Chemistry of Forest Products Branch*, vol. 20, pp. 15–19, 1976.

[16] S. Rastogi, A. Shukla, and S. A. Kolhapure, "Evaluation of the clinical efficacy and safety of RG-01 (Rumalaya gel) in the management of chronic sub-acute inflammatory joint disorder," *Medicine Update*, vol. 12, no. 1, pp. 31–37, 2004.

[17] A. Sharma and S. A. Kolhapure, "Evaluation of the efficacy and safety of Rumalaya gel in the management of acute and chronic inflammatory musculoskeltal disorders: an open, prospective, noncomparative, phase III clinical trial," *Medicine Update*, vol. 12, no. 10, pp. 39–45, 2005.

[18] C. A. Winter, E. A. Risley, and G. W. Nuss, "Carrageenin-induced edema in hind paw of the rat as an assay for antiinflammatory drugs," *Proceedings of the Society for Experimental Biology and Medicine*, vol. 111, pp. 544–547, 1962.

[19] C. A. Winter and C. C. Porter, "Effect of alterations in the side chain upon antiinflammatory and liver glycogen activities of hydrocortisone esters," *Journal of the American Pharmaceutical Association*, vol. 46, pp. 515–519, 1957.

[20] R. Koster, M. Anderson, and J. De Beer, "Acetic acid for analgesic screening," *Federation Proceedings*, vol. 18, pp. 412–417, 1959.

[21] S. Aydin, T. Demir, Y. Ozturk et al., "Analgesic activity of Nepeta italica L.," *Phytotherapy Research*, vol. 13, pp. 20–23, 1999.

[22] M. A. Antônio and A. R. M. Souza Brito, "Oral anti-inflammatory and anti-ulcerogenic activities of a hydroalcoholic extract and partitioned fractions of *Turnera ulmifolia* (Turneraceae)," *Journal of Ethnopharmacology*, vol. 61, no. 3, pp. 215–228, 1998.

[23] J. R. Vane and R. M. Botting, "New insights into the mode of action of anti-inflammatory drugs," *Inflammation Research*, vol. 44, no. 1, pp. 1–10, 1995.

[24] J. B. Perianayagam, S. K. Sharma, and K. K. Pillai, "Anti-inflammatory activity of *Trichodesma indicum* root extract in experimental animals," *Journal of Ethnopharmacology*, vol. 104, no. 3, pp. 410–414, 2006.

[25] K. F. Swingle and F. E. Shideman, "Phases of the inflammatory response to subcutaneous implantation of a cotton pellet and their modification by certain anti-inflammatory agents," *Journal of Pharmacology and Experimental Therapeutics*, vol. 183, no. 1, pp. 226–234, 1972.

[26] C. R. McCurdy and S. S. Scully, "Analgesic substances derived from natural products (natureceuticals)," *Life Sciences*, vol. 78, no. 5, pp. 476–484, 2005.

[27] E. Elisabetsky, T. A. Arnador, R. R. Albuquerque, D. S. Nunes, and A. Do CT Carvalho, "Analgesic activity of *Psychotria colorata* (Willd. ex R. and S.) Muell. Arg. alkaloids," *Journal of Ethnopharmacology*, vol. 48, no. 2, pp. 77–83, 1995.

[28] F. Ahmed, M. H. Hossain, A. A. Rahman et al., "Antinociceptive and sedative effects of the bark of *Cerbera odollam* Gaertn," *International Journal of Oriental Pharmacy and Experimental Medicine*, vol. 6, pp. 344–348, 2006.

[29] R. A. Ribeiro, M. L. Vale, S. M. Thomazzi et al., "Involvement of resident macrophages and mast cells in the writhing nociceptive response induced by zymosan and acetic acid in mice," *European Journal of Pharmacology*, vol. 387, no. 1, pp. 111–118, 2000.

[30] N. Voilley, "Acid-sensing ion channels (ASICs): new targets for the analgesic effects of non-steroid anti-inflammatory drugs (NSAIDs)," *Current Drug Targets*, vol. 3, no. 1, pp. 71–79, 2004.

[31] M. M. Hossain, M. S. Ali, A. Saha et al., "Antinociceptive activity of whole plant extracts of *Paederia foetida*," *Dhaka University Journal of Pharmaceutical Sciences*, vol. 5, pp. 67–69, 2006.

[32] H. V. Annegowda, M. N. Mordi, S. Ramanathan, and S. M. Mansor, "Analgesic and antioxidant properties of ethanolic extract of *Terminalia catappa* L. leaves," *International Journal of Pharmacology*, vol. 6, no. 6, pp. 910–915, 2010.

[33] H. K. Kim, S. K. Park, J. L. Zhou et al., "Reactive oxygen species (ROS) play an important role in a rat model of neuropathic pain," *Pain*, vol. 111, no. 1-2, pp. 116–124, 2004.

[34] T. Okuda, "Flavonoids," in *Chemistry of Organic Natural Products*, H. Mitsuhashi, O. Tanaka, S. Nazoe, and M. Nagai Nankodo, Eds., pp. 219–228, Tokyo, Japan, 1962.

[35] W. R. Sawadogo, R. Boly, M. Lompo et al., "Anti-inflammatory, analgesic and antipyretic activities of *Dicliptera verticillata*," *International Journal of Pharmacology*, vol. 2, no. 4, pp. 435–438, 2006.

[36] C. Jothimanivannan, R. S. Kumar, and N. Subramanian, "Anti-inflammatory and analgesic activities of ethanol extract of aerial parts of *Justicia gendarussa* Burm," *International Journal of Pharmacology*, vol. 6, pp. 278–283, 2010.

[37] J. R. S. Hoult, M. A. Moroney, and M. Paya, "Actions of flavonoids and coumarins on lipoxygenase and cyclooxygenase," *Methods in Enzymology*, vol. 234, pp. 443–454, 1994.

3

Assessment of 5-HT$_7$ Receptor Agonists Selectivity Using Nociceptive and Thermoregulation Tests in Knockout versus Wild-Type Mice

Alex Brenchat,[1] Maria Rocasalbas,[1] Daniel Zamanillo,[1] Michel Hamon,[2] José Miguel Vela,[1] and Luz Romero[1]

[1] *Department of Pharmacology, Drug Discovery and Preclinical Development, ESTEVE, Avenida Mare de Déu de Montserrat 221, 08041 Barcelona, Spain*
[2] *UMR 894 INSERM-CPN/UPMC, Faculté de Médecine Pierre et Marie Curie, Site Pitié-Salpêtrière, 91 boulevard de l'Hôpital, 75634 Paris Cedex 13, France*

Correspondence should be addressed to Luz Romero, lromero@esteve.es

Academic Editor: Karim A. Alkadhi

No study has ever examined the effect of 5-HT$_7$ receptor agonists on nociception by using 5-HT$_7$ receptor knockout mice. Basal sensitivity to noxious heat stimuli and formalin-induced nociception in both phase I and II of the formalin test did not differ in 5-HT$_7$ receptor knockout mice and paired wild-type controls. Similarly, there was no significant difference in basal body temperature between both genotypes. Subcutaneous administration of 5-HT$_7$ receptor agonists AS-19 (10 mg/kg), E-57431 (10 mg/kg), and E-55888 (20 mg/kg) significantly reduced formalin-induced licking/biting behavior during the phase II of the test in wild-type but not in 5-HT$_7$ receptor knockout mice. At these active analgesic doses, none of the three 5-HT$_7$ receptor agonists modified the basal body temperature neither in wild-type nor in 5-HT$_7$ receptor knockout mice. However, a significant decrease in body temperature was observed at a higher dose (20 mg/kg) of AS-19 and E-57431 in both genotypes. Our data strongly suggest that the 5-HT$_7$ receptor agonists AS-19, E-57431, and E-55888 produce antinociception in the formalin test by activating 5-HT$_7$ receptors. These results also strengthen the idea that the 5-HT$_7$ receptor plays a role in thermoregulation, but by acting in concert with other receptors.

1. Introduction

The 5-HT$_7$ receptor has been cloned from different genomes and its binding profile is consistent across species and between cloned and native receptors [1, 2]. In recent years, considerable efforts have focused on the development of selective 5-HT$_7$ receptor agonists and antagonists. To date, the search for 5-HT$_7$ receptor antagonists has led to the discovery of LY215840 [3], SB-258719 [4], DR4004 [5], SB-269970 [6], and SB-656104-A [7]. Regarding 5-HT$_7$ receptor agonists, AS-19 [8, 9], MSD-5a [10], LP-44 [11], LP-211 [12], E-55888 [13], and E-57431 [14] have been developed. However, most of these agonists display rather modest selectivity because their affinity for the 5-HT$_7$ type is only 11-fold higher than for 5-HT$_{1D}$ in case of AS-19 [13], 28.6-fold higher than for 5-HT$_{1A}$ in case of MSD-5a [10], and 33-fold higher than for 5-HT$_{1A}$ in case of MSD-5a [10], and 33-fold higher than for dopamine D2 receptor [15], and 5-14-fold higher than for 5-HT$_{1B}$, 5-HT$_{2B}$, 5-HT$_{2C}$, and 5-HT$_{5A}$ in case of LP-211 [16]. Indeed, among 5-HT$_7$ receptor agonists, only E-55888 and E-57431 seem to have a satisfactory selectivity with affinity for the 5-HT$_7$ receptor 280-fold higher than for 5-HT$_{1A}$ and 112.7-fold higher than for 5-HT$_{1D}$, respectively [13] (see Table 1). When tested in a functional assay, 5-HT$_7$ receptor agonists concentration dependently increased cAMP formation in HEK-293F/h5-HT$_7$ cells. AS-19 has been found to behave as a potent (EC$_{50}$ = 9 ± 1 nM) but partial 5-HT$_7$ receptor agonist, with a maximal effect reaching 77% of that of 5-HT [13]. However, E-55888 and E-57431 behave as full agonists, with efficacies (E_{max} = 99 ± 1% and 94.5 ± 1%, resp.) and potencies (EC$_{50}$ = 16 ± 1 nM and 21.5 ± 1 nM) similar to those of 5-HT, as previously described [13, 14].

TABLE 1: Binding profiles of the 5-HT$_7$ receptor agonists AS-19, E-57431, and E-55888.

Receptor	Affinity (K_i (nM))		
	AS-19	E-57431	E-55888
h5-HT$_{1A}$	89.7 (149.5 x)	n.s.	700 (280 x)
r5-HT$_{1B}$	490 (816.6 x)	n.s.	n.s.
h5-HT$_{1D}$	6.6 (11 x)	53 (112.7 x)	n.s.
h5-HT$_{2A}$	n.s.	560 (1191.5 x)	n.s.
h5-HT$_{2B}$	n.s.	n.s.	n.s.
h5-HT$_{2C}$	n.s.	n.s.	n.s.
h5-HT$_3$	n.s.	n.s.	n.s.
h5-HT$_{4e}$	—	n.s.	n.s.
gp5-HT$_4$	n.s.	n.s.	—
h5-HT$_{5A}$	98.5 (164.2 x)	n.s.	n.s.
h5-HT$_6$	n.s.	n.s.	n.s.
h5-HT$_7$	0.6	0.47	2.5
h5-HT transporter (SERT)	n.s.	n.s.	n.s.
Other receptors	n.s.[a]	n.s.[b]	n.s.[a]

n.s.: not significant (K_i > 1 μM or less than 50% inhibition of specific radioligand binding at 1 μM);
—: data not available.
gp: guinea pig; h: human; r: rat.
Data obtained from Brenchat et al. [13, 14]
Data in parentheses after K_i values represent the affinity ratio versus 5-HT$_7$ receptors calculated as K_i for the tested receptor/K_i for 5-HT$_7$ receptor. It is expressed as number-fold higher (x) for 5-HT$_7$ than for the tested receptor.
[a]See the panel of other receptors assayed [13].
[b]See the panel of other receptors assayed [14].

From data obtained with these pharmacological tools, it has been claimed that 5-HT$_7$ receptors are involved in a number of physiological and pathophysiological phenomena such as nociception and thermoregulation. Data supporting a role for 5-HT$_7$ receptors in pain control mostly suggest an antinociceptive effect of 5-HT$_7$ receptor activation in the CNS and, in contrast, a pronociceptive effect of 5-HT$_7$ receptor activation in the periphery [17–23]. However, an overall antinociceptive effect has been observed following systemic administration of the selective 5-HT$_7$ receptor agonists AS-19, E-57431, and E-55888 to rodents suffering from neuropathic pain [13, 14].

On the other hand, 5-HT$_7$ receptors have been involved in the control of body temperature based on studies using some 5-HT$_7$ receptor agonists (5-CT, 8-OH-DPAT, and LP-211), 5-HT$_7$ receptor antagonists (SB-258719 and SB-269970) and 5-HT$_7$ receptor knockout mice. Activation of 5-HT$_7$ receptors has been reported to decrease body temperature in a complex manner, in concert with other serotonergic receptors such as the 5-HT$_{1A}$ receptor and/or nonserotonergic receptors [16, 24–28].

In addition to pharmacological studies using 5-HT$_7$ receptor agonists and antagonists, the 5-HT$_7$ receptor knockout mice may provide a relevant tool to explore the functions of this receptor, and to assess the specificity of ligands supposed to interact selectively with it. Accordingly, the present study examines the effects of the so-called 5-HT$_7$ receptor agonists AS-19, E-57431, and E-55888 on formalin-induced pain behavior and thermoregulation in 5-HT$_7$ receptor knockout and paired wild-type mice in order to determine the *in vivo* functional selectivity of these ligands at this specific receptor type.

2. Materials and Methods

2.1. Animals. Male, 5- to 8-week-old, 5-HT$_7$ receptor knockout (5-HT$_7$R$^{-/-}$) C57BL/6J mice and their wild-type 5-HT$_7$R$^{+/+}$ siblings used in this study were provided by Deltagen (CA, USA). Embryonic stem cells derived from the 129/OlaHsd mouse substrain were used to generate chimeric mice. F1 mice were generated by breeding with C57BL/6 females. F2 homozygous mutant mice were produced by intercrossing F1 heterozygous males and females. Successive mating of heterozygous progeny to the inbred C57BL/6J strain was performed for at least 8 generations before the knockout and wild-type homozygous offsprings were used in the present study. Genotyping was performed by PCR analysis using a protocol described by The Jackson Laboratory (http://jaxmice.jax.org/protocolsdb/f?p=116:2:24205673177 16723::NO:2:P2_MASTER_PROTOCOL_ID,P2_JRS_CODE: 1854,005769). Animals were housed in groups of five, provided with food and water *ad libitum* and kept in controlled laboratory conditions with ambient temperature maintained at 21 ± 1°C and light in 12 h cycles (on at 07:00 h and off at 19:00 h). Experiments were carried out in a sound-attenuated, air-regulated, experimental room. All experimental procedures and animal husbandry were conducted according to ethical principles for the evaluation of pain in conscious animals [29], and to ethical guidelines of the European Communities Council Directive of November

24, 1986 (86/609/EEC). The experimental work received approval by the Local Ethical Committee.

2.2. Drugs. Formaldehyde (37 wt.% solution) was purchased from Panreac (Spain) and dissolved in physiological saline. Drugs used for treatments were AS-19 (dimethyl-[5-(1,3,5-tri-methyl-1H-pyrazol-4-yl)-1,2,3,4-tetrahydro-naphthalen-2(S)-yl]-amine) [8, 9], E-55888 (dimethyl-{2-[3-(1,3,5-trimethyl-1H-pyrazol-4-yl)-phenyl]-ethyl}-amine dihydro-chloride) [13], and E-57431 (2-(2-(dimethylamino)ethyl)-4-(1,3,5-tri-methyl-1H-pyrazol-4-yl)phenol) [14]. AS-19 is a potent selective 5-HT$_7$ receptor agonist commercially available from Tocris Bioscience (UK), whereas E-55888 and E-57431 are 5-HT$_7$ receptor agonists developed by ESTEVE Laboratories (Barcelona, Spain). All three 5-HT$_7$ receptor agonists were synthesized for the purpose of this study at ESTEVE, dissolved in aqueous solutions containing 0.5% (hydroxypropyl) methyl cellulose (Sigma-Aldrich, Spain) and administered in a volume of 5 ml/kg through the subcutaneous (s.c.) route. Doses of drugs (referred to their salt forms) and time of evaluation were selected based on previous studies [13, 14] and on pilot experiments in models used in this study. All treatments were performed under blind conditions in independent groups of mice and behavioral evaluation was done 30 min after drug administration.

2.3. Nociceptive Behavioral Tests

2.3.1. Tail Flick Test. Animals were placed in a loose plexiglas restrainer with their tail extruding through a hole to perform the tail flick test as previously described [30]. A photobeam was placed on the tail about 4 cm from the tip. The latency to tail flick response was recorded automatically to the nearest 0.1 s. The intensity of the radiant heat source was adjusted to yield baseline latencies between 3 and 5 s in wild-type mice. A cut-off latency of 10 s was imposed to avoid damage of tail tissues.

2.3.2. Tail Immersion Test. Animals were placed in a loose plexiglas restrainer with their tail extending through a hole in the water bath of the apparatus (Stuart Bibby Sterilin Ltd, Water Baths SWB1D, UK), as previously described [31]. The lower 2/3 of the tail was immersed in hot water maintained at a constant temperature of 52.0 ± 0.5°C. The latency between tail immersion and attempts to remove the tail from the hot water bath was recorded. A cut-off latency of 15 s was imposed to avoid damage of tail tissues.

2.3.3. Hot Plate Test. Animals were placed individually on the surface of the hot plate apparatus (PanLab, LE 7406, Spain) surrounded by a plexiglas cylinder (20 cm in diameter, 25 cm high). The temperature of the surface was maintained at 55.0 ± 0.5°C, according to the method previously described [32]. The time between placement and the occurrence of forepaw licking (FPL), hindpaw licking (HPL), or jump was recorded as response latency. A cut-off latency of 240 s was established to avoid damage of paw tissues.

2.3.4. Formalin Test. Formalin (20 µL of a 2.5% formalin solution; 0.92% of formaldehyde) was injected into the dorsal surface on the right hind paw, as previously described [33]. The formalin test is a valid and reliable model of nociception with two distinct periods of high licking activity that have different nociceptive mechanisms, an early phase lasting the first 5 min and a late phase lasting from 15 to 45 min after the injection of formalin. Mice were placed on a paper surface surrounded by a plexiglas cylinder (20 × 25 cm) and the time spent licking and biting the injected paw was measured using a chronometer. A time course of the licking/biting behaviors was monitored during 45 minutes after formalin injection to evaluate possible differences between genotypes. Drug effects were quantified at 0–5 min (phase I) and 15–30 min (phase II) after formalin injection, two periods of time in which the formalin-induced licking and biting time was high enough to test antinociceptive effects of drugs.

2.3.5. Rectal Temperature. The body temperature was recorded using a precision thermometer (YSI 4600) equipped with a flexible probe (YSI 402). This probe was lubricated with vaseline and inserted 2 cm into the rectum. Temperature recordings were made 20 s following insertion of the probe, as previously described [27, 28].

2.4. Data Analysis. Data are presented as mean values ± S.E.M. Statistical analysis to test significant differences among groups was made using ANOVA followed by Bonferroni's post hoc comparison. Unpaired Student's *t*-test was used to test differences between two groups. The level of significance was set at $P < 0.05$. Data analysis and graphing were done using GraphPad Prism software (version 4.0; GraphPad Software Inc., USA).

3. Results

3.1. Similar Response to Noxious Thermal Stimuli and Formalin-Induced Nociception in 5-HT$_7$ Receptor Knockout and Wild-Type Mice. Sensitivity to noxious heat measured as the latency of response to thermal stimulation in the tail flick, tail immersion, and hot plate tests was similar in 5-HT$_7$ receptor knockout mice and paired wild-type mice (Figure 1). No significant differences between the two genotypes were found in tail withdrawal latency in the tail flick ($t_{49} = 1.09$, $P = 0.28$) and tail immersion ($t_{49} = 1.82$, $P = 0.08$) tests (Figure 1(a)). Both genotypes showed also the same latency for all measured behaviors in the hot plate test (Figure 1(b)): forepaw licking ($t_{49} = 1.69$, $P = 0.10$), hindpaw licking ($t_{49} = 0.73$, $P = 0.47$), and jump ($t_{48} = 0.81$, $P = 0.42$), suggesting that 5-HT$_7$ receptor knockout mice perceive and respond normally to acute thermal nociceptive stimuli. In addition, formalin-induced licking and biting of the paw injected with formalin in 5-HT$_7$ receptor knockout mice did not differ from wild-type mice. Repeated measures ANOVA (time × genotype) showed a significant effect of time ($F_{8,162} = 24.30$, $P < 0.001$), but no effect of genotype ($F_{1,162} = 1.76$, $P = 0.19$) and no interaction between these two factors

(a) Tail flick and Tail immersion

(b) Hot plate 55°C

-□- 5-HT$_7$R$^{+/+}$
-■- 5-HT$_7$R$^{-/-}$

(c) Formalin-induced nociception

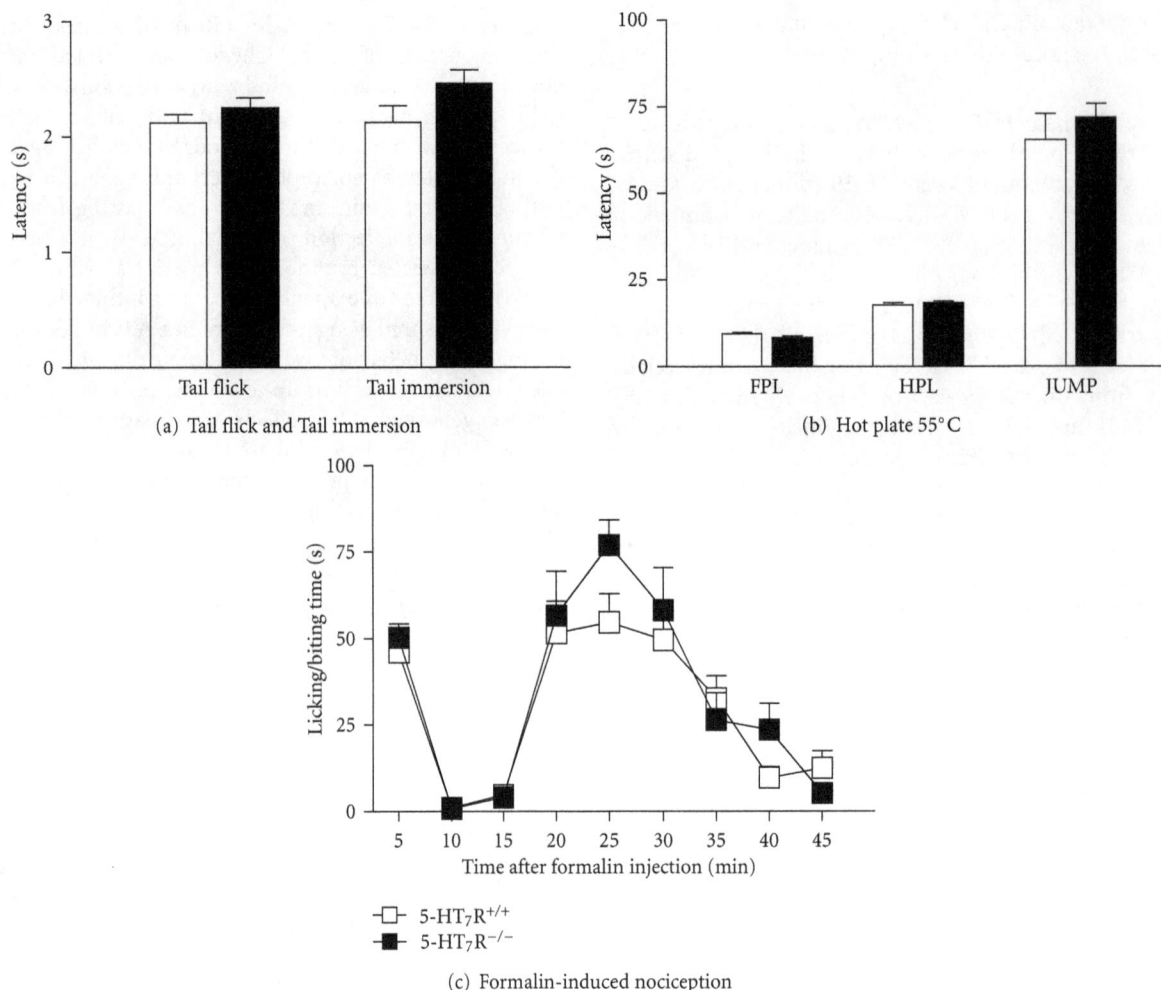

FIGURE 1: Nociceptive behavior of wild-type and 5-HT$_7$ receptor knockout mice in the tail flick and tail immersion tests (a), hot plate 55°C test (b), and formalin test (c). Both genotypes showed similar latency for all measured behaviors in the tail flick, tail immersion, and hot plate tests. Formalin-induced licking and biting of the hind paw injected with formalin in 5-HT$_7$ receptor knockout mice did not significantly differ from those in wild-type mice either in phase I (0–5 min) or in phase II (15–45 min). Only a slight but not significant increase of the licking/biting time was observed 25 min after formalin injection in 5-HT$_7$ receptor knockout mice compared to wild-type mice. Each bar or symbol represents the mean ± S.E.M. (n = 10–12 per group). Forepaw licking: FPL; hindpaw licking: HPL. No significant differences were observed in thermal nociception (unpaired Student's t-test) or formalin-induced nociceptive behaviors (Two-Way ANOVA).

($F_{8,162}$ = 0.90, P = 0.52). A slightly greater licking/biting time was observed 25 min after formalin injection in the 5-HT$_7$ receptor knockout in comparison with wild-type mice, but difference was not significant (Figure 1(c)).

3.2. 5-HT$_7$ Receptor Agonists Inhibited Selectively Phase II of Formalin-Induced Nociceptive Behavior in Wild-Type but Not in 5-HT$_7$ Receptor Knockout Mice. To examine the *in vivo* functional specificity of 5-HT$_7$ receptor agonists, AS-19, E-57431 and E-55888 were subcutaneously administered to wild-type and 5-HT$_7$ receptor knockout mice, and treated animals were then subjected to nociceptive tests. Effective doses of AS-19 (10 mg/kg), E-57431 (10 mg/kg), and E-55888 (20 mg/kg) in reversing allodynia/hyperalgesia following capsaicin sensitization and nerve injury [13, 14] were used in these experiments. The 5-HT$_7$ receptor agonists were

administered in the formalin test at doses devoid of motor disturbing effects which could interfere with licking/biting behaviors, as previously described [14].

No significant effects were exerted by 5-HT$_7$ receptor agonists on the response to thermal stimuli in the tail flick, tail immersion, and hot plate tests, and the formalin-induced phase I nociceptive behavior was not modified when 5-HT$_7$ receptor agonists were administered to wild-type or 5-HT$_7$ receptor knockout mice (data not shown). However, all three 5-HT$_7$ receptor agonists inhibited phase II of the formalin-induced nociceptive behavior in wild-type mice, as evidenced by a reduction in the duration of licking/biting of the hindpaw injected with formalin (Figure 2). Two-way ANOVA (treatment × genotype) showed a significant effect of treatment after AS-19 administration ($F_{1,38}$ = 10.34, P = 0.003), without genotype effect ($F_{1,38}$ = 0.04,

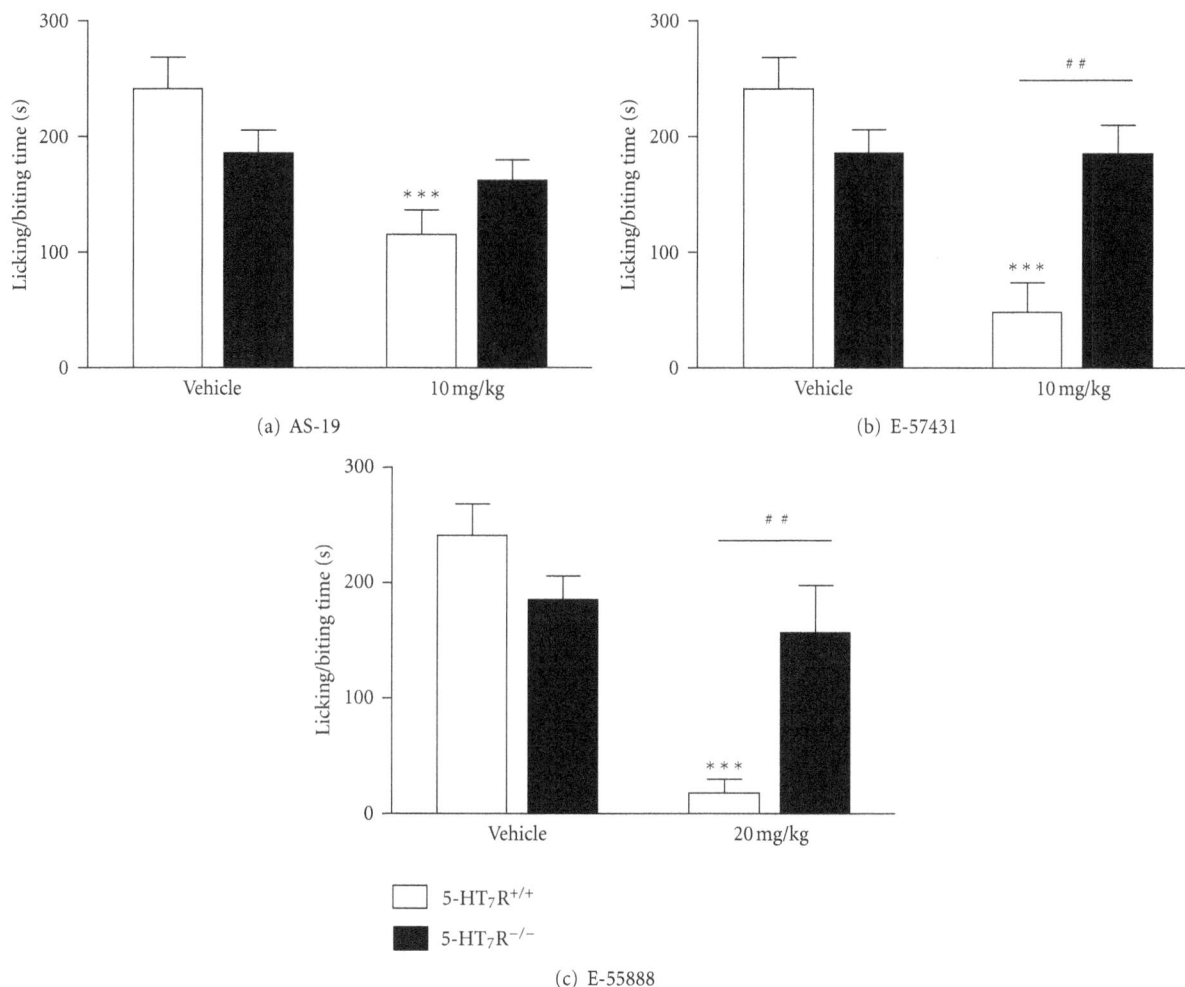

(a) AS-19

(b) E-57431

(c) E-55888

5-HT$_7$R$^{+/+}$

5-HT$_7$R$^{-/-}$

FIGURE 2: Effects of 5-HT$_7$ receptor agonists AS-19 (a), E-57431 (b), and E-55888 (c) on formalin-induced nociceptive behaviors during phase II in wild-type and 5-HT$_7$ receptor knockout mice. Subcutaneous administration of AS-19 (10 mg/kg), E-57431 (10 mg/kg), and E-55888 (20 mg/kg) significantly reduced the licking/biting time of the hind paw injected with formalin in wild-type but not in 5-HT$_7$ receptor knockout mice. Each bar represents the mean ± S.E.M. (n = 7–12). ***P < 0.001 versus vehicle corresponding group; ##P < 0.01 versus corresponding dose in 5-HT$_7$ receptor knockout mice (Bonferroni multiple comparison test after ANOVA).

P = 0.84) and a significant interaction between these two factors ($F_{1,38}$ = 4.86, P = 0.03). The comparison between treatments revealed a significant reduction of licking/biting time after AS-19 administration at 10 mg/kg in wild-type mice (P < 0.001; Figure 2). Two-way ANOVA calculated for E-57431 also showed a significant effect of treatment after E-57431 administration ($F_{1,39}$ = 15.04, P < 0.001), without genotype effect ($F_{1,39}$ = 2.64, P = 0.11) and a significant interaction between these two factors ($F_{1,39}$ = 14.91, P < 0.001). The comparison between treatments revealed a significant reduction of licking/biting time after E-57431 administration at 10 mg/kg in wild-type mice (P < 0.001; Figure 2). In addition, a significant difference was found between genotypes when E-57431 was administered at 10 mg/kg (P < 0.01; Figure 2). In the same way, two-way ANOVA calculated for E-55888 also showed a significant effect of treatment after E-55888 administration ($F_{1,35}$ = 22.3, P < 0.001), without genotype effect ($F_{1,35}$ = 2.42, P = 0.13) and a significant interaction between these two factors

($F_{1,35}$ = 13.32, P < 0.001). The comparison between treatments revealed a significant reduction of licking/biting time after E-55888 administration at 20 mg/kg in wild-type mice (P < 0.001; Figure 2). In addition, a significant difference was found between genotypes when E-55888 was administered at 20 mg/kg (P < 0.01; Figure 2). Interestingly, none of the three 5-HT$_7$ receptor agonists exerted significant effects on formalin phase II nociceptive behavior in 5-HT$_7$ receptor knockout mice (Figure 2).

3.3. Selective Doses of 5-HT$_7$ Receptor Agonists Produced No Effect on Body Temperature in 5-HT$_7$ Receptor Knockout and Wild-Type Mice. The *in vivo* specificity of the 5-HT$_7$ receptor agonists (AS-19, E-57431, and E-55888) was further examined using 5-HT$_7$ receptor knockout and paired wild-type mice in the paradigm based on 5-HT$_7$ receptor-mediated hypothermia [27]. Basal body temperature did not significantly differ in 5-HT$_7$ receptor knockout and

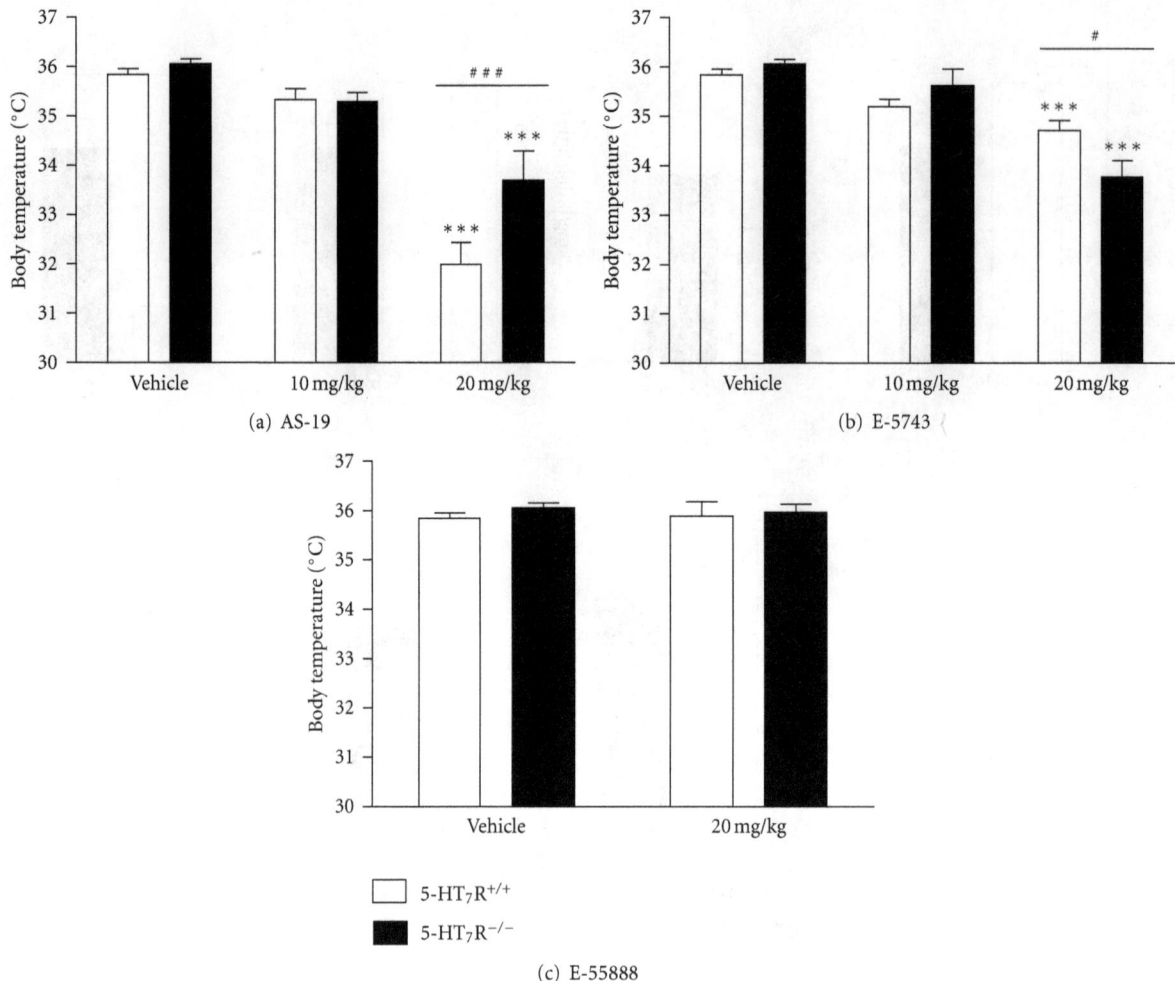

FIGURE 3: Effects of 5-HT$_7$ receptor agonists AS-19 (a), E-57431 (b), and E-55888 (c) on body temperature in wild-type and 5-HT$_7$ receptor knockout mice. Subcutaneous administration of AS-19 and E-57431 at 20 mg/kg significantly reduced body temperature in both wild-type and 5-HT$_7$ receptor knockout mice and showed significant differences between both genotypes. However, E-55888 at 20 mg/kg did not reduce the body temperature neither in wild-type nor in 5-HT$_7$ knockout mice. Each bar represents the mean ± S.E.M. ($n = 8$–12). ***$P < 0.001$ versus vehicle corresponding group; #$P < 0.05$; ###$P < 0.001$ versus corresponding dose in 5-HT$_7$ receptor knockout mice (Bonferroni multiple comparison test post-ANOVA).

paired wild-type mice (36.1 ± 0.1°C and 35.8 ± 0.1°C, resp.; Figure 3).

Two-way ANOVA (treatment × genotype) showed a significant effect of treatment after AS-19 administration ($F_{2,49} = 62.17$, $P < 0.001$), with genotype effect ($F_{1,49} = 6.88$, $P = 0.01$) and a significant interaction between these two factors ($F_{2,49} = 4.77$, $P = 0.01$). The comparison between treatments revealed a significant reduction of body temperature after AS-19 administration at 20 mg/kg in wild-type and 5-HT$_7$ receptor knockout mice ($P < 0.001$; Figure 3). In addition, a significant difference was found between genotypes when AS-19 was administered at 20 mg/kg ($P < 0.001$; Figure 3). Two-way ANOVA calculated for E-57431 also showed a significant effect of treatment after E-57431 administration ($F_{2,49} = 35.85$, $P < 0.001$), without genotype effect ($F_{1,49} = 0.31$, $P = 0.58$) and a significant interaction between these two factors ($F_{2,49} = 5.82$, $P = 0.005$). The comparison between treatments revealed a significant

reduction of body temperature after E-57431 administration at 20 mg/kg in wild-type and 5-HT$_7$ receptor knockout mice ($P < 0.001$; Figure 3). In addition, a significant difference was found between genotypes when E-57431 was administered at 20 mg/kg ($P < 0.05$; Figure 3). However, two-way ANOVA calculated for E-55888 did not show significant differences on treatment after E-55888 administration ($F_{1,35} = 0.02$, $P = 0.89$), neither genotype effect ($F_{1,35} = 0.91$, $P = 0.35$) nor interaction between these two factors ($F_{1,35} = 0.21$, $P = 0.65$). The comparison between treatments and genotypes did not reveal significant reduction of body temperature after E-55888 administration at 20 mg/kg ($P > 0.05$; Figure 3).

Subcutaneous administration of doses of AS-19 (10 mg/kg), E-57431 (10 mg/kg), and E-55888 (20 mg/kg) which exerted analgesic effects in phase II formalin-induced pain, did not significantly change body temperature neither in 5-HT$_7$ receptor wild-type nor in knockout mice (Figure 3). However, administration of a higher dose

(20 mg/kg, s.c.) of the 5-HT$_7$ receptor agonists AS-19 and E-57431 significantly reduced body temperature in both genotypes (Figure 3), suggesting that at such a high dose the selectivity window of AS-19 and E-57431 was overstepped. AS-19 at the 20 mg/kg dose produced a higher body temperature reduction in wild-type than in 5-HT$_7$ receptor knockout mice (3.8 versus 2.4°C, resp.). In contrast, E-57431 at the same high dose (20 mg/kg) produced a lower body temperature reduction in wild-type than in 5-HT$_7$ receptor knockout mice (1.1 versus 2.3°C, resp.) (Figure 3).

4. Discussion

In this study, the *in vivo* target-specific effects of the 5-HT$_7$ receptor agonists AS-19, E-57431, and E-55888 on nociception (i.e., formalin-induced nociception) and thermoregulation were examined using 5-HT$_7$ receptor knockout mice. These 5-HT$_7$ receptor agonists exerted antinociceptive effects in phase II of the formalin test in wild-type but not in 5-HT$_7$ receptor knockout mice, suggesting that their analgesic effect is actually 5-HT$_7$ receptor mediated. Analgesic doses of 5-HT$_7$ receptor agonists did not change body temperature neither in 5-HT$_7$ receptor knockout nor in wild-type mice. However, a reduction in body temperature was observed in both genotypes when the dose of the agonists were increased up to levels exceeding their selectivity window.

The 5-HT$_7$ receptor knockout mice offer a complementary approach to classical pharmacology and might provide insights into the functional implications of 5-HT$_7$ receptors. To date, data obtained with these mutants suggest the involvement of 5-HT$_7$ receptors in depression, schizophrenia, sleep, learning, locomotion, and hypothermia [25, 28, 34–37].

In this work, we demonstrated that sensitivity to noxious heat measured as the latency time of response to thermal stimulation in the tail flick, tail immersion, and hot plate tests did not differ in 5-HT$_7$ receptor knockout compared to wild-type mice, as previously described [38]. In addition, the formalin-induced nociceptive behavior of 5-HT$_7$ receptor knockout mice was not different from wild-type mice as no significant differences in licking/biting time were found between both genotypes, for either phase I or phase II of the formalin test. These results suggest that basic mechanisms for transduction, transmission, and perception of, as well as response to, nociceptive stimuli are intact in mice lacking 5-HT$_7$ receptors. As previously reported, the loss of function of the missing 5-HT$_7$ receptor could induce possible adaptive changes which could compensate for some alterations, thereby resulting in wild-type-like responses [38–40].

Thermal nociception and early phase response in the formalin test are caused predominantly by direct activation of peripheral C-fibers, whereas the late response (phase II) in the formalin test involves functional changes in the dorsal horn of the spinal cord (i.e., central sensitization) [41–43]. In this study, subcutaneous administration of 5-HT$_7$ receptor agonists was devoid of activity in acute nociceptive tests (i.e., thermal- and formalin-induced phase I nociception), but exerted clear-cut antinociceptive effects in phase II of

the formalin test in wild-type mice. These results are in line with previous studies showing that 5-HT$_7$ receptor agonists and antagonists were ineffective in acute thermal nociceptive pain [44–47]. The lack of antinociceptive effects in thermal and phase I formalin-induced nociception, observed when 5-HT$_7$ receptor agonists were administered, suggests no direct modulation by the 5-HT$_7$ receptor subtype of acute nociceptive signals coming from small caliber unmyelinated nociceptive afferents. However, activation of spinal 5-HT$_7$ receptors has been shown to play a role in the antinociceptive effects of opioids [44–47].

Our results on phase II formalin-induced behavior are in line with previous reports describing antinociceptive effects of selective 5-HT$_7$ receptor agonists by systemic or spinal administration in neurogenic and neuropathic pain conditions involving central sensitization [13, 14, 17]. However, a clear-cut pronociceptive (proallodynic) effect was found when a 5-HT$_7$ receptor agonist was administered intraplantarly into the ipsilateral hind paw injected with a low subactive dose of capsaicin [17]. In contrast, data in the literature using the formalin test suggest a pronociceptive role of both peripheral and spinal 5-HT$_7$ receptors. Indeed, intraplantar or spinal administration of 5-carboxamidotryptamine, a nonselective 5-HT$_7$ receptor agonist, increased phase II formalin-induced nociceptive behavior, and these effects were significantly reversed by the selective 5-HT$_7$ receptor antagonist SB-269970 [23]. Differences could be due to species (mice versus rats), primary administration route (systemic versus spinal and local peripheral), selectivity of the 5-HT$_7$ agonists used and animal models.

To further assess the *in vivo* specificity of the 5-HT$_7$ receptor agonists used in this study, we examined in 5-HT$_7$ receptor knockout mice, the effects of the 5-HT$_7$ receptor agonists AS-19, E-57431, and E-55888 on both formalin-induced nociception and body temperature. Under our experimental conditions, 5-HT$_7$ receptor agonists, at doses effective to reduce phase II formalin-induced nociceptive behavior, affected body temperature neither in wild-type mice nor in 5-HT$_7$ knockout mutants. However, AS-19 and E-57431 at the high dose of 20 mg/kg significantly reduced body temperature not only in wild-type but also in 5-HT$_7$ receptor knockout mice, indicating a non-5-HT$_7$ receptor-mediated effect possibly due to interactions of these compounds with other 5-HT receptors when their selectivity window is surpassed. In line with this interpretation, we found that E-55888, the most selective 5-HT$_7$ receptor agonist based on *in vitro* radioligand binding assays (Table 1), even at the dose of 20 mg/kg, did not exert any effect on body temperature in both genotypes. Taken together, the finding that the less selective agonists (AS-19 and E-57431) at high doses reduced body temperature in both wild-type and knockout mice, whereas the most selective one (E-55888) did not, suggests that activation of 5-HT$_7$ receptors alone is not enough to affect body temperature. Our results do not rule out the possibility that 5-HT$_7$ receptors might contribute to the regulation of body temperature by acting in concert with other serotonergic and/or nonserotonergic receptors. Indeed, we found a higher hypothermic effect induced by AS-19 (20 mg/kg) in wild-type compared to 5-HT$_7$ receptor knockout mice, suggesting that 5-HT$_7$ receptors might promote the decrease in body temperature when other mechanisms are also recruited. The *in vitro* binding profile of these ligands (see Table 1) suggests that 5-HT$_{1D}$ and/or 5-HT$_{1A}$ receptors could be involved in the observed hypothermic effects of AS-19 and E-57431, also because activation of these receptor types has been reported to induce hypothermia [16, 28, 48]. Overall, as previously reported, 5-HT$_7$ receptors appear to be involved in a complex manner in thermoregulation, probably through mechanisms implicating direct/indirect interactions between 5-HT$_7$ receptors and other molecular targets.

5. Conclusions

Data obtained in this study strengthen the notion that 5-HT$_7$ receptors play a role in nociceptive control in pain conditions involving central sensitization and add further support to their fine-tuning effects in body temperature homeostasis through possible actions in concert with other molecular targets. In addition, this study provides evidence that formalin-induced nociceptive behaviors and body temperature in 5-HT$_7$ receptor knockout mice are useful models and relatively simple approaches to assess *in vivo* specificity of 5-HT$_7$ receptor agonists.

Authors' Contribution

A. Brenchat and M. Rocasalbas contributed equally to this paper.

Conflict of Interests

There was no conflict of interests with respect to the work reported in the paper.

Acknowledgment

The authors thank Mrs. Mercè Olivet for her administrative assistance.

References

[1] P. B. Hedlund, "The 5-HT$_7$ receptor and disorders of the nervous system: an overview," *Psychopharmacology*, vol. 206, no. 3, pp. 345–354, 2009.

[2] M. Leopoldo, E. Lacivita, F. Berardi, R. Perrone, and P. B. Hedlund, "Serotonin 5-HT$_7$ receptor agents: structure-activity relationships and potential therapeutic applications in central nervous system disorders," *Pharmacology and Therapeutics*, vol. 129, no. 2, pp. 120–148, 2011.

[3] D. J. Cushing, J. M. Zgombick, D. L. Nelson, and M. L. Cohen, "LY215840, a high-affinity 5-HT$_7$ receptor ligand, blocks serotonin-induced relaxation in canine coronary artery," *Journal of Pharmacology and Experimental Therapeutics*, vol. 277, no. 3, pp. 1560–1566, 1996.

[4] I. T. Forbes, S. Dabbs, D. M. Duckworth et al., "(R)-3,N-Dim-ethyl-N-[1-methyl-3-(4-methyl-piperidin-1-yl)propyl] ben-zenesulfonamide: the first selective 5-HT$_7$ receptor

[5] C. Kikuchi, H. Nagaso, T. Hiranuma, and M. Koyama, "Tetrahydrobenzindoles: selective antagonists of the 5-HT$_7$ receptor," *Journal of Medicinal Chemistry*, vol. 42, no. 4, pp. 533–535, 1999.

[6] P. J. Lovell, S. M. Bromidge, S. Dabbs et al., "A novel, potent, and selective 5-HT$_7$ antagonist: (R)-3-(2-(2-(4-methylpiperidin-1-yl)- ethyl)pyrrolidine-1-sulfonyl)phenol (SB-269970)," *Journal of Medicinal Chemistry*, vol. 43, no. 3, pp. 342–345, 2000.

[7] I. T. Forbes, S. Douglas, A. D. Gribble et al., "SB-656104-A: a novel 5-HT$_7$ receptor antagonist with improved in vivo properties," *Bioorganic and Medicinal Chemistry Letters*, vol. 12, no. 22, pp. 3341–3344, 2002.

[8] A. M. Johansson, M. Brisander, A. Sanin, S. Rosqvist, N. Mohell, A. Malmberg et al., "5-Aryl substituted (S)-2-(dimethylamino)-tetralins: novel serotonin 5-HT$_7$ receptor ligands," in *Proceedings of the 226th American Chemical Society National Meeting*, New York, NY, USA, 2003.

[9] A. Sanin, M. Brisander, S. Rosqvist, N. Mohell, A. Malberg, A. Johansson et al., "5-Aryl substituted (S)-2-(dimethylamino)-tetralins novel serotonin 5HT$_7$ receptor ligands," in *Proceedings of the 14th Camerino-Noord Symposium*, Ongoing Progress in the Receptor Chemistry, Camerino, Italy, 2003.

[10] C. G. Thomson, M. S. Beer, N. R. Curtis, H. J. Diggle, E. Handford, and J. J. Kulagowski, "Thiazoles and thiopyridines: novel series of high affinity h5HT$_7$ ligands," *Bioorganic and Medicinal Chemistry Letters*, vol. 14, no. 3, pp. 677–680, 2004.

[11] M. Leopoldo, F. Berardi, N. A. Colabufo et al., "Structure-affinity relationship study on N-(1,2,3,4-tetrahydrona-phthalen-1-yl)-4-aryl-1-piperazinealkylamides, a new class of 5-hydroxytryptamine 7 receptor agents," *Journal of Medicinal Chemistry*, vol. 47, no. 26, pp. 6616–6624, 2004.

[12] M. Leopoldo, E. Lacivita, P. De Giorgio et al., "Structural mod-ifications of N-(1,2,3,4-tetrahydronaphthalen-1-yl)-4-aryl-1-piperazinehexanamides: Influence on lipophilicity and 5-HT$_7$ receptor activity. Part III," *Journal of Medicinal Chemistry*, vol. 51, no. 18, pp. 5813–5822, 2008.

[13] A. Brenchat, L. Romero, M. García et al., "5-HT$_7$ receptor activation inhibits mechanical hypersensitivity secondary to capsaicin sensitization in mice," *Pain*, vol. 141, no. 3, pp. 239–247, 2009.

[14] A. Brenchat, X. Nadal, L. Romero et al., "Pharmacological activation of 5-HT$_7$ receptors reduces nerve injury-induced mechanical and thermal hypersensitivity," *Pain*, vol. 149, no. 3, pp. 483–494, 2010.

[15] M. Leopoldo, E. Lacivita, M. Contino, N. A. Colabufo, F. Berardi, and R. Perrone, "Structure-activity relationship study on N-(1,2,3,4-tetrahydronaphthalen-1- yl)-4-aryl-1-piperazinehexanamides, a class of 5-HT$_7$ receptor agents," *Journal of Medicinal Chemistry*, vol. 50, no. 17, pp. 4214–4221, 2007.

[16] P. B. Hedlund, M. Leopoldo, S. Caccia et al., "LP-211 is a brain penetrant selective agonist for the serotonin 5-HT$_7$ receptor," *Neuroscience Letters*, vol. 481, no. 1, pp. 12–16, 2010.

[17] A. Brenchat, D. Zamanillo, M. Hamon, L. Romero, J. M. Vela et al., "Role of peripheral versus spinal 5-HT$_7$ receptors in the modulation of pain under sensitizing conditions," *European Journal of Pain*, vol. 16, no. 1, pp. 72–81, 2012.

[18] M. I. Diaz-Reval, R. Ventura-Martinez, M. Deciga-Campos, J. A. Terron, F. Cabre, F. J. Lopez-Munoz et al., "Evidence for a

[4] ... antagonist," *Journal of Medicinal Chemistry*, vol. 41, no. 5, pp. 655–657, 1998.

central mechanism of action of S-(+)-ketoprofen," *European Journal of Pharmacology*, vol. 483, no. 2–3, pp. 241–248, 2004.

[19] S. Doly, J. Fischer, M. J. Brisorgueil, D. Vergé, and M. Conrath, "Pre- and postsynaptic localization of the 5-HT$_7$ receptor in rat dorsal spinal cord: immunocytochemical evidence," *Journal of Comparative Neurology*, vol. 490, no. 3, pp. 256–269, 2005.

[20] S. E. Harte, R. G. Kender, and G. S. Borszcz, "Activation of 5-HT$_{1A}$ and 5-HT$_7$ receptors in the parafascicular nucleus suppresses the affective reaction of rats to noxious stimulation," *Pain*, vol. 113, no. 3, pp. 405–415, 2005.

[21] T. Meuser, C. Pietruck, A. Gabriel, G. X. Xie, K. J. Lim, and P. Pierce Palmer, "5-HT$_7$ receptors are involved in mediating 5-HT-induced activation of rat primary afferent neurons," *Life Sciences*, vol. 71, no. 19, pp. 2279–2289, 2002.

[22] J. F. Neumaier, T. J. Sexton, J. Yracheta, A. M. Diaz, and M. Brownfield, "Localization of 5-HT$_7$ receptors in rat brain by immunocytochemistry, in situ hybridization, and agonist stimulated cFos expression," *Journal of Chemical Neuroanatomy*, vol. 21, no. 1, pp. 63–73, 2001.

[23] H. I. Rocha-González, A. Meneses, S. M. Carlton, and V. Granados-Soto, "Pronociceptive role of peripheral and spinal 5-HT$_7$ receptors in the formalin test," *Pain*, vol. 117, no. 1-2, pp. 182–192, 2005.

[24] M. R. Guscott, E. Egan, G. P. Cook et al., "The hypothermic effect of 5-CT in mice is mediated through the 5-HT$_7$ receptor," *Neuropharmacology*, vol. 44, no. 8, pp. 1031–1037, 2003.

[25] M. Guscott, L. J. Bristow, K. Hadingham et al., "Genetic knockout and pharmacological blockade studies of the 5-HT$_7$ receptor suggest therapeutic potential in depression," *Neuropharmacology*, vol. 48, no. 4, pp. 492–502, 2005.

[26] J. J. Hagan, G. W. Price, P. Jeffrey et al., "Characterization of SB-269970-A, a selective 5-HT$_7$ receptor antagonist," *British Journal of Pharmacology*, vol. 130, no. 3, pp. 539–548, 2000.

[27] P. B. Hedlund, P. E. Danielson, E. A. Thomas, K. Slanina, M. J. Carson, and J. G. Sutcliffe, "No hypothermic response to serotonin in 5-HT$_7$ receptor knockout mice," *Proceedings of the National Academy of Sciences of the United States of America*, vol. 100, no. 3, pp. 1375–1380, 2003.

[28] P. B. Hedlund, L. Kelly, C. Mazur, T. Lovenberg, J. G. Sutcliffe, and P. Bonaventure, "8-OH-DPAT acts on both 5-HT$_{1A}$ and 5-HT$_7$ receptors to induce hypothermia in rodents," *European Journal of Pharmacology*, vol. 487, no. 1–3, pp. 125–132, 2004.

[29] M. Zimmermann, "Ethical guidelines for investigations of experimental pain in conscious animals," *Pain*, vol. 16, no. 2, pp. 109–110, 1983.

[30] F. E. D'Amour, D. L. Smith et al., "A method for determining loss of pain sensation," *Journal of Pharmacology and Experimental Therapeutics*, vol. 72, no. 1, pp. 74–79, 1941.

[31] K. Ramabadran, M. Bansinath, H. Turndorf, and M. M. Puig, "Tail immersion test for the evaluation of a nociceptive reaction in mice. Methodological considerations," *Journal of Pharmacological Methods*, vol. 21, no. 1, pp. 21–31, 1989.

[32] G. Woolfe, A. D. MacDonald et al., "The evaluation of the analgesic action of pethidine hydrochloride (Demerol)," *Journal of Pharmacology and Experimental Therapeutics*, vol. 80, no. 3, pp. 300–307, 1944.

[33] S. Hunskaar and K. Hole, "The formalin test in mice: dissociation between inflammatory and non-inflammatory pain," *Pain*, vol. 30, no. 1, pp. 103–114, 1987.

[34] R. Galici, J. D. Boggs, K. L. Miller, P. Bonaventure, and J. R. Atack, "Effects of SB-269970, a 5-HT$_7$ receptor antagonist,

[35] P. B. Hedlund, S. Huitron-Resendiz, S. J. Henriksen, and J. G. Sutcliffe, "5-HT$_7$ receptor inhibition and inactivation induce antidepressantlike behavior and sleep pattern," *Biological Psychiatry*, vol. 58, no. 10, pp. 831–837, 2005.

[36] J. Liu, T. Akay, P. B. Hedlund, K. G. Pearson, and L. M. Jordan, "Spinal 5-HT$_7$ receptors are critical for alternating activity during locomotion: In vitro neonatal and in vivo adult studies using 5-HT$_7$ receptor knockout mice," *Journal of Neurophysiology*, vol. 102, no. 1, pp. 337–348, 2009.

[37] J. Shelton, P. Bonaventure, X. Li, S. Yun, T. Lovenberg, and C. Dugovic, "5-HT$_7$ receptor deletion enhances REM sleep suppression induced by selective serotonin reuptake inhibitors, but not by direct stimulation of 5-HT$_{1A}$ receptor," *Neuropharmacology*, vol. 56, pp. 448–454, 2009.

[38] A. J. Roberts, T. Krucker, C. L. Levy, K. A. Slanina, J. G. Sutcliffe, and P. B. Hedlund, "Mice lacking 5-HT$_7$ receptors show specific impairments in contextual learning," *European Journal of Neuroscience*, vol. 19, no. 7, pp. 1913–1922, 2004.

[39] G. Sarkisyan and P. B. Hedlund, "The 5-HT$_7$ receptor is involved in allocentric spatial memory information processing," *Behavioural Brain Research*, vol. 202, no. 1, pp. 26–31, 2009.

[40] S. Semenova, M. A. Geyer, J. G. Sutcliffe, A. Markou, and P. B. Hedlund, "Inactivation of the 5-HT$_7$ receptor partially blocks phencyclidine-induced disruption of prepulse inhibition," *Biological Psychiatry*, vol. 63, no. 1, pp. 98–105, 2008.

[41] T. J. Coderre and R. Melzack, "The contribution of excitatory amino acids to central sensitization and persistent nociception after formalin-induced tissue injury," *Journal of Neuroscience*, vol. 12, no. 9, pp. 3665–3670, 1992.

[42] A. Tjølsen, O. G. Berge, S. Hunskaar, J. H. Rosland, and K. Hole, "The formalin test: an evaluation of the method," *Pain*, vol. 51, no. 1, pp. 5–17, 1992.

[43] K. Vissers, V. Hoffmann, F. Geenen, R. Biermans, and T. Meert, "Is the second phase of the formalin test useful to predict activity in chronic constriction injury models? A pharmacological comparison in different species," *Pain Practice*, vol. 3, pp. 298–309, 2003.

[44] A. Brenchat, M. Ejarque, D. Zamanillo, J. M. Vela, L. Romero et al., "Potentiation of morphine analgesia by adjuvant activation of 5-HT$_7$ receptors," *Journal of Pharmacological Sciences*, vol. 116, no. 4, pp. 388–391, 2011.

[45] A. Dogrul, M. H. Ossipov, and F. Porreca, "Differential mediation of descending pain facilitation and inhibition by spinal 5HT$_3$ and 5HT$_7$ receptors," *Brain Research*, vol. 1280, pp. 52–59, 2009.

[46] A. Dogrul and M. Seyrek, "Systemic morphine produce antinociception mediated by spinal 5-HT$_7$, but not 5-HT$_{1A}$ and 5-HT$_2$ receptors in the spinal cord," *British Journal of Pharmacology*, vol. 149, no. 5, pp. 498–505, 2006.

[47] O. Yanarates, A. Dogrul, V. Yildirim et al., "Spinal 5-HT$_7$ receptors play an important role in the antinociceptive and antihyperalgesic effects of tramadol and its metabolite, o-desmethyltramadol, via activation of descending serotonergic pathways," *Anesthesiology*, vol. 112, no. 3, pp. 696–710, 2010.

[48] H. O. Kalkman and V. Neumann, "Evidence for a 5-HT$_{1D}$ receptor-mediated hypothermic effect of the α1-adrenoceptor agonist, SDZ NVI-085, in guinea-pigs," *European Journal of Pharmacology*, vol. 285, no. 3, pp. 313–315, 1995.

4

Central Dopaminergic System and Its Implications in Stress-Mediated Neurological Disorders and Gastric Ulcers: Short Review

Naila Rasheed[1] and Abdullah Alghasham[2]

[1] Department of Medical Biochemistry, College of Medicine, Qassim University, P.O. BOX 6655, Buraidah 51452, Saudi Arabia
[2] Department of Pharmacology and Therapeutics, College of Medicine, Qassim University, P.O. BOX 6655, Buraidah 51452, Saudi Arabia

Correspondence should be addressed to Naila Rasheed, naila1381@gmail.com

Academic Editor: Mustafa F. Lokhandwala

For decades, it has been suggested that dysfunction of dopaminergic pathways and their associated modulations in dopamine levels play a major role in the pathogenesis of neurological disorders. Dopaminergic system is involved in the stress response, and the neural mechanisms involved in stress are important for current research, but the recent and past data on the stress response by dopaminergic system have received little attention. Therefore, we have discussed these data on the stress response and propose a role for dopamine in coping with stress. In addition, we have also discussed gastric stress ulcers and their correlation with dopaminergic system. Furthermore, we have also highlighted some of the glucocorticoids and dopamine-mediated neurological disorders. Our literature survey suggests that dopaminergic system has received little attention in both clinical and preclinical research on stress, but the current research on this issue will surely identify a better understanding of stressful events and will give better ideas for further efficient antistress treatments.

1. Introduction

Dopamine (DA) is an important endogenous catecholamine, which exerts widespread effects on both neuronal (as a neurotransmitter) and nonneuronal tissues (as an autocrine or paracrine agent) [1]. Within the central nervous system (CNS), DA binds to specific membrane receptors presented by neurons, and it plays a key role in the control of locomotion, learning, working memory, cognition, and emotion [2, 3]. The brain DA system is involved in various neurological and psychiatric disturbances including Parkinson's disease, schizophrenia, amphetamine, and cocaine addiction [1, 3]. Therefore, it is considered to be a major target for drug designing applied in the treatment of neurological diseases. Stress has been shown to alter normal dopaminergic neurotransmission [4], and exposure to stress profoundly increases the dopaminergic activity [4, 5] and induces relevant adaptive response of DA receptors in specific brain regions [6]. Stress also activates the hypothalamus-pituitary-adrenal

(HPA) axis and releases glucocorticoids (GCs). The interplay between GCs and the dopaminergic system is linked with various neurological disorders such as schizophrenia, bipolar depressive disorder and major depressive disorder, addiction, and Parkinson's disease [7, 8]. A number of reports showed the involvement of GCs on DA-mediated behavioral responsiveness by the modulatory effects of corticosterone [8–10]. Many reports suggest the involvement of DA system in locomotors alterations under different stressful conditions [9–11]. The stress-induced adaptation of brain DA function involves receptors, and it has also been demonstrated that DA receptor densities are affected by altered extracellular DA levels [10, 12, 13]. It is also demonstrated that stress manipulations induced the alteration in motor activity of experimental animals, and dopaminergic pathways are crucial to neural substrates for the control of spontaneous locomotor activity [3, 11]. These studies clearly indicated that DA plays an essential role in locomotion via neural transmission.

Dopaminergic system is also known to play a regulatory role in gastric ulcers under various stressful conditions [14, 15]. Patients with Parkinson's disease have higher rate of ulcer, where DA becomes deficient. But in patients with schizophrenia, DA level usually becomes high, and the rate of gastric ulcer becomes very less [15]. This indicates that DA levels must have a link with gastric pathology. Studies also suggested that modulation of dopaminergic transmission induced by DA drugs facilitates the gastric cytomodulatory effects [15, 16]. Furthermore, administration of DA or related agents attenuated stress ulcerogenesis, whereas opposite effects have been also seen with DA-lytic drugs [15–17]. Not only this, but it is also reported that DA mediates gastric cytoprotective effects on other neurotransmitters [18, 19]. Now, it is well established that stress induced ulcerogenesis is governed by activation of the mesocorticolimbic DA systems [15–20]. Alterations of DA levels and total ulcer score in acute and chronic unpredictable stress models have been summarized in Table 1. All this debate clearly indicates that DA plays an important role in ulcerogenesis during stress. This paper provides an update on DA activities in stressful events that represent, in our opinion, the optimal utility as future therapeutic target for neurodegenerative disorders.

2. Interplay between Stressful Events and Central Dopaminergic System

In 1950, Hns Selye borrowed the term "stress" from physics and hypothesized that a constellation of stereotypic psychological and physiological events occurring in seriously ill patients represented the consequences of a severe, prolonged application of adaptation responses. He recognized that stress plays a very significant role in the development of all types of diseases [21]. Selye believed that daily lives are influenced by two different kinds of stress: pleasant stress contributing to "wellness" and unpleasant stress contributing to disease and sickness [21]. Mesocortical and mesolimbic (M-L) dopaminergic systems are known to mediate HPA axis-induced GC release and other CNS effects [8, 22, 23]. Various neurological disorders are linked with GCs and the dopaminergic system [7, 8, 23]. Evidence shows that central dopaminergic system exerts positive effects on the HPA axis and the sympathetic nervous system (SNS), and reciprocally, glucocorticoids and catecholamines mediated stress-induced alterations [24, 25]. Modulations of DA in major brain regions are mediated by dopaminergic receptors, which are classified as D_1 and D_2 types. Classification of these DA receptors is based on the mechanism that links these G-protein-coupled receptors (GPCRs) to the second messenger system [26]. Thus, D_1-like receptors stimulate the adenylate cyclase activity via Gs subunit leading to an increased cyclic adenosine monophosphate (cAMP) concentration [27]. On the other hand, D_2-like receptors are negatively coupled via the Gi subunit to the adenylate cyclase, which leads to a decline in the cAMP concentration. Both D_1 and D_2 of receptors are abundantly expressed in major brain areas such as nucleus accumbens, striatum, frontal cortex, amygdala, and hippocampus [27]. Furthermore, both D_1 and D_2 are also involved in vigilance, hormonal homeostasis, and locomotor

activities. It is reported that stressful experiences alter DA metabolism through D_1 and D_2 receptors and release in the M-L system [28–30]. Furthermore, it is also reported that exposure to a single unavoidable/uncontrollable aversive experience may lead to inhibition of DA release in the nucleus accumbens as well as to impair the response to both rewarding and aversive stimuli [25, 31]. The effects of stressful experiences on DA functioning in the M-L system can be very different or even opposite depending on situation, the genetic background of the organism, and its life history [24]. We and the others have shown that stress differentially increases the dynamics of DA depending on the brain regions involved [9, 30]. Reports also stated that stressful stimuli tend to cause the largest increase in DA levels in the PFC (prefrontal cortex) region, with markedly smaller changes in the limbic and dorsal striatal regions [32, 33]; however, this relationship is altered by lesions of different nuclei. Thus, stress causes release of DA in the amygdala, and lesions of the amygdala tend to block stress-induced increases in PFC DA levels [34]. Lesions of the PFC also affect this response. Studies in which the PFC DA innervations are lesioned show that subsequent stressors cause a much larger increase in DA levels within the nucleus accumbens, particularly with respect to the duration of the response [31, 34]. This suggested that PFC DA released in response to stress actually blunts the responsiveness of the subcortical limbic DA system. In contrast, 6-OHDA lesions of PFC DA levels were found to decrease the basal electrophysiologic activity of ventral tegmental area (VTA) DA neurons [35]. Repeated stress also has important clinical implications in regard to the DA system. A recent study examined how chronic stress in the form of cold exposure affects the discharge of VTA DA neurons. Thus, after exposing rats to cold, there was a 64% decrease in the number of spontaneously active DA neurons, with no significant alteration in their average firing rate. Nonetheless, there was a subpopulation of neurons that exhibited excessive burst activity in the exposed rats [36]. Unlike acute exposure to stressful or noxious stimuli, chronic stress actually attenuates DA neuron baseline activity.

The interplay between glucocorticoids (GCs) and the dopaminergic systems has been reported in many human diseases [37]. GCs are released as a result of HPA-axis activation in stressful condition [7, 8, 38]. Mesocortical and M-L dopaminergic neuronal systems are hypothesized to mediate some of the CNS effects of glucocorticoids [7, 22, 38]. Our previous study favors this hypothesis, in which we found elevated levels of corticosterone and alteration in GCs receptor in different brain regions during stress [39, 40]. The fact that both corticosterone and DA are sensitive to both psychological and physical environmental stimuli suggests that the interaction between these two chemical messengers may be involved in mediating the differential responding to positively reinforcing drugs following a single or repeated stressful experience. This is further supported by various other investigators that provide evidence for a decreased prefrontal dopaminergic transmission. Adrenalectomy impaired working memory resulted in decreased dopaminergic transmission in the PFC [41]. Furthermore, addition of GCs can increase dopaminergic activity in PFC,

TABLE 1: Acute and chronic unpredictable stress-induced alterations in dopamine, prostaglandin E_2 levels, histopathological changes, and mean ulcer score in gastric tissues.

Parameters in gastric tissues	Models		
	Nonstress	Acute stress	Chronic unpredictable stress
Dopamine levels	0	↓	↓↓
Prostaglandin E_2	0	0	↓
Histopathological changes	0	↑	↑↑
Mean ulcer score	0	↑	↑↑
Plasma corticosterone	0	↑↑	↑

This information was obtained from our previous paper [39]. Plasma corticosterone was shown as stress marker. Symbols represent the following: 0: no effect, ↓: small decrease, ↓↓: large decrease, ↑: small increase, and ↑↑: large increase.

suggesting a crosstalk between the GCs receptor and the dopaminergic system. Taken all together, these data suggest that, both GCs and DA systems represent attractive therapeutic targets for stress-induced neurological disorders and should be investigated further. Modulations of dopaminergic pathways and their associated changes of dopamine levels in neurological disorders have been shown in Table 2.

Here, we have discussed some of the DA- and GCs-mediated neurological diseases.

2.1. Schizophrenia. Millions of people suffer from schizophrenia at some point in their life, making it one of the most common health problems in the whole world [8]. This biological disorder of the brain is a result of abnormalities, which arise early in life and disrupt the normal development of the brain. These abnormalities involve structural differences between a schizophrenic brain and a healthy brain [14]. The role of HPA axis changes in patients with schizophrenia is currently a matter of debate. Now, it is well established that hyperactivity of HPA axis is one of the parts for pathogenesis of schizophrenia. First, reduced GR gene expression levels, studied mainly by *in situ* hybridization assays, have been described in the frontal cortex and throughout all the hippocampus subfields of schizophrenic patients [8, 52, 53]. Second, neuropathological brain changes observed in schizophrenia are similar as changes caused by increased GC levels [54]. Conclusions should be made with caution as quantitative mRNA versus protein expression studies do not always result in a GR signal change of the same magnitude. Furthermore, it is also possible that these findings may be a downstream effect of the primary etiology or could be epiphenomena or even the effect of a drug treatment. One of the negative symptoms of schizophrenia is an impairment of working memory (the short-term storage needed for certain tasks). Several research groups have reported that HPA disruption leads to working memory impairment [55–57]. Furthermore, addition of GCs can increase dopaminergic activity in PFC, which suggests a crosstalk between the GR and the dopaminergic system [41].

Schizophrenic brains under stressful conditions tend to have larger lateral ventricles and a smaller volume of tissue in the left temporal lobe in comparison to healthy brains [58], and the chemical nature of a schizophrenic brain is different in the manner the brain handles DA in stressful (GC

secretion) events [8]. Thousands of chemical processes take place in a functioning neuron. The transfer of information is mediated by neurotransmitters that interact with certain receptors [8]. A study was conducted in which presynaptic DA function (measured by the uptake of fluorodopa) was observed by positron emission tomography (PET) in the brains of seven schizophrenic patients and eight healthy people (controls). The fluorodopa influx constant was higher in the schizophrenic patients. Their receptors took up more fluorodopa [58]. In conclusion, these alterations in presynaptic DA function during stressful conditions constituted a part of the disrupted neural circuits that predispose people to schizophrenia [58–60]. The DA receptors involved in these processes can be separated into the D_1 and D_2 families. The D_1 family contains the receptors D_1 and D_5. The D_1 receptors in the brain are linked to episodic memory, emotion, and cognition. These functions are disturbed in schizophrenic patients during stressful conditions. In addition, D_1 binding of DA was found to be lower in schizophrenic patients as compared to healthy subjects of the same age. The binding was lower as a result of fewer D_1 receptors. Certain antipsychotic drugs stimulate D_1-regulated pathways, which increases the D_1 to D_2 activity balance in the brain. This balance can also be regained by the release of DA. Not much is known about D_5 due to the lack of drugs that are selective for it. The D_2 family contains the receptors D_2, D_3, and D_4. D_2 is the second most abundant DA receptor in the brain. D_2 receptor blockade is the main target for antipsychotic drugs, because there is a higher density of D_2 in schizophrenic brains under stressful conditions [8, 58–60]. Studies have shown a selective loss of D_3 mRNA expression in the parietal and motor cortices of postmortem, schizophrenic brains [61]. This phenomenon may be due to either the course of the disease or therapy given to the patients. Studies have also found that the density of D_4 receptors was elevated sixfold in schizophrenic patients. These DA receptors are affected by alterations in the neural cell membranes, which could disrupt communication between cells. Abnormalities in two long-chain fatty acids in the blood cells of people with negative symptoms have been discovered. These substances break down into products that are involved in the DA system [59]. DA is secreted by cells in the midbrain that send their axons to the basal ganglia and frontal lobe. Certain drugs used for schizophrenia bind to the DA receptors. This blocks DA binding to the receptor. This deactivates the biochemical

TABLE 2: Modulation of dopaminergic pathways and their associated changes of dopamine levels in neurological disorders.

DA pathways	DA alterations	Disorders	References
Nigrostriatal	DA decrease	Parkinson's disease	[42–45]
		Huntington's disease	[43, 44]
		ADHD	[46]
	DA increase	Schizophrenia	[43]
		Tourette's syndrome	[47]
		ADHD	[43]
Mesocortical	DA increase	Schizophrenia	[43]
		Tourette's syndrome	[43]
	DA decrease	Epilepsy	[48, 49]
Mesolimbic		Drug addiction	[43, 50]
	DA increase	Obesity	[43, 50]
		Depression	[50]
Tuberoinfundibular	DA decrease	Pituitary tumors	[51]

There are four major dopaminergic pathways: (1) nigrostriatal pathway, in which substantia nigra neurons innervate the stratum; (2) nesocortical pathway, which links the ventral tegmental area to medial prefrontal, cingulate, and entorhinal cortices; (3) nesolimbic pathway, composed of ventral tegmental area cells projecting to the nucleus accumbens and other limbic areas; (4) tuberoinfundibular, which projects from arcuate and periventricular nuclei of the hypothalamus to the pituitary gland. Abbreviations: DA: dopamine; ADHD: attention-deficit hyperactivity disorder.

processes normally initiated by DA binding. First, DA binds to the receptor, and then the receptor autophosphorylates. By phosphorylation, this receptor activates adenylate cyclase, which then makes cAMP. These processes involve the synthesis of cAMP and synaptic action at synapses using DA as a transmitter. The DA synapses are incapacitated by antipsychotic drugs. DA antagonists are drugs that block DA receptors. The brain responds to this receptor blockade by making extra DA receptors. This is the postsynaptic cells' attempt to compensate for the weakening of synaptic transmission, which is caused by the drugs. These extra receptors restore the cell's sensitivity to DA. The brain also compensates by increasing DA synthesis. The increase in DA synthesis lasts one to two weeks of medication from the start of therapy, which is the same time required for the medication to become effective. Drugs have been discovered to alleviate the upregulation of receptors and the increased synthesis of DA [62]. Antischizophrenic drugs are called neuroleptics. A DA antagonist is chlorpromazine (Thorazine), and reserpine operates by depleting transmitter stores. Ligand-binding techniques, which use neuroleptic drugs labeled with radioisotopes, demonstrate that such drugs bind to DA receptors. A correlation exists between this ability to bind DA and the dosage required to improve schizophrenic symptoms in patients. This effect could also be directly observed by PET in living subjects [58]. Controlling DA and DA receptors is essential for the treatment of schizophrenia. Because schizophrenia is hereditary, it is important to see progress for the next generation [59]. In the future, there will be more sophisticated drugs that do not merely suppress symptoms but also allow for normal cognitive functioning. Although schizophrenics or stressful events may never be normal, they can be made tolerable.

2.2. Parkinson's Disease. Parkinson's disease (PD) is a devastating neurodegenerative disorder affecting several million people worldwide. It inflicts a tremendous social and economic burden on modern society where the incidence of the disease increases with age [8]. Currently, the mean age of onset is around 55 years. In all cases, the clinical features which characterize PD, including resting tremor, bradykinesia, and postural instability, are progressive [63]. Distinct among the pathological features of PD is the significant loss of dopaminergic neurons in the substantia nigra leading to a dramatic depletion of DA in the striatum. Although neurological disorders are present in every population and PD is one of them, treatment of PD is still limited to a few drugs such as levodopa. The etiology of PD is still not completely understood, but neuroinflammation is an important contributor to the neuronal loss in the disease [64]. Indeed, few drugs have been reported to partially inhibit microglial reaction, to decrease the production of proinflammatory cytokines and NO, and thus to attenuate the degeneration of DA-containing neurons in *in vivo* PD models [8, 65, 66]. While in humans these drugs provide relief from symptoms, however, none of them has been shown to inhibit disease progress; they also have varying degrees of side effects [67]. Therefore, there is an urgent need for novel neuroprotective agents for the treatment of PD patients.

It is not obvious if an immediate pathological link exists between the dopaminergic and the GCs systems in this disorder. Affecting these systems can relieve some of the symptoms of Parkinson's disease, for example, raising the DA levels in patients improves their working memory deficit [68, 69]. Evidence for an interaction between GR and DA pathways in the region of the brain, involved in PD, comes from studies with transgenic mice, expressing less GR [70]. These mice show increased concentrations of DA, DA D_1, and D_2 receptor ligand binding in the striatum and decreased binding to dopamine transporter in the substantia nigra resulting in a sensitization of dopaminergic functions [70]. The foregoing discussion indicates that it is not clear to what extent the pathological link exists between the GCs and DA systems in PD and its utility as monotherapy in this disorder, but data clearly suggests their roles in PD and supports further studies.

2.3. Bipolar Depressive and Major Depressive Disorders. Depressive disorders present another example of a connection between stress axis dysregulations and a psychiatric illness [70–73]. It has been reported that in psychotic major depression (PMD), the psychotic symptoms may be due to an increase in DA activity and synthesis secondary to HPA axis over activity [8, 74]. Numerous reports suggest interactions between the HPA axis and the central dopaminergic system contributing to the development of delusions and cognitive deficits in psychotic major depression [55, 75]. In experiments with depressed and schizophrenic patients, assessing the effect of DA receptor agonists on multiple hormone levels, some investigators [76] could not find a causal link between HPA axis hyperactivity and DA dysregulation to explain psychotic symptoms in psychotic major depression. However, other symptoms of depression, such as impaired cognitive functions, can be related with DA neurotransmission [77]. Several antidepressants are also reported to enhance DA transmission and improve working memory impairment in patients [78], suggesting a link between HPA axis and DA in PMD. In addition, the use of mifepristone such as RU486, the morning-after pill, a GC antagonist which primarily blocks GRs in the PFC of the brain, has been reported to ameliorate psychosis and depression in patients with Cushing's disease [79, 80] and even turned out to be quickly effective to treat PMD in cases of little responsiveness to combination therapies of antipsychotics and antidepressants [81, 82]. These results strongly suggest that the psychosis observed in PMD is caused by HPA axis over activation. Some mood stabilizers are also reported to inhibit the transcriptional activity of GR and thus inhibit the detrimental effect of excess GCs on the central nervous system [83]. Reciprocally, transgenic mice overexpressing GR specifically in the forebrain display a significant increase in anxiety-like and depressive behaviors. They are also supersensitive to antidepressants and show enhanced sensitization to cocaine. This phenotype is associated in specific brain regions with increased expression of genes relevant to emotionality [84].

In view of these data, this indicates a crosstalk with the dopaminergic system and supports the general hypothesis that GC hormonal disturbances can indeed lead to the development of disorders. Furthermore, it indicates that natural variations in GR gene expression can contribute to the fine tuning of emotional stability or liability and play a role in bipolar disorder and may represent an attractive therapeutic target in patients with these disorders.

2.4. Addiction. Stress is known to facilitate the psychostimulant self-administration, which represents an indication for the degree of addiction. Adrenalectomized animals studies have shown a consistently lower drug intake as compared to control animals. Subsequent administration of corticosterone up to hormonal stress levels resulted in a restoration of

DA receptor agonist responses in a dose-dependent manner. Importantly, the effect of GC (stress) abolishment on self-administration cannot be attributed to nonspecific decreases in motivation or motor behavior, respectively, as seeking behavior for food is not affected [85]. It is also reported that adrenalectomy reduces the extracellular concentrations of DA in the shell of the accumbens (Acb), both basally and after psychostimulant administration, providing evidence for an interaction between GCs and DA [86, 87]. These effects were most probably GR dependent, because GR antagonists also induced a drop in DA Acb shell levels, whereas the usage of MR antagonists had no effect [88]. Deletion of GR in the nervous system, using the Cre-loxP recombination system, also results in a loss of sensitization after cocaine treatment, confirming the important role for GR signaling in DA-related emotional behavior [89]. GC-activated GR thus enhances drug responding by selectively facilitating dopaminergic transmission in the shell of the Acb. Studies monitoring DA levels after stress-induced GC secretion, exogenous GC administration, or in a background of high endogenous GC levels are more controversial. For example, the group of Chrousos found that chronic hypercortisolemia rather inhibits dopamine synthesis and turnover in the Acb [90]. It is clear, however, by using the same tools (adrenalectomy or pharmacological blockade of GC production) that GCs are implicated in stress-induced sensitization to psychostimulants as well as in the relapse to drug-seeking behavior induced by stress [91]. Of importance, the key for developing stress-induced sensitization is possibly a long-term exposure to high levels of corticosterone as opposed to an acute treatment.

Stress is a contributing factor, and DA is a fundamental regulator of neurological diseases including substance use disorders, anxiety, depression, and schizophrenia. Therefore, DA or its receptors should be therapeutic targets for controlling the stress and for prevention of the onset of stress-related neurological disorders. Now, it is well established that GCs and DA have an important role in maintaining normal brain functions and the molecular and mechanistic aspects of GC effects on normal functioning of brain and behavior with the specific reference to DA signaling. Therefore, GCs, DA and DA signaling are emerging therapeutic targets for interdisciplinary research field that addresses the interplay between neuronal and endocrine signaling in psychiatric disorders. Figure 1 summarizes an overview on stress-induced modulations in dopaminergic system and its associated pathological conditions. In addition, possible therapeutic targets have also been mentioned.

3. Dopamine and Gastric Stress Ulcers

Among the various neurotransmitters, the dopaminergic system, in particular, plays an important regulatory role in stress-induced gastric ulcers [6–10]. Interestingly, in DA deficiency diseases (such as Parkinson's disease), the degree of ulceration was found to be higher [92, 93]; whereas in patients having DA excess amount (such as Schizophrenia), the degree of ulceration was found to be lower [92, 93], this clearly indicate a link between DA levels and gastric

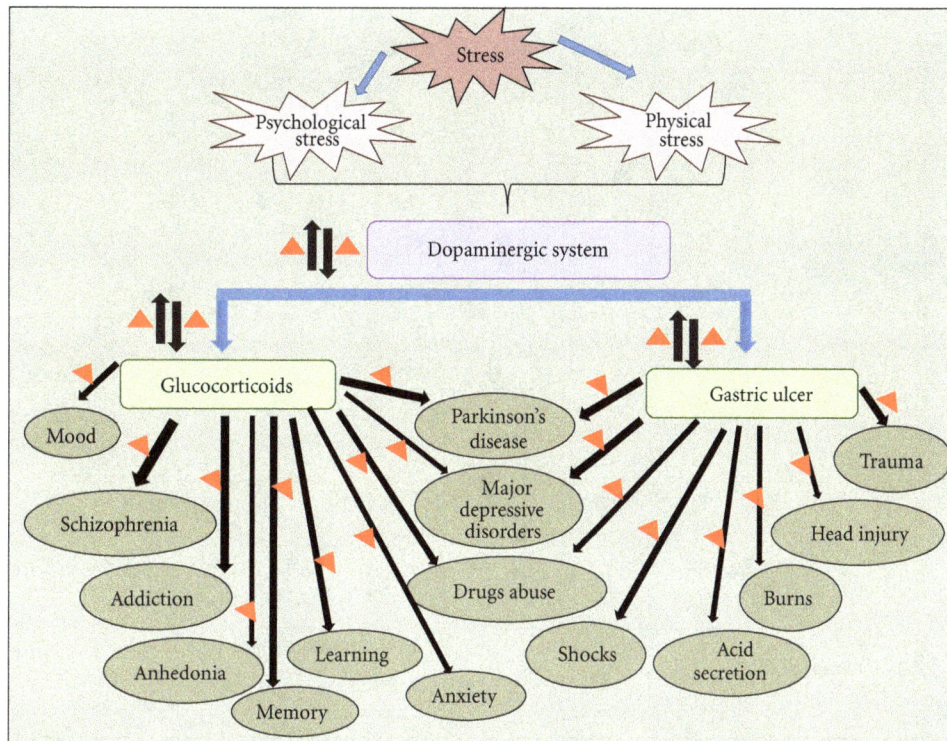

FIGURE 1: Overview of stress-induced dopaminergic modulations and their associated changes in glucocorticoid and gastric ulcer. Stressful stimuli lead to dopamine release in the brains of animals or humans. The number of neurological disorders has been linked to the dopaminergic modulated response due to physiological or psychological stressors via perturbations in glucocorticoids and gastric ulcer. Up and down arrows together indicate modulations, and triangles indicate possible therapeutic targets.

pathology. The modulation in dopaminergic transmission by specific DA drugs is also known to affect on gastric cytomodulatory functions [94]. Other contributing factors of DA system to stress ulcers are increased gastric motility, vagal overactivity, decreased gastric mucosal blood flow, and various other neuroendocrinological factors [95–97]. Elevated corticosteroid level is also known to modulate gastric glands to secrete acid and pepsin, which further deteriorate gastric mucosal integrity [97–100]. Stress-mediated peptic ulcer has been involved in various neuropathological conditions [97]. Brain-gut axis plays an important role in controlling gastric functions for various brain neurochemical factors during stress ulcer disease [15]. As early as 1965, Strang [101] noted an apparent association between central DA and peripheral gastric disease in those Parkinson's disease patients, characterized by central DA deficiency, exhibited a higher-than-expected incidence of ulcer disease. Later, Szabo [102] confirmed a protective role for DA in an experimental model of duodenal ulcer. Now, connection between DA activity and gastroduodenal ulcer disease is well established [18, 103]. A number of pharmacological agents have now been designed and tested that showed protective role against brain dysfunctioning [104, 105], but whether they have antiulcer activity that remains to be investigated other than our paper [39]. Previously, we have shown that a drug A68930 has antistress activity in acute and chronic unpredictable stress models [39]. In the same paper, we

have shown that stimulated dopaminergic receptors (D_1/D_2) modulate the activity gastric H^+K^+-ATPase and PGE_2 levels in acute and chronic unpredictable stress models, and the stress-induced gastric ulceration could be attributed to the stimulation of paraventricular nucleus of hypothalamus, increased intestinal motility, acid secretion, and so forth [39, 106, 107]. This has been summarized in Figure 2.

Elevated corticosteroid levels are known to modulate gastric glands to secrete acid and pepsin [108], which can further deteriorate gastric mucosal integrity. It is well known that the gastric tissue is under reciprocal control of cholinergic (stimulatory) and adrenergic (inhibitory) autonomic fibers, and an intimate connection exists between the sympathoadrenal system and mucosal integrity, suggesting that the decrease in gastric dopamine levels during stress may be associated with the disruption of normal tone of sympathetic and parasympathetic actions. Gastric cytomodulatory effects are also proposed through the modulation of dopaminergic transmission by specific DA drugs. For example, both central and peripheral administration of DA and related agents attenuated stress ulcerogenesis, whereas opposite effects were observed with DA-lytic drugs [16–19]. DA is also reported to mediate gastric cytoprotective effects of other neurotransmitters [18, 19]. In 1981, Willems et al. [109] suggested that there exist two distinct DA receptor subtypes in the periphery (DA_1 and DA_2). Glavin [110] tested several of these compounds for their ability

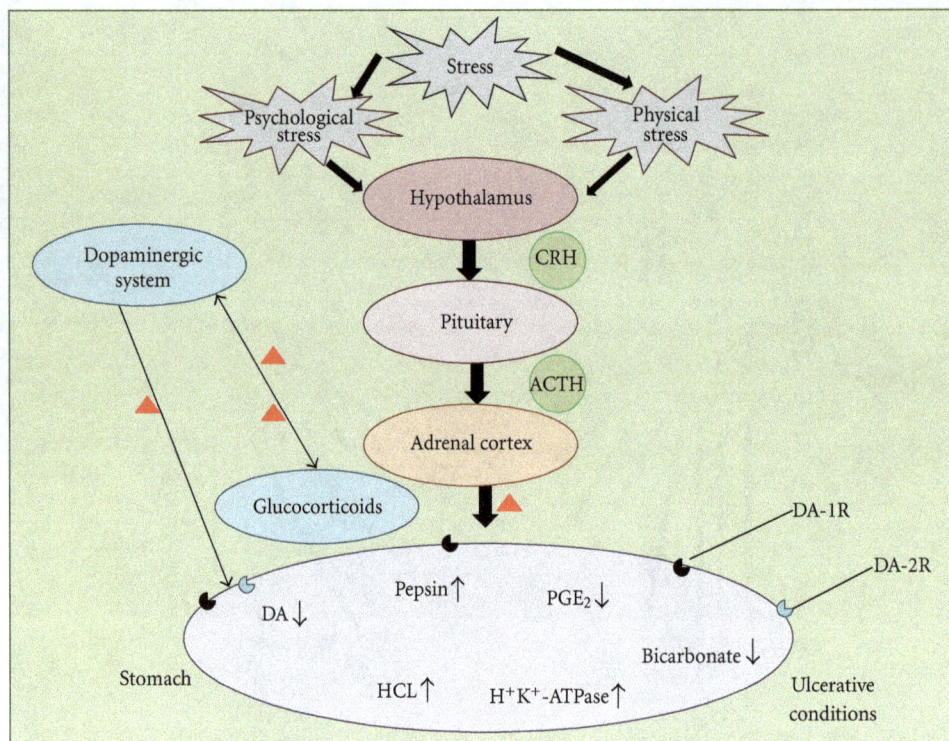

FIGURE 2: Stress-induced modulations in dopaminergic system and gastric ulcer. Hormonal pathways by which psychological and physical stress induce modulations in stomach functioning, resulting in an increase production of gastric ulceration and modulation of dopaminergic system. Up arrows indicate increased response, down arrows indicate decreased response, triangles indicate possible therapeutic targets. Abbreviations: CRH: corticotrophin-releasing hormone; ACTH: adrenocorticotrophin-releasing factor; PGE_2 and prostaglandin E_2; HCL: hydrochloric acid; H^+K^+-ATPase: hydrogen-potassium ATPase: DA: dopamine; DA-1R: DA receptor 1; DA-2R: DA receptor 2.

to influence restraint stress ulcerogenesis. The selective DA_1 agonist SKF38393,markedly reduced restraint stress-induced ulcers as well as ethanol-induced gastric lesions and basal gastric acid secretion. The selective DA_1 antagonist SCH23390 worsened stress ulcers, ethanol ulcers, and augmented gastric secretion. DA_2 selective compounds (N-0434, N-0437, quinpirole, eticlopride) were inactive against stress ulcer formation. Additional support for mesolimbic DA as a critical site in mediating gastrointestinal responses to stress challenge comes from Kauffman's group [111], who showed that neurotensin-induced protection against stress ulcerogenesis requires intact mesolimbic DA for the full expression of this effect DA antagonist administered into terminal fields of the mesolimbic DA tract significantly obtund the antiulcer activity of neurotensin. These results, together with those of Henke, strongly implicate central DA, and in particular mesolimbic DA acting through D_1 receptors, as an important endogenous gastroprotective system [112]. There exists a significant role for DA as an endogenous protective element against stress-related gastro-duodenal mucosal injury. Both central and peripheral DA contributes to this effect, likely through D_1/DA_1 receptors. It also appears likely that mesolimbic DA, preferentially activated by stress challenge, is primary mediator of central component of DA-induced gastroprotection.

Data revealed herein may gather importance in respect of several facts. The results provide insights into the role of dopaminergic system in modulating various aspects of stress and gastric pathology through the stimulation of specific dopamine receptors. Gastroprotective effects of antistress drugs may have clinical relevance, as stress-induced gastric injury and bleeding are the major causes for death of patients suffering from shock, trauma, and massive burns [113, 114].

4. Conclusion

Despite the power of modern molecular or pharmacological approaches and persisting investigative efforts, the complete interaction between the mesocorticolimbic dopaminergic system and stress activation remains to be identified. Recent advancements have contributed to the recognition of dopaminergic innervation as a useful system for determining reactions to perturbations in environmental conditions, for selective information processing and for controlling emotional behavior, all of which play an essential role in the ability (or failure) to cope with the external world. Now, it is well established that stressful events provoke major behavioral, neurochemical, and gastric ulcerative effects involving mesocorticolimbic DA functioning, but the type of alterations induced by these experiences remains highly controversial, but it may depend on the behavioural situation and genetic makeup of the organism. Exposure to uncontrollable aversive experiences leads to inhibition of DA release in the mesoaccumbens DA system as well as impaired responding to rewarding and aversive stimuli. Repeated and chronic stressful experiences can reduce the capability of stressors to disrupt behavior, induce behavioral sensitization to psychostimulants, and to promote adaptive changes of mesolimbic DA functioning. For the last two decades, studies aimed to develop new pharmacological approaches to search for drugs devoid of behaviorally sensitizing effects and capable of protecting the organism against the devastating effects of adaptation to stress. This paper updates the current knowledge on the physiological regulation of DA neurons by glucocorticoids, and gastric ulcer suggests that the blockade of these conditions surely opens new therapeutic strategies for the treatment of neurological disorders.

Acknowledgment

This work was supported by funds from College of Medicine, Qassim University.

References

[1] C. Sarkar, B. Basu, D. Chakroborty, P. S. Dasgupta, and S. Basu, "The immunoregulatory role of dopamine: an update," *Brain, Behavior, and Immunity*, vol. 24, no. 4, pp. 525–528, 2010.

[2] A. Nieoullon and A. Coquerel, "Dopamine: a key regulator to adapt action, emotion, motivation and cognition," *Current Opinion in Neurology*, vol. 16, supplement 2, pp. S3–S9, 2003.

[3] N. Benturquia, C. Courtin, F. Noble, and C. Marie-Claire, "Involvement of D1 dopamine receptor in MDMA-induced locomotor activity and striatal gene expression in mice," *Brain Research*, vol. 1211, pp. 1–5, 2008.

[4] L. Pani, A. Porcella, and G. L. Gessa, "The role of stress in the pathophysiology of the dopaminergic system," *Molecular Psychiatry*, vol. 5, no. 1, pp. 14–21, 2000.

[5] J. Varga, A. Domokos, I. Barna, R. Jankord, G. Bagdy, and D. Zelena, "Lack of vasopressin does not prevent the behavioural and endocrine changes induced by chronic unpredictable stress," *Brain Research Bulletin*, vol. 84, no. 1, pp. 45–52, 2011.

[6] J. Brunelin, T. d'Amato, J. van Os, A. Cochet, M. F. Suaud-Chagny, and M. Saoud, "Effects of acute metabolic stress on the dopaminergic and pituitary-adrenal axis activity in patients with schizophrenia, their unaffected siblings and controls," *Schizophrenia Research*, vol. 100, no. 1–3, pp. 206–211, 2008.

[7] S. S. Daftary, J. Panksepp, Y. Dong, and D. B. Saal, "Stress-induced, glucocorticoid-dependent strengthening of glutamatergic synaptic transmission in midbrain dopamine neurons," *Neuroscience Letters*, vol. 452, no. 3, pp. 273–276, 2009.

[8] K. V. Craenenbroeck, K. D. Bosscher, W. V. Berghe, P. Vanhoenacker, and G. Haegeman, "Role of glucocorticoids in dopamine-related neuropsychiatric disorders," *Molecular and Cellular Endocrinology*, vol. 245, no. 1-2, pp. 10–22, 2006.

[9] S. Cabib and S. Puglisi-Allegra, "The mesoaccumbens dopamine in coping with stress," *Neuroscience and Biobehavioral Reviews*, vol. 36, no. 1, pp. 79–89, 2012.

[10] N. Rasheed, A. Ahmad, C. P. Pandey, R. K. Chaturvedi, M. Lohani, and G. Palit, "Differential response of central dopaminergic system in acute and chronic unpredictable stress models in rats," *Neurochemical Research*, vol. 35, no. 1, pp. 22–32, 2010.

[11] L. A. Pohorecky, A. Sweeny, and P. Buckendahl, "Differential sensitivity to amphetamine's effect on open field behavior of psychosocially stressed male rats," *Psychopharmacology*, vol. 218, no. 1, pp. 281–292, 2011.

[12] J. D. Salamone, M. Correa, S. M. Mingote, and S. M. Weber, "Beyond the reward hypothesis: alternative functions of nucleus accumbens dopamine," *Current Opinion in Pharmacology*, vol. 5, no. 1, pp. 34–41, 2005.

[13] S. B. Floresco, "Dopaminergic regulation of limbic-striatal interplay: 2006 CCNP Young Investigator Award," *Journal of Psychiatry and Neuroscience*, vol. 32, no. 6, pp. 400–411, 2007.

[14] D. J. Lodge and A. A. Grace, "Developmental pathology, dopamine, stress and schizophrenia," *International Journal of Developmental Neuroscience*, vol. 29, no. 3, pp. 207–213, 2011.

[15] V. Ozdemir, M. M. Jamal, K. Osapay et al., "Cosegregation of gastrointestinal ulcers and schizophrenia in a large national inpatient discharge database: revisiting the "brain-gut axis" hypothesis in ulcer pathogenesis," *Journal of Investigative Medicine*, vol. 55, no. 6, pp. 315–320, 2007.

[16] T. Brzozowski, P. C. Konturek, S. J. Konturek et al., "Exogenous and endogenous ghrelin in gastroprotection against stress-induced gastric damage," *Regulatory Peptides*, vol. 120, no. 1–3, pp. 39–51, 2004.

[17] J. Landeira-Fernandez and C. V. Grijalva, "Participation of the substantia nigra dopaminergic neurons in the occurrence of gastric mucosal erosions," *Physiology and Behavior*, vol. 81, no. 1, pp. 91–99, 2004.

[18] K. Nishikawa, K. Amagase, and K. Takeuchi, "Effect of dopamine on the healing of acetic acid-induced gastric ulcers in rats," *Inflammopharmacology*, vol. 15, no. 5, pp. 209–213, 2007.

[19] S. F. Saad, A. M. Agha, and A. E. N. S. Amrin, "Effect of bromazepam on stress-induced gastric ulcer in rats and its relation to brain neurotransmitters," *Pharmacological Research*, vol. 44, no. 6, pp. 495–501, 2001.

[20] S. B. Degen, E. J. W. Geven, F. Sluyter, M. W. P. Hof, M. C. J. van der Elst, and A. R. Cools, "Apomorphine-susceptible and apomorphine-unsusceptible Wistar rats differ in their recovery from stress-induced ulcers," *Life Sciences*, vol. 72, no. 10, pp. 1117–1124, 2003.

[21] H. Selye, "Stress and the general adaptation syndrome," *British Medical Journal*, vol. 1, no. 4667, pp. 1383–1392, 1950.

[22] J. J. Radley, K. L. Gosselink, and P. E. Sawchenko, "A discrete GABAergic relay mediates medial prefrontal cortical inhibition of the neuroendocrine stress response," *Journal of Neuroscience*, vol. 29, no. 22, pp. 7330–7340, 2009.

[23] M. Asanuma, I. Miyazaki, and N. Ogawa, "Dopamine- or L-DOPA-induced neurotoxicity: the role of dopamine quinone formation and tyrosinase in a model of Parkinson's disease," *Neurotoxicity Research*, vol. 5, no. 3, pp. 165–176, 2003.

[24] J. D. Steketee and P. W. Kalivas, "Drug wanting: behavioral sensitization and relapse to drug-seeking behavior," *Pharmacological Reviews*, vol. 63, no. 2, pp. 348–365, 2011.

[25] S. Cabib and S. Puglisi-Allegra, "Stress, depression and the mesolimbic dopamine system," *Psychopharmacology*, vol. 128, no. 4, pp. 331–342, 1996.

[26] M. Jaber, S. W. Robinson, C. Missale, and M. G. Caron, "Dopamine receptors and brain function," *Neuropharmacology*, vol. 35, no. 11, pp. 1503–1519, 1996.

[27] C. Missale, S. R. Nash, S. W. Robinson, M. Jaber, and M. G. Caron, "Dopamine receptors: from structure to function," *Physiological Reviews*, vol. 78, no. 1, pp. 189–225, 1998.

[28] A. Imperato, L. Angelucci, P. Casolini, A. Zocchi, and S. Puglisi-Allegra, "Repeated stressful experiences differently affect limbic dopamine release during and following stress," *Brain Research*, vol. 577, no. 2, pp. 194–199, 1992.

[29] X. Belda and A. Armario, "Dopamine D1 and D2 dopamine receptors regulate immobilization stress-induced activation of the hypothalamus-pituitary-adrenal axis," *Psychopharmacology*, vol. 206, no. 3, pp. 355–365, 2009.

[30] J. W. Jahng, V. Ryu, S. B. Yoo, S. J. Noh, J. Y. Kim, and J. H. Lee, "Mesolimbic dopaminergic activity responding to acute stress is blunted in adolescent rats that experienced neonatal maternal separation," *Neuroscience*, vol. 171, no. 1, pp. 144–152, 2010.

[31] S. L. Broom and B. K. Yamamoto, "Effects of subchronic methamphetamine exposure on basal dopamine and stress-induced dopamine release in the nucleus accumbens shell of rats," *Psychopharmacology*, vol. 181, no. 3, pp. 467–476, 2005.

[32] J. J. Radley and P. E. Sawchenko, "A common substrate for prefrontal and hippocampal inhibition of the neuroendocrine stress response," *Journal of Neuroscience*, vol. 31, no. 26, pp. 9683–9695, 2011.

[33] T. Uehara, T. Sumiyoshi, T. Matsuoka, H. Itoh, and M. Kurachi, "Effect of prefrontal cortex inactivation on behavioral and neurochemical abnormalities in rats with excitotoxic lesions of the entorhinal cortex," *Synapse*, vol. 61, no. 6, pp. 391–400, 2007.

[34] G. D. Stuber, D. R. Sparta, A. M. Stamatakis et al., "Excitatory transmission from the amygdala to nucleus accumbens facilitates reward seeking," *Nature*, vol. 475, no. 7356, pp. 377–380, 2011.

[35] D. G. Harden, D. King, J. M. Finlay, and A. A. Grace, "Depletion of dopamine in the prefrontal cortex decreases the basal electrophysiological activity of mesolimbic dopamine neurons," *Brain Research*, vol. 794, no. 1, pp. 96–102, 1998.

[36] H. Moore, H. J. Rose, and A. A. Grace, "Chronic cold stress reduces the spontaneous activity of ventral tegmental dopamine neurons," *Neuropsychopharmacology*, vol. 24, no. 4, pp. 410–419, 2001.

[37] F. L. Groeneweg, H. Karst, E. R. de Kloet, and M. Joëls, "Rapid non-genomic effects of corticosteroids and their role in the central stress response," *Journal of Endocrinology*, vol. 209, no. 2, pp. 153–167, 2011.

[38] G. E. Tafet and R. Bernardini, "Psychoneuroendocrinological links between chronic stress and depression," *Progress in Neuro-Psychopharmacology and Biological Psychiatry*, vol. 27, no. 6, pp. 893–903, 2003.

[39] N. Rasheed, A. Ahmad, N. Singh et al., "Differential response of A 68930 and sulpiride in stress-induced gastric ulcers in rats," *European Journal of Pharmacology*, vol. 643, no. 1, pp. 121–128, 2010.

[40] N. Rasheed, A. Ahmad, M. Al Sheeha, A. Alghasham, and G. Palit, "Neuroprotective and anti-stress effect of A 68930 in acute and chronic unpredictable stress model in rats," *Neuroscience Letters*, vol. 504, no. 2, pp. 151–155, 2011.

[41] K. Mizoguchi, A. Ishige, S. Takeda, M. Aburada, and T. Tabira, "Endogenous glucocorticoids are essential for maintaining prefrontal cortical cognitive function," *Journal of Neuroscience*, vol. 24, no. 24, pp. 5492–5499, 2004.

[42] S. Gandhi, A. Vaarmann, Z. Yao, M. R. Duchen, N. W. Wood, and A. Y. Abramov, "Dopamine induced neurodegeneration in a PINK1 model of Parkinson's disease," *PLoS ONE*, vol. 7, no. 5, Article ID e37564, 2012.

[43] Y. Bozzi and E. Borrelli, "Dopamine in neurotoxicity and neuroprotection: what do D2 receptors have to do with it?" *Trends in Neurosciences*, vol. 29, no. 3, pp. 167–174, 2006.

[44] C. Bédard, M. J. Wallman, E. Pourcher, P. V. Gould, A. Parent, and M. Parent, "Serotonin and dopamine striatal innervation in Parkinson's disease and Huntington's chorea," *Parkinsonism and Related Disorders*, vol. 17, no. 8, pp. 593–598, 2011.

[45] L. H. Shen, M. H. Liao, and Y. C. Tseng, "Recent advances in imaging of dopaminergic neurons for evaluation of neuropsychiatric disorders," *Journal of Biomedicine and Biotechnology*, vol. 2012, Article ID 259349, 14 pages, 2012.

[46] B. K. Madras, G. M. Miller, and A. J. Fischman, "The dopamine transporter and attention-deficit/hyperactivity disorder," *Biological Psychiatry*, vol. 57, no. 11, pp. 1397–1409, 2005.

[47] H. S. Singer, "Tourette's syndrome: from behaviour to biology," *The Lancet Neurology*, vol. 4, no. 3, pp. 149–159, 2005.

[48] M. J. O'Neill, C. A. Hicks, M. A. Ward et al., "Dopamine D2 receptor agonists protect against ischaemia-induced hippocampal neurodegeneration in global cerebral ischaemia," *European Journal of Pharmacology*, vol. 352, no. 1, pp. 37–46, 1998.

[49] Y. Bozzi, D. Vallone, and E. Borrelli, "Neuroprotective role of dopamine against hippocampal cell death," *Journal of Neuroscience*, vol. 20, no. 22, pp. 8643–8649, 2000.

[50] S. K. Park, M. D. Nguyen, A. Fischer et al., "Par-4 links dopamine signaling and depression," *Cell*, vol. 122, no. 2, pp. 275–287, 2005.

[51] C. Iaccarino, T. A. Samad, C. Mathis et al., "Control of lactotrop proliferation by dopamine: essential role of signalling through D2 receptors and ERKs," *Proceeding of the National Academy of Sciences USA*, vol. 99, pp. 14530–14535, 2002.

[52] M. J. Webster, M. B. Knable, J. O'Grady, J. Orthmann, and C. S. Weickert, "Regional specificity of brain glucocorticoid receptor mRNA alterations in subjects with schizophrenia and mood disorders," *Molecular Psychiatry*, vol. 7, no. 9, pp. 985–994, 2002.

[53] W. R. Perlman, M. J. Webster, J. E. Kleinman, and C. S. Weickert, "Reduced glucocorticoid and estrogen receptor alpha messenger ribonucleic acid levels in the amygdala of patients with major mental illness," *Biological Psychiatry*, vol. 56, no. 11, pp. 844–852, 2004.

[54] D. Cotter and C. M. Pariante, "Stress and the progression of the developmental hypothesis of schizophrenia," *British Journal of Psychiatry*, vol. 181, pp. 363–365, 2002.

[55] J. W. Newcomer, G. Selke, A. K. Melson et al., "Decreased memory performance in healthy humans induced by stress-level cortisol treatment," *Archives of General Psychiatry*, vol. 56, no. 6, pp. 527–533, 1999.

[56] A. K. Heffelfinger and J. W. Newcomer, "Glucocorticoid effects on memory function over the human life span," *Development and Psychopathology*, vol. 13, no. 3, pp. 491–513, 2001.

[57] B. Roozendaal and D. J. F. de Quervain, "Glucocorticoid therapy and memory function: lessons learned from basic research," *Neurology*, vol. 64, no. 2, pp. 184–185, 2005.

[58] G. Sedvall and L. Farde, "Chemical brain anatomy in schizophrenia," *The Lancet*, vol. 346, no. 8977, pp. 743–749, 1995.

[59] P. Brown, "Understanding the inner voices," *New Scientist*, vol. 143, no. 1933, pp. 26–31, 1994.

[60] J. Hietala, E. Syvalahti, K. Vuorio et al., "Presynaptic dopamine function in striatum of neuroleptic-naive

schizophrenic patients," *The Lancet*, vol. 346, no. 8983, pp. 1130–1131, 1995.

[61] C. Schmauss, V. Haroutunian, K. L. Davis, and M. Davidson, "Selective loss of dopamine D3-type receptor mRNA expression in parietal and motor cortices of patients with chronic schizophrenia," *Proceedings of the National Academy of Sciences of the United States of America*, vol. 90, no. 19, pp. 8942–8946, 1993.

[62] M. Lickey and B. Gordon, *Medicine and Mental Illness*, W. H. Freeman, New York, NY, USA, 1990.

[63] S. Fahn and D. Sulzer, "Neurodegeneration and neuroprotection in Parkinson disease," *Neurotherapeutics*, vol. 1, no. 1, pp. 139–154, 2004.

[64] H. M. Gao, B. Liu, W. Zhang, and J. S. Hong, "Novel anti-inflammatory therapy for Parkinson's disease," *Trends in Pharmacological Sciences*, vol. 24, no. 8, pp. 395–401, 2003.

[65] I. Kurkowska-Jastrzębska, T. Litwin, I. Joniec et al., "Dexamethasone protects against dopaminergic neurons damage in a mouse model of Parkinson's disease," *International Immunopharmacology*, vol. 4, no. 10-11, pp. 1307–1318, 2004.

[66] A. Castaño, A. J. Herrera, J. Cano, and A. Machado, "The degenerative effect of a single intranigral injection of LPS on the dopaminergic system is prevented by dexamethasone, and not mimicked by rh-TNF-α IL-1β IFN-γ," *Journal of Neurochemistry*, vol. 81, no. 1, pp. 150–157, 2002.

[67] A. Kanthasamy, H. Jin, S. Mehrotra, R. Mishra, A. Kanthasamy, and A. Rana, "Novel cell death signaling pathways in neurotoxicity models of dopaminergic degeneration: relevance to oxidative stress and neuroinflammation in Parkinson's disease," *NeuroToxicology*, vol. 31, no. 5, pp. 555–561, 2010.

[68] K. W. Lange, T. W. Robbins, C. D. Marsden, M. James, A. M. Owen, and G. M. Paul, "L-Dopa withdrawal in Parkinson's disease selectively impairs cognitive performance in tests sensitive to frontal lobe dysfunction," *Psychopharmacology*, vol. 107, no. 2-3, pp. 394–404, 1992.

[69] K. W. Lange, G. M. Paul, M. Naumann, and W. Gsell, "Dopaminergic effects on cognitive performance in patients with Parkinson's disease," *Journal of Neural Transmission, Supplement*, no. 46, pp. 423–432, 1995.

[70] M. Cyr, M. Morissette, N. Barden, S. Beaulieu, J. Rochford, and T. Di Paolo, "Dopaminergic activity in transgenic mice underexpressing glucocorticoid receptors: effect of antidepressants," *Neuroscience*, vol. 102, no. 1, pp. 151–158, 2001.

[71] C. A. Caamaño, M. I. Morano, and H. Akil, "Corticosteroid receptors: a dynamic interplay between protein folding and homeostatic control. Possible implications in psychiatric disorders," *Psychopharmacology Bulletin*, vol. 35, no. 1, pp. 6–23, 2001.

[72] K. Mizoguchi, M. Yuzurihara, M. Nagata, A. Ishige, H. Sasaki, and T. Tabira, "Dopamine-receptor stimulation in the prefrontal cortex ameliorates stress-induced rotarod impairment," *Pharmacology Biochemistry and Behavior*, vol. 72, no. 3, pp. 723–728, 2002.

[73] C. M. Pariante and A. H. Miller, "Glucocorticoid receptors in major depression: relevance to pathophysiology and treatment," *Biological Psychiatry*, vol. 49, no. 5, pp. 391–404, 2001.

[74] S. K. Fleming, C. Blasey, and A. F. Schatzberg, "Neuropsychological correlates of psychotic features in major depressive disorders: a review and meta-analysis," *Journal of Psychiatric Research*, vol. 38, no. 1, pp. 27–35, 2004.

[75] D. M. Lyons, J. M. Lopez, C. Yang, and A. F. Schatzberg, "Stress-level cortisol treatment impairs inhibitory control of behavior in monkeys," *Journal of Neuroscience*, vol. 20, no. 20, pp. 7816–7821, 2000.

[76] F. Duval, M. C. Mokrani, M. A. Crocq et al., "Dopaminergic function and the cortisol response to dexamethasone in psychotic depression," *Progress in Neuro-Psychopharmacology and Biological Psychiatry*, vol. 24, no. 2, pp. 207–225, 2000.

[77] D. J. F. de Quervain, B. Roozendaal, and J. L. McGaugh, "Stress and glucocorticoids impair retrieval of long-term spatial memory," *Nature*, vol. 394, no. 6695, pp. 787–790, 1998.

[78] J. R. Calabrese and P. J. Markovitz, "Treatment of depression: new pharmacologic approaches," *Primary Care*, vol. 18, no. 2, pp. 421–433, 1991.

[79] A. J. van der Lely, K. Foeken, R. C. van der Mast, and S. W. J. Lamberts, "Rapid reversal of acute psychosis in the Cushing syndrome with the cortisol-receptor antagonist mifepristone (RU 486)," *Annals of Internal Medicine*, vol. 114, no. 2, pp. 143–144, 1991.

[80] O. Sartor and G. B. Cutler Jr., "Mifepristone: treatment of Cushing's syndrome," *Clinical Obstetrics and Gynecology*, vol. 39, no. 2, pp. 506–510, 1996.

[81] J. K. Belanoff, A. J. Rothschild, F. Cassidy et al., "An open label trial of C-1073 (mifepristone) for psychotic major depression," *Biological Psychiatry*, vol. 52, no. 5, pp. 386–392, 2002.

[82] J. W. Chu, D. F. Matthias, J. Belanoff, A. Schatzberg, A. R. Hoffman, and D. Feldman, "Successful long-term treatment of refractory Cushing's disease with high-dose mifepristone (RU 486)," *Journal of Clinical Endocrinology and Metabolism*, vol. 86, no. 8, pp. 3568–3573, 2001.

[83] A. Basta-Kaim, B. Budziszewska, L. Jaworska-Feil et al., "Mood stabilizers inhibit glucocorticoid receptor function in LMCAT cells," *European Journal of Pharmacology*, vol. 495, no. 2-3, pp. 103–110, 2004.

[84] Q. Wei, X. Y. Lu, L. Liu et al., "Glucocorticoid receptor overexpression in forebrain: a mouse model of increased emotional lability," *Proceedings of the National Academy of Sciences of the United States of America*, vol. 101, no. 32, pp. 11851–11856, 2004.

[85] P. V. Piazza and M. Le Moal, "The role of stress in drug self-administration," *Trends in Pharmacological Sciences*, vol. 19, no. 2, pp. 67–74, 1998.

[86] P. V. Piazza, M. Barrot, F. Rougé-Pont et al., "Suppression of glucocorticoid secretion and antipsychotic drugs have similar effects on the mesolimbic dopaminergic transmission," *Proceedings of the National Academy of Sciences of the United States of America*, vol. 93, no. 26, pp. 15445–15450, 1996.

[87] P. V. Piazza, V. Deroche-Gamonent, F. Rouge-Pont, and M. Le Moal, "Vertical shifts in self-administration dose-response functions predict a drug-vulnerable phenotype predisposed to addiction," *Journal of Neuroscience*, vol. 20, no. 11, pp. 4226–4232, 2000.

[88] M. Marinelli, B. Aouizerate, M. Barrot, M. Le Moal, and P. V. Piazza, "Dopamine-dependent responses to morphine depend on glucocorticoid receptors," *Proceedings of the National Academy of Sciences of the United States of America*, vol. 95, no. 13, pp. 7742–7747, 1998.

[89] V. Deroche-Gamonet, I. Sillaber, B. Aouizerate et al., "The glucocorticoid receptor as a potential target to reduce cocaine abuse," *Journal of Neuroscience*, vol. 23, no. 11, pp. 4785–4790, 2003.

[90] K. Pacak, O. Tjurmina, M. Palkovits et al., "Chronic hypercortisolemia inhibits dopamine synthesis and turnover in the nucleus accumbens: an in vivo microdialysis study," *Neuroendocrinology*, vol. 76, no. 3, pp. 148–157, 2002.

[91] I. E. M. de Jong and E. R. de Kloet, "Glucocorticoids and vulnerability to psychostimulant drugs: toward substrate and mechanism," *Annals of the New York Academy of Sciences*, vol. 1018, pp. 192–198, 2004.

[92] Y. Taché, H. Yang, M. Miampamba, V. Martinez, and P. Q. Yuan, "Role of brainstem TRH/TRH-R1 receptors in the vagal gastric cholinergic response to various stimuli including sham-feeding," *Autonomic Neuroscience: Basic and Clinical*, vol. 125, no. 1-2, pp. 42–52, 2006.

[93] P. Ericsson, R. Håkanson, J. F. Rehfeld, and P. Norlén, "Gastrin release: antrum microdialysis reveals a complex neural control," *Regulatory Peptides*, vol. 161, no. 1–3, pp. 22–32, 2010.

[94] G. B. Glavin, "Activity of selective dopamine DA1 and DA2 agonists and antagonists on experimental gastric lesions and gastric acid secretion," *Journal of Pharmacology and Experimental Therapeutics*, vol. 251, no. 2, pp. 726–730, 1989.

[95] S. I. Chandranath, S. M. A. Bastaki, A. D'Souza, A. Adem, and J. Singh, "Attenuation of stress-induced gastric lesions by lansoprazole, PD-136450 and ranitidine in rats," *Molecular and Cellular Biochemistry*, vol. 349, no. 1-2, pp. 205–212, 2011.

[96] T. Brzozowski, P. C. Konturek, S. Chlopicki et al., "Therapeutic potential of 1-methylnicotinamide against acute gastric lesions induced by stress: role of endogenous prostacyclin and sensory nerves," *Journal of Pharmacology and Experimental Therapeutics*, vol. 326, no. 1, pp. 105–116, 2008.

[97] M. Yigiter, Y. Albayrak, B. Polat, B. Suleyman, A. B. Salman, and H. Suleyman, "Influence of adrenal hormones in the occurrence and prevention of stress ulcers," *Journal of Pediatric Surgery*, vol. 45, no. 11, pp. 2154–2159, 2010.

[98] R. S. Choung and N. J. Talley, "Epidemiology and clinical presentation of stress-related peptic damage and chronic peptic ulcer," *Current Molecular Medicine*, vol. 8, no. 4, pp. 253–257, 2008.

[99] G. Fink, "Stress controversies: post-traumatic stress disorder, hippocampal volume, gastroduodenal ulceration," *Journal of Neuroendocrinology*, vol. 23, no. 2, pp. 107–117, 2011.

[100] M. L. Schubert, "Gastric exocrine and endocrine secretion," *Current Opinion in Gastroenterology*, vol. 25, no. 6, pp. 529–536, 2009.

[101] R. R. Strang, "The association of gastro-duodenal ulceration and Parkinson's disease," *The Medical Journal of Australia*, vol. 310, pp. 842–843, 1965.

[102] S. Szabo, "Dopamine disorder in duodenal ulceration," *The Lancet*, vol. 2, no. 8148, pp. 880–882, 1979.

[103] E. S. Chung, Y. C. Chung, E. Bok et al., "Fluoxetine prevents LPS-induced degeneration of nigral dopaminergic neurons by inhibiting microglia-mediated oxidative stress," *Brain Research*, vol. 1363, pp. 143–150, 2010.

[104] A. Kumar, A. Prakash, and D. Pahwa, "Galantamine potentiates the protective effect of rofecoxib and caffeic acid against intrahippocampal Kainic acid-induced cognitive dysfunction in rat," *Brain Research Bulletin*, vol. 85, no. 3-4, pp. 158–168, 2011.

[105] M. Roghani, A. Niknam, M. R. Jalali-Nadoushan, Z. Kiasalari, M. Khalili, and T. Baluchnejadmojarad, "Oral pelargonidin exerts dose-dependent neuroprotection in 6-hydroxydopamine rat model of hemi-parkinsonism," *Brain Research Bulletin*, vol. 82, no. 5-6, pp. 279–283, 2010.

[106] G. B. Glavin, "Dopamine and gastroprotection. The brain-gut axis," *Digestive Diseases and Sciences*, vol. 36, no. 12, pp. 1670–1672, 1991.

[107] E. A. Mayer, "The neurobiology of stress and gastrointestinal disease," *Gut*, vol. 47, no. 6, pp. 861–869, 2000.

[108] S. J. Gray, J. A. Benson, and R. W. Reifenstein, "Chronic stress and peptic ulcer. I. Effect of corticotropin (ACTH) and cortisone on gastric secretion," *The Journal of the American Medical Association*, vol. 147, no. 16, pp. 1529–1537, 1951.

[109] J. L. Willems, W. A. Buylaert, R. A. Lefebvre, and M. G. Bogaert, "Neuronal dopamine receptors on autonomic ganglia and sympathetic nerves and dopamine receptors in the gastrointestinal system," *Pharmacological Reviews*, vol. 37, no. 2, pp. 165–216, 1985.

[110] G. B. Glavin, "Dopamine: a stress modulator in the brain and gut," *General Pharmacology*, vol. 23, no. 6, pp. 1023–1026, 1992.

[111] L. P. Xing, C. Balaban, J. Seaton, J. Washington, and G. Kauffman, "Mesolimbic dopamine mediates gastric mucosal protection by central neurotensin," *American Journal of Physiology*, vol. 260, no. 1, pp. G34–G38, 1991.

[112] P. G. Henke, "Limbic lesions and the energizing, aversive, and inhibitory effects of non-reward in rats," *Canadian Journal of Psychology*, vol. 33, no. 3, pp. 133–140, 1979.

[113] W. Hoogerwerf and P. J. Pasricha, "Pharmacotherapy of gastric acidity, peptic ulcers, and gastroesophageal reflux disease," in *The Pharmacological Basis of Therapeutics*, L. L. Brunton, J. S. Lazo, and K. L. Parker, Eds., pp. 967–981, Mc Graw Hill, New York, NY, USA, 2006.

[114] J. D. Valle, "Peptic ulcer disease and related disorders," in *Harrison's Principles of Internal Medicine*, A. S. Fauci, E. Braunwald, D. L. Kasper et al., Eds., pp. 1855–1871, Mc Graw Hill, New York, NY, USA, 2008.

5

Drug-Eluting Stents in Multivessel Coronary Artery Disease: Cost Effectiveness and Clinical Outcomes

Kanaiya Panchal,[1] Snehal Patel,[1] and Parloop Bhatt[2]

[1] Department of Pharmacology, Nirma University, Ahmedabad, Gujarat 382 481, India
[2] Department of Pharmacology, L. M. College of Pharmacy, Ahmedabad, Gujarat 380009, India

Correspondence should be addressed to Parloop Bhatt, parloop72@gmail.com

Academic Editor: Alex Chen

Multivessel coronary artery disease is more often treated either with coronary artery bypass surgery (CABG) or percutaneous coronary intervention (PCI) with stenting. The advent of drug-eluting stent (DES) has changed the revascularization strategy, and caused an increase in the use of DES in multivessel disease (MVD), with reduced rate of repeat revascularization compared to conventional bare metal stent. The comparative studies of DES-PCI over CABG have shown comparable safety; however, the rate of major adverse cerebrovascular and cardiac events and repeat revascularization was significantly higher with DES-PCI at long term. In diabetic patients with MVD, concern of repeat revascularization with DES-PCI is persistent. More recent, one-year economic outcomes have reported that the CABG is favored among patients with high angiographic complexity. The higher rate of repeat revascularization with DES-PCI in MVD would lead to increased economic burden on patient at long term besides bearing high cost of DES. In diabetic MVD patients, CABG is associated with having better clinical outcomes and being more cost-effective approach when compared to DES-PCI at long term.

1. Introduction

Coronary Artery Disease (CAD) is a major public health and medical concern in both developed and developing countries [1]. CAD, characterized by reduced blood supply to the heart muscle, is the most common cause of death in Western countries. The current treatment modalities for the coronary artery revascularization are Balloon Angioplasty, Percutaneous Coronary Intervention (PCI) with coronary stenting, and Coronary Artery Bypass Grafting (CABG) [2]. The choice of treatment modality is based on a various clinical characteristics, including patient age, comorbidities, extent and severity of disease, and number of diseased vessel, besides importantly lesion characteristics [3]. The optimal revascularization strategy for patients with multivessel coronary vessel disease remains a subject of debate.

Earlier treatment of multivessel disease (MVD) was limited to balloon angioplasty or CABG, which then was managed with coronary stenting using Bare Metal Stent (BMS) with favorable clinical outcomes [4, 5]. Despite the benefits, use of BMS was hindered by the problem of restenosis owing to neointimal hyperplasia requiring repeat revascularization. In an effort to overcome the higher rate of restenosis with BMS, drug-eluting stents (DES) were developed [6]. The safety and efficacy of DES over BMS has been extensively investigated in a number of clinical trials and observational studies with reduced rate of redo interventions [7]. Although the indication of DES in MVD remains off-label and nonapproved by regulatory authorities (Per the Company DES Instructions for Use), the clinical safety of DES-PCI in MVD is increasingly evident. However, the significant higher cost of DES-PCI has raised the concern about its cost effectiveness over CABG in MVD patients. In light of the above facts, this paper summarizes the outcomes of contributing important clinical and pharmaco-economic coronary intervention studies comparing use of DES-PCI with CABG in MVD patients.

TABLE 1: Death and repeat revascularization at five years with CABG and stenting.

| Study Name | CABG versus Stenting | |
	Rate of repeat revascularization	Death
ERACI-II	7.2% versus 28.4%, $P = 0.0002$	11.5% versus 7.1%, $P = 0.182$
ARTS	8.8% versus 30.3%, $P < 0.001$	7.6% versus 8.0%; $P = 0.83$
SOS	6.0% versus 20.7%, $P < 0.001^*$	4.3% versus 8.1%; $P = 0.016$

*Clinical outcomes at median followup of 02 years.

2. Balloon Angioplasty/Coronary Stenting versus CABG

(a) A number of studies have established the benefits associated with BMS over balloon angioplasty, prompting its use worldwide and by 1999, 84.2% of all interventions involved use of BMS [8, 9]. As compared to balloon angioplasty, BMS-PCI reduced the rate of repeat revascularization in MVD from 54% to 28% as reported in several studies like BARI, ERACI II, and ARTS trials [10–12]. These studies established the safety and effectiveness of BMS-PCI in MVD and encouraged its use in interventional practice.

(b) Several studies (Table 1) comparing BMS-PCI with CABG in MVD have shown favorable clinical outcomes with CABG, with lower rate of repeat revascularization at long term [11–13].

(c) Long-term safety profile, expressed by death, stroke, and myocardial infarction, was similar to that of CABG at 5 years (16.7% versus 16.9%, $P < 0.69$), but repeat revascularization were reported significantly more frequent after BMS-PCI than CABG (29.0% versus 7.9%, $P < 0.001$) in a pooled analysis of 4 randomized trials (ARTS, ERACI-II, MASS-II, and SOS Trials) [14].

(d) Long-term mortality at 5 years was similar after CABG and PCI (8.4% versus 10.0%) from collaborative analysis of individual patients with MVD, from six balloon angioplasty and four BMS trials. However, in subsets of patients older than 65 year and diabetic patients, reduced rate of mortality was reported following CABG as compared to PCI [15].

(e) Many studies have compared the cost effectiveness of both treatments in patients with MVD [16]. The incremental cost of CABG remained substantial when revascularization procedures were excluded from the cost analysis. In addition, the initial cost saving of 4,212 € with BMS compared to CABG decreased to 2,779 € after one year, 1,798 € after three years, and costs were similar after five years [17–19].

Thus, in MVD patients BMS-PCI reduces rate of repeat revascularization as compared to balloon angioplasty but has higher repeat revascularization as compared to CABG accounting for increased follow-up cost with similar long-term safety profile.

3. Drug-Eluting Stent in Real-World Setting

Substantial change in the revascularization practice of MVD was noted after the introduction of DES [7]. Structurally, DES combines different stent platforms (Stainless Steel, Cobalt Chromium) with various drugs (antiproliferative) and/or polymers having different elution rates and actions. The superiority of DES over BMS has been extensively studied in the form of Sirolimus Eluting Stent (SES) and Paclitaxel Eluting Stent in a number of studies [7, 20–22]. The second-generation DES, Zotarolimus (ENDEAVOR, Medtronic), and Everolimus (XIENCE, Abbott Vascular) also have been thoroughly investigated thereafter and confirmed superiority over BMS [23, 24]. By 2005 this resulted in use of DES in 80% to 90% of all revascularization procedures within United States [25]. However, it also warned against the risk of late stent thrombosis associated with DES [26], leading the US regulatory authorities to address the off-label use of DES [27]. Several individual reports and meta-analysis then confirmed the safety of DES in off-label indication in real-world practice [28, 29]. Newer DES with biodegradable polymer or DES that is polymer-free and completely biodegradable has been developed reporting exciting results. However, the clinical and cost effectiveness of newer DES in MVD is not adequately reported [30–33].

4. Drug-Eluting Stent in Multivessel Disease: Clinical Outcomes

Although historically CABG has been the treatment of choice in MVD, DES-PCI has been increasingly used in MVD as an off-label indication. The clinical safety and efficacy of DES-PCI over CABG have been examined in several studies in MVD patients mentioned below.

(a) Early studies like ARTS II and ERACI III have reported that DES-PCI was comparable to CABG with lower rate of repeat revascularization when compared with BMS cohort; however, the rate of repeat revascularization was reported higher as compared to CABG cohort [34, 35].

(b) In a meta-analysis of 24,268 patients with multivessel CAD treated with CABG or DES-PCI, overall Major Adverse Cerebrovascular and Cardiac Events (MACCE) were higher after DES-PCI due to excess of redo-revascularization compared with CABG at mean follow-up time of 20 months [36].

(c) More recent, results from multivessel revascularization registry of 5 years outcome of DES-PCI reported significantly higher rates of revascularization in DES-PCI group as compared to CABG, with similar rates of mortality and of the composite safety outcomes. This was also observed for diabetic subgroup [37].

(d) Comparision between PCI using Paclitaxel coated eluting stent and CABG (SYNTAX trial) was the largest randomized trial in 1800 patients, which assessed the optimal revascularization strategy in patients with three-vessel or left main coronary artery disease and enrolled more than 70% of multivessel CAD patients with or without left main disease. In MVD subset, the trial concluded that rate of MACCE was significantly higher in DES-PCI compared with CABG (28.8% versus 18.8%, $P < 0.001$), with significant difference in rate of revascularization (19.4% versus 10.0%, $P < 0.001$) at 3 years. The study also reported that in patients with less complex multivessel disease (low SYNTAX score), DES-PCI is an acceptable revascularization procedure (MACCE; PCI 28.8% versus CABG 22.2%, $P = 0.45$) [38, 39]. Extended followup at 4 years also reported lower rate of MACCE with CABG (PCI 33.5% versus CABG 23.6%, $P < 0.001$) in the overall cohort [40].

5. Diabetic Patients with MVD

(a) Diabetic subgroup trials reported that mortality and safety composite were comparable between the treatments, whereas revascularization was significantly higher in the DES-PCI as compared to CABG [41, 42]. Similar trend towards higher rate of repeat revascularization (28.0% versus 12.9%, $P = 0.001$) and MACCE (37.0% versus 22.9%, $P = 0.002$) with comparable safety endpoints (16.3% versus 14.0%, $P = 0.53$) was observed with DES-PCI in diabetic subgroup analysis of SYNTAX trial at 3 years [39].

(b) In 5-year followup of ARTS trial, results reported that CABG has comparable safety and superior efficacy compared to BMS and SES in diabetic patients with MVD, with significantly lower rate of repeat revascularization (SES 33.2% versus CABG 10.7%, $P < 0.001$) [43].

(c) Meta-analysis of studies comparing CABG with DES-PCI in diabetic patients with MVD have concluded that DES-PCI is safe, which may represent a viable alternative to CABG for selected diabetic MVD patients [44].

(d) FREEDOM trial was designed to determine the optimal revascularization strategy most recent to contemporary practice for the diabetic MVD patients and have addressed the clinical and cost effectiveness of DES-PCI over CABG at long term [45]. The results revealed the superiority of CABG over DES-PCI with reduced rates of death and myocardial infarction and higher rate of stroke in diabetic MVD patients at 5 year [46].

6. DES-PCI over CABG in Multivessel Disease: Cost Effectiveness

There has been continuous debate about which revascularization strategy amongst CABG and DES-PCI is more promising, as measured by overall cost effectiveness. The cost of a DES ($1,800 to $2,100) is at least three times higher than the price of a conventional BMS ($600 to $700) and most authors reported implantation of 3-4 DES per patient treated for MVD, leading to a significant increase in the initial total procedural cost [34, 38]. Numerous studies have established the cost effectiveness of DES over BMS in real practice [47–51], besides the favorable clinical outcomes with DES. These studies revealed significant reduction in the need for repeat revascularization procedures, leading to a decrease in the follow-up costs, in spite of higher cost of index procedure with DES as compared to BMS.

Economic benefits of DES-PCI over CABG have been examined in very few studies that have enrolled MVD patients.

(a) A prospectively designed health economic evaluation embedded within the SYNTAX trial revealed that PCI using DES is an economically attractive strategy over the first year for patients with low and moderate angiographic complexity, while CABG is favored among patients with high angiographic complexity. The detailed cost analysis demonstrated that the procedural cost in PCI using DES were significantly higher ($14,509), owing to number of DES used (average 4.5 Stent), guide wires, balloon catheter, and medication cost, while overall initial hospitalization cost was $5,693/patient higher with CABG. At 1 year, follow-up cost was $2,282/patient higher with DES-PCI, mainly due to more frequent revascularization procedures. Finally, the total 1 year costs remained $3,590/patient higher with CABG, while quality-adjusted life expectancy was slightly higher with PCI. In a subset of patients with triple vessel disease, cost analysis revealed that the cost difference was 1,768/patient higher in CABG, with mean difference of repeat revascularization of 12.01 events/100 patients, and the incremental cost effectiveness ratio for CABG was reported $14,664 per repeat revascularization avoided. In addition, the complexity of MVD measured by SYNTAX score demonstrated that in patients with high angiographic complexity, total 1-year costs were similar for CABG and DES-PCI (difference of $466/patient), and the incremental cost-effectiveness ratio for CABG was $43,486 per quality-adjusted life-year gained [52].

(b) Besides, clinical outcomes and cost effectiveness, relief from angina and quality of life, may play a critical role in selecting a revascularization strategy. A sub-study of SYNTAX trial demonstrated that among patients with three-vessel or left main CAD, there was greater relief from angina after CABG than after DES-PCI at 6 and 12 months, although the extent of the benefit was small. The proportion of patients who were free from angina was similar in the two groups at 1 month and 6 months and was higher in CABG group than in the PCI group at 12 months (76.3% versus 71.6%, $P = 0.05$) [53].

(c) At 4-year followup it has been reported that, CABG is a more cost-effective strategy than DES-PCI in terms of preventing repeat revascularization, myocardial infarction and death, hence saving costs [54]. A cost effectiveness study of MVD in real-world setting reported a moderately higher rate of repeat revascularization and composite MACCE in DES-PCI compared to CABG, with significantly less costs over 5 years [55].

(d) According to very recent data, CABG was associated with higher initial cost (difference of \$8,622) than PCI which subsequently reduced to \$3,600 at 5 years due to higher follow-up cost with PCI in diabetic MVD patients [56].

7. Conclusion

According to most studies, the incidence of death/stroke/ myocardial infarction in patients with MVD at long term was similar in CABG and DES-PCI. At long term, rates of repeat revascularization and MACCE are higher with DES-PCI than CABG. In diabetic MVD patients, similar outcomes were observed. However, the critical determining factor in MVD patients is the angiographic complexity. Based on current evidences, DES-PCI is an economically dominant strategy for patients with low and intermediate complexities while CABG is favored among patients with high angiographic complexities over first year in consideration of the clinical and cost effective outcomes.

Abbreviations

ARTS: Arterial revascularization therapies study
ERACI II: Argentine randomized study: coronary angioplasty with stenting versus coronary bypass surgery in multivessel disease
BARI: Bypass angioplasty revascularization investigation
CARDia: Coronary artery revascularization in diabetes
FREEDOM: Future revascularization evaluation in patients with diabetes mellitus: optimal management of multivessel disease
MASS-II: The medicine, angioplasty, or surgery study
SOS: The stent or surgery trial
SYNTAX: Synergy between PCI with TAXUS and cardiac surgery.

References

[1] V. L. Roger, A. S. Go, D. M. Lloyd-Jones et al., "Heart disease and stroke statistics-2012 update: a report from the American heart association," *Circulation*, vol. 125, no. 1, pp. e2–e220, 2012.

[2] G. N. Levine, E. R. Bates, J. C. Blankenship et al., "2011 ACCF/AHA/SCAI guideline for percutaneous coronary intervention a report of the American College of Cardiology Foundation/American Heart Association Task Force on Practice Guidelines and the Society for Cardiovascular Angiography and Interventions," *Circulation*, vol. 124, no. 23, pp. e574–e651, 2011.

[3] A. Moustapha and H. V. Anderson, "Revascularization interventions for ischemic heart disease," *Current Opinion in Cardiology*, vol. 15, no. 6, pp. 463–471, 2000.

[4] R. H. Stables, "Coronary artery bypass surgery versus percutaneous coronary intervention with stent implantation in patients with multivessel coronary artery disease (the Stent or Surgery trial): a randomised controlled trial," *The Lancet*, vol. 360, no. 9338, pp. 965–970, 2002.

[5] A. Rodriguez, V. Bernardi, J. Navia et al., "Argentine randomized study: coronary angioplasty with stenting versus coronary bypass surgery in patients with multiple-vessel disease (ERACI II): 30-day and one-year follow-up results," *Journal of the American College of Cardiology*, vol. 37, no. 1, pp. 51–58, 2001.

[6] J. Schofer, M. Schlüter, A. H. Gershlick et al., "Sirolimus-eluting stents for treatment of patients with long atherosclerotic lesions in small coronary arteries: double-blind, randomised controlled trial (E-SIRIUS)," *The Lancet*, vol. 362, no. 9390, pp. 1093–1099, 2003.

[7] A. Kastrati, J. Mehilli, J. Pache et al., "Analysis of 14 trials comparing sirolimus-eluting stents with bare-metal stents," *The New England Journal of Medicine*, vol. 356, no. 10, pp. 1030–1039, 2007.

[8] F. Versaci, A. Gaspardone, F. Tomai, F. Crea, L. Chiariello, and P. A. Gioffrè, "A comparison of coronary-artery stenting with angioplasty for isolated stenosis of the proximal left anterior descending coronary artery," *The New England Journal of Medicine*, vol. 336, no. 12, pp. 817–822, 1997.

[9] P. W. Serruys, M. J. B. Kutryk, and A. T. L. Ong, "Coronary-artery stents," *The New England Journal of Medicine*, vol. 354, no. 5, pp. 483–495, 2006.

[10] R. L. Frye, E. L. Alderman, K. Andrews et al., "Comparison of coronary bypass surgery with angioplasty in patients with multivessel disease: the Bypass Angioplasty Revascularization Investigation (BARI) investigators," *The New England Journal of Medicine*, vol. 335, no. 4, pp. 217–225, 1996.

[11] A. E. Rodriguez, J. Baldi, C. F. Pereira et al., "Five-year follow-up of the Argentine randomized trial of coronary angioplasty with stenting versus coronary bypass surgery in patients with multiple vessel disease (ERACI II)," *Journal of the American College of Cardiology*, vol. 46, no. 4, pp. 582–588, 2005.

[12] P. W. Serruys, A. T. L. Ong, L. A. Van Herwerden et al., "Five-year outcomes after coronary stenting versus bypass surgery for the treatment of multivessel disease: the final analysis of the arterial revascularization therapies study (ARTS) randomized trial," *Journal of the American College of Cardiology*, vol. 46, no. 4, pp. 575–581, 2005.

[13] J. Booth, T. Clayton, J. Pepper et al., "Randomized, controlled trial of coronary artery bypass surgery versus percutaneous coronary intervention in patients with multivessel coronary artery disease: six-year follow-up from the Stent or Surgery Trial (SoS)," *Circulation*, vol. 118, no. 4, pp. 381–388, 2008.

[14] J. Daemen, E. Boersma, M. Flather et al., "Long-term safety and efficacy of percutaneous coronary intervention with stenting and coronary artery bypass surgery for multivessel coronary artery disease: a meta-analysis with 5-year patient-level data from the ARTS, ERACI-II, MASS-II, and SoS trials," *Circulation*, vol. 118, no. 11, pp. 1146–1154, 2008.

[15] M. A. Hlatky, D. B. Boothroyd, D. M. Bravata et al., "Coronary artery bypass surgery compared with percutaneous coronary interventions for multivessel disease: a collaborative analysis of individual patient data from ten randomised trials," *The Lancet*, vol. 373, no. 9670, pp. 1190–1197, 2009.

[16] K. T. Stroupe, D. A. Morrison, M. A. Hlatky et al., "Cost-effectiveness of coronary artery bypass grafts versus percutaneous coronary intervention for revascularization of high-risk patients," *Circulation*, vol. 114, no. 12, pp. 1251–1257, 2006.

[17] D. J. Cohen, B. Dulisse, J. Zhang et al., "Cost-effectiveness of PCI with or without drug-eluting stents vs bypass surgery for treatment of multivessel coronary disease: 1-year results from the ARTS I and ARTS II trials," *Circulation*, vol. 112, supplement 2, article II-550, 2005, Abstract no. 2611.

[18] V. M. G. Legrand, P. W. Serruys, F. Unger et al., "Three-year outcome after coronary stenting versus bypass surgery for the treatment of multivessel disease," *Circulation*, vol. 109, no. 9, pp. 1114–1120, 2004.

[19] P. B. Berger, M. H. Sketch Jr., and R. M. Califf, "Choosing between percutaneous coronary intervention and coronary artery bypass grafting for patients with multivessel disease: what can we learn from the Arterial Revascularization Therapy Study (ARTS)?" *Circulation*, vol. 109, no. 9, pp. 1079–1081, 2004.

[20] C. Stettler, S. Wandel, S. Allemann et al., "Outcomes associated with drug-eluting and bare-metal stents: a collaborative network meta-analysis," *The Lancet*, vol. 370, no. 9591, pp. 937–948, 2007.

[21] C. Spaulding, J. Daemen, E. Boersma, D. E. Cutlip, and P. W. Serruys, "A pooled analysis of data comparing sirolimus-eluting stents with bare-metal stents," *The New England Journal of Medicine*, vol. 356, no. 10, pp. 989–997, 2007.

[22] G. W. Stone, J. W. Moses, S. G. Ellis et al., "Safety and efficacy of sirolimus- and paclitaxel-eluting coronary stents," *The New England Journal of Medicine*, vol. 356, no. 10, pp. 998–1008, 2007.

[23] E. L. Eisenstein, M. B. Leon, D. E. Kandzari et al., "Long-term clinical and economic analysis of the Endeavor zotarolimus-eluting stent versus the Cypher sirolimus-eluting stent: 3-year results from the ENDEAVOR III trial," *JACC*, vol. 2, no. 12, pp. 1199–1207, 2009.

[24] P. W. Serruys, P. Ruygrok, J. Neuzner et al., "A randomised comparison of an everolimus-eluting coronary stent with a Paclitaxel eluting coronary stent: the SPIRIT II trial," *EuroIntervention*, vol. 2, pp. 286–294, 2006.

[25] A. Jeremias and A. Kirtane, "Balancing efficacy and safety of drug-eluting stents in patients undergoing percutaneous coronary intervention," *Annals of Internal Medicine*, vol. 148, no. 3, pp. 234–238, 2008.

[26] A. A. Bavry, D. J. Kumbhani, T. J. Helton, P. P. Borek, G. R. Mood, and D. L. Bhatt, "Late thrombosis of drug-eluting stents: a metaanalysis of randomized clinical trials," *American Journal of Medicine*, vol. 119, no. 12, pp. 1056–1061, 2006.

[27] A. Farb and A. B. Boam, "Stent thrombosis redux—the FDA perspective," *The New England Journal of Medicine*, vol. 356, no. 10, pp. 984–987, 2007.

[28] D. T. Ko, M. Chiu, H. Guo et al., "Safety and effectiveness of drug-eluting and bare-metal stents for patients with off- and on-label indications," *Journal of the American College of Cardiology*, vol. 53, no. 19, pp. 1773–1782, 2009.

[29] A. J. Kirtane, A. Gupta, S. Iyengar et al., "Safety and efficacy of drug-eluting and bare metal stents: comprehensive meta-analysis of randomized trials and observational studies," *Circulation*, vol. 119, no. 25, pp. 3198–3206, 2009.

[30] J. A. Bittl, "Editorial: bioresorbable stents: the next revolution," *Circulation*, vol. 122, no. 22, pp. 2236–2238, 2010.

[31] P. W. Serruys, Y. Onuma, J. A. Ormiston et al., "Evaluation of the second generation of a bioresorbable everolimus drug-eluting vascular scaffold for treatment of de novo coronary artery stenosis: six-month clinical and imaging outcomes," *Circulation*, vol. 122, no. 22, pp. 2301–2312, 2010.

[32] P. W. Serruys, Y. Onuma, D. Dudek et al., "Evaluation of the second generation of a bioresorbable everolimus-eluting vascular scaffold for the treatment of de Novo Coronary Artery stenosis: 12-month clinical and imaging outcomes," *Journal of the American College of Cardiology*, vol. 58, no. 15, pp. 1578–1588, 2011.

[33] D. Dudek, Y. Onuma, J. A. Ormiston, L. Thuesen, K. Miquel-Hebert, and P. W. Serruys, "Four-year clinical follow-up of the ABSORB everolimus-eluting bioresorbable vascular scaffold in patients with de novo coronary artery disease: The ABSORB trial," *EuroIntervention*, vol. 7, no. 9, pp. 1060–1061, 2012.

[34] P. W. Serruys, Y. Onuma, S. Garg et al., "5-year clinical outcomes of the ARTS II (Arterial Revascularization Therapies Study II) of the sirolimus-eluting stent in the treatment of patients with multivessel de novo coronary artery lesions," *Journal of the American College of Cardiology*, vol. 55, no. 11, pp. 1093–1101, 2010.

[35] A. E. Rodriguez, A. O. Maree, J. Mieres et al., "Late loss of early benefit from drug-eluting stents when compared with bare-metal stents and coronary artery bypass surgery: 3 Years follow-up of the ERACI III registry," *European Heart Journal*, vol. 28, no. 17, pp. 2118–2125, 2007.

[36] U. Benedetto, G. Melina, E. Angeloni et al., "Coronary artery bypass grafting versus drug-eluting stents in multivessel coronary disease. A meta-analysis on 24,268 patients," *European Journal of Cardio-thoracic Surgery*, vol. 36, no. 4, pp. 611–615, 2009.

[37] D. W. Park, Y. H. Kim, H. G. Song et al., "Long-term comparison of drug-eluting stents and coronary artery bypass grafting for multivessel coronary revascularization: 5-year outcomes from the asan medical center-multivessel revascularization registry," *Journal of the American College of Cardiology*, vol. 57, no. 2, pp. 128–137, 2011.

[38] P. W. Serruvs, M. C. Morice, A. P. Kappetein et al., "Percutaneous coronary intervention versus coronary-artery bypass grafting for severe coronary artery disease," *The New England Journal of Medicine*, vol. 360, no. 10, pp. 961–972, 2009.

[39] A. P. Kappetein, T. E. Feldman, M. J. MacK et al., "Comparison of coronary bypass surgery with drug-eluting stenting for the treatment of left main and/or three-vessel disease: 3-year follow-up of the SYNTAX trial," *European Heart Journal*, vol. 32, no. 17, pp. 2125–2134, 2011.

[40] "Four years follow up of the SYNTAX trial: optimal revascularization strategy in patients with three vessel disease and/or left main disease," *Journal of the American College of Cardiology*, vol. 58, article 61, 2011.

[41] A. Kapur, R. J. Hall, I. S. Malik et al., "Randomized comparison of percutaneous coronary intervention with coronary artery bypass grafting in diabetic patients. 1-year results of the CARDia (Coronary Artery Revascularization in Diabetes) trial," *Journal of the American College of Cardiology*, vol. 55, no. 5, pp. 432–440, 2010.

[42] A. P. Banning, S. Westaby, M. C. Morice et al., "Diabetic and nondiabetic patients with left main and/or 3-vessel coronary artery disease: comparison of outcomes with cardiac surgery and paclitaxel-eluting stents," *Journal of the American College of Cardiology*, vol. 55, no. 11, pp. 1067–1075, 2010.

[43] Y. Onuma, J. J. Wykrzykowska, S. Garg, P. Vranckx, and P. W. Serruys, "5-year follow-up of coronary revascularization in diabetic patients with multivessel coronary artery disease: insights from ARTS (Arterial revascularization therapy study)-II and ARTS-I trials," *JACC*, vol. 4, no. 3, pp. 317–323, 2011.

[44] M. S. Lee, T. Yang, J. Dhoot, Z. Iqbal, and H. Liao, "Meta-analysis of studies comparing coronary artery bypass grafting with drug-eluting stenting in patients with diabetes mellitus and multivessel coronary artery disease," *American Journal of Cardiology*, vol. 105, no. 11, pp. 1540–1544, 2010.

[45] M. E. Farkouh, G. Dangas, M. B. Leon et al., "Design of the future revascularization evaluation in patients with diabetes mellitus: optimal management of multivessel disease (FREEDOM) trial," *American Heart Journal*, vol. 155, no. 2, pp. 215–223, 2008.

[46] M. E. Farkouh, M. Domanski, L. A. Sleep et al., "Strategies for multivessel revascularization in patients with diabetes," *The New England Journal of Medicine*. In press.

[47] D. J. Cohen, A. Bakhai, C. Shi et al., "Cost-effectiveness of sirolimus-eluting stents for treatment of complex coronary stenoses: results from the sirolimus-eluting balloon expand-able stent in the treatment of patients with de novo native coronary artery lesions (SIRIUS) trial," *Circulation*, vol. 110, no. 5, pp. 508–514, 2004.

[48] C. Kaiser, H. P. Brunner-La Rocca, P. T. Buser et al., "Incre-mental cost-effectiveness of drug-eluting stents compared with a third-generation bare-metal stent in a real-world setting: randomised Basel Stent Kosten Effektivitäts Trial (BASKET)," *The Lancet*, vol. 366, no. 9489, pp. 921–929, 2005.

[49] S. Rinfret, D. J. Cohen, A. A. Tahami Monfared, J. LeLorier, J. Mireault, and E. Schampaert, "Cost effectiveness of the sirolimus-eluting stent in high-risk patients in Canada: an analysis from the C-SIRIUS trial," *American Journal of Cardio-vascular Drugs*, vol. 6, no. 3, pp. 159–168, 2006.

[50] A. Bakhai, G. W. Stone, E. Mahoney et al., "Cost effectiveness of Paclitaxel eluting stents for patients undergoing percuta-neous coronary revascularization. Results from the TAXUS-IV trial," *Journal of the American College of Cardiology*, vol. 48, no. 2, pp. 253–261, 2006.

[51] D. G. Sionis and I. T. Iakovou, "Cost-effectiveness of drug-eluting stents," *Hellenic Journal of Cardiology*, vol. 47, no. 5, pp. 292–297, 2006.

[52] D. J. Cohen, T. A. Lavelle, B. Van Hout et al., "Economic out-comes of percutaneous coronary intervention with drug-eluting stents versus bypass surgery for patients with left main or three-vessel coronary artery disease: one-year results from the SYNTAX trial," *Catheterization and Cardiovascular Interventions*, vol. 79, no. 2, pp. 198–209, 2012.

[53] D. J. Cohen, B. Van Hout, P. W. Serruys et al., "Quality of life after PCI with drug-eluting stents or coronary-artery bypass surgery," *The New England Journal of Medicine*, vol. 364, no. 11, pp. 1016–1026, 2011.

[54] A. Perikhanyan, "Effectiveness and cost-effectiveness of coro-nary artery bypass surgery versus drug eluting stents in Armenia: a feasibility study," *Georgian Medical News*, no. 195, pp. 44–51, 2011.

[55] M. Gyoengyoesi, L. Krenn, D. Glogarand et al., "Cost-effectiveness of percutaneous coronary intervention with taxus stents in patients with multivessel coronary artery dis-ease compared with aortocoronary bypass surgery 5 years after intervention," *Journal of the American College of Cardiology*, vol. 59, no. 13, supplement, Article ID E1442, 2012.

[56] E. A. Magnuson, *Late-Breaking Clinical Trials: Health Eco-nomics and Quality of Life in Contemporary Trials*, American Heart Association Scientific Sessions, Los Angeles, NY, USA, 2012.

6

Antinociceptive, Anti-Inflammatory, and Antipyretic Activity of Mangrove Plants: A Mini Review

J. A. Shilpi,[1] M. E. Islam,[2] M. Billah,[2] K. M. D. Islam,[2] F. Sabrin,[3] S. J. Uddin,[4] L. Nahar,[5] and S. D. Sarker[6]

[1] Pharmacy Discipline, Khulna University, Khulna 9208, Bangladesh
[2] Biotechnology and Genetics Discipline, Khulna University, Khulna 9208, Bangladesh
[3] Department of Biotechnology and Genetic Engineering, Mawlana Bhashani Science and Technology University, Santosh, Tangail 1902, Bangladesh
[4] School of Pharmacy, Griffith University, QLD 4222, Australia
[5] Leicester School of Pharmacy, De Montfort University, The Gateway, Leicester LE1 9BH, UK
[6] Department of Pharmacy, School of Applied Sciences, University of Wolverhampton, MA Building, Wulfruna Street, Wolverhampton WV1 1LY, UK

Correspondence should be addressed to S. D. Sarker, s.sarker@wlv.ac.uk

Academic Editor: Esra Küpeli Akkol

Mangrove plants are specialised plants that grow in the tidal coasts of tropic and subtropic regions of the world. Their unique ecology and traditional medicinal uses of mangrove plants have attracted the attention of researchers over the years, and as a result, reports on biological activity of mangrove plants have increased significantly in recent years. This review has been set out to compile and appraise the results on antinociceptive, anti-inflammatory, and antipyretic activity of mangrove plants. While the Web of Knowledge, Google Scholar, and PubMed were the starting points to gather information, other pieces of relevant published literature were also adequately explored for this purpose. A total of 29 reports on 17 plant species have been found to report such activities. While 19 reports were on the biological activity of the crude extracts, 10 reports identified the active compound(s) of various chemical classes of natural products including terpenes, steroids, and flavonoids. This review finds that antinociceptive, anti-inflammatory, and antipyretic activity appears to be widespread in mangrove plants.

1. Introduction

Mangrove forests are a special type of vegetation found in the coastal regions of the tropical and subtropical parts of the world. Global area that comprises mangrove forest is about 181000 square km. Majority of the mangrove forests is confined to the South East Asia and Australia, which accounts for 43% of the worldwide mangrove area (Table 1) [1, 2]. About 70 plant species of 27 genera have been reported from mangrove forests [2]. However, it should be noted that mangrove forests generally support the growth of non-mangrove plant species as well. For example, 334 plant species of 245 genera have been reported so far from the Sundarbans [3]. Flora of mangrove forests is unique from others in that their habitat extends along the border where the fresh and sea water merge. Therefore, unlike common terrestrial plants, they can withstand high salt concentration, can remain submerged in water, and maintain an efficient nutrient retention mechanism [1].

Mangrove forests are still quite unfamiliar to a vast population due to their limited distribution. However, the people inhabiting areas near mangrove forests heavily depend on these forests to meet their needs including their healthcare. During the early stage of human civilization, mangrove forests drew very little or no attention. This is to some extent because of the difficulty to access these areas. As the population continued to grow, people had to find new and unexplored sources including mangrove forests. In some parts of the world, mangrove forests are over utilised. As a result, human establishment grew in close proximity of

TABLE 1: Distribution of major mangrove forests around the world [2].

Region	Country
South and South East Asia	The Sundarbans, Bangladesh and India; Pichavaram, India; Balochistan, Pakistan; Estuarine mangroves, Thailand; Srilanka; The Philippines; East China, Taiwan; Japan; Malaysia; Borneo, Java and Eastern Indonesia
Middle East	Arabian Peninsula; Red Sea; Gulf including Bahrain, Qatar, UAE and Oman
Australasia	Western and Eastern Australia; South Pacific Islands; Papua New Guinea; Solomons Island
North and South America and the Caribbean	Florida and Bahamas, USA; Mexico; Puerto Rico; Eastern Venezuela; Trinidad; Guiana, Brazil
Africa	North West of Africa stretching from Mauritania to Sierra Leone; West of Africa from Liberia to Nigeria; South West Africa from Nigeria to Angola; East of Africa from Somalia to Tanzania; Mozambique; Madagascar and South Africa

these forests. For example, the density of population near the Sundarbans is as high as >500 per sq km [2]. Most of these people are directly or indirectly rely on the Sundarbans for their livelihood. In addition, natural disasters are putting these forests under the threat of extinction. For example, the mangrove forest in Tamil Nadu State of India was declared Reserve forests in 1880, but its protection ultimately failed [2].

Like other terrestrial plants, many mangrove plants have ethnopharmacological relevance and have also been exploited by the local people in the search for remedies for various ailments. However, only a few of the mangrove plants have so far been included in any books listing medicinal plants. This may be due to the difficulty in collecting and identifying these plant species and lack of adequate information available about their uses. As a part of our INSPIRE Project, funded by the British Council, a recent visit to the Sundarbans and subsequent interviews with people living nearby villages have revealed that the local people use a number of plants from the Sundarbans to treat various medical conditions.

With the introduction of rapid and reliable screening methods, researchers around the world have picked plant species of various origins including mangrove plants in the search for new medicine. This review aims to compile and appraise reports on the antinociceptive, anti-inflammatory, and antipyretic activity of mangrove plants.

2. Methodology

Web of knowledge, Google Scholar, and PubMed were used to search for the published reports since 1950. Other relevant publications, for example, books and journal articles, were also consulted. A total of 57 mangrove species were searched for the activity. The results are presented in three different tables; Table 2 gives a general outline of works that have been carried out so far on various mangrove plants for antinociceptive, anti-inflammatory, and antipyretic activity. It also describes the plant species, family, plant part used for the investigation, reported activity, and the screening method. Table 3 deals with those reports reporting the identification of active compound(s).

3. Antinociceptive, Anti-Inflammatory, and Antipyretic Activity

From the search, 29 hits were found with different mangrove species reporting one or more of these activities: antinociceptive, anti-inlfammatory, and antipyretic activity (Tables 2 and 3) [4–32]. Some of the reports coincide for a given species, and, therefore, a total of 17 plants were reported to have such activity. However, only one plant, *Pongamia pinnata* was studied for antipyretic activity. In nine cases, further phytochemical studies were carried out to find out the active constituent(s). One of the studies justified that the activity might be due to betulinic acid since betulinic acid is known for its anti-inflammatory activity and was present in the extract [8]. According to chemical classification, the active compounds, isolated from the mangrove plants, can be classified into diterpenes [11, 15], flavonoids [24], isoflavonoids [25, 29], monoterpenes [30], phenolics [30], steroids [32], triterpenes [29], xanthones [14], and a compound with unidentified structure [13] (Table 3).

The diterpenoids reported by Yodsaoue et al. [11] from the root extract of *Caesalpinia mimosoides* showed anti-inflammatory activity in micromolar range. The most potent activity was observed with mimosol D (Figure 1), which showed an IC_{50} for the inhibition of nitric oxide production at $3\,\mu M$ and TNF-α production at $6.5\,\mu M$. Among the diterpenoids from the stems and twigs of the Chinese mangrove plant, *Excoecaria agallocha*, agallochaol O (Figure 2) at $100\,\mu M$ showed 52.6% inhibition of interleukin-6 (IL-6) and other proinflammatory cytokines induced by lipopolysaccharide (LPS) [15]. Bio-assay guided phytochemical investigation of *Ipomoea-pes-caprae* resulted in the isolation of eugenol (Figure 3), a well-known analgesic, anti-inflammatory natural product [31, 33]. Some studies resulted in the isolation of steroids and triterpenes as the active compounds (Table 3) [32].

Plants often produce secondary metabolites under stressful conditions. Therefore, it is not surprising that mangrove plants, facing various ecological and environmental stresses, biosynthesise a wide range secondary metabolites of potential medicinal importance. The present literature survey has revealed that mangrove plants contain a wide range

TABLE 2: Antinociceptive, anti-inflammatory, and antipyretic activity of mangrove plant species.

No	Plant name	Family	Plant part tested	Observed activity	Test method	Refs
1	*Acanthus hirsutus* Boiss.	Acanthaceae	Aqueous extract	Antinociceptive	Acetic-acid-induced in mice	[4]
2	*Acanthus ilicifolius* Linn.		MeOH fraction of leaf extract	Anti-inflammatory	Carrageenan-induced rat paw oedema, COX (1 and 2) and 5-LOX activity	[5]
3	*Aegiceras corniculatum* (Linn.) Blanco.		*n*-Hexane, EtOAc and MeOH extracts of stem	Antinociceptive, Anti-inflammatory	Acetic-acid-induced, formalin-induced paw licking and hot plate test in mice	[6]
4	*Aegiceras corniculatum* (Linn.) Blanco.	Myrsinaceae	MeOH extract of stem	Anti-inflammatory	Rat paw oedema and peritonitis models were employed for *in vivo* studies. For *in vitro* studies, human platelets and rat neutrophils were stimulated with Ca(2+)-ionophore A23187 leading to the production of various proinflammatory metabolites, that is, 12-HTT, 12-HETE and LTB(4), and 5-HETE	[7]
5	*Avicennia officinalis* Linn.	Avicenniaceae	MeOH extract of leaves	Anti-inflammatory	Freunds adjuvant-induced arthritis, carrageenan-, and formalin-induced rat paw oedema	[8]
6	*Barringtonia racemosa* Linn.	Lecythidaceae	98% *n*-Hexane, 98% $CHCl_3$ and 95% EtOH extracts of leaf	Anti-inflammatory	Inhibition of nitric oxide formation in RAW 264.7 cells by Griess assay Amount of lipid peroxidation by ferric thiocyanate method	[9]
7	*Barringtonia racemosa* Linn.		Aqueous bark extract	Antinociceptive	Tail flick, hot plate, and formalin tests in rat	[10]
8	*Caesalpinia mimosoides* Lamk.	Leguminosae	CH_2Cl_2 and acetone extracts, pure compounds	Anti-inflammatory	Inhibition of lipopolysaccharide (LPS) induced nitric oxide (NO) production in RAW 264.7 cell lines	[11]
9	*Ceriops decandra* (Griff.) W. Theob.	Rhizophoraceae	EtOH extract of leaf and pneumatophore	Antinociceptive	Acetic-acid-induced in mice	[12]
10	*Calophyllum inophyllum* Linn.		EtOH extract of nut kernel	Anti-inflammatory	Carrageenan- and formalin-induced rat paw oedemas, cotton pellet implantation	[13]
11	*Calophyllum inophyllum* Linn.	Clusiaceae	(Pure compounds tested)	Anti-inflammatory	Carrageenan-induced hind paw oedema, cotton pellet granuloma and granuloma pouch techniques, in normal and adrenalectomized rats	[14]
12	*Excoecaria agallocha* Linn.	Euphorbiaceae	(Pure compounds tested)	Anti-inflammatory	Suppression of the expression of NF-κB and AP-1 targeted genes including TNF-alpha- and IL-6-induced by lipopolysaccharide (LPS) in mouse macrophages Raw 264.7 cells	[15]
13	*Nypa fruticans* Wurmb.	Arecaceae	MeOH extract of leaf and stem	Antinociceptive	Acetic-acid-induced in mice	[16]
14	*Pandanus foetidus* Roxb.	Pandanaceae	MeOH extract of leaf	Antinociceptive	Acetic-acid-induced in mice	[17]
15	*Pongamia pinnata* (L.) Pierre		70% EtOH extract of leaf	Antinociceptive and antipyretic activity	Hotplate and tail flick, acetic acid writhing and Randall-Selitto nociceptive tests in mice and brewer's yeast-induced pyrexia in rats	[18]
16	*Pongamia pinnata* (L.) Pierre	Fabaceae	70% EtOH extract of leaf	Anti-inflammatory	Carrageenin, histamine, 5-hydroxytryptamine and prostaglandin E-2-induced hind paw edema, kaolin-carrageenan and formaldehyde-induced hind paw oedema, cotton pellet granuloma models of inflammation	[19]

TABLE 2: Continued.

No	Plant name	Family	Plant part tested	Observed activity	Test method	Refs
17	*Pongamia pinnata* (L.) Pierre		70% EtOH extract of seed	Antinociceptive, Anti-inflammatory	Carrageenan-induced hind paw oedema and Randall-Selitto nociceptive test in rat	[20]
18	*Pongamia pinnata* (L.) Pierre		PE, CHCl₃, acetone and EtOH extracts of seed	Antinociceptive, Anti-inflammatory		[21]
19	*Pongamia pinnata* (L.) Pierre		70% EtOH extract of seed	Anti-inflammatory	Bradykinin and PGE-1-induced inflammation, histamine and 5-HT-induced inflammation	[22]
20	*Tamarix indica* Willd.	Tamaricaceae	80% MeOH extract of root	Antinociceptive, Anti-inflammatory	Acetic-acid-induced in mice, using carrageenan induced rat paw oedema	[23]
21	*Derris scandens* (Roxb.) Benth.		CHCl₃ extracts of leaf and root and pure compounds	Anti-inflammatory	Carrageenan-induced paw oedema in rats	[24]
22	*Derris scandens* (Roxb.) Benth.	Fabaceae	Aqueous extract of stem and pure compounds	Anti-inflammatory	Eicosanoid inhibition	[25]
23	*Ipomoea imperati* (Vahl) Griseb.		EtOH extract of whole plant	Antinociceptive	Acetic-acid-induced and hot plate test in mice	[26]
24	*Ipomoea imperati* (Vahl) Griseb.		MeOH-water extract of leaf	Anti-inflammatory	Mouse ear oedema induced by croton oil, arachidonic acid, cotton pellet-induced granulomas, inhibition of Phospholipase A(2) purified from *Apis mellifera* bee venom	[27]
25	*Ipomoea pes-caprae* (L.) R-Br.	Convolvulaceae	MeOH extract and two fractions of aerial part	Antinociceptive	Acetic-acid-induced and formalin test in mice	[28]
26	*Ipomoea pes-caprae* (L.) R-Br.		Pure compounds	Antinociceptive	Acetic-acid-induced and formalin test in mice	[29]
27	*Ipomoea pes-caprae* (L.) R-Br.		Crude extract and pure compounds	Anti-inflammatory	Inhibition of prostaglandin synthesis *in vitro*	[30]
28	*Ipomoea pes-caprae* (L.) R-Br.		Crude extract	Anti-inflammatory	Carrageenan-induced paw oedema and ear oedema induced in rats by arachidonic acid or ethyl phenylpropiolate, inhibition of prostaglandin synthesis *in vitro*	[31]
29	*Heritiera littoralis* Aiton	Sterculiaceae	Pure compounds	Anti-inflammatory	Nitric oxide (NO) inhibitory effects using RAW 264.7 macrophage cells	[32]

TABLE 3: Analgesic, anti-inflammatory compounds from mangrove plants.

No	Pure compound related to the observed activity	Refs
5	The anti-inflammatory activity of methanolic extract of *Avicennia officinalis* may be due to the presence of the phytoconstituent, betulinic acid	[8]
8	Mimosol D, taepeenin D, taepeenin L, (*E*)-7-hydroxy-3-(4-methoxybenzyl)chroman-4-one, (*E*)-7,8-dihydroxy-3-(4-methoxybenzyl)chroman-4-one, (*E*)-7-hydroxy-8-methoxy-3-(4-methoxybenzyl)chroman-4-one	[11]
10	Calophyllolide	[13]
11	Dehydrocycloguanandin and calophyllin-B	[14]
12	Agallochaol K, agallochaol O, agallochaol P, agallochaol Q, *ent*-17-hydroxykaur-15-en-3-one, *ent*-kaur-15-en-3b,17-diol, *ent*-15,18-dihydroxylabd-8,13E-diene	[15]
21	Ovaliflavanone and lupinifolin	[24]
22	3-γ,γ-dimethylallylweighteone, scandenin and genistein	[25]
26	Glochidone, betulinic acid, α-amyrin acetate, β-amyrin acetate, isoquercitrin	[29]
27	Eugenol and 4-vinyl-guaiacol	[30]
29	Ergosterol peroxide, 6-α-hydroxystigmast-4-en-3-one and stigmast-4-en-3-one	[32]

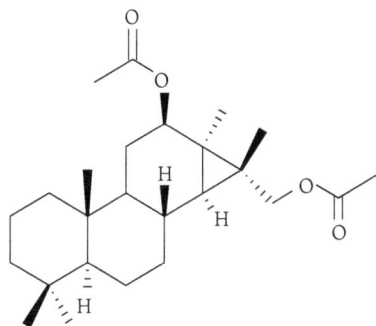

FIGURE 1: Mimosol D, an anti-inflammatory diterpene from the roots of *Caesalpinia mimosoides*.

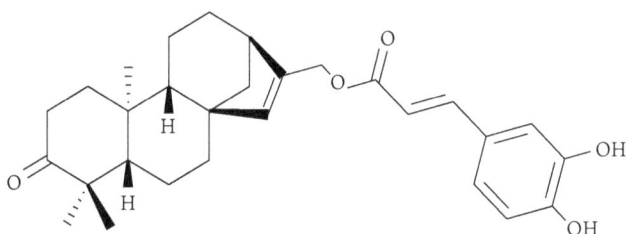

FIGURE 2: Agallochaol O, an anti-inflammatory diterpene from the stems and twigs of *Excoecaria agallocha*.

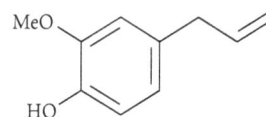

FIGURE 3: Eugenol, an analgesic and anti-inflammatory compound, from *Ipomoea-pes-caprae*.

of compounds showing antinociceptive, anti-inflammatory and or antipyretic activity (Tables 2 and 3).

Pain itself is not any disease. It is manifested in certain disease or pathological conditions. Use of natural products in the management of pain goes back to thousands of years. Use of poppy by various civilizations or the use of willow bark to cure fever led to the isolation of morphine and salicylic acid, respectively [34]. These two drugs are still used extensively in modern medical practice. Present trend of the researchers to focus on mangrove plants has opened up an arena to find bioactive compounds from a source that has long been ignored or less explored. It is expected that research on mangrove plants will continue to rise in the coming days.

4. Possible Mechanism of Actions

It must be stressed that there are no or a few reports available on the possible mechanisms of action of the extracts or isolated compounds from the mangrove plants. However, exploring the methods applied in the published reports on evaluation of antinociceptive, anti-inflammatory, and/or antipyretic activity of mangrove plants [4–34], the following assumptions can be made about the possible mechanisms of actions. The sensation of pain can be initiated either peripherally or through the central nervous system. Peripherally mediated pain can be inhibited by NSAIDs which blocks the anti-inflammatory pathways responsible for pain. On the other hand, opioid analgesics are useful for the management of centrally acting pain in which opioid analgesics act by inhibition of opioid receptors. Acetic-acid-induced and formalin-induced paw licking represents peripherally acting pain sensation. Intraperitoneal administration of acetic acid

or formalin mediates pain response through the release of inflammatory mediators, mainly prostacycline (PGI_2) [35, 36]. The hot plate test, the tail flick test, and the Randall-Selitto nociceptive test represent nociception through central mechanism [35, 37]. The rat paw oedema is an anti-inflammatory model that can be induced by carrageenan, formalin, kaolin, cotton pellet granuloma and granuloma, pouch. Inflammation of the rat paw can also be stimulated by administration of inflammatory mediators like histamine, or eicosanoids like 5-hydroxytryptamine and prostaglandin E-2 [22, 25]. Other anti-inflammatory models that have been used in the assessment include nitric oxide, TNF-α, and IL-6 induction by the administration of lipopolysaccharides in cell culture [14].

A wide range of methods were adopted by different research groups for the study of antinociceptive activity of mangrove plants. All these methods can be summed up to two major mechanisms, that is, centrally acting and peripherally mediated pain sensation. Different mangrove plants were able to inhibit pain sensation of both types. Therefore, it is possible to find opioid analgesics as well as analgesics in mangrove plants that act by inhibition of inflammatory pathways responsible for pain. Only in few cases, plants were investigated by methods that represent both of the mechanisms. Interestingly, articles that report the isolation of active compounds used methods representing peripherally acting pain sensation.

5. Conclusions

This review has revealed that antinociceptive, anti-inflammatory, and antipyretic activity appears to be widespread among mangrove plants, and thorough and systematic phytochemical and pharmacological studies are much needed to discover new antinociceptive, anti-inflammatory, and antipyretic medicinal entities from mangrove plants.

Acknowledgment

A part of this study was supported by an INSPIRE grant (no. SP_137, 2011–2013) from the British Council.

References

[1] D. M. Alongi, "Present state and future of the world's mangrove forests," *Environmental Conservation*, vol. 29, no. 3, pp. 331–349, 2002.

[2] M. Spalding, F. Blasco, and C. Field, *World Mangrove Atlas*, The International Society for Mangrove Ecosystems, Okinawa, Japan, 1997.

[3] S. Sarker, K. C. Kuri, M. S. M. Chowdhury, and M. T. Rahman, "Mangrove: a livelihood option for coastal community of Bangladesh," *Bangladesh Research Publications Journal*, vol. 3, no. 4, pp. 1187–1192, 2010.

[4] U. S. Harput, O. Arihan, A. B. Iskit, A. Nagatsu, and I. Saracoglu, "Antinociceptive, free radical-scavenging, and cytotoxic activities of *Acanthus hirsutus* Boiss," *Journal of Medicinal Food*, vol. 14, no. 7-8, pp. 767–774, 2011.

[5] M. S. Kumar, B. Gorain, D. K. Roy et al., "Anti-inflammatory activity of *Acanthus ilicifolius*," *Journal of Ethnopharmacology*, vol. 120, no. 1, pp. 7–12, 2008.

[6] T. Roome, A. Dar, and A. Naqvi, "Evaluation of antinociceptive effect of Aegiceras corniculatum stems extracts and its possible mechanism of action in rodents," *Journal of Ethnopharmacology*, vol. 135, no. 2, pp. 351–358, 2011.

[7] T. Roome, A. Dar, S. Naqvi, S. Ali, and M. I. Choudhary, "Aegiceras corniculatum extract suppresses initial and late phases of inflammation in rat paw and attenuates the production of eicosanoids in rat neutrophils and human platelets," *Journal of Ethnopharmacology*, vol. 120, no. 2, pp. 248–254, 2008.

[8] M. Sumithra, V. K. Janjanam, and V. S. Kancharana, "Influence of methanolic extract of Avicennia officinalis leaves on acute, subacute and chronic inflammatory models," *International Journal of PharmTech Research*, vol. 3, no. 2, pp. 763–768, 2011.

[9] M. Behbahani, A. M. Ali, R. Muse, and N. B. Mohd, "Anti-oxidant and anti-inflammatory activities of leaves of Barringtonia racemosa," *Journal of Medicinal Plants Research*, vol. 1, no. 5, pp. 95–102, 2011.

[10] S. A. Deraniyagala, W. D. Ratnasooriya, and C. L. Goonasekara, "Antinociceptive effect and toxicological study of the aqueous bark extract of Barringtonia racemosa on rats," *Journal of Ethnopharmacology*, vol. 86, no. 1, pp. 21–26, 2003.

[11] O. Yodsaoue, C. Karalai, C. Ponglimanont, S. Tewtrakul, and S. Chantrapromma, "Potential anti-inflammatory diterpenoids from the roots of *Caesalpinia mimosoides* Lamk," *Phytochemistry*, vol. 71, no. 14-15, pp. 1756–1764, 2010.

[12] S. J. Uddin, J. A. Shilpi, J. Barua, and R. Rouf, "Antinociceptive activity of *Ceriops decandra* leaf and pneumatophore," *Fitoterapia*, vol. 76, no. 2, pp. 261–263, 2005.

[13] T. N. Bhalla, R. C. Saxena, S. K. Nigam, G. Misra, and K. P. Bhargava, "Calophyllolide: a new non-steroidal anti-inflammatory agent," *Indian Journal of Medical Research*, vol. 72, no. 5, pp. 762–765, 1980.

[14] C. Gopalakrishnan, D. Shankaranarayanan, and S. K. Nazimudeen, "Anti inflammatory and central nervous system depressant activities of xanthones from *Calophyllum inophyllum* and *Mesua ferrea*," *Indian Journal of Pharmacology*, vol. 12, no. 3, pp. 181–192, 1980.

[15] Y. Li, J. Liu, S. Yu, P. Proksch, J. Gu, and W. Lin, "TNF-α inhibitory diterpenoids from the Chinese mangrove plant *Excoecaria agallocha* L," *Phytochemistry*, vol. 71, no. 17-18, pp. 2124–2131, 2010.

[16] H. Reza, W. M. Haq, A. K. Das, S. Rahman, R. Jahan, and M. Rahmatullah, "Anti-hyperglycemic and antinociceptive activity of methanol leaf and stem extract of *Nypa Fruticans* Wurmb," *Pakistan Journal of Pharmaceutical Sciences*, vol. 24, no. 4, pp. 485–488, 2011.

[17] S. J. Uddin, J. A. Shilpi, M. T. Rahman, M. Ferdous, R. Rouf, and S. D. Sarker, "Assessment of neuropharmacological activities of *Pandanus foetidus* (Pandanaceae) in mice," *Pharmazie*, vol. 61, no. 4, pp. 362–364, 2006.

[18] K. Srinivasan, S. Muruganandan, J. Lal et al., "Antinociceptive and antipyretic activities of *Pongamia pinnata* leaves," *Phytotherapy Research*, vol. 17, no. 3, pp. 259–264, 2003.

[19] K. Srinivasan, S. Muruganandan, J. Lal, S. Chandra, S. K. Tandan, and V. Ravi Prakash, "Evaluation of anti-inflammatory activity of *Pongamia pinnata* leaves in rats," *Journal of Ethnopharmacology*, vol. 78, no. 2-3, pp. 151–157, 2001.

[20] S. Muruganandan, K. Srinivasan, S. K. Tandan, J. Lal, S. Chandra, and V. Raviprakash, "Anti-inflammatory and antinociceptive activities of some medicinal plants," *Journal of Medicinal and Aromatic Plant Sciences*, vol. 22-23, no. 4A-1A, pp. 56–58, 2000.

[21] R. K. Singh, V. K. Joshi, R. K. Goel, S. S. Gambhir, and S. B. Achaiya, "Pharmacological actions of *Pongamia pinnata* seeds—a preliminary study," *Indian Journal of Experimental Biology*, vol. 34, no. 12, pp. 1204–1207, 1996.

[22] R. K. Singh and B. L. Pandey, "Anti-inflammatory activity of seed extracts of *Pongamia pinnata* in rat," *Indian Journal of Physiology and Pharmacology*, vol. 40, no. 4, pp. 355–358, 1996.

[23] M. A. Rahman, E. Haque, M. Hasanuzzaman, and I. Z. Shahid, "Antinociceptive, antiinflammatory and antibacterial properties of *Tamarix indica* roots," *International Journal of Pharmacology*, vol. 7, no. 4, pp. 527–531, 2011.

[24] S. Ganapaty, J. S. Josaphine, and P. S. Thomas, "Anti-inflammatory activity of *Derris scandens*," *Journal of Natural Remedies*, vol. 6, no. 1, pp. 73–76, 2006.

[25] P. Laupattarakasem, P. J. Houghton, and J. R. S. Hoult, "Anti-inflammatory isoflavonoids from the stems of *Derris scandens*," *Planta Medica*, vol. 70, no. 6, pp. 496–501, 2004.

[26] A. C. B. De Paula-Zurron, N. M. M. A. Petraglia, C. R. Aur et al., "Antinociceptive activity of *Ipomoea imperati* (Vahl) Griseb., Convolvulaceae," *Revista Brasileira de Farmacognosia-Brazilian Journal of Pharmacognosy*, vol. 20, no. 2, pp. 180–185, 2010.

[27] A. C. B. Paula, L. S. S. Hayashi, and J. C. Freitas, "Anti-inflammatory and antispasmodic activity of *Ipomoea imperati* (Vahl) Griseb (Convolvulaceae)," *Brazilian Journal of Medical and Biological Research*, vol. 36, no. 1, pp. 105–112, 2003.

[28] M. M. de Souza, A. Madeira, C. Berti, R. Krogh, R. A. Yunes, and V. Cechinel, "Antinociceptive properties of the methanolic extract obtained from *Ipomoea pes-caprae* (L.) R. Br," *Journal of Ethnopharmacology*, vol. 69, no. 1, pp. 85–90, 2000.

[29] R. Krogh, R. Kroth, C. Berti et al., "Isolation and identification of compounds with antinociceptive action from *Ipomoea pes-caprae* (L.) R. Br," *Pharmazie*, vol. 54, no. 6, pp. 464–466, 1999.

[30] U. Pongprayoon, P. Baeckstrom, U. Jacobsson, M. Lindstrom, and L. Bohlin, "Compounds inhibiting prostaglandin synthesis isolated from *Ipomoea pes-caprae*," *Planta Medica*, vol. 57, no. 6, pp. 515–518, 1991.

[31] U. Pongprayoon, L. Bohlin, P. Soonthornsaratune, and S. Wasuwat, "Antiinflammatory activity of *Ipomoea pes-caprae* (L.) R. Br," *Phytotherapy Research*, vol. 5, no. 2, pp. 63–66, 1991.

[32] S. Tewtrakul, P. Tansakul, C. Daengrot, C. Ponglimanont, and C. Karalai, "Anti-inflammatory principles from *Heritiera littoralis* bark," *Phytomedicine*, vol. 17, no. 11, pp. 851–855, 2010.

[33] K. Pramod, S. H. Ansari, and J. Ali, "Eugenol: a natural compound with versatile pharmacological actions," *Natural Product Communications*, vol. 5, no. 12, pp. 1999–2006, 2010.

[34] W. Sneader, *Drug Discovery: A History*, John Wiley & Sons, England, UK, 2005.

[35] M. T. Rahman, J. A. Shilpi, M. Ahmed, and C. F. Hossain, "Preliminary pharmacological studies on *Piper chaba* stem bark," *Journal of Ethnopharmacology*, vol. 99, no. 2, pp. 203–209, 2005.

[36] E. Elisabetsky, T. A. Arnador, R. R. Albuquerque, D. S. Nunes, and A. D. T. Carvalho, "Analgesic activity of *Psychotria colorata* (Willd. ex R. and S.) Muell. Arg. alkaloids," *Journal of Ethnopharmacology*, vol. 48, no. 2, pp. 77–83, 1995.

[37] X. G. Dong and L. C. Yu, "Alterations in the substance P-induced anti-nociception in the central nervous system of rats after morphine tolerance," *Neuroscience Letters*, vol. 381, no. 1-2, pp. 47–50, 2005.

7

Methanolic Root Extract of *Rauwolfia serpentina* Benth Improves the Glycemic, Antiatherogenic, and Cardioprotective Indices in Alloxan-Induced Diabetic Mice

Muhammad Bilal Azmi[1, 2] and Shamim A. Qureshi[1]

[1] *Department of Biochemistry, University of Karachi, Karachi 75270, Pakistan*
[2] *Quality Enhancement Cell, Dow University of Health Sciences, Karachi 74200, Pakistan*

Correspondence should be addressed to Shamim A. Qureshi, qureshi29@live.com

Academic Editor: Owen L. Woodman

The aim of the study was to evaluate the phytochemistry and the effect of methanolic root extract (MREt) of *Rauwolfia serpentina* on alloxan-induced diabetic *Wister* male mice. Mice were divided in control (distilled water at 1 mL/kg) and alloxan-induced diabetic mice which subdivided into diabetic (distilled water at 1 mL/kg), negative (0.05% dimethyl sulfoxide at 1 mL/kg), positive (glibenclamide at 5 mg/kg) controls, and three test groups (MREt at 10, 30, and 60 mg/kg). All treatments were given orally for 14 days. Qualitatively MREt showed the presence of alkaloids, carbohydrates, flavonoids, glycosides, cardiac glycosides, phlobatannins, resins, saponins, steroids, tannins, and triterpenoids, while quantitatively extract was rich in total phenols. The flavonoids, saponins and alkaloids were also determined in root powder. MREt found effective in improving the body weights, glucose and insulin levels, insulin/glucose ratio, glycosylated and total hemoglobin in test groups as compared to diabetic control. Similarly, significantly decreased levels of total cholesterol, triglycerides, low-density lipoprotein (LDL-c), and very low-density lipoprotein (VLDL-c) cholesterols were found in test groups. Significant lipolysis with improved glycogenesis was also found in liver tissues of all test groups. ALT levels were found normal in all groups. Thus, MREt improves the glycemic, antiatherogenic, coronary risk, and cardioprotective indices in alloxan-induced diabetic mice.

1. Introduction

Today more than 385 million people are suffering from diabetes worldwide and forecasted that 439 million adults will develop this disease in 2030 with high prevalence in developing countries [1]. Similarly, Pakistan is facing the same problem, and it will be ranked fourth among countries with 14.5 million people having diabetes in 2025 [2]. Therefore, diabetes due to absolute or relative insulin deficiency or insulin resistance becomes a widespread endocrine disorder that not only affects the glucose homeostasis but also chronically alters lipid and protein metabolisms with increase in cellular oxidative stress [3].

Commercially available pharmaceutical formulations used for the treatment of diabetes are not entirely free from side effects and do not completely restore normal glucose homeostasis [3]. On the contrary, plant-based medicines are water soluble with no side effect. It has been reported that over 80%, world population is dependent on herbal medicine for their therapeutic benefits [4], and more than 800 plant species have been mentioned in the literature with significant hypoglycemic activity [5]. However, searching for new antidiabetic drug from natural sources including herbs is still an attractive research aspect as these are cost effective substances with no side effect. Most of herbal medicines contain glycosides, alkaloids, terpenoids, flavonoids, carotenoids, and so forth that have significant hypoglycemic effect [6, 7]. Therefore, plant kingdom has become a target for multinational drug companies and research institutes for the discovery of new biologically active compounds that could be potential antidiabetic drug with few or no side effects.

Medicinally important herb *Rauwolfia serpentina* Benth (family: Apocynaceae) has an extensive spectrum of valuable therapeutic actions with mainly effective in the treatment of hypertension and psychotic disorders like schizophrenia, anxiety, insomnia, insanity, and so forth [8, 9]. It has also reported in the treatment of skin cancers, burns, eczema, and snake bite [10, 11]. Various indole alkaloids and related constituents have been isolated from the roots of this plant which have significant biological activities [12]. The root extract was found effective in the treatment of gastrointestinal disorders like diarrhea, dysentery, cholera, and so forth and also in breast cancer [11, 13]. An *in vitro* study described the antimicrobial and antioxidant activities of leaf extract of this plant [11]. The hypotensive action of *R. serpentina*, in terms of reserpine one of its major constituents that is commonly used as a natural tranquilizer, has been well scientifically investigated and documented [14] as compared to other briefly described activities such as hypoglycemic activity. Though, therapeutic effects of *Rauwolfia* with incomplete hypoglycemic action in diabetic patients, diabetic hypertensive patients and in anesthetized cats were brief [15–17]. A preliminary study related to its hypoglycaemic and hypolipidemic activities in alloxan-induced diabetic rats has been published in 2009 by using a single dose of methanolic root extract of *R. serpentina* [18] which was further elaborated by determining the acute toxicity and median lethal dose (LD_{50}) of same extract [19]. Therefore, in continuation of this research idea, the present study was designed to evaluate the phytochemistry and long-term therapeutic effect of methanolic root extract of *R. serpentina* on glycemic, antiatherogenic, and cardioprotective indices in alloxan-induced diabetic mice.

2. Materials and Methods

2.1. Plant Material. Roots of *Rauwolfia serpentina* were purchased from Hamdard Dawakhana, Saddar, Karachi and identified by expert in Botany Department, University of Karachi, Karachi-75270, Pakistan. The voucher specimen has been kept in our department (KU/BCH/SAQ/02).

2.2. Preparation of Methanolic Root Extract (MREt). Forty grams of ground powder of roots of *R. serpentina* was extracted with methanol (1 L; 95%) overnight and filtered through Whatman no. 1 filter paper twice. The filtrate was then concentrated till dryness by using rotary vacuum evaporator (Eylea-18) to obtain brown residue that referred as methanolic root extract [18].

2.3. Phytochemical Analyses

2.3.1. Qualitative Phytochemical Analysis of MREt. The MREt of *R. serpentina* was tested for the presence of different phytoconstituents like alkaloids, flavonoids, and so forth by standard methods [20–22].

(1) *Tests for Alkaloids*

    (i) *Hager's Test.* MREt (1 mL) was taken in the test tube and few drops of Hager's reagent were added, resulted

in the formation of yellow precipitate which confirmed the presence of alkaloids.

    (ii) *Wagner's Test.* MREt (1 mL) was acidified with hydrocholoric acid, to this few drops of Wagner's reagent was added. A yellow or brown precipitate indicated the presence of alkaloids.

(2) *Test for Anthraquinones (Borutrager's Test).* To MREt (1 mL), 10% $FeCl_3$ (1 mL) and concentrated HCl (0.5 mL) were added. Boiled in a water bath for few minutes, filtered it and the filtrate was treated with diethyl ether and concentrated ammonia. Appearnce of pink or deep colour indicated the presence of anthraquinones.

(3) *Tests for Carbohydrates*

    (i) *Benedict's Test.* MREt (2 mg) was shaken with distilled water (10 mL), filtered and filtrate was concentrated, then Benedict's reagent (5 mL) was added to this and boiled for 5 minutes, resulted in the formation of the brick red color precipitate within 5 minutes and indicated the presence of carbohydrates.

    (ii) *Fehling's Test.* MREt (2 mg) was shaken with distilled water (10 mL), filtered and filtrate was concentrated, to this mixture of the equal parts of the Fehling's solution A and B (1 mL) were added and boiled for few minutes, resulted in the formation of red or brick color precipitate which indicated the presence of the reducing sugar.

    (iii) *Mohlisch's Test.* MREt (2 mg) was shaken with distilled water (10 mL), filtered and filtrate was concentrated, to this 2 drops of freshly prepared alcoholic solution of α- naphthol (20%) and concentrated sulphuric acid (2 mL) were added to observe a layer below the mixture. Red violet ring appeared that indicated the presence of carbohydrates which disappeared on the addition of the excess alkali. The same test was also used to detect the presence of glycosides in extract.

(4) *Test for Flavonoids (Ammonia Test).* A small piece of filter paper was dipped in MREt (1 mL) and exposed to ammonia vapours that resulted in the formation of yellow spot on filter paper indicated the presence of flavonoids.

(5) *Test for Cardiac Glycosides (Keller-Killani Test).* MREt (5 mL) was treated with glacial acetic acid (2 mL) mixed with one drop of ferric chloride solution. To this concentrated sulphuric acid (1 mL) was added. A brown ring appeared at the interface indicated a deoxy sugar characteristic of cardenolides, followed by the formation of a violet ring below that brown ring.

(6) *Test for Resins.* MREt (1 mL) was dissolved in acetone (1 mL), and the solution was poured in distilled water (2 mL). Turbidity indicated the presence of resins.

(7) *Test for Steroids (Liebermann-Burchard's Test).* MREt (0.5 mL) was dissolved in acetic anhydride, heated to boiling, cooled, and then concentrated sulphuric acid (1 mL) was added along the sides of test tube that resulted in the formation of green color indicated the presence of the steroids.

(8) *Test for Saponins.* MREt (5 mL) was taken in test tube and a drop of the sodium bicarbonate solution was added, shaked vigorously, and left for 3 minutes. Formation of the honeycomb like froth indicated the presence of saponins.

(9) *Test for Triterpenoids (Salkowski's Test).* MREt (5 mL) was shaken with chloroform (2 mL) followed by the addition of sulphuric acid (3 mL) slowly by the sides of the test tube. Formation of the reddish brown color indicated the presence of the steroids.

(10) *Test for Tannins.* To MREt (1–2 mL), few drops of $FeCl_3$ (5%) solution was added resulted in the formation of green colour indicated the presence gallotannins, while brown color indicated the presence of pseudotannins.

(11) *Test for Phlobatannins.* MREt (1 mL) was boiled with hydrochloric acid (1%) resulted in the formation of red precipitate which indicated the presence of phlobatannins.

2.3.2. Quantitative Phytochemical Analysis

(1) *Determination of Alkaloids.* Ground root powder (5 g) of *R. serpentina* was weighed and taken into a beaker (250 mL). To this 10% acetic acid in ethanol (200 mL) was added, covered, and allowed to stand for 4 hours. This was filtered and the extract was concentrated on a water bath to 1/4 of its original volume. Concentrated ammonium hydroxide was added drop wise to the extract until the precipitation was completed. The whole solution was allowed to settle and the precipitate was collected and washed with dilute ammonium hydroxide and then filtered. The residue is the alkaloid, which was oven-dried and weighed [23].

(2) *Determination of Flavonoid.* Ground root powder (10 g) of *R. serpentina* was extracted repeatedly with 80% aqueous methanol (100 mL) at room temperature. The whole solution was filtered through Whatman filter paper no. 42 (125 mm). The filtrate was later transferred into a crucible and evaporated into dryness over a water bath and weighed untill a constant weight was achieved [24].

(3) *Determination of Saponin.* Ground root powder (20 g) of *R. serpentina* was taken into a conical flask and 20% aqueous ethanol was added. The sample was heated over a hot water bath for 4 hours with continuous stirring at about 55°C. The mixture was filtered and the residue reextracted with another 200 mL of same 20% ethanol. The combined extracts were reduced to 40 mL over water bath at about 90°C. The concentrate was transferred into a 250 mL separatory

funnel and 20 mL of diethyl ether was added and shaken vigorously. The aqueous layer was recovered while the diethyl ether layer was discarded. The purification process was repeated. 60 mL of n-butanol was added. The combined n-butanol extracts were washed twice with 5% aqueous sodium chloride (10 mL). The remaining solution was heated in a water bath. After evaporation, the sample was dried in the oven to a constant weight [25].

(4) *Determination of Total Phenolic Content.* Total phenolic content was determined using Folin-Ciocalteu reagent. Test, having 0.1 mg of the plant extract, was prepared and mixed with 1 mL of Folin-Ciocalteu reagent (1 : 10 diluted with distilled water) after 3 minutes, 2% sodium carbonate (3 mL) was added, shaken for few seconds, and then incubated for 2 hours at room temperature with intermittent shaking. The absorbance was read at 760 nm against a reagent blank. The standard curve was prepared using 0.01–0.1 mg of gallic acid. The total phenolic content was expressed in mg/g of MREt [26].

2.4. Alloxan Monohydrate (Sigma).
Diabetes was induced in overnight fasted mice by a single intraperitoneal injection of alloxan monohydrate (150 mg/kg). After 72 hours of this injection fasting blood glucose levels were monitored from tail vein of mice with the help of glucometer (*Optium Xceed*, Diabetes Monitoring system by Abbott), mice showed glucose level ≥190 mg/dL were selected, grouped, and each group subjected to its respective treatment.

2.5. Glibenclamide.
Antidiabetic drug glibenclamide (*Doanil*) purchased from Sanofi-Aventis Pakistan Ltd. and used as positive control (5 mg/kg).

2.6. Dimethyl Sulphoxide (DMSO).
An analytical grade DMSO was purchased from Fisher Scientific (UK), and its 0.05% concentration was used as vehicle for administering the doses of MREt in test mice.

2.7. Experimental Mice and Treatment Groups.
Male albino Wister mice (25–35 grams) were purchased from the breeding house of Dow University of Health Sciences (DUHS), Karachi. Experimental mice were acclimatized and maintained individually in cages in an air conditioned room with temperature not more than 23 ± 2°C (relative humidity 55%) for one week prior to the experiment in the conventional animal house of same university. The care and handling of these mice were in accordance to the internationally accepted standard guidelines for animal handling. Mice were given standard laboratory diet with free access to water *ad libitum* and during the experimental period no physical stress was provided. The experimental protocol was approved by the Institutional Ethical Review Board (IERB) of DUHS in June 2010 (Authority letter Reference Number: IRB-186/DUHS-10).

Overnight (12–14 hours) fasted mice (blood glucose level ≥190 mg/dL) were randomly divided into seven groups (6 mice/group) in the following manner.

(1) Group I: control: normal mice treated with distilled water (1 mL/kg).

(2) Group II: diabetic control: alloxan-induced diabetic mice treated with distilled water (1 mL/kg).

(3) Group III: negative control: alloxan-induced diabetic mice treated with 0.05% DMSO (1 mL/kg).

(4) Group IV: positive control: alloxan-induced diabetic mice treated with glibenclamide (5 mg/kg).

(5) Group V: test group: alloxan-induced diabetic mice treated with MREt (10 mg/kg).

(6) Group VI: test group: alloxan-induced diabetic mice treated with MREt (30 mg/kg).

(7) Group VII: test group: alloxan-induced diabetic mice treated with MREt (60 mg/kg).

Each treatment was given to its respective group orally once in a day for 14 days consecutively. At the end of animal trial, mice were sacrificed to collect whole blood, serum and liver tissues that were used to analyze hematological and biochemical parameters.

2.8. Determination of Body Weight. Body weights of animals of each group were measured at initial (0 day) and final (14 day) days of trial by using balance (Kitchen scale 1800) and calculate percentage of body weight gain or loss with the following formula [27]:

$$\% \text{ Body weight change} = \frac{\text{Final weight} - \text{initial weight}}{\text{initial weight}} \times 100. \quad (1)$$

2.9. Determination of Biochemical Parameters. Fasting blood glucose levels were monitored in each group by glucometer at initial (0 day) and final day (14 day) of trial to determine percent glycemic change by using the following formula [28]. Where G_o = blood glucose level at 0 day and G_x = blood glucose level at 14 day:

$$\% \text{ Glycemic change} = \frac{G_x - G_o}{G_o} \times 100. \quad (2)$$

Other parameters including serum alanine aminotransferase (ALT), total cholesterol (TC), triglycerides (TG), high density lipoprotein-cholesterol (HDL-c) concentrations were determined by commercially available enzymatic assay kits (*Randox*, United Kingdom). Whereas low density lipoprotein-cholesterol (LDL-c) and very low density lipoprotein-cholesterol (VLDL-c) were calculated by Friedewald formulae [29]. Estimation of total lipids and glycogen contents in liver homogenate was done by gravemetric and colorimetric methods, respectively [30, 31].

2.10. Determination of Serum Insulin Level and Insulin/Glucose (I/G) Ratio. The serum insulin levels were determined by cobas e411 analyzer, Hitachi (Roche Diagnostics GmbH, Mannheim, Germany) and expressed as μU/mL. Whereas I/G ratio was determined as fasting insulin (μU/mL)/glucose (mg/dL) and expressed as μU/mg [32].

2.11. Determination of Hematological Parameters. Total hemoglobin (Hb) and glycosylated hemoglobin level (HbA1$_c$) levels were evaluated by Automated Analyzer, Sysmex (XS-1000i) and commercially available Kit (Nycocard Kit, USA), respectively.

2.12. Determination of Antiatherogenic, Cardioprotective, and Coronary Risk Indices. Cardioprotective index (CPI) was estimated in term of HDL-c to LDL-c and TG to HDL-c ratios [33, 34]. Where as antiatherogenic (AAI) and coronary risk indices (CRI) were calculated by the following formulae [35, 36]:

$$AAI = 100 \times \left[\frac{\text{HDL-c}}{\text{Total cholesterol} - \text{HDL-c}} \right],$$
$$CRI = \frac{\text{Total cholesterol}}{\text{HDL-cholesterol}}. \quad (3)$$

2.13. Statistical Analysis. Results of the present study are expressed as mean ± SEM (standard error mean). The data were analyzed with statistical package for social sciences (SPSS version 18) by using *one-way* ANOVA followed by LSD (least significant difference) test at $P < 0.05$. The differences were considered significant at $P < 0.05$, $P < 0.01$, $P < 0.001$, and $P < 0.0001$ when compared with respective controls.

3. Results

3.1. Total Yield of MREt of R. serpentina. Total yield of MREt of *R. serpentina* was 5% g/g of dry root powder. The quality of extract was maintained by kept in an air-tight container and stored in refrigerator below 10°C until used.

3.2. Phytochemical Profile of MREt. Qualitative analysis of MREt showed the presence of alkaloids, carbohydrates, flavonoids, glycosides, cardiac glycosides, phlobatannins, resins, saponins, steroids, tannins, and triterpenoids. Whereas quantitatively the amount of alkaloids, saponins, flavonoids in root powder and total phenols in MREt were found as 7, 97, 20 and 233 mg/gm respectively (Table 1).

3.3. Effect of MREt on Body Weight. In diabetic and negative controls marked reduction in percent body weight was observed up to −11.08 and −9.25%, respectively as compared to control mice. Whereas +8.45% gain in body weight was observed in mice treated with glibenclamide as compared to diabetic and negative controls ($P < 0.0001$). Though all three doses of MREt slightly reduced ($P < 0.05$ and $P < 0.01$) the body weight in test mice but it was not as high as it was observed in diabetic and negative controls (Table 2).

3.4. Effect of MREt on Blood Glucose Level. Significant percent glycemic change was found as −51, −46, and −49% in test mice treated with MREt at 10, 30, and 60 mg/kg, respectively as compared to diabetic and negative controls ($P < 0.0001$). Similarly −40% reduction in blood glucose level was also observed in positive control group (Table 3).

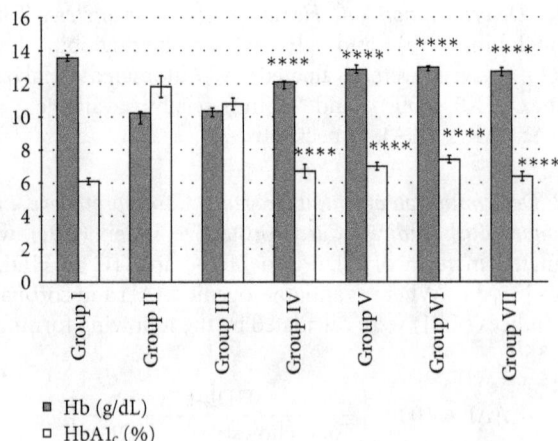

FIGURE 1: Effect of MREt on hemoglobin (g/dL) and glycosylated hemoglobin (HbA1$_c$) levels. Each bar represents the mean ± SEM ($n = 6$). ****$P < 0.0001$, when compared with group II and III.

TABLE 1: Phytochemical analysis of MREt of *R. serpentina*.

Phytoconstituent	Qualitative analysis	Quantitative analysis (mg/gm)
Alkaloids	Positive	7*
Anthraquinones	Negative	—
Carbohydrates	Positive	—
Flavonoids	Positive	97*
Glycosides	Positive	—
Cardiac glycosides	Positive	—
Phlobatannins	Positive	—
Resins	Positive	—
Saponins	Positive	20*
Steroids	Positive	—
Tanins	Positive	—
Triterpenoids	Positive	—
Total phenols	Positive	233

*mg/gm of root powder.

3.5. Effect of MREt on Hb and HbA1$_c$. Glibenclamide andall three doses of MREt significantly ($P < 0.0001$) improved the total Hb level from 12.10 to 12.98 g/dL in positive control and test groups as compared to diabetic and negative control mice that showed 10 g/dL (Figure 1). Similarly significantly improved percentage of HbA1$_c$ from 6.3 to 7.4% was observed in all test groups ($P < 0.0001$) and positive control as compared to same controls that showed its value from 10.78 to 11.83% (Figure 1).

3.6. Effect of MREt on Lipid Profile. MREt at 10, 30, and 60 mg/kg in test mice induced significant ($P < 0.0001$) decrease in serum TC levels up to 146.19, 129.33, and 138.50 mg/dL, respectively as compared to diabetic and negative controls which showed TC levels up to 260.42 and 254.11 mg/dL, respectively. Glibenclamide treated group also showed significant ($P < 0.0001$ & $P < 0.001$) decrease up to 178.40 mg/dL as compared to same controls (Table 4). A

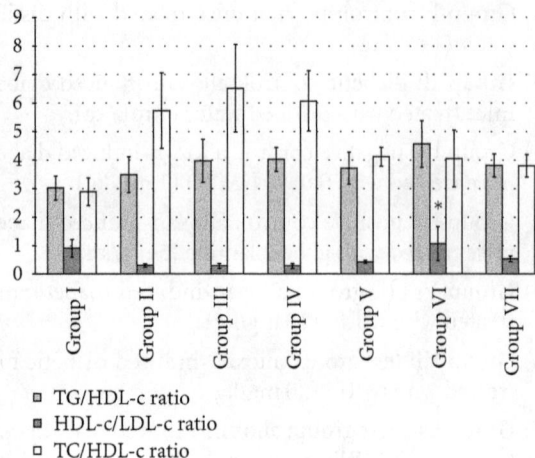

FIGURE 2: Effect of MREt on cardioprotective indices. Each bar represents the mean ± SEM ($n = 6$). *$P < 0.05$, when compared with group II and III.

significant decrease was also found in serum TG levels up to 128.27 and 138.75 mg/dL in test mice treated with same extract at 10 and 60 mg/kg, respectively as compared to diabetic and negative control groups that showed the same parameter up to 161.33 and 173.50 mg/dL ($P < 0.05$ and $P < 0.01$). Though MREt at 30 mg/kg also decreased the TG level in its respective group as compared to same control groups but it was not statistically significant. Prominent fall ($P < 0.05$ and $P < 0.01$) was also observed in same parameter of positive control group (Table 4). LDL-c levels in diabetic test mice treated with MREt at 10, 30 and 60 mg/kg were significantly decreased ($P < 0.01$, $P < 0.001$ and $P < 0.0001$) up to 83.83, 63.46, and 73.30 mg/dL, respectively as compared to diabetic and negative controls that showed very high levels of same parameter (Table 4). Decrease ($P < 0.05$ and $P < 0.01$) levels of VLDL ranging from 24 to 29 mg/dL was also observed in positive control and three test groups (Table 4). However, decreased levels of HDL-c were observed in test mice as compared to control, diabetic, and negative control groups but that decrease was in relation of low levels of TC that were observed in test mice (Table 4).

3.7. Effect of MREt on CPI, AAI, and CRI. In case of CPI, TG/HDL-c ratio was found reduced from 3.71 to 4.56 in positive control and test groups treated with glibenclamide and MREt, respectively (Figure 2). Similarly improved HDL-c/LDL-c ratio was observed in test groups from 0.43 to 1.07 compared with diabetic and negative controls which showed reduced same ratio from 0.29 to 0.3 (Figure 2). CRI in term of TC/HDL-c ratio was observed decrease in test groups treated with MREt from 3.8 to 4.11 as compared to same control groups which showed marked increase from 5.73 to 6.52 in the same ratio. Even positive control group showed high value of same index (Figure 2). An improvement was also found in values of AAI from 33 to 53% in test groups as compared to diabetic, negative, and positive controls that showed the same AAI from 23 to 24% (Table 4).

TABLE 2: Effect of MREt of *R. serpentina* on body weights of mice.

Groups	Treatments	Body weight (gm)		Weight change (%)
		Initial weight at 0 day	Final weight at 14 day	
Group I	Distilled water (1 mL/ kg)	28.25 ± 0.85	31.25 ± 0.85	+10.68 ± 1.49
Group II	Alloxan treated (150 mg/kg)	29.25 ± 1.6	26 ± 1.41	−11.08 ± 1.48
Group III	0.05% DMSO (1 mL/kg)	29.5 ± 0.87	26.75 ± 0.63	−9.25 ± 0.62
Group IV	Glibenclamide (5 mg/kg)	29.5 ± 0.5	32 ± 0.71	+8.45 ± 0.89****a,b
Group V	MREt (10 mg/kg)	30.75 ± 1.31	29 ± 1.22	−5.69 ± 0.78*a
Group VI	MREt (30 mg/kg)	28.50 ± 1.55	26.75 ± 1.65	−6.25 ± 1.05*a
Group VII	MREt (60 mg/kg)	27.50 ± 1.5	26.75 ± 1.89	−2.94 ± 2.37****a,**b

Values are expressed as mean ± SEM ($n = 6$). $*P < 0.05$, $**P < 0.01$, and $****P < 0.0001$, when compared with respective group II (a) and III (b). Negative (−)/positive (+) signs represent loss/gain in weights of mice at 14th day.

TABLE 3: Effect of MREt of *R. serpentina* on fasting blood glucose level in mice.

Groups	Treatments	Initial day (G_0)	Final day (G_x)	Glycemic change (%)
Group I	Distilled water (1 mL/ kg)	102.25 ± 2.72	98 ± 5.84	−4.16
Group II	Alloxan treated (150 mg/kg)	198.25 ± 4.91	245.50 ± 20.66	23.83
Group III	0.05% DMSO (1 mL/kg)	199.50 ± 5.62	257.25 ± 22.68	28.95
Group IV	Glibenclamide (5 mg/kg)	195.25 ± 3.12	116.50 ± 14.46****	−40.46
Group V	MREt (10 mg/kg)	198.25 ± 5.01	96.25 ± 4.94****	−51.45
Group VI	MREt (30 mg/kg)	197.50 ± 6.2	105 ± 12.39****	−46.84
Group VII	MREt (60 mg/kg)	195.2 ± 5.66	98 ± 6.54****	−49.80

Values are expressed as mean ± SEM ($n = 6$). $****P < 0.0001$, when compared with group II and III at respective day. Negative (−)/positive (+) signs represent decrease/increase in percent glycemic change at 14th day.

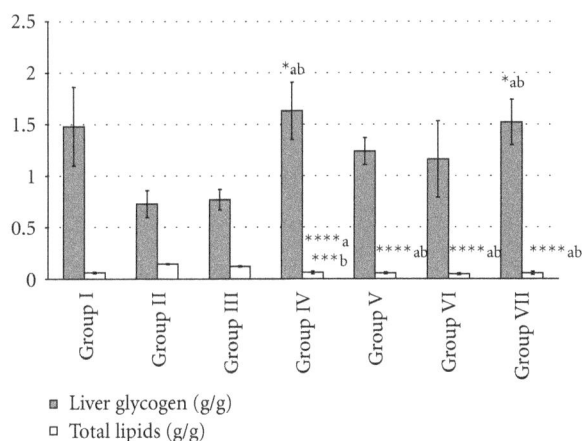

FIGURE 3: Effect of MREt on hepatic glycogen and total lipids (g/g). Each bar represents the mean ± SEM ($n = 6$). $*P < 0.05$ and $****P < 0.0001$, when compared with group II (a) and (b) III.

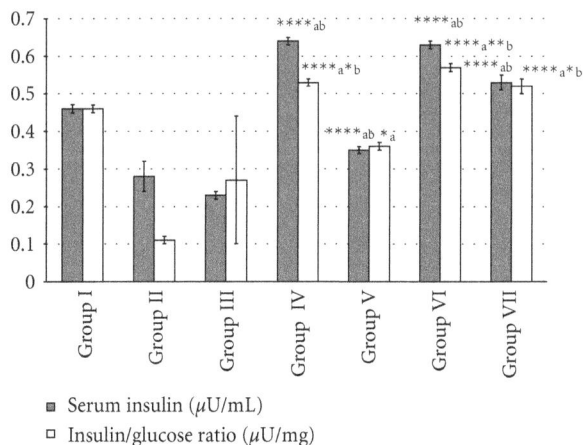

FIGURE 4: Effect of MREt on serum insulin level and insulin/glucose ratio. Each bar represents the mean ± SEM ($n = 6$). $*P < 0.05$, $**P < 0.01$, and $****P < 0.0001$, when compared with group II (a) and III (b).

3.8. Effect of MREt on ALT. Normal serum ALT levels were observed in all experimental controls and test groups (Table 4).

3.9. Effect of MREt on Liver Glycogen and Total Lipids. The liver glycogen amount was found improved in positive control and test groups from 1.16 to 1.63 g/g of tissue as compared to diabetic and negative control groups that showed its decrease amount from 0.73 to 0.77 g/g tissue (Table 4). Whereas total lipid content in liver tissue was increased in

diabetic and negative control groups (0.145 ± 0.005 and 0.12 ± 0.007 g/g tissue) as compared to MREt treated mice and positive control group that showed significantly reduced ($P < 0.0001$) level of total lipids in their livers from 0.045–0.06 g/g of tissue (Figure 3).

3.10. Effect of MREt on Serum Insulin Level and Insulin/Glucose (I/G) Ratio. Serum insulin levels and I/G ratio were significantly improved ($P < 0.05$, $P < 0.001$ and $P < 0.0001$)

TABLE 4: Effect of MREt on lipid profile, alanine transaminase (ALT), and antiatherogenic index in mice.

Parameters	Group I	Group II	Group III	Group IV	Group V	Group VI	Group VII
Cholesterol (mg/dL)	141.65 ± 13.05	260.42 ± 10.18	254.11 ± 14.94	178.40 ± 15.95****a,***b	146.19 ± 10.01****a,b	129.33 ± 19.34****a,b	138.50 ± 9.29***a,b
TG (mg/dL)	148.86 ± 2.08	161.33 ± 3.83	173.50 ± 19.05	121.15 ± 3.38*a,**b	128.27 ± 6.59*a,**b	149.12 ± 15.46	138.75 ± 10.66*b
HDL-c (mg/dL)	53.08 ± 8.47	50.69 ± 7.93	45.63 ± 10.01	31.20 ± 3.59	36.72 ± 5.39	36.07 ± 7.06	37.45 ± 4.03
LDL-c (mg/dL)	66.56 ± 9.61	175.09 ± 15.76	164.64 ± 19.70	122.98 ± 18.34*a	83.83 ± 7.09*a,b	63.46 ± 23.68****a,b	73.30 ± 8.96****a,***b
VLDL-c (mg/dL)	29.77 ± 0.41	32.27 ± 0.77	34.70 ± 3.81	24.23 ± 0.68*a,**b	25.65 ± 1.32*a,*b	29.82 ± 3.09	27.75 ± 2.13*b
AAI (%)	37.31 ± 6.43	24.98 ± 4.62	23.67 ± 6.68	23.56 ± 6.39	33.34 ± 3.83	53.29 ± 24.04	37.54 ± 4.59
ALT (U/L)	15.63 ± 0.38	16.93 ± 0.35	16.26 ± 0.19	9.82 ± 0.11***a,b	7.68 ± 0.4***a,b	6.75 ± 0.21***a,b	7.25 ± 0.23***a,b

Values are expressed as mean ± SEM ($n = 6$). $*P < 0.05$, $**P < 0.01$, $***P < 0.001$, and $****P < 0.0001$, when compared with respective group II (a) and III (b).

in all test and positive control groups and found 0.35–0.64 μU/mL and 0.36–0.57 μU/mg, respectively as compared to diabetic and negative controls that showed low levels of serum insulin and I/G ratios (Figure 4).

4. Discussion

The frequency of diabetes increases day by day with rapid rise in mortality burden that establishes threat of this disease as one of the leading cause of death globally [1]. Beside the presence of commercially available oral antidiabetic drugs and insulin injections for the treatments of both type I and II diabetes, a vast scientific data is available which describe that variety of herbs are used as effective hypoglycemic agents with different modes of action [37]. Today investigating a hypoglycemic herb with potent hypotensive and hypolipidemic activities is a strong and interesting research aspect of ethanopharmacology. The detailed spectrum of *Rauwolfia serpentina* in the management of diabetic dyslipidemia has not been reported yet. Therefore the present study was designed to identify the phytochemical profile of MREt of *R. serpentina* and its long-term hypoglycemic, hypolipidemic effects and weight improving pattern in alloxan-induced daibetic *Wister* male mice.

The present study demonstrates the presence of alkaloids, carbohydrates, flavonoids, glycosides, cardiac glycosides, phlobatannins, resins, saponins, steroids, tannins, and triterpenoids in MREt. The quantitative profile of the same extract clearly illustrates the presence of high magnitude of antioxidant compounds like total phenols 233 mg/gm of extract. Similarly, flavonoids, alkaloids, and saponins were found as 97, 7, and 20 mg/gm in root powder of same herb. A vast literature provides scientific evidence that plants rich in flavonoids possess potent antidiabetic, hypolipidemic, hypotensive, anti-inflammatory, and antioxidative activities [5, 38].

Alloxan is a pyrimidine derivative and commonly used as universal toxin that causes the irreversible destruction of β-cells in the islets of Langerhans, which not only induced diabetes by inhibiting the release of insulin but also act as a good enhancer of oxidative stress by elevating the production of reactive oxygen species (ROS) that directly associated with the weight loss in diabetic mice [39]. However, in the present investigation, the percent change in body weights of alloxan-induced diabetic mice treated with the doses of MREt of *R. serpentina* showed less reduction than diabetic control groups at 14 day of animal trial. Of which, MREt in a dose of 60 mg/kg showed marked improvement in body weight whereas the body weights recovered slowly in the other two test groups treated with 10 and 30 mg/kg of same extract. In diabetic condition, body utilized triglycerides as an alternate source of energy which is also accompanied by catabolism of tissue protein that results in loss of both fat and lean mass which in turn induce a significant reduction in total body weight [40]. It has been reported that this unhealthy loss in total body weight is more accelerated due to polyuria induced by dehydration because of hyperglycemia, one of the characteristic symptoms of diabetes [41]. The MREt (10, 30, and 60 mg/kg) induced a significant percent glycemic

reduction in fasting blood glucose levels of all three test groups at 14 day from −46 to −51% as compared to marked increase in percent glycemic change from 23 to 28% that was observed in diabetic and negative control groups. This observation also supports our previous finding that MREt of *R. serpentina* improves the glucose tolerance in *Wister* mice [19].

The antidiabetic effect of MREt of *R. serpentina* is more strengthened by observing the fair control of $HbA1_c$ levels in all three test groups treated with the same extract and interestingly, the $HbA1_c$ levels in test groups at 14 day of trial were found almost equal to its level observed in normal (control) and positive control mice. However, the high percentage of $HbA1_c$ was found in diabetic and negative controls that represents poor glycemic control. It has been reported that in diabetes, increased amount of blood glucose nonezymatically combines with hemoglobin to form glycated (glycosylated) hemoglobin ($HbA1_c$), and hence the $HbA1_c$ level reflects the average amount of glucose in blood [42]. Increased concentration of $HbA1_c$ in diabetes also affects the total Hb level in blood besides the contribution of other chronic causes such as renal dysfunction, and in this regard several studies reported the presence of unrecognized anemia in diabetic patients [43]. In the present study, MREt significantly improved the total Hb levels in all test groups and brought it back to the level that was observed in control mice, as compared to diabetic and negative controls that showed low levels of same parameter.

The elevated serum levels of TC, TG, and LDL-c provide a high risk for the development of atherosclerosis and other cardiovascular diseases (CVD) whereas increased HDL-c level associated with the decrease in this risk [40]. In alloxan-induced diabetes, hyperglycemia is associated with hypertriglyceridemia and hypercholesterolemia [18]. In the present study, MREt of *R. serpentina* significantly decreases the levels of TC, TG, LDL-c, and VLDL-c in all test groups as compared to the diabetic and negative control groups. Both lipoproteins including LDL-c and VLDL are involved in depositing TC and TG on walls of coronary arteries and initiate the process of atherosclerotic plaques [44]. Reduced serum levels of LDL-c and VLDL-c found in test mice groups treated with doses (10, 30, and 60 mg/kg) of MREt, is among one of the beneficial aspects of this current research and proved the antiatherosclerotic potential of this extract. However, a decrease in HDL-c levels was also observed in test mice, which actually reflects the significantly lower levels of TC found in test groups as only 30% cholesterol transported by HDL-c in blood from peripheral tissues to liver for its metabolism and excretion [45]. Scientific evidence described that many plant extract or herbal products possess lipid lowering potential by producing the decrease in all cholesterol-associated lipoprotein levels including HDL-c but improving the cardioprotective indices [46]. Hypocholesterolemic and hypotriglyceridemic effects of MREt are actually the result of its potent hypoglycemic effect that is probably due to an increase in glucose utilization by peripheral tissues [18] or inhibiting the activity of rate-limiting enzyme 3-hydroxy-3-methyl glutaryl CoA reductase (HMG-CoA reductase) of cholesterol biosynthesis. The experimentally obtained hypotriglceridemic effect of MREt may also be due to the improvement in lipolysis by reducing the activity of hormone-sensitive lipase [40, 47].

To support lipid lowering potential of MREt of *Rauwolfia*, the antiatherogenic index (AAI) was also evaluated and found increased from 33 to 53% in test groups mice treated with extract (10, 30, and 60 mg/kg) as compared to diabetic controls which again represents the antiatherosclerotic significance of *Rauwolfia*. Slight improvement has also been observed in cardioprotective index of test groups in terms of TG/HDL-c and HDL-c/LDL-c ratios as compared to diabetic control. TG/HDL-c ratio is preferable under 4 and ideal under 2 whereas HDL-c/LDL-c ratio is preferable over 0.3 and ideal over 0.4 [48]. Out of these ratios, HDL-c/LDL-c ratio was found ideal in the present study. It has been reported that an increase in TG/HDL-c and a decrease in HDL-c/LDL-c ratios are good predictors of CVD and insulin resistance in subjects [49]. Similarly coronary risk index (CRI) in term of TC/HDL-c ratio significantly decreased in all MREt treated test mice, which provides further strength to the present study. According to the past findings, the value of CRI greater than 5 indicates that subject is on high risk of CVD while under 3.5 is ideal for biochemical functioning [33, 34]; hence, CRI is highly improved in MREt treated test mice.

Attention-grabbing point of the present study is that the oral antidiabetic drug glibenclamide, one of the well-known sulfonylureas, also produced significant antidiabetic effect in alloxan-induced diabetic mice though this drug is classified as secretagogues and it requires alive β-cells of pancreas to enhance the release of insulin [3]. It was also proved by observing the increase in serum insulin level and insulin/glucose (I/G) ratio in positive control group which constitutes alloxan-induced diabetic mice treated with glibenclamide at 5 mg/kg, it tells that may be few β-cells were still alive. Though, extrapancreatic effects of sulfonylureas in type-II diabetes have also been reported [50]. Similarly, the serum insulin level and I/G ratio were gradually improved in all MREt treated mice (test groups) and become better than its levels found in diabetic control group that showed decreased insulin level and increased I/G ratio. Interestingly this improvement provides another possibility of antidiabetic mechanism of action of MREt that besides having extrapancreatic action, it may also has some pancreatic action as same as glibenclamide through which it could enhance the release of insulin via activating few alive β-cells as a result of which insulin in turn produce its anabolic action by improving the ability of body to utilize glucose as a source of energy. This possibility was also supported by observing the gradual improvement in liver glycogen in all test mice treated with MREt from 10 to 60 mg/kg and even the highest experimental dose of extract gave same amount of hepatic glycogen that was observed in control group whereas its low amount was observed in diabetic and negative control groups. This finding clearly proved that the process of glycogenesis has been improved in all test mice by *Rauwolfia*. Similarly the total lipids in liver tissue were significantly recovered in MREt treated test groups as compared to diabetic and negative controls which indicate the

hepatoprotective effect of this medicinal plant as reduction in liver lipid content improves the liver functioning [51].

ALT is liver-specific enzyme that provides a deep insight about the hepatic functioning, it elevates in case of hepatic injuries or malfunctioning [44]. The pharmacological basis of therapeutics clearly states that orally administrated drug must pass through hepatic metabolism so it should not be toxic to liver [18]. Therefore, to investigate any toxic effect of MREt on liver, serum ALT level was measured. Though, the decreased levels of ALT were observed in all test groups treated with MREt (10, 30, and 60 mg/kg) as compared to normal, diabetic and negative controls but considered normal levels of this enzyme. As scientific literature states that normal ALT level range from 0 to 37 U/L [52, 53].

The obtained significant antidiabetic and hypolipidemic effects of MREt of *R. serpentina* may be due to the presences of high quantity of total polyphenolic compounds in the same extract as compared to other constituents. Therefore, total flavonoids could be targeted, isolated, and studied as an active fraction involved in antidiabetic activity of same extract in future.

5. Conclusion

The present study concludes that MREt of *R. serpentina* is an effective antidiabetic agent as it improves glycemic, antiatherogenic, and cardioprotective indices in alloxan-induced diabetic mice.

Conflict of Interests

The auothers declare that they have no conflict of interests.

Acknowledgments

The authors are highly thankful to University of Karachi for providing Dean Research Grant for conducting this experimental work. They also appreciate the technical assistance provided by Mr. Ali Zia, Application Specialist of Roche Diagnostic, Ms. Tooba Lateef, Lecturer in the Department of Biochemistry, Jinnah University for Women, and Ms. Shaima Hasnat, MS Scholar, Department of Biochemistry, University of Karachi, Karachi, Pakistan throughout the entire period of this study.

References

[1] J. E. Shaw, R. A. Sicree, and P. Z. Zimmet, "Global estimates of the prevalence of diabetes for 2010 and 2030," *Diabetes Research and Clinical Practice*, vol. 87, no. 1, pp. 4–14, 2010.

[2] Z. A. Shaikh, M. Z. Shaikh, and G. Ali, "Diabetic patients, awareness about life style modifications," *Professional Medical Journal*, vol. 18, no. 2, pp. 265–268, 2011.

[3] H. P. Rang, M. M. Dale, J. M. Ritter, and P. K. Moore, "The Endocrine Pancreas and the control of blood glucose," in *Pharmacology*, J. G. Hardman and L. E. Limbird, Eds., p. 385, Churchill Livingstone, New York, NY, USA, 5th edition, 2003.

[4] S. Tiwari, "Plant: a rich source of herbal medicine," *Journal of Natural Product*, vol. 1, pp. 27–35, 2008.

[5] N. Aggarwal and Shishu, "A review of recent investigations on medicinal herbs possessing anti-diabetic properties," *Journal of Nutrition Disorder Therapy*, vol. 1, no. 1, p. 102, 2011.

[6] D. Pitchai, R. Manikkam, S. R. Rajendran, and G. Pitchai, "Database on pharmacophore analysis of active principles, from medicinal plants," *Bioinformation*, vol. 5, no. 2, pp. 43–45, 2010.

[7] L. W. Singh, "Traditional medicinal plants of Manipur as anti-diabetics," *Journal of Medicinal Plant Research*, vol. 5, no. 5, pp. 677–687, 2011.

[8] S. A. Qureshi and S. K. Udani, "Hypolipidaemic activity of *Rauwolfia serpentina* Benth," *Pakistan Journal of Nutrition*, vol. 8, no. 7, pp. 1103–1106, 2009.

[9] N. H. Mashour, G. I. Lin, and W. H. Frishman, "Herbal medicine for the treatment of cardiovascular disease: clinical considerations," *Archives of Internal Medicine*, vol. 158, no. 20, pp. 2225–2234, 1998.

[10] R. Harisaranraj, K. Suresh, S. Saravana Babu, and V. Vaira Achundahan, "Phytochemical based strategies for pathogen control and antioxidant capacities of *Rauwolfia serpentina* extracts," *Recent Research Science Technology*, vol. 1, no. 2, pp. 67–78, 2009.

[11] A. Dey and J. N. De, "Ethnobotanical aspects of *Rauwolfia serpentina* (L). Benth. ex Kurz. in India, Nepal and Bangladesh," *Journal of Medicinal Plant Research*, vol. 5, no. 2, pp. 144–150, 2011.

[12] A. Itoh, T. Kumashiro, M. Yamaguchi et al., "Indole alkaloids and other constituents of *Rauwolfia serpentina*," *Journal of Natural Products*, vol. 68, no. 6, pp. 848–852, 2005.

[13] J. L. Stanford, E. J. Martin, L. A. Brinton, and R. N. Hoover, "Rauwolfia use and breast cancer: a case-control study," *Journal of the National Cancer Institute*, vol. 76, no. 5, pp. 817–822, 1986.

[14] R. J. Vakil, "*Rauwolfia serpentina* in the treatment of high blood pressure; a review of the literature," *Circulation*, vol. 12, no. 2, pp. 220–229, 1955.

[15] L. Cazzaroli and D. Dall'Oglio, "Effect of *Rauwolfia serpentina* on the glycemic curve of the glucose tolerance in normal subject and diabetics," *Progresso Medicine*, vol. 14, no. 2, pp. 52–56, 1958.

[16] A. S. Cohen, N. S. Stearns, H. Levitin, and D. Hurwitz, "Studies on *Rauwolfia alkaloids* in diabetic hypertensive patients," *Annals of Internal Medicine*, vol. 51, pp. 238–247, 1959.

[17] M. L. Chatterjee, M. S. De, and D. Setb, "Effect of different fractions of *Rauwolfia serpentina* alkaloids on blood sugar levels in anaesthetized cats," *Bulletin of the Calcutta School of Tropical Medicine*, vol. 8, pp. 152–153, 1960.

[18] S. A. Qureshi, A. Nawaz, S. K. Udani, and B. Azmi, "Hypoglycaemic and hypolipidemic activities of *Rauwolfia serpentina* in alloxan-induced diabetic rats," *International Journal of Pharmacology*, vol. 5, no. 5, pp. 323–326, 2009.

[19] M. B. Azmi and S. A. Qureshi, "Methanolic root extract of *Rauwolfia serpentina* Benth improves the glucose tolerance in Wister mice," *Journal of Food Drug Analysis*, vol. 20, no. 2, pp. 54–58, 2012.

[20] K. S. Chandrashekar, H. Vignesh, and K. S. Prasanna, "Phytochemical studies of Stem Bark of *Michelia Champaca* Linn," *International Research Journal of Pharmacy*, vol. 1, no. 1, pp. 243–246, 2010.

[21] H. O. Edeoga, D. E. Okwu, and B. O. Mbaebie, "Phytochemical constituents of some Nigerian medicinal plants," *African Journal of Biotechnology*, vol. 4, no. 7, pp. 685–688, 2005.

[22] S. Shanmugam, T. S. Kumar, and K. P. Selvam, *Laboratory Handbook on Biochemistry*, PHI Learning Private Limited, New Delhi, India, 2010.

[23] J. B. Harborne, *Phytochemical Methods*, Chapman and Hall, London, UK, 1973.

[24] B. A. Boham and A. R. Kocipai, "Flavonoids and condensed tannins from leaves of Hawaiian *vaccinium vaticulatum* and *V. calycinium*," *Pacific Science*, vol. 48, pp. 458–463, 1974.

[25] B. O. Obdoni and P. O. Ochuko, "Phytochemicals studies and comparative efficacy of the crude extracts of the some Homostatic plants in Edo and Delta States of Nigeria," *Global Journal of Pure Applied Science*, vol. 8, pp. 203–208, 2001.

[26] M. Sengul, H. Yildiz, N. Gungor, B. Cetin, Z. Eser, and S. Ercisli, "Total phenolic content, antioxidant and antimicrobial activities of some medicinal plants," *Pakistan Journal of Pharmaceutical Sciences*, vol. 22, no. 1, pp. 102–106, 2009.

[27] A. B. Saba, A. A. Oyagbemi, and O. I. Azeez, "Antidiabetic and haematinic effects of *Parquetina nigrescens* on alloxan induced type-1 diabetes and normocytic normochromic anaemia in Wistar rats," *African Health Sciences*, vol. 10, no. 3, pp. 276–282, 2010.

[28] M. Perfumi and R. Tacconi, "Antihyperglycemic effect of fresh *Opuntia dillenii* fruit from Tenerife (Canary Islands)," *International Journal of Pharmacognosy*, vol. 34, no. 1, pp. 41–47, 1996.

[29] W. T. Friedewald, R. I. Levy, and D. S. Fredrickson, "Estimation of the concentration of low-density lipoprotein cholesterol in plasma, without use of the preparative ultracentrifuge," *Clinical Chemistry*, vol. 18, no. 6, pp. 499–502, 1972.

[30] J. Folch, M. Lees, and G. H. S. Stanley, "A simple method for the isolation and purification of total lipides from animal tissues," *The Journal of Biological Chemistry*, vol. 226, no. 1, pp. 497–509, 1956.

[31] M. Dubois, K. A. Gilles, J. K. Hamilton, P. A. Rebers, and F. Smith, "Colorimetric method for determination of sugars and related substances," *Analytical Chemistry*, vol. 28, no. 3, pp. 350–358, 1956.

[32] A. M. M. Jalil, A. Ismail, P. P. Chong, M. Hamid, and S. H. S. Kamaruddin, "Effects of cocoa extract containing polyphenols and methylxanthines on biochemical parameters of obese-diabetic rats," *Journal of the Science of Food and Agriculture*, vol. 89, no. 1, pp. 130–137, 2009.

[33] P. Barter, A. M. Gotto, J. C. LaRosa et al., "HDL cholesterol, very low levels of LDL cholesterol, and cardiovascular events," *The New England Journal of Medicine*, vol. 357, no. 13, pp. 1301–1310, 2007.

[34] H. T. Kang, J. K. Kim, J. Y. Kim, J. A. Linton, J. H. Yoon, and S. B. Koh, "Independent association of TG/ HDL-c with urinary albumin excretion in normotensive subjects in a rural Korean population," *Clinica Chimica Acta*, vol. 413, pp. 319–324, 2012.

[35] M. A. Waqar and Y. Mahmmod, "Anti- Platelet, Anti- hypercholesterolemia and anti-oxidant effects of Ethanolic extract of *Brassica oleracea* in high fat diet provided rats," *World Applied Sciences Journal*, vol. 8, no. 1, pp. 107–112, 2010.

[36] A. A. Adeneye and J. A. Olagunju, "Preliminary hypoglycemic and hypolipidemic activities of the aqueous seed extract of *Carica papaya* Linn. in Wistar rats," *Biology and Medicine*, vol. 1, no. 1, pp. 1–10, 2009.

[37] P. K. Prabhakar and M. Doble, "Mechanism of action of natural products used in the treatment of diabetes mellitus," *Chinese Journal of Integrative Medicine*, vol. 17, no. 8, pp. 563–574, 2011.

[38] A. A. Adeneye, T. I. Adeleke, and A. K. Adeneye, "Hypoglycemic and hypolipidemic effects of the aqueous fresh leaves

extract of *Clerodendrum capitatum* in Wistar rats," *Journal of Ethnopharmacology*, vol. 116, no. 1, pp. 7–10, 2008.

[39] J. E. Sun, Z. H. Ao, Z. M. Lu et al., "Antihyperglycemic and antilipidperoxidative effects of dry matter of culture broth of Inonotus obliquus in submerged culture on normal and alloxan-diabetes mice," *Journal of Ethnopharmacology*, vol. 118, no. 1, pp. 7–13, 2008.

[40] M. L. Bishop, E. P. Fody, and L. Schoeff, *Clinical Chemistry: Principles, Procedures, Correlations*, Lippincott Williams & Wilkins, 6th edition, 2010.

[41] S. D. Wolfsthal, R. Manno, and E. Fontanilla, "Emergencies in diabetic patients in the primary care setting," *Primary Care*, vol. 33, no. 3, pp. 711–725, 2006.

[42] R. A. Silverman, U. Thakker, T. Ellman et al., "Hemoglobin A1c as a screen for previously undiagnosed prediabetes and diabetes in an acute-care setting," *Diabetes Care*, vol. 34, no. 9, pp. 1908–1912, 2011.

[43] M. C. Thomas, R. J. MacIsaac, C. Tsalamandris, D. Power, and G. Jerums, "Unrecognized anemia in patients with diabetes: a cross-sectional survey," *Diabetes Care*, vol. 26, no. 4, pp. 1164–1169, 2003.

[44] S. A. Qureshi, M. Kamran, M. Asad, A. Zia, T. Lateef, and M. B. Azmi, "A preliminary study of Santalum album on serum lipids and enzymes," *Global Journal of Pharmacology*, vol. 4, no. 2, pp. 71–74, 2010.

[45] P. O. Kwiterovich, "The metabolic pathways of high-density lipoprotein, low-density lipoprotein, and triglycerides: a current review," *American Journal of Cardiology*, vol. 86, no. 12, pp. 5–10, 2000.

[46] A. Aissaoui, S. Zizi, Z. H. Israili, and B. Lyoussi, "Hypoglycemic and hypolipidemic effects of *Coriandrum sativum* L. in Meriones shawi rats," *Journal of Ethnopharmacology*, vol. 137, no. 1, pp. 652–661, 2011.

[47] D. L. Nelson and M. M. L. Cox, *Lehninger Principles of Biochemistry*, W.H. Freeman and Company, New York, NY, USA, 5th edition, 2008.

[48] J. M. Gaziano, C. H. Hennekens, C. J. O'Donnell, J. L. Breslow, and J. E. Buring, "Fasting triglycerides, high-density lipoprotein, and risk of myocardial infarction," *Circulation*, vol. 96, no. 8, pp. 2520–2525, 1997.

[49] T. Marotta, B. F. Russo, and L. A. Ferrara, "Triglyceride-to-HDL-cholesterol ratio and metabolic syndrome as contributors to cardiovascular risk in overweight patients," *Obesity*, vol. 18, no. 8, pp. 1608–1613, 2010.

[50] K. Kaku, Y. Inoue, and T. Kaneko, "Extrapancreatic effects of sulfonylurea drugs," *Diabetes Research and Clinical Practice*, vol. 28, pp. S105–S108, 1995.

[51] S. Rigazio, H. R. Lehto, H. Tuunanen et al., "The lowering of hepatic fatty acid uptake improves liver function and insulin sensitivity without affecting hepatic fat content in humans," *American Journal of Physiology-Endocrinology and Metabolism*, vol. 295, no. 2, pp. E413–E419, 2008.

[52] D. W. Moss and A. R. Henderson, "Enzymes," in *Tietz Fundamental of Clinical Chemistry*, C. A. Burtis and E. R. Ashwood, Eds., WB Sunders Company, 4th edition, 1996.

[53] S. Reitman and S. Frankel, "A colorimetric method for the determination of serum glutamic oxalacetic and glutamic pyruvic transaminases," *American Journal of Clinical Pathology*, vol. 28, no. 1, pp. 56–63, 1957.

8

Memory-Enhancing Activity of Palmatine in Mice Using Elevated Plus Maze and Morris Water Maze

Dinesh Dhingra and Varun Kumar

Department of Pharmaceutical Sciences, Guru Jambheshwar University of Science and Technology, Haryana, Hisar 125001, India

Correspondence should be addressed to Dinesh Dhingra, din_dhingra@rediffmail.com

Academic Editor: Karim A. Alkadhi

The present study was designed to evaluate the effect of palmatine on memory of Swiss young male albino mice. Palmatine (0.1, 0.5, 1 mg/kg, *i.p.*) and physostigmine (0.1 mg/kg, *i.p.*) per se were administered for 10 successive days to separate groups of mice. Effect of drugs on learning and memory of mice was evaluated using elevated plus maze and Morris water maze. Brain acetylcholinesterase activity was also estimated. Effect of palmatine on scopolamine- and diazepam-induced amnesia was also investigated. Palmatine (0.5 and 1 mg/kg) and physostigmine significantly improved learning and memory of mice, as indicated by decrease in transfer latency using elevated plus maze, and decrease in escape latency during training and increase in time spent in target quadrant during retrieval using Morris water maze. The drugs did not show any significant effect on locomotor activity of the mice. Memory-enhancing activity of palmatine (1 mg/kg) was comparable to physostigmine. Palmatine (1 mg/kg) significantly reversed scopolamine- and diazepam-induced amnesia in mice. Palmatine and physostigmine also significantly reduced brain acetylcholinesterase activity of mice. Thus, palmatine showed memory-enhancing activity in mice probably by inhibiting brain acetylcholinesterase activity, through involvement of GABA-benzodiazepine pathway, and due to its antioxidant activity.

1. Introduction

Dementia, the commonest form (accounting for approximately 60% of all cases) of which is Alzheimer's disease (AD), mainly affects older people and it is estimated that, by 2050, more than 115 million people will have dementia [1]. AD is a neurodegenerative disorder characterized by cognitive and memory deterioration, progressive impairment of activities of daily living, and a multiplicity of behavioural and psychological disturbances [2]. The primary causes of AD appear to be (i) decreased cholinergic activity; (ii) deposition of amyloid-beta peptides in the brain; (iii) oxidative stress. Acetylcholinesterase (AChE) plays a key role in the regulation of the cholinergic system and hence, inhibition of AChE has emerged as one of the most promising strategies for the treatment of AD. One of the major therapeutic strategies is to inhibit the AChE, and hence, to increase the acetylcholine level in the brain [3]. The imbalance between the generation of free radicals and antioxidants has also been claimed to be a cause of AD [4].

Palmatine is a quaternary protoberberine alkaloid. It is typically yellow in color and is an active constituent of a number of plants, such as *Coptidis rhizoma* [5], and so forth. Palmatine has been reported to possess sedative [6] and antioxidant activities [5]. It has been also shown to be inhibitor of beta-site amyloid precursor protein-cleaving enzyme 1 (BACE 1), acetyl- and butyrylcholinesterases [5]. Thus, palmatine has potential for the management of dementia. So the present study was designed to investigate the effect of palmatine on the learning and memory of mice by employing behavioral models.

2. Materials and Methods

2.1. Experimental Animals. Swiss male albino mice, weighing around 20–25 g, were purchased from Disease Free Small Animal House, Lala Lajpat Rai University of Veterinary and Animal Sciences, Hisar (Haryana). Since estrogens (female sex hormones) have been found to have effect on memory, we excluded female mice and used only male mice for the study

[7]. Animals were housed separately in groups of 8 per cage (Polycarbonate cage size: $29 \times 22 \times 14$ cm) under laboratory conditions with alternating light and dark cycle of 12 h each. The animals had free access to food and water. The animals were kept fasted 2 h before and 2 h after drug administration. The animals were acclimatized for at least five days before behavioural experiments which were carried out between 09:00 and 17:00 h. The experimental protocol was approved by Institutional Animals Ethics Committee (IAEC) and animal care was taken as per the guidelines of Committee for the Purpose of Control and Supervision of Experiments on Animals (CPCSEA), Ministry of Environment and Forests, Government of India (Registration no. 0436).

2.2. Drugs and Chemicals. Palmatine and scopolamine hydrobromide (Sigma-Aldrich, St. Louis, USA); physostigmine, acetylcholine iodide, acetylthiocholine iodide, and 5,5'-dithiobis-2-nitrobenzoic acid (Hi-Media Laboratories, Mumbai); diazepam (Calmpose injection, Ranbaxy Laboratories Ltd., Gurgaon, India).

2.3. Selection of Doses. Doses of various drugs were selected on the basis of literature, that is, 0.4 mg/kg for scopolamine, 1 mg/kg for diazepam [8], 0.1 mg/kg for physostigmine [9], 0.1 and 1 mg/kg for palmatine [8].

2.4. Vehicle. Palmatine was suspended in 10% Tween 80 in normal saline. Scopolamine hydrobromide was dissolved in normal saline. Injection of diazepam was diluted in normal saline.

2.5. Models Employed for Evaluation of Memory Enhancing Activity in Mice

2.5.1. Elevated Plus Maze. The procedure, technique, and end point for testing learning and memory were followed as per the parameters described earlier [8, 10, 11]. The elevated plus maze for mice consisted of two open arms (16 cm $\times$ 5 cm) and two covered arms (16 cm $\times$ 5 cm $\times$ 15 cm) extended from a central platform (5 cm $\times$ 5 cm) and the maze was elevated to a height of 25 cm from the floor. On the first day, each mouse was placed at the end of an open arm, facing away from the central platform. Transfer latency (TL) was defined as the time taken by the animal to move from the open arm into one of the covered arms with all its four legs. TL was recorded on the first day (i.e., 10th day of drug administration) for each animal. If the animal did not enter into one of the covered arm within 90 sec, it was gently pushed into one of the two covered arms and TL was assigned as 90 sec. The mouse was allowed to explore the maze for another 2 minutes and then returned to its home cage. Retention of this learned-task (memory) was examined 24 h (11th day) after the first day trial.

2.5.2. Morris Water Maze. The procedure, technique, and end point for testing memory were followed as per the parameters described earlier [12, 13]. Briefly, Morris water maze-(MWM) for mice consisted of a circular pool (60 cm in diameter, 25 cm in height) filled to a depth of 20 cm with water maintained at 25°C. The water was made opaque with nontoxic white colored dye. The tank was divided into four equal quadrants with the help of two threads, fixed at right angle to each other on the rim of the pool. A submerged platform (with top surface 6 cm $\times$ 6 cm and painted in white) was placed inside the target quadrants (Q4 in present study) of this pool 1 cm below surface of water. The position of platform was kept unaltered throughout the training session. Each animal was subjected to four consecutive trials each day with a gap of 5 min for four consecutive days (starting from 6th day of drug administration to 9th day), during which they were allowed to escape on to the hidden platform and to remain there for 20 s. During the training session, the mouse was gently placed in the water between quadrants, facing the wall of pool with drop location changing for each trial, and allowed 120 sec to locate submerged platform. If the mouse failed to find the platform within 120 s, it was guided gently on to the platform and allowed to remain there for 20 s. Escape latency (EL) is the time taken by the animal to move from the starting quadrant to find the hidden plateform in the target quadrant. EL was recorded on the 6th day to 9th day for each animal. Each animal was subjected to training trials for four consecutive days, the starting position was changed with each exposure as mentioned below and target quadrant (Q4 in the present study) remained constant throughout the training period.

Day1 Q1 Q2 Q3 Q4.

Day2 Q2 Q3 Q4 Q1.

Day3 Q3 Q4 Q1 Q2.

Day4 Q4 Q1 Q2 Q3.

On the fifth day (i.e., 10th day of drug administration), the platform was removed and mouse was placed in any of the three quadrants and allowed to explore the target quadrant for 300 s. Mean time spent in all the three quadrants that is, Q1, Q2, and Q3 was recorded. The mean time spent in the target quadrant in search of the missing platform was noted as index of retrieval or memory. The observer always stood at the same position. Care was taken not to disturb the relative location of water maze with respect to other objects in the laboratory.

2.5.3. Measurement of Locomotor Activity. To rule out the effects of the drugs on motor activity, horizontal locomotor activities of control and test animals were recorded for a period of 5 min using Medicraft Photoactometer, Model number 600-4D (INCO, Ambala, India). The photoactometer consisted of a square arena (30 $\times$ 30 $\times$ 25 cm) with wire mesh bottom, in which the animal moves. Six lights and six photocells placed in the outer periphery of the bottom in such a way that a single mouse can block only one beam. Technically its principle is that a photocell is activated when the rays of light falling on the photocells are cut off by animals crossing the beam of light. As the photocell is activated, a count is recorded. The photocells are connected to an electronic automatic counting device which counts the number of "cut offs."

2.6. Biochemical Estimation

2.6.1. Collection of Brain Sample. Immediately after behavioural testing (retrieval) on elevated plus maze, animals were sacrificed by cervical dislocation under light anaesthesia with diethylether. The whole brain was carefully removed from the skull. For preparation of brain homogenate, the fresh whole brain was weighed and transferred to a glass homogenizer and homogenized in an ice bath after adding 10 volumes of phosphate buffer (pH 8, 0.1 M). The homogenate was centrifuged using refrigerated centrifuge at 3000 rpm for 10 min at 4°C and the resultant cloudy supernatant liquid was used for the estimation of brain acetylcholinesterase activity.

2.6.2. Brain Acetylcholinesterase Activity. Brain acetylcholinesterase was estimated using the method of Ellman et al. [14]. Briefly, 0.4 mL of brain homogenate was added to a test tube containing 2.6 mL of phosphate buffer. 0.1 mL DTNB reagent was added to the above mixture and absorbance was noted at 412 nm. 0.02 mL of acetylcholine iodide solution was added and again absorbance was noted 15 min thereafter. Change in absorbance per min was calculated.

The rate of hydrolysis of substrate was calculated using following formula:

$$R = \text{change in absorbance/min} \times 5.74 \times 10^{-4}/C0,$$

R = rate of hydrolysis of acetylcholine iodide/min/mg tissue,

$C0$ = weight of tissue homogenate in mg/mL.

2.7. Experimental Design

2.7.1. Groups for Elevated Plus Maze

Group 1 to 5. Normal saline, palmatine (0.1, 0.5 and 1 mg/kg, *i.p.*), and physostigmine (0.1 mg/kg, *i.p.*), respectively, were administered for 11 successive days. TL was recorded 30 minutes after the drug administration on 10th day (learning) and retention was examined on 11th day.

Group 6 and 7. Normal saline and palmatine (1 mg/kg, *i.p.*), respectively, were injected for 11 successive days. On 10th day, TL was recorded 45 min after the injection. On the 11th day, scopolamine was injected (0.4 mg/kg, *i.p.*) 30 min after injection of palmatine and TL was recorded 45 min after the injection of scopolamine.

Group 8 and 9. Normal saline and palmatine (1 mg/kg, *i.p.*), respectively, were injected for 11 successive days. On 10th day, TL was recorded 45 min after the injection. On the 11th day, diazepam was injected (0.4 mg/kg, *i.p.*) 30 min after injection of palmatine and TL was recorded 45 min after the injection of diazepam.

2.7.2. Groups for Morris Water Maze

Groups 10 to 14. Normal saline, palmatine (0.1, 0.5 and 1 mg/kg, *i.p.*), and physostigmine (0.1 mg/kg, *i.p.*), respectively, were administered for 10 successive days. Escape latency (EL) was recorded 45 min after drug administration from 6th day to 9th day. On 10th day, time spent in target quadrant (TSTQ) was noted 45 min after the drug administration.

Group 15 and 16. Normal saline and palmatine (1 mg/kg, *p.o.*), respectively, were injected for 10 successive days. EL was recorded 45 min after drug administration from 6th day to 9th day. On 10th day, scopolamine was injected 30 min after injection of palmatine and TSTQ was noted 45 min after the injection of scopolamine.

Group 17 and 18. Normal saline, palmatine (1 mg/kg, *p.o.*), respectively, were injected for 10 successive days. EL was 45 min after drug administration from 6th day to 9th day. On 10th day, diazepam (1 mg/kg, *i.p.*) was injected 30 min after injection of palmatine and TSTQ was noted 45 min after the injection of diazepam.

2.7.3. Measurement of Locomotor Activity. Locomotor activity was measured 24 h after performing water maze test in mice of groups 10 to 14 using photoactometer (INCO, Ambala).

2.8. Statistical Analysis. All the results are expressed as Mean ± S.E.M. Data were analyzed by analysis of variance (ANOVA) followed by Tukey's post hoc test in Graph Pad Instat package, version 3.05. $P < 0.05$ was considered as significant.

3. Results

3.1. Effect of Palmatine and Other Drugs Employed on Transfer Latency (TL) of Mice. Palmatine and physostigmine administered for 10 successive days did not significantly affect TL of mice on 10th day (learning) as compared to the control group. But palmatine (0.5 and 1 mg/kg, *i.p.*) and physostigmine (0.1 mg/kg, *i.p.*) significantly decreased TL in mice on 11th day (memory) as compared to the control group, thus showed significant memory enhancing activity. The lowest dose of palmatine (0.1 mg/kg, *i.p.*) did not significantly decrease TL of mice on 11th day as compared to vehicle treated control group. Scopolamine (0.4 mg/kg, *i.p.*) and diazepam (1 mg/kg, *i.p.*) significantly increased TL in mice, indicating its amnesic effect. Palmatine (1 mg/kg, *i.p.*) significantly reversed scopolamine-induced and diazepam-induced memory impairment in mice as compared to respective scopolamine and diazepam treated groups (Table 1).

3.2. Effect of Palmatine and Other Drugs Employed on Escape Latency (EL) and Time Spent in Target Quadrant (TSTQ) of Mice Using Morris Water Maze. Palmatine (0.5 and 1 mg/kg, *i.p.*) and physostigmine (0.1 mg/kg, *i.p.*) significantly

TABLE 1: Effect of palmatine and other drugs employed on transfer latency (TL) of mice using elevated plus maze.

Treatments	Dose $(kg)^{-1}$	TL (sec) on 10th day	TL (sec) on 11th day
Control (vehicle) for 10 days	10 mL	20.25 ± 2.27	17.13 ± 1.24
Physostigmine for 10 days	0.1 mg	16.38 ± 1.39	8.25 ± 0.88^b
Scopolamine	0.4 mg	19.25 ± 2.16	28.25 ± 1.85^b
Diazepam	1 mg	19.14 ± 2.11	24.57 ± 2.30^a
Palmatine for 10 days	0.1 mg	18.37 ± 1.73	14.13 ± 1.73
Palmatine for 10 days	0.5 mg	15.87 ± 1.72	9.88 ± 0.83^a
Palmatine for 10 days	1 mg	15.75 ± 2.30	8.75 ± 0.75^b
Palmatine for 10 days + scopolamine on 10th day	1 mg + 0.4 mg	15.14 ± 1.98	15.57 ± 1.2^c
Palmatine for 10 days + diazepam on 10th day	1 mg + 1 mg	20.75 ± 2.20	17 ± 1.50^d

$n = 8$ in each group. Values are expressed as Mean ± SEM. Data was analyzed by one-way ANOVA followed by Tukey's post-hoc test.
$F(8, 60) = 1.417$; $P = 0.02079$ (10th day);
$F(8, 60) = 21.034$; $P < 0.0001$ (11th day);
[a] $P < 0.05$ as compared to control;
[b] $P < 0.01$ as compared to control;
[c] $P < 0.001$ as compared to scopolamine treated group;
[d] $P < 0.01$ as compared to diazepam treated group.

TABLE 2: Effect of palmatine and other drugs employed on escape latency (EL) of mice using Morris water maze.

Treatments	Dose $(kg)^{-1}$	EL (sec) Day-6	EL (sec) Day-7	EL (sec) Day-8	EL (sec) Day-9
Control (vehicle) for 10 days	10 mL	105.90 ± 3.28	96.34 ± 3.44	78.38 ± 3.70	54.19 ± 3.44
Physostigmine for 10 days	0.1 mg	104.31 ± 3.06	101.25 ± 2.51	74.09 ± 2.45	33.5 ± 2.66^c
Scopolamine	0.4 mg	106.62 ± 18.16	87.66 ± 3.75	69.63 ± 3.49	44.44 ± 2.81^b
Diazepam	1 mg	105.96 ± 2.59	91.66 ± 2.48	69.47 ± 3.21	42.56 ± 2.52^a
Palmatine for 10 days	0.1 mg	103.93 ± 2.95	100.93 ± 3.13	78.09 ± 4.01^b	44.22 ± 2.98
Palmatine for 10 days	0.5 mg	100 ± 3.25	88.38 ± 3.84	61.56 ± 2.98^c	32.09 ± 2.4^b
Palmatine for 10 days	1 mg	99.75 ± 2.80	75.43 ± 3.54^b	49.78 ± 2.31	26.06 ± 1.54^c
Palmatine for 10 days + scopolamine on 10th day	1 mg + 0.4 mg	107.29 ± 3.01	83.69 ± 3.48	54.75 ± 2.26	28.13 ± 1.33^d
Palmatine for 10 days + diazepam on 10th day	1 mg + 1 mg	109.90 ± 2.23	85.21 ± 2.84	55.81 ± 3.39	29.91 ± 1.59^e

$n = 8$. Values are expressed as Mean ± SEM. Data was analyzed by one-way ANOVA followed by Tukey's post-hoc test.
$F(8, 279) = 1.264$; $P = 0.2625$ (day 6);
$F(8, 279) = 7.147$; $P < 0.0001$ (day 7);
$F(8, 279) = 11.079$; $P < 0.0001$ (day 8);
$F(8, 279) = 14.251$; $P < 0.0001$ (day 9);
[a] $P < 0.05$ as compared to control;
[b] $P < 0.01$ as compared to control;
[c] $P < 0.001$ as compared to control;
[d] $P < 0.001$ as compared to scopolamine treated group;
[e] $P < 0.01$ as compared to diazepam treated group.

decreased EL of mice on 9th day and increased TSTQ by mice on 10th day as compared to the control group, thus showed significant improvement of learning and memory. The lowest dose of palmatine (0.1 mg/kg, *i.p.*) did not significantly decrease EL or increase TSTQ as compared to vehicle treated control group. Scopolamine (0.4 mg/kg, *i.p.*) and diazepam (1 mg/kg, *i.p.*) significantly increased EL and decreased TSTQ by mice, indicating their amnesic effects. Palmatine (1 mg/kg, *i.p.*) significantly reversed scopolamine-induced and diazepam-induced learning and memory impairment in mice as compared to respective scopolamine and diazepam treated groups (Tables 2 and 3).

3.3. Effect of Palmatine and Physostigmine on Brain Acetyl Cholinesterase (AChE) Activity in Mice. Administration of palmatine (0.5 mg/kg and 1 mg/kg) and physostigmine for

11 consecutive days produced a significant decrease in brain AChE activity as compared to control group. The lowest dose of palmatine 0.1 mg/kg did not produce significantly decrease in AChE activity as compared to control group (Figure 1).

3.4. Effect of Palmatine and Physostigmine on Locomotor Activity of Mice. Palmatine and physostigmine used in the present study did not significantly affect the spontaneous locomotor activities of mice as compared to the respective control groups (Table 4).

4. Discussion

In the present study, palmatine (0.5 and 1 mg/kg, *i.p.*) administered for 10 successive days showed significant memory

TABLE 3: Effect of palmatine and other drugs employed on time spent in target quadrant of mice using Morris water maze.

Treatments	Dose $(kg)^{-1}$	Time spent (sec) in target quadrant (10th day)
Control (vehicle) for 10 days	10 mL	94.38 ± 4.50
Physostigmine for 10 days	0.1 mg	125.88 ± 6.98^a
Scopolamine	0.4 mg	65.50 ± 4.04^a
Diazepam	1 mg	68.13 ± 5.16^a
Palmatine for 10 days	0.1 mg	85.25 ± 4.07
Palmatine for 10 days	0.5 mg	119.63 ± 5.33^a
Palmatine for 10 days	1 mg	124.12 ± 5.26^b
Palmatine for 10 days + scopolamine on 10th day	1 mg + 0.4 mg	109 ± 7.78^c
Palmatine for 10 days + diazepam on 10th day	1 mg + 1 mg	96.5 ± 5.29^d

$n = 8$. Values are expressed as Mean $\pm$ SEM. Data was analyzed by one-way ANOVA followed by Tukey's post-hoc test.
$F(8, 63) = 17.197; P < 0.0001;$
[a]$P < 0.05$ as compared to control;
[b]$P < 0.01$ as compared to control;
[c]$P < 0.001$ as compared to scopolamine treated group;
[d]$P < 0.05$ as compared to diazepam treated group.

TABLE 4: Effect of palmatine and physostigmine on locomotor activity of mice.

Treatment for 10 days	Dose $(kg)^{-1}$	Locomotor activity counts/5 min
Control	10 mL	297.43 ± 9.5
Physostigmine	0.1 mg	310.14 ± 10.64
Palmatine	0.1 mg	281.38 ± 12.41
Palmatine	0.5 mg	294 ± 10.69
Palmatine	1 mg	302.75 ± 5.12

$n = 8$ in each group. Values are expressed as Mean $\pm$ SEM. Data was analyzed by one-way ANOVA followed by Tukey's post-hoc test.
$F(4, 33) = 1.152; P = 0.3497.$

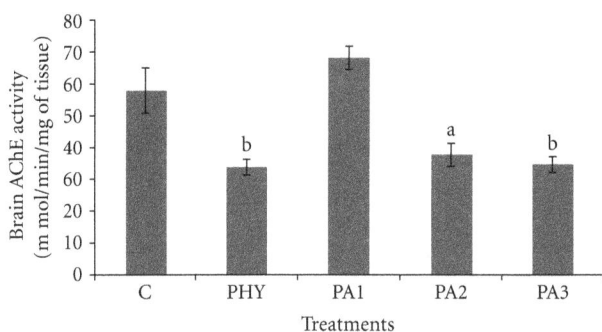

FIGURE 1: Effect of palmatine and physostigmine on brain AChE activity of mice. $n = 8$ in each group. Values are expressed as Mean $\pm$ SEM. Data was analyzed by one-way ANOVA followed by Tukey's Post-hoc test. $F(4, 33) = 14.736; P < 0.0001;$ [a]$P < 0.05$ as compared to control; [b]$P < 0.01$ as compared to control; C = Control; PHY = Physostigmine (0.1 mg/kg); PA1 = Palmatine (0.1 mg/kg); PA2 = Palmatine (0.5 mg/kg); PA3 = Palmatine (1 mg/kg).

enhancing effect in mice. This is the first study showing memory enhancing activity of palmatine in mice. Elevated plus maze and Morris water maze were employed as behavioral models for evaluation of learning and memory. These models are widely employed for evaluating the effect of drugs on learning and memory [10, 12]. In elevated plus maze, decrease in transfer latency on 2nd day (i.e.,

24 h after the first trial) indicated improvement of memory and viceversa. In Morris water maze, a decrease in escape latency during training and increase in time spent in target quadrant during retrieval indicated improvement of learning and memory respectively; and vice versa. Palmatine did not show any significant change in locomotor functions of mice as compared to the vehicle treated control, so this did not produce any motor effects. Thus, memory enhancing effect of palmatine is specific and not false positive. Out of the two effective doses of palmatine (0.5 and 1 mg/kg, i.p.), higher dose (1 mg/kg) produced better memory enhancing effect in mice ($P < 0.01$) as compared to the lower dose ($P < 0.05$) in both the behavioural models employed, hence the higher dose (1 mg/kg) was employed for elucidating the probable mechanisms of memory enhancing activity.

Central cholinergic system plays a major role in regulation of cognitive function [15]. Drugs that reduce cholinergic function such as muscarinic receptor antagonist scopolamine produce amnesia in laboratory animals. In the present study, scopolamine and diazepam significantly impaired memory of mice. Memory impairment effect of diazepam has been reported in the literature [11]. Palmatine (1 mg/kg, i.p.) administered for 10 successive days to separate groups of mice significantly reversed scopolamine-induced amnesia and diazepam-induced amnesia in mice. Benzodiazepines produce amnesia in laboratory animals by activation of benzodiazepine receptors and GABAergic system [16, 17]. Flumazenil (benzodiazepine-receptor antagonist) and beta-carbolines (benzodiazepine inverse agonist) have been demonstrated to reverse benzodiazepine-induced amnesia [18]. Reversal of scopolamine- and diazepam-induced amnesia by palmatine indicated the possible facilitation of cholinergic transmission or GABA-benzodiazepine pathway. Palmatine (1 mg/kg) also significantly reduced brain AChE activity in mice as compared to the control group. This suggests that the memory enhancing effect of palmatine might be due to inhibition of AChE, leading to increase in brain levels of acetylcholine. This is supported by an earlier study where palmatine showed inhibition of acetylcholinesterase activity [5]. Acetylcholine is considered to be one of the important neurotransmitter involved in the regulation of cognitive functions. Cognitive dysfunction has been shown to be associated with impaired cholinergic transmission and the facilitation of central cholinergic transmission resulting in improved memory. Moreover, selective loss of cholinergic neurons in certain brain parts appeared to be a characteristic feature of senile dementia [19]. The degeneration and dysfunction of cortical cholinergic neurons is closely associated with cognitive deficits of AD [20]. Thus, the drugs which enhance cholinergic function can be used for treatment of dementia closely related to AD. Physostigmine (0.1 mg/kg, *i.p.*) injected for 10 successive days significantly improved memory of mice. Memory enhancement activity of physostigmine has been well reported in the literature. Physostigmine, a cholinesterase inhibitor, could improve memory in normal subjects [21] as well as in patients with dementia [22].

The memory enhancing activity of palmatine is also supported by its beta-site amyloid precursor protein-cleaving enzyme 1 (BACE 1) inhibiting property [5]. BACE1 is the major beta-secretase to cleave the beta-amyloid precursor protein to generate beta-amyloid. Oxidative stress has been shown to affect amyloid-beta generation in the AD pathogenesis. Upregulation of BACE 1 gene transcription by oxidative stress may contribute to the pathogenesis of AD [23]. Palmatine has also been reported to possess antioxidant activity [5]. Thus, palmatine produced significant memory enhancing effect in mice probably due to its antioxidant property by virtue of which susceptible brain cells get exposed to less oxidative stress resulting in reduced brain damage and improvement of neuronal function.

In conclusion, palmatine showed memory enhancing activity in mice probably by inhibiting brain acetylcholinesterase activity, through involvement of GABA-benzodiazepine pathway and due to its antioxidant activity.

Conflict of Interests

The authors do not have any conflict of interests with the content of the paper.

References

[1] A. Sosa, E. Albanese, C. Blossom et al., "Prevalence, distribution, and impact of mild cognitive impairment in Latin America, China, and India: a 10/66 population-based study," *PLoS Medicine*, vol. 9, no. 2, pp. 1–11, 2012.

[2] C. P. Ferri, M. Prince, C. Brayne et al., "Global prevalence of dementia: a Delphi consensus study," *The Lancet*, vol. 366, no. 9503, pp. 2112–2117, 2005.

[3] S. H. Lu, J. W. Wu, H. L. Liu et al., "The discovery of potential acetylcholinesterase inhibitors: a combination of pharmacophore modeling, virtual screening, and molecular docking studies," *Journal of Biomedical Science*, vol. 18, no. 1, article 8, 2011.

[4] M. Guglielmotto, E. Tamagno, and O. Danni, "Oxidative stress and hypoxia contribute to Alzheimer's disease pathogenesis: two sides of the same coin," *The Scientific World Journal*, vol. 9, pp. 781–791, 2009.

[5] H. A. Jung, B. S. Min, T. Yokozawa, J. H. Lee, Y. S. Kim, and J. S. Choi, "Anti-Alzheimer and antioxidant activities of coptidis rhizoma alkaloids," *Biological and Pharmaceutical Bulletin*, vol. 32, no. 8, pp. 1433–1438, 2009.

[6] M. T. Hsieh, S. H. Su, H. Y. Tsai, W. H. Peng, C. C. Hsieh, and C. F. Chen, "Effects of palmatine on motor activity and the concentration of central monoamines and its metabolites in rats," *Japanese Journal of Pharmacology*, vol. 61, no. 1, pp. 1–5, 1993.

[7] L. L. Harburger, J. C. Bennett, and K. M. Frick, "Effects of estrogen and progesterone on spatial memory consolidation in aged females," *Neurobiology of Aging*, vol. 28, no. 4, pp. 602–610, 2007.

[8] D. Dhingra, M. Parle, and S. K. Kulkarni, "Memory enhancing activity of Glycyrrhiza glabra in mice," *Journal of Ethnopharmacology*, vol. 91, no. 2-3, pp. 361–365, 2004.

[9] N. Singh, A. Sharma, and M. Singh, "Effects of BN-50730 (PAF receptor antagonist) and physostigmine (AChE inhibitor) on learning and memory in mice," *Methods and Findings in Experimental and Clinical Pharmacology*, vol. 19, no. 9, pp. 585–588, 1997.

[10] J. Itoh, T. Nabeshima, and T. Kameyama, "Utility of an elevated plus-maze for the evaluation of memory in mice: effects of nootropics, scopolamine and electroconvulsive shock," *Psychopharmacology*, vol. 101, no. 1, pp. 27–33, 1990.

[11] M. Parle and D. Dhingra, "Ascorbic acid: a promising memory-enhancer in mice," *Journal of Pharmacological Sciences*, vol. 93, no. 2, pp. 129–135, 2003.

[12] R. Morris, "Developments of a water-maze procedure for studying spatial learning in the rat," *Journal of Neuroscience Methods*, vol. 11, no. 1, pp. 47–60, 1984.

[13] M. Parle and N. Singh, "Reversal of memory deficits by atorvastatin and simvastatin in rats," *Yakugaku Zasshi*, vol. 127, no. 7, pp. 1125–1137, 2007.

[14] G. L. Ellman, K. D. Courtney, V. Andres, and R. M. Featherstone Jr., "A new and rapid colorimetric determination of acetylcholinesterase activity," *Biochemical Pharmacology*, vol. 7, no. 2, pp. 88–IN1, 1961.

[15] A. Blokland, "Acetylcholine: a neurotransmitter for learning and memory?" *Brain Research Reviews*, vol. 21, no. 3, pp. 285–300, 1995.

[16] N. Singh, A. Sharma, and M. Singh, "Possible mechanism of alprazolam-induced amnesia in mice," *Pharmacology*, vol. 56, no. 1, pp. 46–50, 1998.

[17] M. R. Zarrindast, H. Haidari, M. R. Jafari, and B. Djahanguiri, "Influence of β-adrenoceptor agonists and antagonists on baclofen-induced memory impairment in mice," *Behavioural Pharmacology*, vol. 15, no. 4, pp. 293–297, 2004.

[18] L. H. Jensen, D. N. Stephens, M. Sarter, and E. N. Petersen, "Bidirectional effects of β-carbolines and benzodiazepines on cognitive processes," *Brain Research Bulletin*, vol. 19, no. 3, pp. 359–364, 1987.

[19] T. Watanabe, N. Yamagata, K. Takasaki et al., "Decreased acetylcholine release is correlated to memory impairment in the Tg2576 transgenic mouse model of Alzheimer's disease," *Brain Research*, vol. 1249, pp. 222–228, 2009.

[20] R. T. Bartus, R. L. Dean, B. Beer, and A. S. Lippa, "The cholinergic hypothesis of geriatric memory dysfunction," *Science*, vol. 217, no. 4558, pp. 408–414, 1982.

[21] K. L. Davis, R. C. Mohs, J. R. Tinklenberg, A. Pfefferbaum, L. E. Hollister, and B. S. Kopell, "Physostigmine: improvement of long-term memory processes in normal humans," *Science*, vol. 201, no. 4352, pp. 272–274, 1978.

[22] K. L. Davis and R. C. Mohs, "Enhancement of memory by physostigmine," *The New England Journal of Medicine*, vol. 301, no. 17, pp. 946–947, 1979.

[23] Y. Tong, W. Zhou, V. Fung et al., "Oxidative stress potentiates BACE1 gene expression and Aβ generation," *Journal of Neural Transmission*, vol. 112, no. 3, pp. 455–469, 2005.

9

The Anti-Inflammatory, Phytoestrogenic, and Antioxidative Role of *Labisia pumila* in Prevention of Postmenopausal Osteoporosis

M. E. Nadia, A. S. Nazrun, M. Norazlina, N. M. Isa, M. Norliza, and S. Ima Nirwana

Department of Pharmacology, Faculty of Medicine, The National University of Malaysia, Kuala Lumpur campus, 50300 Kuala Lumpur, Malaysia

Correspondence should be addressed to A. S. Nazrun, anazrun@yahoo.com

Academic Editor: Satya Sarker

Osteoporosis is characterized by skeletal degeneration with low bone mass and destruction of microarchitecture of bone tissue which is attributed to various factors including inflammation. Women are more likely to develop osteoporosis than men due to reduction in estrogen during menopause which leads to decline in bone-formation and increase in bone-resorption activity. Estrogen is able to suppress production of proinflammatory cytokines such as IL-1, IL-6, IL-7, and TNF-α. This is why these cytokines are elevated in postmenopausal women. Studies have shown that estrogen reduction is able to stimulate focal inflammation in bone. *Labisia pumila* (LP) which is known to exert phytoestrogenic effect can be used as an alternative to ERT which can produce positive effects on bone without causing side effects. LP contains antioxidant as well as exerting anti-inflammatory effect which can act as free radical scavenger, thus inhibiting TNF-α production and COX-2 expression which leads to decline in RANKL expression, resulting in reduction in osteoclast activity which consequently reduces bone loss. Hence, it is the phytoestrogenic, anti-inflammatory, and antioxidative properties that make LP an effective agent against osteoporosis.

1. Introduction

Plant has been one of the sources of medicine to treat various illnesses and diseases since ancient time. In the early 19th century, when chemical analysis first became available, scientists began to extract and modify the active ingredients from plants which later led to wide development of natural or traditional medicine that was mostly passed on orally from one generation to another. More than 35,000 plant species have been reported to be used in various human cultures around the world for their medical purposes [1]. Traditional medicine has been defined by the World Health Organization (WHO) as "health practices, approaches, knowledge and beliefs incorporating plant, animal and mineral-based medicines, spiritual therapies, manual techniques and exercises, applied singularly or in combination, to treat, diagnose and prevent illnesses or maintain well-being" [2].

Currently in Malaysia, over 2,000 species of lower plants with medicinal and therapeutic properties have been identified, and most of them have been used for many generations in various health care systems. About 17.1% of Malaysians used herbs to treat their health problems while 29.6% of them consumed herbs for their health maintenance [3]. The earliest report on medicinal plant research in Malaysia was carried out by Arthur in 1954 [4]. Subsequently, more plants were screened chemically for alkaloids, saponins, triterpenes, and steroids in the 90s [5, 6].

Amongst the famous herbs that are widely used in Malaysia by the locals are *Labisia pumila* (Kacip Fatimah), *Eurycoma longifolia Jack* (Tongkat Ali), *Orthosiphon stamineus* (Misai Kucing), *Quercus infectoria* (Manjakani), and *Piper sarmentosum* (daun kaduk). These plants are similar in terms of exhibiting phytochemical properties that are protective against various diseases. These herbs are known to exert antibacterial, antioxidant, and anti-inflammatory properties that make them beneficial against many types of diseases such as fever, asthma, joint pains, gastrointestinal diseases, bone disorders, and inflammatory disorders. [7–9]. This paper is a review which will be focusing on the content and health benefits of one of the famous Malaysian herbs, Kacip Fatimah.

Kacip Fatimah or its scientific name *Labisia pumila* (LP) is a member of small genus of slightly woody plants of the family Myrsinaceae. There are four known varieties of *Labisia pumila* found in Malaysia but only three of them are widely used by the locals, which are recognized as *Labisia pumila* var. *pumila*, *Labisia pumila* var. *alata*, and *Labisia pumila* var. *lanceolata* [10, 11]. LP is found mainly in the lowland and hillforests of peninsular Malaysia at an altitude between 300 and 700 metres. It is also known by the locals as Selusuh Fatimah, Rumput Siti Fatimah, Akar Fatimah, Pokok Pinggang, and Belangkas Hutan [12, 13]. Of all the subtypes, *Labisia pumila* var. *alata* is the most widely used by the locals [10]. Its water extract is traditionally consumed especially by the Malay women to treat menstrual irregularities and painful menstruation, help contracting birth channel after delivery, and to promote sexual health function [14, 15]. It has also been used to treat dysentery, gonorrhoea, rheumatism, and sickness in bones [16, 17].

It is the phytoestrogen, anti-inflammatory, and antioxidative properties that make LP effective against various illnesses. LP was reported to exert estrogenic properties [18–20]. Theoretically, phytoestrogens can act as anti-estrogenic agents by blocking the estrogen receptors and exerting weaker estrogenic effect compared with the hormone [21]. The water extract of LP has been found to inhibit estradiol binding to antibodies raised against estradiol, suggesting the presence of estrogen-like compounds in the extract [22]. It also contains triterpene and saponins, including the compound ardisiacrispin A which were thought to be the reason behind the phytoestrogenic activity of LP [23].

LP has been widely used by the locals in Malaysia not only to ease menstrual pain, induce labor, and promote healthy sexual function but it is also used as an alternative to estrogen replacement therapy in postmenopausal women [24, 25]. Postmenopausal women are prone to osteoporosis due to the reduction in estrogen level. Estrogen acts on estrogen receptor-α (ERα) and receptor-β (ERβ) which has high affinity towards osteoblasts and osteoclasts [26]. Activation of estrogen-receptor complex is vital in maintaining bone remodelling processes [27]. Estrogen can induce osteoclasts apoptosis and inhibit osteoblasts apoptosis, which indirectly will reduce bone resorption and increase bone-formation activity [28]. Hence, reduction in estrogen is highly associated with bone loss. Dietary phytoestrogens such as LP can be an alternative to synthetic estrogen for hormone therapy to reduce side effects of prolonged hormone therapy such as risk of breast cancer, endometrial cancer, and cardiovascular diseases [29, 30]. This paper will focus on the role of *Labisia pumila* in offering protection against postmenopausal osteoporosis via its anti-inflammatory properties.

2. Anti-Inflammatory Role of *Labisia pumila*

Osteoporosis is characterized by skeletal degeneration with low bone mass and destruction of microarchitecture of bone tissue. According to the National Institute of Health, osteoporosis is a skeletal disease which involves decline in mass and density which later leads to fracture [31]. Women, especially postmenopausal women, are more likely to develop osteoporosis than men due to tremendous decline in estrogen during menopause which will lead to decline in bone formation and increase in bone-resorption activity [32]. Osteoporosis is attributed to various factors, and there are evidences that inflammation also exerts significant influence on bone turnover, inducing osteoporosis [33, 34]. According to studies by Lorenzo and Manolagas and Jilka, certain pro-inflammatory cytokines play potential critical roles both in the normal bone remodeling process and in the pathogenesis of osteoporosis [34, 35]. For example, interleukin- (IL-) 6 promotes osteoclasts differentiation and activation [36]. IL-1 is another potent stimulator of bone resorption [37] that has been linked to the accelerated bone loss seen in postmenopausal osteoporosis [38].

Various epidemiologic studies reported an increase in the risk of developing osteoporosis in various inflammatory conditions such as rheumatoid arthritis, haematological diseases, and inflammatory bowel disease [39, 40]. Proinflammatory cytokines such as tumor necrosis factor (TNF)-α, IL-6, IL-1, IL-11, IL-15, and IL-17 are elevated in these conditions [41]. IL-6 and IL-1 may influence osteoclastogenesis by stimulating self-renewal and inhibiting the apoptosis of osteoclasts progenitors [42, 43]. They promote osteoclasts differentiation which is an important stimulator of bone resorption that has been linked to accelerated bone loss seen in postmenopausal women [36]. Receptor activator of NF-$\kappa\beta$ ligand (RANKL) is a membrane-bound molecule of TNF ligand family which plays a crucial role in osteoclasts formation [44]. TNF is a cytokine that is involved in inflammation and is an important cofactor in bone resorption because this cytokine supports osteoclasts activation mediated by RANKL and c-Fms/macrophage colony-stimulating factor.

Estrogen is able to suppress the production of these proinflammatory cytokines [45, 46]. This is why estrogen withdrawal following menopause will lead to increase in these cytokines as proven in many studies. Studies on bone resorption demonstrated that the fall of estrogen level in postmenopausal women was able to stimulate local inflammation in the bone. Ovariectomy in rats was accompanied by increased production of IL-1 and TNF-α which later resulted in decrease in bone density. Hence, it is suggested that estrogen withdrawal can be associated with an increase in production of proinflammatory cytokines, which in turn increases osteoclasts activity resulting in profound bone loss [47]. Estrogen will stimulate production of osteoprotegerin (OPG), which is a potent antiosteoclastogenic factor. OPG acts as a decoy, blocking the binding of the RANK expressed in osteoblasts progenitors, to RANKL which is expressed in committed preosteoblastic cells [48]. This estrogen deficiency leads to upregulation of cytokines [49] and downregulation of OPG which will result in increase in inflammatory responses and increase in bone-resorption activity. In a study by Collin-Osdoby et al., [50] increases in RANKL and OPG mRNA expression were seen in endothelial cells following an inflammatory stimulus. Therefore, suppression of these potent inflammatory mediators has been proposed to explain the deleterious effects of estrogen deficiency on the human skeletal system at menopause.

3. Phytoestrogenic Role of *Labisia pumila*

LP which has been opposed to exert phytoestrogen property can be used as an alternative to estrogen replacement therapy (ERT) in postmenopausal inflammation-induced osteoporosis. In contrast to ERT which can cause many harmful side effects, LP which originated from natural resources will not cause any side effect, if taken within its safe therapeutic dose. Toxicity testing of LP which was done by the Herbal Medicine Research Centre of Institute of Medical Research has shown that LD50 is safe at more than 5.0 g/kg [51]. LP extract was found to exhibit no-adverse-effect level (NOAEL) at the dose of 50 mg/kg in subacute toxicity study [52], 1000 mg/kg in subchronic toxicity study [53], and 800 mg/kg in reproductive toxicity study [51]. Therefore, LP is safe to be given at high dose as long as it does not outweigh the toxic dose.

Studies have shown that production of proinflammatory cytokines in response to estrogen withdrawal at menopause is responsible to the stimulation of osteoclastic bone resorption [54–56]. A study done by Choi et al. [57] indicated that the LP extract may have good potential to be developed as novel anti-inflammatory drug due to an experimental finding of treatment with LP extract which has markedly inhibited the TNF-α production and the expression of cyclooxygenase (COX)-2. COX-2 is an enzyme that is responsible for the production of mediators involved in inflammation. In vitro experiments have revealed increased COX-2 expression after stimulation with proinflammatory cytokines, such as IL-1 and TNF-α [58].

Pharmacological inhibition of COX can provide a relief from the symptoms of inflammation and pain. Studies have shown that COX-2 plays an important role in pathophysiology of osteoporosis by stimulating the production of prostaglandin (PGE$_2$). Excessive PGE$_2$ production might lead to increase in bone resorption, while deficient of its production might impair the bone-formation response, both to mechanical loading and remodelling [59]. Consequently, inhibition of the COX-2 enzyme in postmenopausal women may prevent menopausal bone loss [60]. Inhibition of the main proinflammatory cytokines has proven that LP extract could be a good material for the regulation of anti-inflammation process. TNF has been shown to stimulate osteoclast differentiation, increase its activation, inhibit its apoptosis, and inhibit osteoblast differentiation [61–63]. It also reduces bone formation in cultured osteoblast *in vitro* [64]. Similar to IL-1, TNF-stimulated induction of osteoclast-like-cell formation in bone marrow culture is mediated by increases in RANKL expression. However, in addition to increasing RANKL expression, TNF also inhibits OPG in an osteoblastic model [65]. Hence, inhibition of TNF will indirectly help in reducing bone loss.

4. Antioxidative Role of *Labisia pumila*

Based on previous studies, LP has been shown to exhibit antioxidative properties due to the presence of flavanoids, ascorbic acid, beta-carotene, anthocyanin, and phenolic compounds [66, 67]. According to Norhaiza et al. [68], there were positive correlations between the antioxidant capacities and the antioxidant compounds of LP extract with β-carotene having the best correlation, followed by flavonoid, ascorbic acid, anthocyanin, and phenolic content. β-carotene is one of the basic constituent of antioxidative effect. The chemical abilities of β-carotene to quench singlet oxygen and to inhibit peroxyl free radical actions are well established [69]. Flavonoid has been shown to be highly effective scavenger of free radicals that are involved in diseases such as osteoporosis and rheumatism which is associated with aging due to oxidative stress [70]. Anthocyanin and phenolic on the other hand, not only play a role as antioxidative agents, but also as anti-inflammatory agents [71–73]. These antioxidative and anti-inflammatory properties of LP extract explained the effectiveness of this medicinal plant against various diseases such as osteoporosis, rheumatism, and women sexual function.

Osteoporosis in postmenopausal women can also be explained in terms of oxidative stress mechanism. Ovariectomy has been proposed by many studies as a model of postmenopausal osteoporosis. Following ovariectomy, decline in estrogen level will result in significant bone loss due to bone resorption outweighing bone-formation activity [74]. Estrogen can be considered as an antioxidant as it was found to exhibit antioxidant protection of lipoproteins in the aqueous system [75] and was also shown to increase the expression of glutathione peroxidase in osteoclasts [76]. That is why decline in estrogen will lead to increase in osteoclasts activity resulting in bone loss. Free radicals are continuously produced in the body, mostly by biochemical redox reactions involving oxygen, which occur as part of normal cell metabolism. Free radicals, mainly reactive oxygen species (ROS), are efficiently scavenged, but oxidative stress occurs when there is an imbalance between increased ROS and inadequate antioxidant activity [77] which consequently accelerates aging process and leads to degenerative diseases such as osteoporosis, rheumatism, and cardiovascular disease.

ROS alter mitochondrial and nuclear DNA integrity by increasing the risk of mutations. When DNA repair mechanisms are overwhelmed, cells undergo apoptosis which will lead to tissue damage [78]. This can be applicable in postmenopausal osteoporosis mechanism. When body is subjected to high oxidative stress following estrogen reduction, lipid accumulation will occur. Lipid peroxidation will promote osteoblast apoptosis and simultaneously upregulating ROS production [79, 80]. ROS was shown to promote osteoclast resorption activity either directly or mimicking RANK signalling and stimulating osteoclast differentiation, or indirectly, by stimulating osteoblast/osteoclast coupling and subsequent osteoclast differentiation [81]. Oxidative stress has been acceded as a major contributor to the immune response. Activation of immune response mechanism is characterized by establishment of an inflammatory response. Thus, osteoporosis can be associated with inflammatory mechanism.

Estrogen can prevent osteoblast cell death and RANKL stimulation by suppressing ROS. Estrogen deficiency is a key step in ROS-mediated stimulation of bone loss via TNF-α signalling pathway. Stimulation of this proinflammatory cytokine will induce bone resorption by indirectly affecting production of essential osteoclast differentiation factor, thereby enhancing proliferation of osteoclast lineage [82]. Glutathione peroxide (GPx) and superoxide dismutase (SOD) are the main antioxidative enzymes that play a pivotal role in counteracting oxidative stress [83]. These enzymes were found to be lowered in postmenopausal women with osteoporosis. This failure of antioxidant defences will result in deleterious effect of hydrogen peroxide on bone health [84]. Studies of antioxidant supplementation such as vitamin E on postmenopausal rat model have shown that lipid peroxidation was successfully inhibited and antioxidative enzymes were restored to acceptable level. In study by Norazlina et al. (2007), IL-6 level was high in ovariectomised rats showing high bone resorption rate, and this level was significantly reduced after three months of tocotrienol (vitamin E) supplementation. In the same study, vitamin E-deficient rats given palm vitamin E showed an improvement in bone calcium content and reduced bone resorption marker [85]. Hence, it is shown that antioxidant is effective in reducing bone-resorption activity as well as improving bone calcium content.

Main antioxidative compound in LP such as flavonoid and β-carotene has been shown in previous studies to inhibit production of nitric oxide and expression of inducible nitric oxide synthase (iNOS) [86] most likely by suppression of NF-κB [87]. NF-kB is an oxidative stress-responsive transcription factor which is activated by free radicals, inflammatory stimuli, and other cytokines. Thus, free radicals may increase bone resorption through activation of NF-kB. It has previously been shown in vitro and in rodents that free radicals are involved in osteoclastogenesis and in bone resorption [88]. Oxidative stress may increase bone resorption through activation of NF-κB which plays an important role in osteoclastogenesis [89, 90]. Hence, supplementation of LP which contains antioxidative properties can reduce oxidative stress level which indirectly prevents bone loss.

According to a recent study by Nazrun et al. (2011), osteocalcin, a bone formation marker, was found to be lowered in ovariectomised rats. After being treated with LP results showed an increase in osteocalcin to the level seen in sham-operated group indicating normalisation of bone formation. Bone resorption marker, CTX on the other hand, was found to be reduced after the rats were treated with LP [91]. CTX is sensitive and specific in detection of osteoporosis [92]. This result showed that LP was as effective as estrogen in preventing changes in bone markers induced by ovariectomy.

Based on its positive effects on the bone markers of ovariectomised rats which are comparable to estrogen and its safety profile, LP has the potential to be used as an alternative treatment for postmenopausal osteoporosis. All in all, it is the anti-inflammatory, phytoestrogenic, and antioxidative properties of LP that make it an effective natural medicine in treatment and prevention of osteoporosis.

Acknowledgment

One of the authors would like to thanks University Kebangsaan Malaysia (UKM) for the grants and the Pharmacology Department staffs for their technical support.

References

[1] A. Lewington, *Medicinal Plants and Plant Extracts: A Review of Their Importation into Europe*, Traffic International, Cambridge, UK, 1993.

[2] WHO, *Traditional Medicine*, WHO, Geneva, Switzerland, 2003.

[3] S. Elliot, *Pharmacy Needs Tropical Forests*, Manufacturing Chemist, 1986.

[4] H. R. Arthur, "A phytochemical survey of some plants of north Borneo," *Journal of Pharmacy and Pharmacology*, vol. 6, no. 1, pp. 66–72, 1954.

[5] L. E. Teo, G. Pachiaper, K. C. Chan et al., "A new phytochemical survey of Malaysia V. Preliminary screening and plant chemical studies," *Journal of Ethnopharmacology*, vol. 28, no. 1, pp. 63–101, 1990.

[6] A. L. Mohamed, A. Zainudin, G. H. Petol et al., "Phytochemical and toxicity screening of plants from Fraser Hill, Pahang," in *Chemical Prospecting in the Malaysian Forest*, G. Ismail, M. Mohamaed, and L. B. Din, Eds., pp. 1–8, Pelanduk, Petaling Jaya, Malaysia, 1995.

[7] G. Kaur, H. Hamid, A. Ali, M. S. Alam, and M. Athar, "Antiinflammatory evaluation of alcoholic extract of galls of *Quercus infectoria*," *Journal of Ethnopharmacology*, vol. 90, no. 2-3, pp. 285–292, 2004.

[8] Z. A. Zakaria, H. Patahuddin, A. S. Mohamad, D. A. Israf, and M. R. Sulaiman, "In vivo anti-nociceptive and anti-inflammatory activities of the aqueous extract of the leaves of Piper *sarmentosum*," *Journal of Ethnopharmacology*, vol. 128, no. 1, pp. 42–48, 2010.

[9] C. L. Hsu, B. O. H. Hong, Y. U. Shan, and G. C. Yen, "Antioxidant and Anti-Inflammatory effects of orthosiphon aristatus and its bioactive compounds," *Journal of Agricultural and Food Chemistry*, vol. 58, no. 4, pp. 2150–2156, 2010.

[10] B. C. Stone, "Notes on the genus Labisia Lindl (Myrsinaceae)," *Malayan Nature Journal*, vol. 42, pp. 43–51, 1988.

[11] A. J. Jamia, P. J. Houghton, S. R. Milligan, and J. Ibrahim, "The Oestrogenic and Cytotoxic Effects of the Extracts of Labisia pumila var. alata and Labisia pumila var. pumila In Vitro," *Malaysian Journal of Health Sciences*, vol. 1, pp. 53–60, 1988.

[12] I. H. Burkill, *Dictionary of the Economic Products of the Malay Peninsula*, Publisher Crown Agents for the Colonies, London, UK, 1935.

[13] M. A. Rasadah and A. S. Zainon, *Database on ASEAN Herbal and Medicinal Plants*, vol. 1, ASEAN Publication, 2003.

[14] M. Zakaria and M. A. Mohd, *Traditional Malay Medicinal Plants*, vol. 8, Penerbit Fajar Bakti, Kuala Lumpur, Malaysia, 1994.

[15] G. Bodeker, *Health and Beauty from the Rainforest: Malaysian Traditions of Ramuan*, Editions Didier Millet Pty, Kuala Lumpur, Malaysia, 1999.

[16] A. Fasihuddin, A. H. Rahman, and R. Hasmah, "Medicinal plants used by bajau community in sabah," in *Trends in*

Traditional Medicine Research, K. L. Chan et al., Ed., pp. 493–504, The School of Pharmaceutical Sciences, University of Science Malaysia, Penang, Malaysia, 1995.

[17] J. A. Jamal, P. J. Houghton, and S. R. Milligan, "Testing of labisia pumila for oestrogenic activity using a recombinant yeast screen," *Journal of Pharmacy and Pharmacology*, vol. 50, p. 79, 1998.

[18] Institute for Medical Research, *Estrogenic and Androgenic Activities of Kacip Fatimah (Labisia Pumila)*, Abstracts of Research Projects, Ministry of Health Malaysia, Kuala Lumpur, Malaysia, 2002.

[19] L. Manneras, M. Fazliana, W. M. Wan Nazaimoon et al., "Beneficial metabolic effects of the Malaysian herb Labisia pumila var. alata in a rat model of polycystic ovary syndrome," *Journal of Ethnopharmacology*, vol. 127, pp. 346–351, 2010.

[20] M. Fazliana, W. M. Wan Nazaimoon, H. F. Gu, and C. G. Östenson, "*Labisia pumila* extract regulates body weight and adipokines in ovariectomized rats," *Maturitas*, vol. 62, no. 1, pp. 91–97, 2009.

[21] IFST, *Current Hot Topics. Phytoestrogens*, Institute of Food Science and Technology, London, UK, 2001.

[22] H. Husniza, *Estrogenic and Androgenic Activities of Kacip Fatimah (Labisia pumila)*, Abstracts of Research Projects, Institute of Medical Research, Ministry of Health ·Malaysia, Kuala Lumpur, Malaysia, 2002.

[23] B. Avula, Y. H. Wang, Z. Ali, T. J. Smillie, and I. A. Khan, "Quantitative determination of triperpene saponins and alkenated-phenolics from Labisia pumila by LCUV/ELSD method and confirmation by LC-ESI-TOF," *Planta Medica*, vol. 76, p. 25, 2010.

[24] V. Beral, E. Banks, and G. Reeves, "Evidence from randomised trials on the long-term effects of hormone replacement therapy," *Lancet*, vol. 360, no. 9337, pp. 942–944, 2002.

[25] R. T. Chlebowski, J. A. Kim, and N. F. Col, "Estrogen deficiency symptom management in breast cancer survivors in the changing context of menopausal hormone therapy," *Seminars in Oncology*, vol. 30, no. 6, pp. 776–88, 2003.

[26] B. Komm and P. V. N. Bodine, "Regulation of bone cell function by estrogens," in *Osteoporosis*, R. Marcus, D. Feldman, and J. Kelsey, Eds., pp. 305–337, Academic Press, San Diego, Calif, USA, 2001.

[27] S. C. Manolagas, S. Kousteni, and R. L. Jilka, "Sex steroids and bone," *Recent Progress in Hormone Research*, vol. 57, pp. 385–409, 2002.

[28] S. C. Manolagas, "Birth and death of bone cells: basic regulatory mechanisms and implications for the pathogenesis and treatment of osteoporosis," *Endocrine Reviews*, vol. 21, no. 2, pp. 115–137, 2000.

[29] N. E. Lane, *The Osteoporosis Book: A Guide for Patients and Their Families*, Oxford University Press, New York, NY, USA, 2001.

[30] E. Amir, O. C. Freedman, B. Seruga, and D. G. Evans, "Assessing women at high risk of breast cancer: a review of risk assessment models," *Journal of the National Cancer Institute*, vol. 102, no. 10, pp. 680–691, 2010.

[31] NIH, *Osteoporosis and Related Bone Disease*, National Resource Centre, 2011.

[32] J. P. Bilezikian, "Osteoporosis in men," *Journal of Clinical Endocrinology and Metabolism*, vol. 84, no. 10, pp. 3431–3434, 1999.

[33] J. R. Arron and Y. Choi, "Bone versus immune system," *Nature*, vol. 408, no. 6812, pp. 535–536, 2000.

[34] J. Lorenzo, "Interactions between immune and bone cells: new insights with many remaining questions," *Journal of Clinical Investigation*, vol. 106, no. 6, pp. 749–752, 2000.

[35] S. C. Manolagas and R. L. Jilka, "Mechanisms of disease: bone marrow, cytokines, and bone remodeling. Emerging insights into the pathophysiology of osteoporosis," *The New England Journal of Medicine*, vol. 332, no. 5, pp. 305–311, 1995.

[36] S. C. Manolagas, "Birth and death of bone cells: basic regulatory mechanisms and implications for the pathogenesis and treatment of osteoporosis," *Endocrine Reviews*, vol. 21, no. 2, pp. 115–137, 2000.

[37] S. Wei, H. Kitaura, P. Zhou, F. Patrick Ross, and S. L. Teitelbaum, "IL-1 mediates TNF-induced osteoclastogenesis," *Journal of Clinical Investigation*, vol. 115, no. 2, pp. 282–290, 2005.

[38] R. Pacifici, L. Rifas, R. McCracken et al., "Ovarian steroid treatment blocks a postmenopausal increase in blood monocyte interleukin 1 release," *Proceedings of the National Academy of Sciences of the United States of America*, vol. 86, no. 7, pp. 2398–2402, 1989.

[39] D. Mitra, D. M. Elvins, D. J. Speden, and A. J. Collins, "The prevalence of vertebral fractures in mild ankylosing spondylitis and their relationship to bone mineral density," *Rheumatology*, vol. 39, no. 1, pp. 85–89, 2000.

[40] T. Jensen, M. Klarlund, M. Hansen, K. E. Jensen, H. Skjodt, and L. Hydlldstrup, "Connective tissue metabolism in patients with unclassified polyarthritis and early rheumatoid arthritis. Relationship to disease activity, bone mineral density, and radiographyc outcome," *Journal of Rheumatology*, vol. 31, pp. 1698–1708, 2004.

[41] K. Ishihara and T. Hirano, "IL-6 in autoimmune disease and chronic inflammatory proliferative disease," *Cytokine and Growth Factor Reviews*, vol. 13, no. 4-5, pp. 357–368, 2002.

[42] G. Girasole, G. Passeri, R. L. Jilka, and S. C. Manolagas, "Interleukin-11: a new cytokine critical for osteoclast development," *Journal of Clinical Investigation*, vol. 93, no. 4, pp. 1516–1524, 1994.

[43] R. L. Jilka, R. S. Weinstein, T. Bellido, A. M. Parfitt, and S. C. Manolagas, "Osteoblast programmed cell death (apoptosis): modulation by growth factors and cytokines," *Journal of Bone and Mineral Research*, vol. 13, no. 5, pp. 793–802, 1998.

[44] K. Fuller, B. Wong, S. Fox, Y. Choi, and T. J. Chambers, "TRANCE is necessary and sufficient for osteoblast-mediated activation of bone resorption in osteoclasts," *Journal of Experimental Medicine*, vol. 188, no. 5, pp. 997–1001, 1998.

[45] R. L. Jilka, "Cytokines, bone remodeling, and estrogen deficiency," *Bone*, vol. 23, no. 2, pp. 75–81, 1998.

[46] D. A. Papanicolaou, R. L. Wilder, S. C. Manolagas, and G. P. Chrousos, "The pathophysiologic roles of interleukin-6 in human disease," *Annals of Internal Medicine*, vol. 128, no. 2, pp. 127–137, 1998.

[47] R. B. Kimble, A. B. Matayoshi, J. L. Vannice, V. T. Kung, C. Williams, and R. Pacifici, "Simultaneous block of interleukin-1 and tumor necrosis factor is required to completely prevent bone loss in the early postovariectomy period," *Endocrinology*, vol. 136, no. 7, pp. 3054–3061, 1995.

[48] L. C. Hofbauer, S. Khosla, C. R. Dunstan, D. L. Lacey, T. C. Spelsberg, and B. L. Riggs, "Estrogen stimulates gene expression and protein production of osteoprotegerin in human osteoblastic cells," *Endocrinology*, vol. 140, no. 9, pp. 4367–4370, 1999.

[49] S. Cenci, M. N. Weitzmann, C. Roggia et al., "Estrogen deficiency induces bone loss by enhancing T-cell production

of TNF-α," *Journal of Clinical Investigation*, vol. 106, no. 10, pp. 1229–1237, 2000.

[50] P. Collin-Osdoby, L. Rothe, F. Anderson, M. Nelson, W. Maloney, and P. Osdoby, "Receptor activator of NF-κB and osteoprotegerin expression by human microvascular endothelial cells, regulation by inflammatory cytokines, and role in human osteoclastogenesis," *Journal of Biological Chemistry*, vol. 276, no. 23, pp. 20659–20672, 2001.

[51] M. F. Wan Ezumi, S. Siti Amrah, A. W. M. Suhaimi, and S. S. J. Mohsin, "Evaluation of the female reproductive toxicity of aqueous extract of Labisia pumila var. alata in rats," *Indian Journal of Pharmacology*, vol. 39, no. 1, pp. 30–32, 2007.

[52] G. D. Singh, M. Ganjoo, M. S. Youssouf et al., "Sub-acute toxicity evaluation of an aqueous extract of Labisia pumila, a Malaysian herb," *Food and Chemical Toxicology*, vol. 47, no. 10, pp. 2661–2665, 2009.

[53] S. C. Taneja, *Sub-Chronic (90 days) Oral Toxicity Studies of Aqueous Extract of Labisia pumila in Wistar Rats (250, 500&1000 mg/kg b. wt. only)*, Indian Institute of Integrative Medicine, Jammu, India, 2004.

[54] B. L. Riggs, S. Khosla, and L. J. Melton, "Sex steroids and the construction and conservation of the adult skeleton," *Endocrine Reviews*, vol. 23, no. 3, pp. 279–302, 2002.

[55] F. Syed and S. Khosla, "Mechanisms of sex steroid effects on bone," *Biochemical and Biophysical Research Communications*, vol. 328, no. 3, pp. 688–696, 2005.

[56] R. T. Turner, B. L. Riggs, and T. C. Spelsberg, "Skeletal effects of estrogen," *Endocrine Reviews*, vol. 15, no. 3, pp. 275–300, 1994.

[57] H. K. Choi, D. H. Kim, J. W. Kim, S. Ngadiran, M. R. Sarmidi, and C. S. Park, "Labisia pumila extract protects skin cells from photoaging caused by UVB irradiation," *Journal of Bioscience and Bioengineering*, vol. 109, no. 3, pp. 291–296, 2010.

[58] L. J. Crofford, "COX-1 and COX-2 tissue expression: Implications and predictions," *Journal of Rheumatology*, vol. 24, no. 49, pp. 15–19, 1997.

[59] H. Yasuda, N. Shima, N. Nakagawa et al., "Osteoclast differentiation factor is a ligand for osteoprotegerin/osteoclastogenesis-inhibitory factor and is identical to TRANCE/RANKL," *Proceedings of the National Academy of Sciences of the United States of America*, vol. 95, no. 7, pp. 3597–3602, 1998.

[60] J. H. M. Feyen and L. G. Raisz, "Prostaglandin production by calvariae from sham operated and oophorectomized rats: effect of 17β-estradiol in vivo," *Endocrinology*, vol. 121, no. 2, pp. 819–821, 1987.

[61] M. R. Forwood, "Inducible cyclo-oxygenase (COX-2) mediates the induction of bone formation by mechanical loading in vivo," *Journal of Bone and Mineral Research*, vol. 11, no. 11, pp. 1688–1693, 1996.

[62] K. Fuller, C. Murphy, B. Kirstein, S. W. Fox, and T. J. Chambers, "TNFα potently activates osteoclasts, through a direct action independent of and strongly synergistic with RANKL," *Endocrinology*, vol. 143, no. 3, pp. 1108–1118, 2002.

[63] S. E. Lee, W. J. Chung, H. B. Kwak et al., "Tumor necrosis factor-α supports the survival of osteoclasts through the activation of Akt and ERK," *Journal of Biological Chemistry*, vol. 276, no. 52, pp. 49343–49349, 2001.

[64] L. Gilbert, X. He, P. Farmer et al., "Inhibition of osteoblast differentiation by tumor necrosis factor-α," *Endocrinology*, vol. 141, no. 11, pp. 3956–3964, 2000.

[65] S. Kumar, B. J. Votta, D. J. Rieman, A. M. Badger, M. Gowen, and J. C. Lee, "IL-1- and TNF-induced bone resorption is mediated by p38 mitogen activated protein kinase," *Journal of Cellular Physiology*, vol. 187, no. 3, pp. 294–303, 2001.

[66] L. C. Hofbauer, C. R. Dunstan, T. C. Spelsberg, B. L. Riggs, and S. Khosla, "Osteoprotegerin production by human osteoblast lineage cells is stimulated by vitamin D, bone morphogenetic protein-2, and cytokines," *Biochemical and Biophysical Research Communications*, vol. 250, no. 3, pp. 776–781, 1998.

[67] J. Huang, H. Zhang, N. Shimizu, and T. Takeda, "Triterpenoid saponins from Ardisia mamillata," *Phytochemistry*, vol. 54, no. 8, pp. 817–822, 2000.

[68] M. Norhaiza, M. Maziah, and M. Hakiman, "Antioxidative properties of leaf extracts of a popular Malaysian herb, Labisia pumila," *Journal of Medicinal Plant Research*, vol. 3, no. 4, pp. 217–223, 2009.

[69] G. G. Duthie, P. T. Gardner, and J. A. M. Kyle, "Plant polyphenols: are they the new magic bullet?" *Proceedings of the Nutrition Society*, vol. 62, no. 3, pp. 599–603, 2003.

[70] H. Sies and W. Stahl, "Vitamins E and C, β-carotene, and other carotenoids as antioxidants," *American Journal of Clinical Nutrition*, vol. 62, no. 6, pp. 1315S–121S, 1995.

[71] L. Bravo, "Polyphenols: chemistry, dietary sources, metabolism, and nutritional significance," *Nutrition Reviews*, vol. 56, no. 11, pp. 317–333, 1998.

[72] S. Y. Wang and H. Jiao, "Scavenging capacity of berry crops on superoxide radicals, hydrogen peroxide, hydroxyl radical's, and singlet oxygen," *Journal of Agricultural and Food Chemistry*, vol. 48, no. 11, pp. 5677–5684, 2000.

[73] A. Cassidy, B. Hanley, and R. M. Lamuela-Raventos, "Isoflavones, lignans and stilbenes: origins, etabolism and potential importance tohuman health," *Journal of the Science of Food and Agriculture*, vol. 80, no. 7, pp. 1044–1062, 2000.

[74] P. P. Lelovas, T. T. Xanthos, S. E. Thorma, G. P. Lyritis, and I. A. Dontas, "The laboratory rat as an animal model for osteoporosis research," *Comparative Medicine*, vol. 58, no. 5, pp. 424–430, 2008.

[75] M. Badeau, H. Adlercreutz, P. Kaihovaara, and M. J. Tikkanen, "Estrogen A-ring structure and antioxidative effect on lipoproteins," *Journal of Steroid Biochemistry and Molecular Biology*, vol. 96, no. 3-4, pp. 271–278, 2005.

[76] J. M. Lean, C. J. Jagger, B. Kirstein, K. Fuller, and T. J. Chambers, "Hydrogen peroxide is essential for estrogen-deficiency bone loss and osteoclast formation," *Endocrinology*, vol. 146, no. 2, pp. 728–735, 2005.

[77] B. Halliwell and J. M. C. Gutteridge, *Free Radicals in Biology and Medicine*, Oxford University Press, New York, NY, USA, 2007.

[78] K. Naka, T. Muraguchi, T. Hoshii, and A. Hirao, "Regulation of reactive oxygen species and genomic stability in hematopoietic stem cells," *Antioxidants and Redox Signaling*, vol. 10, no. 11, pp. 1883–1894, 2008.

[79] D. Maggio, M. Barabani, M. Pierandrei et al., "Marked decrease in plasma antioxidants in aged osteoporotic women: results of a cross-sectional study," *Journal of Clinical Endocrinology and Metabolism*, vol. 88, no. 4, pp. 1523–1527, 2003.

[80] M. Almeida, L. Han, M. Martin-Millan et al., "Skeletal involution by age-associated oxidative stress and its acceleration by loss of sex steroids," *Journal of Biological Chemistry*, vol. 282, no. 37, pp. 27285–27297, 2007.

[81] F. Wauquier, L. Leotoing, V. Coxam, J. Guicheux, and Y. Wittrant, "Oxidative stress in bone remodelling and disease," *Trends in Molecular Medicine*, vol. 15, no. 10, pp. 468–477, 2009.

[82] Y. Hayase, Y. Muguruma, and M. Y. Lee, "Osteoclast development from hematopoietic stem cells: apparent divergence

of the osteoclast lineage prior to macrophage commitment," *Experimental Hematology*, vol. 25, no. 1, pp. 19–25, 1997.

[83] N. K. Lee, Y. G. Choi, J. Y. Baik et al., "A crucial role for reactive oxygen species in RANKL-induced osteoclast differentiation," *Blood*, vol. 106, no. 3, pp. 852–859, 2005.

[84] A. N. Sontakke and R. S. Tare, "A duality in the roles of reactive oxygen species with respect to bone metabolism," *Clinica Chimica Acta*, vol. 318, no. 1-2, pp. 145–148, 2002.

[85] M. Norazlina, P. L. Lee, H. I. Lukman, A. S. Nazrun, and S. Ima-Nirwana, "Effects of vitamin E supplementation on bone metabolism in nicotine-treated rats," *Singapore Medical Journal*, vol. 48, no. 3, pp. 195–199, 2007.

[86] J. Gonzalez-Gallego, S. Sanchez-Campoz, and M. J. Tunon, "Anti-inflammatory properties of dietary flavonoids," *Nutricion Hospitalaria*, vol. 22, no. 3, pp. 287–293, 2007.

[87] Y. L. Lin and J. K. Lin, "Epigallocatechin-3-gallate blocks the induction of nitric oxide synthase by down-regulating lipopolysaccharide-induced activity of transcription factor nuclear factor-kappaB," *Molecular Pharmacology*, vol. 52, no. 3, pp. 465–472, 1997.

[88] N. Mody, F. Parhami, T. A. Sarafian, and L. L. Demer, "Oxidative stress modulates osteoblastic differentiation of vascular and bone cells," *Free Radical Biology and Medicine*, vol. 31, no. 4, pp. 509–519, 2001.

[89] J. H. E. Fraser, M. H. Helfrich, H. M. Wallace, and S. H. Ralston, "Hydrogen peroxide, but not superoxide, stimulates bone resorption in mouse calvariae," *Bone*, vol. 19, no. 3, pp. 223–226, 1996.

[90] R. Kitazawa, R. B. Kimble, J. L. Vannice, V. T. Kung, and R. Pacifici, "Interleukin-1 receptor antagonist and tumor necrosis factor binding protein decrease osteoclast formation and bone resorption in ovariectomized mice," *Journal of Clinical Investigation*, vol. 94, no. 6, pp. 2397–2406, 1994.

[91] A. S. Nazrun, P. L. Lee, M. Norliza, M. Norazlina, and N. S. Ima, "The effects of Labisia pumila var. alata on bone markers and bone calcium in a rat model of post-menopausal osteoporosis," *Journal of Ethnopharmacology*, vol. 133, pp. 538–542, 2011.

[92] H. N. Rosen, A. C. Moses, J. Garber et al., "Serum CTX: a new marker of bone resorption that shows treatment effect more often than other markers because of low coefficient of variability and large changes with bisphosphonate therapy," *Calcified Tissue International*, vol. 66, no. 2, pp. 100–103, 2000.

10

Molecular Mechanisms Underlying Anti-Inflammatory Actions of 6-(Methylsulfinyl)hexyl Isothiocyanate Derived from Wasabi (*Wasabia japonica*)

Takuhiro Uto,[1] De-Xing Hou,[2] Osamu Morinaga,[1] and Yukihiro Shoyama[1]

[1] *Department of Pharmacognosy, Faculty of Pharmaceutical Sciences, Nagasaki International University, 2825-7 Huis Ten Bosch, Sasebo, Nagasaki 859-3298, Japan*
[2] *Course of Biological Science and Technology, United Graduate School of Agricultural Sciences, Kagoshima University, Korimoto 1-21-24, Kagoshima 890-0065, Japan*

Correspondence should be addressed to Takuhiro Uto, uto@niu.ac.jp

Academic Editor: Alessandra Bitto

6-(Methylsulfinyl)hexyl isothiocyanate (6-MSITC) is a major bioactive compound in wasabi (*Wasabia japonica*), which is a typical Japanese pungent spice. Recently, *in vivo* and *in vitro* studies demonstrated that 6-MSITC has several biological properties, including anti-inflammatory, antimicrobial, antiplatelet, and anticancer effects. We previously reported that 6-MSITC strongly suppresses cyclooxygenase-2 (COX-2), inducible nitric oxide synthase (iNOS), and cytokines, which are important factors that mediate inflammatory processes. Moreover, molecular analysis demonstrated that 6-MSITC blocks the expressions of these factors by suppressing multiple signal transduction pathways to attenuate the activation of transcriptional factors. Structure-activity relationships of 6-MSITC and its analogues containing an isothiocyanate group revealed that methylsulfinyl group and the length of alkyl chain of 6-MSITC might be related to high inhibitory potency. In this paper, we review the anti-inflammatory properties of 6-MSITC and discuss potential molecular mechanisms focusing on inflammatory responses by macrophages.

1. Introduction

Isothiocyanates (ITCs) are a group of naturally occurring sulfur compounds containing –N=C=S functional group, available often abundantly from many cruciferous vegetables. ITCs are stored as glucosinolate precursors in the plants. The damage of plant tissue such as chopping and mastication activates myrosinase which hydrolyses the glucosinolate (myrosinase-glucosinolate system), and the resultant ITCs play a key role in the defense against herbivores and pathogens [1, 2]. There are a significant number of naturally occurring and synthetic ITCs, and numerous studies have demonstrated the chemopreventive and anti-inflammatory properties of ITCs *in vitro* and *in vivo* [3–5]. Accumulating evidence suggests that ITCs exert their effects through a variety of signaling pathways involved in detoxification, inflammation, apoptosis, and cell cycle regulation, among others [4–6].

Wasabi (*Wasabia japonica*) is a member of the Brassicaceae family of vegetables, and its rhizome is a very popular pungent spice in Japan. Several studies have shown that wasabi has multiple physiological functions, such as appetite enhancement [7], antimicrobial activity [8], inhibition of platelet aggregation [9], and the suppression of N-methyl-N'-nitro-N-nitrosoguanidine-induced rat gastric carcinogenesis [10]. Wasabi differs from other Brassicaceae species in that it contains higher concentration of ITCs, especially long-chain ITCs. The bioactive components of wasabi have been identified as a series of ITC analogues, of which 6-(methylsulfinyl)hexyl isothiocyanate (6-MSITC or 6-MITC) (Figure 1) is a major active compound in wasabi. Several lines of evidence demonstrated the pharmacological potencies of 6-MSITC, such as anti-inflammatory [11–13], antimicrobial [14], antiplatelet [15], and anticancer [16–18] effects. We previously reported that 6-MSITC strongly suppresses inflammatory mediators by regulating

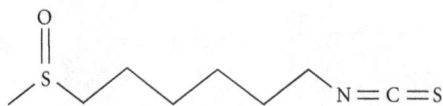

FIGURE 1: Chemical structure of 6-MSITC. 6-MSITC contains methyl sulfoxide group and ITC group linked by alkyl chain.

the signaling pathways [11–13]. In this paper, we describe the anti-inflammatory properties of 6-MSITC and discuss potential molecular mechanisms with special attention to several inflammatory factors in macrophages.

2. Chemistry and Extraction of 6-MSITC

A number of analogues of ITCs are isolated from wasabi, and the main pungent compound of wasabi is allyl ITC. Ina et al. [19] and Etoh et al. [20] reported that the characteristic flavor of wasabi depends on the methylthioalkyl ITCs and methylsulfinylalkyl ITCs. The methylthioalkyl ITCs are found in wasabi alone, whereas methylsulfinylalkyl ITCs are found in both wasabi and horseradish. Wasabi contains much higher levels of all methylsulfinylalkyl ITCs than horseradish [19]. One of the methylsulfinylalkyl ITCs is 6-MSITC, and the chemical structure of 6-MSITC contains methyl sulfoxide group and ITC group linked by alkyl chain (Figure 1). Although the ITCs are generated throughout the entire plant of wasabi, the root is the predominant site of storage. Hara et al. [21] found the myrosinase-glucosinolate composition of wasabi is in the epidermis and vascular cambium of the root. Indeed, wasabi root is particularly rich in most ITCs [19].

Several groups isolated 6-MSITC from wasabi root by monitoring the cellular bioactivities. Ono et al. [22] purified 6-MSITC from the water-soluble fractions of wasabi by monitoring the growth inhibition of MKN-28 cells. The water-soluble fraction of wasabi roots was fractionated by Sephadex G-15 gel filtration and reverse-phase HPLC successfully, and active compound was finally collected by preparative HPLC. The spectroscopic data, including fast atom bombardment mass spectrometry (FAB-MS) and electron ionization mass spectrometry (EI-MS), determined a molecular ion peak at $[M]^+$ m/z 205 and the molecular formula of $C_8H_{15}NOS_2$. Furthermore, IR and NMR completely confirmed that an active compound is 6-MSITC. Morimitsu et al. [23] extracted the smashed wasabi root to give an active ethyl acetate fraction, resulting in 6-MSITC as the major active compound of glutathione S-transferase (GST) activity after purification by silica gel column chromatography and preparative HPLC. The content of 6-MSITC in wasabi is ∼550–556 μg/g wet body weight of wasabi root.

3. Effect of 6-MSITC on Inflammatory Factors

Inflammation is one of the most important host defense systems against tissue injuries and pathogen invasion [24]. In the inflammatory process, macrophages play a central role in induction of inflammatory enzymes, cytokines, chemokines, and other inflammatory factors. Overexpression of these inflammatory factors by macrophages has been implicated in the pathophysiology of many inflammatory diseases, such as rheumatoid arthritis, atherosclerosis, chronic hepatitis, pulmonary fibrosis, and inflammatory brain diseases [25, 26]. Lipopolysaccharide (LPS), a component of Gram-negative bacterial cell wall, activates macrophages to produce prostaglandin E_2 (PGE$_2$) by cyclooxygenase-2 (COX-2), nitric oxide (NO) by inducible NO synthase (iNOS), and inflammatory cytokines through the activating multiple signaling pathways [27, 28]. Thus, the biological reduction of LPS-inducible inflammatory factors is considered to be an effective strategy for inflammatory diseases.

3.1. COX-2. COXs catalyze the synthesis of prostaglandins from arachidonic acid. There are two isoforms of COX, designated COX-1 and COX-2, which are encoded by different genes. COX-1 is constitutively expressed in most tissues and believed to be responsible for normal physiological functions [29]. In contrast, COX-2 is not detectable in normal tissues or resting immune cells, but it could be induced by LPS, inflammatory cytokines, growth factors, and carcinogens [30, 31].

6-MSITC suppressed LPS-induced COX-2 expression and PGE$_2$ release in murine macrophage cell lines RAW264 and human U937 monocytic cells without affecting the constitutive COX-1 expression [11]. Molecular analysis demonstrated that 6-MSITC blocked LPS-induced COX-2 expression in transcriptional level. In the COX-2 gene, cis-acting elements including nuclear factor κB (NF-κB), CCAAT/enhancer-binding protein (C/EBP), and cyclic AMP-response element (CRE) have been identified to play a critical role in regulating transcription [32–36]. Moreover, single site of NF-κB, C/EBP, or CRE cannot sufficiently respond to induce COX-2 transcription activity, and two of these cis-acting elements are at least recruited to achieve maximal induction of transcription [32]. 6-MSITC inhibited LPS-induced COX-2 expression by suppressing transcriptional factors binding to the first 327 base pairs in the 5′ flanking regions of COX-2 gene [11]. Moreover, mutation of a single NF-κB, C/EBP, or CRE promoter element did not abrogate the effect of 6-MSITC. Thus, the inhibition of at least two of these cis-elements is required to achieve the maximal inhibitory action of 6-MSITC on COX-2 gene expression, suggesting that the inhibitory effect of 6-MSITC on COX-2 expression could be obtained by targeting the signaling pathways leading to at least two promoter elements including NF-κB, C/EBP, and CRE sites.

In mouse RAW264 macrophages, COX-2 expression was activated by interferon (IFN)-γ and 12-O-tetradecanonoylphorbol-13-acetate (TPA) in the same manner as LPS [13]. Interestingly, 6-MSITC downregulated COX-2 expression induced by LPS and IFN-γ but did not suppress that induced by TPA. These data indicated that LPS, IFN-γ, and TPA regulate COX-2 expression through different pathways, and 6-MSITC acts as a potent inhibitor against LPS- or IFN-γ-induced COX-2 expression.

3.2. iNOS. NO is produced endogenously during arginine metabolism by isoforms of NOS [37, 38]. NO has a number of important biological functions, including tumor cell killing, host defense against intracellular pathogens, neurotransmission, and inhibition of platelet aggregation [39]. However, excess NO is a potent mediator and regulator of inflammatory responses [40, 41] and also has a multifaceted role in process of cancer [42]. NO is synthesized from L-arginine by NOS, which exists as three distinct isoforms of NOSs, including endothelial nitric oxide synthase (eNOS), neuronal nitric oxide synthase (nNOS), and iNOS [43]. iNOS is induced by various inflammatory stimuli such as LPS and inflammatory cytokines in macrophages, hepatocytes, and endothelial cells [44–46]. A large amount of NO catalyzed by iNOS plays a key role in the various forms of inflammation and carcinogenesis [46–48].

Noshita et al. [49] investigated the inhibitory activities of 6-MSITC and other synthesized ITCs against LPS-induced NO production using mouse peritoneal macrophages and mouse J774.1 macrophage-like cells. Among the tested ITCs, 6-MSITC indicated the strongest inhibition of NO production. We also reported that 6-MSITC reduced NO production, and this inhibition depends on the suppression of iNOS expression at the transcriptional level as well as COX-2 expression [12].

3.3. Inflammatory Cytokines/Chemokines. Inflammatory cytokines such as interleukin (IL), interferon (IF), and tumor necrosis factor (TNF) play important roles in the regulation of the immune system [50]. Similar to PGE$_2$ and NO, overproduction of inflammatory cytokines from macrophages causes oxidative stress, systemic inflammation, and cell dysfunction. In addition, chemokines, which are chemotactic cytokines, are well known as multifunctional mediators of gene transcription, cell proliferation, and leukocyte recruitment to inflamed tissues [50]. Chen et al. [51] performed gene expression profiling by DNA microarray in macrophages. Among a total of 22,050 gene probes, LPS upregulated the expression level of 406 genes (1.8% of the total gene probes) and downregulated 717 genes (3.2% of the total genes probes) by ≥3-fold. The number of genes affected by 6-MSITC consisted of 58% of downregulated genes by LPS and 47% of upregulated genes by LPS. Gene ontology analysis revealed that the gene groups highly affected by 6-MSITC were associated with "inflammatory responses, signal transduction, cytokine activities, hydrolase activity, kinase activity, receptor activity, transferase activity, nucleic acid binding and apoptosis." According to gene profiling and real-time PCR for further confirmation, the upregulation of inflammatory cytokine genes, such as IL-1β, IL-6, and TNF, by LPS was reduced by 6-MSITC. 6-MSITC attenuated the expression of IF-inducible genes (IFI1 and IFI47), which are involved in IF-mediated cell proliferation and differentiation. The inductions of IL receptors (IL10ra, IL23ra, and IL4ra) by LPS were also reduced by 6-MSITC. These results suggested 6-MSITC inhibition of various inflammatory genes may explain its strong anti-inflammatory effects. On the other hand, 6-MSITC restored the expression levels of LPS-reduced CC chemokines (CCL11 and CCL25), IL-3, and receptors (IL1ra12, IL8ra, TNFRSF23, and TNFRSF4) to control levels. Overall, these data suggest that 6-MSITC might regulate the expression of inflammatory and anti-inflammatory cytokines.

4. Effect of 6-MSITC on Transcriptional Regulation Involved in Inflammatory Factors

4.1. Mitogen-Activated Protein Kinase (MAPK). MAPK signaling pathways play a critical role in the regulation of inflammatory response and coordinate the induction of many genes encoding inflammatory factors [52–54]. MAPK has three major subfamily members including extracellular-regulated protein kinase (ERK), p38 kinase, and c-Jun NH$_2$-protein kinase (JNK). The activated form of each MAPK phosphorylates and activates other kinases or transcriptional factors, thereby altering the expression of the target genes such as COX-2, iNOS, and inflammatory cytokines [3, 34, 54]. Our data demonstrated that 6-MSITC blocked LPS-induced phosphorylation of all MAPKs and MAPK kinases (MAPKKs) [11]. Furthermore, MAPK-specific inhibitors (U0126 for MEK1/2, SB203580 for p38 kinase, and SP600125 for JNK) demonstrated that LPS-induced COX-2 expression was partially suppressed by the treatment with single inhibitor. However, the combination treatment of two inhibitors markedly reduced COX-2 expression. In particular, cotreatment with three inhibitors completely inhibited COX-2 expression. Thus, these data indicated that three MAPK pathways cooperatively activated COX-2 expression, and 6-MSITC attenuated COX-2 expression by blocking all of three MAPK pathways. On the other hand, only JNK-specific inhibitor SP600125 suppressed LPS-induced iNOS expression, while ERK-specific inhibitor U0126 and p38-specific inhibitor SB203580 did not, suggesting that only JNK pathway required iNOS expression, and 6-MSITC might suppress iNOS expression by blocking JNK phosphorylation.

4.2. Activator Protein-1 (AP-1). AP-1, a heterodimer of Jun (c-Jun, Jun B, and JunD) and Fos (cFos, Fos B, Fra-1, and Fra-2), plays an important role in inflammatory responses [54, 55]. AP-1 is minimally activated under normal physiologic conditions, but is dramatically activated by inflammatory stimuli, like LPS [55]. The activated AP-1 binds to the promoter elements, which regulate the transcription of inflammatory genes such as COX-2, iNOS, TNF-α, IL-1β, and IL-6 [55]. 6-MSITC completely inhibited LPS-induced phosphorylation of c-Jun, which is a major component of AP-1 in c-Jun/c-Fos heterodimer form [11, 12]. MAPK inhibitors revealed that ERK and JNK signaling pathways cooperatively regulate COX-2 expression by activating AP-1 because SP600125 and U0126, but not SB203580, inhibited c-Jun phosphorylation [11]. Moreover, SP600125 suppressed c-Jun phosphorylation and iNOS expression, suggesting that 6-MSITC might inhibit iNOS expression by blocking JNK-mediated AP-1 activation (Figure 2) [12].

4.3. CREB and C/EBP. The promoter region of COX-2 gene contains binding sites for CREB and C/EBP. LPS-induced

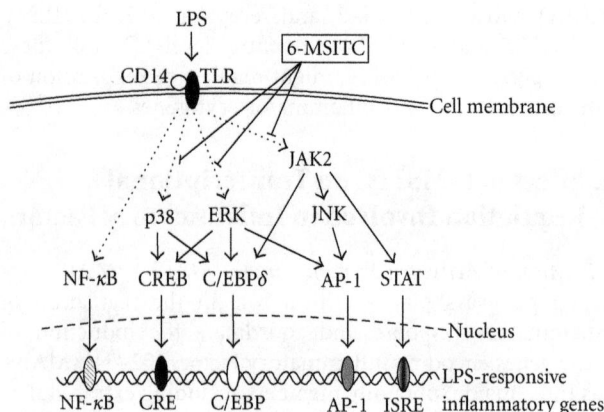

FIGURE 2: Schematic molecular model of 6-MSITC on the suppression of LPS-induced inflammatory factors.

phosphorylation of CREB and nuclear translocation of C/EBP can regulate COX-2 gene expression through CRE site and C/EBP site, respectively [56–58]. Several lines of studies have shown that the binding of CREB to CRE site depends on the phosphorylation of CREB [33, 59, 60], and the binding of C/EBP to COX-2 promoter is preceded by nuclear translocation of C/EBP [28, 56, 61]. 6-MSITC inhibited LPS-induced phosphorylation of CREB [11]. Moreover, LPS-induced expression and nuclear translocation of C/EBPδ, but not C/EBPβ, were blocked by 6-MSITC [11]. The analysis by MAPK inhibitors demonstrated that ERK and p38 kinase pathways cooperatively regulate COX-2 expression by activating CREB and C/EBPδ because ERK-specific inhibitor U0126 and p38 kinase-specific inhibitor SB203580 suppressed CREB phosphorylation and C/EBPδ expression, but JNK-specific inhibitor SP600125 did not. Therefore, 6-MSITC blocked LPS-induced COX-2 expression by suppressing ERK and p38 kinase signaling cascades leading to the activation of CREB and C/EBPδ (Figure 2). The promoter region of iNOS gene also contains binding site for C/EBP. Although 6-MSITC inhibited ERK and p38 kinase signaling cascades leading to C/EBPδ, U0126 and SB203580 had no influence on LPS-induced iNOS expression [12]. Hecker et al. reported that C/EBPβ may involve iNOS gene expression synergistically with NF-κB in primary rat hepatocytes [62]. Our data showed that LPS had no influence on the nuclear translocation of C/EBPβ [11]. These data suggest that LPS-induced iNOS expression, which was reduced by 6-MSITC, was not involved in C/EBP binding site of iNOS gene promoter.

4.4. NF-κB. NF-κB is involved in the induction of inflammatory genes and activated by the inflammatory responses during viral and bacterial infections [63, 64]. Previous analysis has demonstrated that a number of natural occurring compounds suppressed LPS-induced expression of COX-2, iNOS, and inflammatory cytokines by blocking degradation of inhibitor κB (IκB)-α in mouse macrophage cells [56, 65, 66]. However, 6-MSITC had no influence on phosphorylation and degradation of IκB-α and nuclear translocation

of p65 [11, 12]. Thus, 6-MSITC may inhibit inflammatory factors without the suppression of IκB degradation.

4.5. Janus Kinase- (JAK-) Signal Transducers and Activators of Transcription (STAT). The JAK-STAT pathway is an important inflammatory signaling pathway. JAK family, a protein tyrosine kinase (PTK), contains four members, JAK1, JAK2, JAK3, and tyrosine kinase 2 (TYK2), which are differentially regulated in response to various cytokines [67]. Binding of ligands to its receptors activates the phosphorylation of JAK, which subsequently leads to STAT phosphorylation. Phosphorylated STATs translocate to nuclear and regulate the transcription of target genes such as iNOS and COX-2 and inflammatory cytokines/chemokines [68–70]. Our data demonstrated that AG490 (JAK2-specific inhibitor) abolished LPS-induced expression of COX-2 (unpublished data) and iNOS [12]. Furthermore, AG490 reduced LPS-induced c-Jun phosphorylation, a major component of AP-1, and C/EBPδ activation. Molecular analysis with AG490 and SP600125 demonstrated that JAK2 acts upstream of JNK leading to AP-1 activation, and JNK cannot regulate the C/EBPδ activation. Moreover, 6-MSITC blocked LPS-induced JAK2 phosphorylation and its downstream pathways. Taken together, JAK2 might upregulate the expression of inflammatory factors through the induction of STAT phosphorylation, C/EBPδ expression, and JNK-mediated AP-1 activation. Moreover, 6-MSITC suppresses LPS-induced JAK2 phosphorylation leading to the induction of inflammatory factors (Figure 2).

5. Structure-Activity Relationship

Depending on the length of the alkyl chain of MSITC, there are a number of analogues of MSITC (Figure 3). 4-MSITC, also known as sulforaphane, is a major ITC of broccoli [71], and 2-MSITC and 8-MSITC are artificially synthesized [72]. The inhibitory potency on COX-2 and iNOS expression is increased depending on the alkyl chain elongation [11, 12], suggesting that the alkyl chain length is important for the inhibitory activity.

Noshita et al. [49] synthesized a series of ITCs (Figure 3) based on 6-MSITC to check the inhibitory activity against NO production in LPS-induced macrophages. Substitution of ITC group in 6-MSITC with thiocyanate group (1-(methylsulfinyl)-6-thiocyanatohexane, [49]) had no inhibitory effect, indicating the inhibitory action may entirely depend on its ITC group. The alkyl chain elongation in allyl ITCs also increases their lipophilicity (log P value), suggesting that the inhibitory potency of inflammatory factors by ITCs may be related to their log P values. Furthermore, substitution of the methylsulfinyl group in 6-MSITC with a formyl (6-isothiocyanatohexanal [49, 73]), a methylsulfanyl (1-isothiocyanato-6-(methylthio)hexane [49, 74]), or a methyl (n-hexyl ITC [49]), attenuated the inhibitory activity. Polar surface area (PSA) value of these analogues is lower than that of 6-MSITC. In addition, the inhibitory potencies of ITCs showed better correlation with their PSA values rather than their log P values. Taken

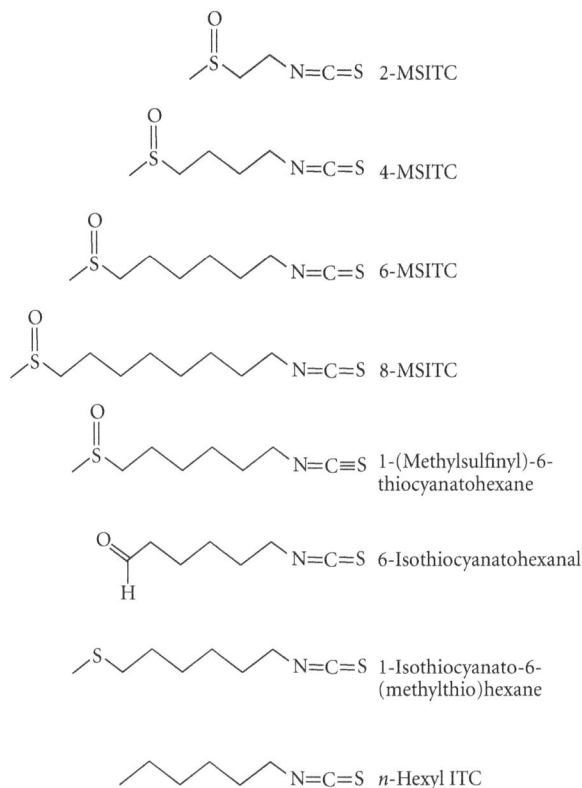

FIGURE 3: Chemical structures of analogues of 6-MSITC. 4-MSITC (sulforaphane), 2-MSITC, and 8-MSITC are analogues of 6-MSITC containing the different length of alkyl chain. 1-(Methylsulfinyl)-6-thiocyanatohexane substituted ITC group in 6-MSITC with thiocyanate group. 6-Isothiocyanatohexanal, 1-isothiocyanato-6-(methylthio)hexane, and n-hexyl ITC substituted the methylsulfinyl group in 6-MSITC with formyl group, methylsulfinyl group, and methyl group, respectively.

together, 6-MSITC has potent biological activity because of its higher PSA value and some degree of log P value [49].

6. Cellular Uptake of 6-MSITC

We investigated the effect of 6-MSITC on the binding of fluorescein-labeled LPS to the LPS receptor by a flow cytometry analysis, and the data suggested that 6-MSITC could not affect the binding of LPS to the receptor in plasma membrane in RAW264 cells (unpublished data). Thus, 6-MSITC has no influence on the interaction of LPS receptors. Several studies have revealed the metabolism of ITCs in several cell lines [4, 70, 75–77]. ITCs appear to penetrate cellular membrane by diffusion and rapidly conjugate with intracellular reduced glutathione (GSH) via their ITC group (–N=C=S). The methylsulfinyl group (CH_3–S(=O)–) and the length of alkyl chain of 6-MSITC might contribute to the cell membrane permeability [49]. GSH is an important intracellular redox buffer that exits as a reduced predominant form, as a disulfide form (GSSG), or as mixed disulfide (GSSR) with protein thiols [78]. The redox status within the cells, reflected by GSH/GSSG [79], has been shown to

be relevant for the regulation of inflammatory genes [80]. However, the detailed relationship between GSH-conjugated ITCs and signaling pathways involved in inflammatory factors is not clear. Future studies are needed to elucidate the role of GSH-conjugated 6-MSITC in LPS-induced cellular signaling pathways.

7. Conclusions

We have demonstrated that 6-MSITC has inhibited several inflammatory factors such as COX-2, iNOS, and inflammatory cytokines at the transcription factor/promoter levels. MAPK signaling pathways are one of the important pathways involved in inflammatory responses, and 6-MSITC suppresses all of three MAPK pathways leading to activation of transcriptional factors. Molecular analysis by MAPK inhibitors revealed the relationship between the transcriptional factors and MAPKs inhibited by 6-MSITC. 6-MSITC blocks LPS-induced COX-2 expression by suppressing ERK and p38 kinase signaling cascades leading to the activation of CREB and C/EBPδ, and by inhibiting JNK cascade leading to AP-1 activation. On the other hand, 6-MSITC attenuates iNOS expression mainly by blocking AP-1 activation. In addition, 6-MSITC inhibits JAK2 signaling pathway, which upregulates the expression of inflammatory factors through STAT phosphorylation, C/EBPδ expression, and JNK-mediated AP-1 activation. We also clarified the structure-activity relationship of MSITC analogues. 6-MSITC has potential usefulness as an anti-inflammatory agent because of its higher PSA value and some degree of log P value.

In recent years, numerous epidemiological and experimental animal studies have shown strong anti-inflammatory and chemopreventive effects of natural products. The elucidation of molecular mechanisms underlying the action of natural compounds may provide further insights into their potential usefulness as anti-inflammatory agents. The further studies on anti-inflammatory properties of 6-MSITC in clinical trial will greatly expand the development of 6-MSITC as an anti-inflammatory agent.

Acknowledgments

This work was funded by "Science and Technology Research Partnership for Sustainable Development (SATREPS)" supported by the Japan Science and Technology Agency (JST), the Japan International Cooperation Agency (JICA), and Japan-China Medical Communication Program from JSPS.

References

[1] L. Rask, E. Andréasson, B. Ekbom, S. Eriksson, B. Pontoppidan, and J. Meijer, "Myrosinase: gene family evolution and herbivore defense in Brassicaceae," Plant Molecular Biology, vol. 42, no. 1, pp. 93–113, 2000.

[2] R. J. Hopkins, N. M. Van Dam, and J. J. A. Van Loon, "Role of glucosinolates in insect-plant relationships and multitrophic interactions," Annual Review of Entomology, vol. 54, pp. 57–83, 2009.

[3] K. J. Woo and T. K. Kwon, "Sulforaphane suppresses lipopolysaccharide-induced cyclooxygenase-2 (COX-2) expression through the modulation of multiple targets in COX-2 gene promoter," *International Immunopharmacology*, vol. 7, no. 13, pp. 1776–1783, 2007.

[4] Y. Zhang, "The molecular basis that unifies the metabolism, cellular uptake and chemopreventive activities of dietary isothiocyanates," *Carcinogenesis*, vol. 33, no. 1, pp. 2–9, 2012.

[5] S. L. Navarro, F. Li, and J. W. Lampe, "Mechanisms of action of isothiocyanates in cancer chemoprevention: an update," *Food & Function*, vol. 2, no. 10, pp. 579–587, 2011.

[6] K. L. Cheung and A. N. Kong, "Molecular targets of dietary phenethyl isothiocyanate and sulforaphane for cancer chemoprevention," *AAPS Journal*, vol. 12, no. 1, pp. 87–97, 2010.

[7] M. Kojima, "Pungent components and functional ingredient of wasabi," *Food Process*, vol. 23, pp. 32–35, 1988.

[8] K. Isshiki and K. Tokuoka, "Allyl isothiocyanate and wholesomeness of food," *Japanese Journal of Food Microbiology*, vol. 12, pp. 1–6, 1993.

[9] H. Kumagai, N. Kashima, T. Seki, H. Sakurai, K. Ishii, and T. Ariga, "Analysis of volatile components in essential oil of upland Wasabi and their inhibitory effects on platelet aggregation," *Bioscience, Biotechnology and Biochemistry*, vol. 58, no. 12, pp. 2131–2135, 1994.

[10] N. Tanida, A. Kawaura, A. Takahashi, K. Sawada, and T. Shimoyama, "Suppressive effect of Wasabi (pungent Japanese spice) on gastric carcinogenesis induced by MNNG in rats," *Nutrition and Cancer*, vol. 16, no. 1, pp. 53–58, 1991.

[11] T. Uto, M. Fujii, and D. X. Hou, "Inhibition of lipopolysaccharide-induced cyclooxygenase-2 transcription by 6-(methylsulfinyl) hexyl isothiocyanate, a chemopreventive compound from *Wasabia japonica* (Miq.) Matsumura, in mouse macrophages," *Biochemical Pharmacology*, vol. 70, no. 12, pp. 1772–1784, 2005.

[12] T. Uto, M. Fujii, and D. X. Hou, "6-(Methylsulfinyl)hexyl isothiocyanate suppresses inducible nitric oxide synthase expression through the inhibition of Janus kinase 2-mediated JNK pathway in lipopolysaccharide-activated murine macrophages," *Biochemical Pharmacology*, vol. 70, no. 8, pp. 1211–1221, 2005.

[13] T. Uto, M. Fujii, and D. X. Hou, "Effects of 6-(methylsulfinyl) hexyl isothiocyanate on cyclooxygenase-2 expression induced by lipopolysaccharide, interferon-gamma and 12-O-tetradecanoylphorbol-13-acetate," *Oncology Reports*, vol. 17, no. 1, pp. 233–238, 2007.

[14] N. Hasegawa, Y. Matsumoto, A. Hoshino, and K. Iwashita, "Comparison of effects of *Wasabia japonica* and allyl isothiocyanate on the growth of four strains of Vibrio parahaemolyticus in lean and fatty tuna meat suspensions," *International Journal of Food Microbiology*, vol. 49, no. 1-2, pp. 27–34, 1999.

[15] Y. Morimitsu, K. Hayashi, Y. Nakagawa et al., "Antiplatelet and anticancer isothiocyanates in Japanese domestic horseradish, Wasabi," *Mechanisms of Ageing and Development*, vol. 116, no. 2-3, pp. 125–134, 2000.

[16] D. X. Hou, M. Fukuda, M. Fujii, and Y. Fuke, "Induction of NADPH:quinone oxidoreductase in murine hepatoma cells by methylsulfinyl isothiocyanates: methyl chain length-activity study," *International Journal of Molecular Medicine*, vol. 6, no. 4, pp. 441–444, 2000.

[17] D. X. Hou, M. Fukuda, M. Fujii, and Y. Fuke, "Transcriptional regulation of nicotinamide adenine dinucleotide phosphate: quinone oxidoreductase in murine hepatoma cells by 6-(methylsufinyl)hexyl isothiocyanate, an active principle of

wasabi (*Eutrema wasabi* Maxim)," *Cancer Letters*, vol. 161, no. 2, pp. 195–200, 2000.

[18] D. X. Hou, Y. Korenori, S. Tanigawa et al., "Dynamics of Nrf2 and Keap1 in ARE-mediated NQO1 expression by wasabi 6-(methylsulfinyl)hexyl isothiocyanate," *Journal of Agricultural and Food Chemistry*, vol. 59, no. 22, pp. 11975–11882.

[19] K. Ina, H. Ina, M. Ueda, A. Yagi, and I. Kishima, "ω-Methylthioalkyl isothiocyanates in Wasabi," *Agricultural Biology and Chemistry*, vol. 53, no. 2, pp. 537–538, 1989.

[20] H. Etoh, A. Nishimura, R. Takasawa et al., "ω-Methylsulfinylalkyl isothiocyanates in wasabi, *Wasabia japonica* Matsum," *Agricultural Biology and Chemistry*, vol. 54, no. 6, pp. 1587–1589, 1990.

[21] M. Hara, K. Mochizuki, S. Kaneko et al., "Changes in pungent components of two *Wasabia japonica* Matsum. cultivars during the cultivation period," *Food Science and Technology Research*, vol. 9, no. 3, pp. 288–291, 2003.

[22] H. Ono, K. Adachi, Y. Fuke, and K. Shinohara, "Purification and structural analysis of substances in wasabi (*Eutrema wasabi* maxim.) that suppress the growth of MKN-28 human stomach cancer cells," *Nippon Shokuhin Kagaku Kogaku Kaishi*, vol. 43, no. 10, pp. 1092–1097, 1996.

[23] Y. Morimitsu, Y. Nakagawa, K. Hayashi et al., "A sulforaphane analogue that potently activates the Nrf2-dependent detoxification pathway," *The Journal of Biological Chemistry*, vol. 277, no. 5, pp. 3456–3463, 2002.

[24] M. D. Maines, "The heme oxygenase system: a regulator of second messenger gases," *Annual Review of Pharmacology and Toxicology*, vol. 37, pp. 517–554, 1997.

[25] L. Boscá, M. Zeini, P. G. Través, and S. Hortelano, "Nitric oxide and cell viability in inflammatory cells: a role for NO in macrophage function and fate," *Toxicology*, vol. 208, no. 2, pp. 249–258, 2005.

[26] Z. Zhu, S. Zhong, and Z. Shen, "Targeting the inflammatory pathways to enhance chemotherapy of cancer," *Cancer Biology and Therapy*, vol. 12, no. 2, pp. 95–105, 2011.

[27] B. Hinz and K. Brune, "Cyclooxygenase-2–0 years later," *Journal of Pharmacology and Experimental Therapeutics*, vol. 300, no. 2, pp. 367–375, 2002.

[28] R. G. Molloy, J. A. Mannick, and M. L. Rodrick, "Cytokines, sepsis and immunomodulation," *British Journal of Surgery*, vol. 80, no. 3, pp. 289–297, 1993.

[29] C. D. Funk, L. B. Funk, M. E. Kennedy, A. S. Pong, and G. A. Fitzgerald, "Human platelet/erythroleukemia cell prostaglandin G/H synthase: cDNA cloning, expression, and gene chromosomal assignment," *FASEB Journal*, vol. 5, no. 9, pp. 2304–2312, 1991.

[30] S. L. Hempel, M. M. Monick, and G. W. Hunninghake, "Lipopolysaccharide induces prostaglandin H synthase-2 protein and mRNA in human alveolar macrophages and blood monocytes," *Journal of Clinical Investigation*, vol. 93, no. 1, pp. 391–396, 1994.

[31] L. J. Crofford, R. L. Wilder, A. P. Ristimaki et al., "Cyclooxygenase-1 and -2 expression in rheumatoid synovial tissues. Effects of interleukin-1β, phorbol ester, and corticosteroids," *Journal of Clinical Investigation*, vol. 93, no. 3, pp. 1095–1101, 1994.

[32] J. R. Mestre, P. J. Mackrell, D. E. Rivadeneira, P. P. Stapleton, T. Tanabe, and J. M. Daly, "Redundancy in the signaling pathways and promoter elements regulating cyclooxygenase-2 gene expression in endotoxin-treated macrophage/monocytic cells," *The Journal of Biological Chemistry*, vol. 276, no. 6, pp. 3977–3982, 2001.

[33] M. Caivano, B. Gorgoni, P. Cohen, and V. Poli, "The induction of cyclooxygenase-2 mRNA in macrophages is biphasic and requires both CCAAT enhancer-binding protein beta (C/EBP beta) and C/EBP delta transcription factors," *The Journal of Biological Chemistry*, vol. 276, no. 52, pp. 48693–48701, 2001.

[34] H. Inoue, C. Yokoyama, S. Hara, Y. Tone, and T. Tanabe, "Transcriptional regulation of human prostaglandin-endoperoxide synthase-2 gene by lipopolysaccharide and phorbol ester in vascular endothelial cells. Involvement of both nuclear factor for interleukin-6 expression site and cAMP response element," *The Journal of Biological Chemistry*, vol. 270, no. 42, pp. 24965–24971, 1995.

[35] H. Inoue, T. Nanayama, S. Hara, C. Yokoyama, and T. Tanabe, "The cyclic AMP response element plays an essential role in the expression of the human prostaglandin-endoperoxide synthase 2 gene in differentiated U937 monocytic cells," *FEBS Letters*, vol. 350, no. 1, pp. 51–54, 1994.

[36] H. Inoue and T. Tanabe, "Transcriptional role of the nuclear factor κB site in the induction by lipopolysaccharide and suppression by dexamethasone of cyclooxygenase-2 in U937 cells," *Biochemical and Biophysical Research Communications*, vol. 244, no. 1, pp. 143–148, 1998.

[37] S. Moncada, R. M. J. Palmer, and E. A. Higgs, "Nitric oxide: physiology, pathophysiology, and pharmacology," *Pharmacological Reviews*, vol. 43, no. 2, pp. 109–142, 1991.

[38] W. K. Alderton, C. E. Cooper, and R. G. Knowles, "Nitric oxide synthases: structure, function and inhibition," *Biochemical Journal*, vol. 357, no. 3, pp. 593–615, 2001.

[39] K. D. Kröncke, K. Fehsel, and V. Kolb-Bachofen, "Inducible nitric oxide synthase in human diseases," *Clinical and Experimental Immunology*, vol. 113, no. 2, pp. 147–156, 1998.

[40] R. B. Lorsbach, W. J. Murphy, C. J. Lowenstein, S. H. Snyder, and S. W. Russell, "Expression of the nitric oxide synthase gene in mouse macrophages activated for tumor cell killing. Molecular basis for the synergy between interferon-γ and lipopolysaccharide," *The Journal of Biological Chemistry*, vol. 268, no. 3, pp. 1908–1913, 1993.

[41] R. Korhonen, A. Lahti, H. Kankaanranta, and E. Moilanen, "Nitric oxide production and signaling in inflammation," *Current Drug Targets*, vol. 4, no. 4, pp. 471–479, 2005.

[42] H. Ohshima and H. Bartsch, "Chronic infections and inflammatory processes as cancer risk factors: possible role of nitric oxide in carcinogenesis," *Mutation Research*, vol. 305, no. 2, pp. 253–264, 1994.

[43] R. M. J. Palmer, D. S. Ashton, and S. Moncada, "Vascular endothelial cells synthesize nitric oxide from L-arginine," *Nature*, vol. 333, no. 6174, pp. 664–666, 1988.

[44] C. Nathan and Q. W. Xie, "Nitric oxide synthases: roles, tolls, and controls," *Cell*, vol. 78, no. 6, pp. 915–918, 1994.

[45] Y. Kobayashi, "The regulatory role of nitric oxide in proinflammatory cytokine expression during the induction and resolution of inflammation," *Journal of Leukocyte Biology*, vol. 88, no. 6, pp. 1157–1162, 2010.

[46] J. MacMicking, Q. W. Xie, and C. Nathan, "Nitric oxide and macrophage function," *Annual Review of Immunology*, vol. 15, pp. 323–350, 1997.

[47] H. Maeda and T. Akaike, "Nitric oxide and oxygen radicals in infection, inflammation and cancer," *Biochemistry (Moscow)*, vol. 63, no. 7, pp. 854–865, 1998.

[48] P. K. Lala and C. Chakraborty, "Role of nitric oxide in carcinogenesis and tumour progression," *The Lancet Oncology*, vol. 2, no. 3, pp. 149–156, 2001.

[49] T. Noshita, Y. Kidachi, H. Funayama, H. Kiyota, H. Yamaguchi, and K. Ryoyama, "Anti-nitric oxide production activity of isothiocyanates correlates with their polar surface area rather than their lipophilicity," *European Journal of Medicinal Chemistry*, vol. 44, no. 12, pp. 4931–4936, 2009.

[50] A. D. Luster, "Mechanisms of disease: chemokines—chemotactic cytokines that mediate inflammation," *The New England Journal of Medicine*, vol. 338, no. 7, pp. 436–445, 1998.

[51] J. Chen, T. Uto, S. Tanigawa, T. Yamada-Kato, M. Fujii, and D. X. Hou, "Microarray-based determination of anti-inflammatory genes targeted by 6-(methylsulfinyl)hexyl isothiocyanate in macrophages," *Experimental and Therapeutic Medicine*, vol. 1, no. 1, pp. 33–40, 2010.

[52] C. Tsatsanis, A. Androulidaki, M. Venihaki, and A. N. Margioris, "Signalling networks regulating cyclooxygenase-2," *International Journal of Biochemistry and Cell Biology*, vol. 38, no. 10, pp. 1654–1661, 2006.

[53] P. Huang, J. Han, and L. Hui, "MAPK signaling in inflammation-associated cancer development," *Protein and Cell*, vol. 1, no. 3, pp. 218–226, 2010.

[54] S. K. Dower and E. E. Qwarnstrom, "Signalling networks, inflammation and innate immunity," *Biochemical Society Transactions*, vol. 31, no. 6, pp. 1462–1471, 2003.

[55] T. C. Hsu, M. R. Young, J. Cmarik, and N. H. Colburn, "Activator protein 1 (AP-1)- and nuclear factor κB (NF-κB)-dependent transcriptional events in carcinogenesis," *Free Radical Biology and Medicine*, vol. 28, no. 9, pp. 1338–1348, 2000.

[56] A. K. Lee, S. H. Sung, Y. C. Kim, and S. G. Kim, "Inhibition of lipopolysaccharide-inducible nitric oxide synthase, TNF-α and COX-2 expression by sauchinone effects on I-κBα phosphorylation, C/EBP and AP-1 activation," *British Journal of Pharmacology*, vol. 139, no. 1, pp. 11–20, 2003.

[57] B. Thomas, F. Berenbaum, L. Humbert et al., "Critical role of C/EBPδ and C/EBPβ factors in the stimulation of the cyclooxygenase-2 gene transcription by interleukin-1β in articular chondrocytes," *European Journal of Biochemistry*, vol. 267, no. 23, pp. 6798–6809, 2000.

[58] F. D'Acquisto, T. Iuvone, L. Rombolà, L. Sautebin, M. Di Rosa, and R. Carnuccio, "Involvement of NF-κB in the regulation of cyclooxygenase-2 protein expression in LPS-stimulated J774 macrophages," *FEBS Letters*, vol. 418, no. 1-2, pp. 175–178, 1997.

[59] K. Subbaramaiah, P. A. Cole, and A. J. Dannenberg, "Retinoids and carnosol suppress cyclooxygenase-2 transcription by CREB-binding protein/p300-dependent and -independent mechanisms," *Cancer Research*, vol. 62, no. 9, pp. 2522–2530, 2002.

[60] A. G. Eliopoulos, C. D. Dumitru, C. C. Wang, J. Cho, and P. N. Tsichlis, "Induction of COX-2 by LPS in macrophages is regulated by Tpl2-dependent CREB activation signals," *EMBO Journal*, vol. 21, no. 18, pp. 4831–4840, 2002.

[61] Y. H. Cho, C. H. Lee, and S. G. Kim, "Potentiation of lipopolysaccharide-inducible cyclooxygenase 2 expression by C2-ceramide via c-Jun N-terminal kinase-mediated activation of CCAAT/enhancer binding protein β in macrophages," *Molecular Pharmacology*, vol. 63, no. 3, pp. 512–523, 2003.

[62] M. Hecker, C. Preiß, and V. B. Schini-Kerth, "Induction by staurosporine of nitric oxide synthase expression in vascular smooth muscle cells: role of NF-κB, CREB and C/EBPβ," *British Journal of Pharmacology*, vol. 120, no. 6, pp. 1067–1074, 1997.

[63] J. Marks-Konczalik, S. C. Chu, and J. Moss, "Cytokine-mediated transcriptional induction of the human inducible nitric oxide synthase gene requires both activator protein 1 and nuclear factor κB-binding sites," *The Journal of Biological Chemistry*, vol. 273, no. 35, pp. 22201–22208, 1998.

[64] Q. W. Xie, Y. Kashiwabara, and C. Nathan, "Role of transcription factor NF-κB/Rel in induction of nitric oxide synthase," *The Journal of Biological Chemistry*, vol. 269, no. 7, pp. 4705–4708, 1994.

[65] C. S. Kim, T. Kawada, B. S. Kim et al., "Capsaicin exhibits anti-inflammatory property by inhibiting IκB-α degradation in LPS-stimulated peritoneal macrophages," *Cellular Signalling*, vol. 15, no. 3, pp. 299–306, 2003.

[66] Y. C. Liang, Y. T. Huang, S. H. Tsai, S. Y. Lin-Shiau, C. F. Chen, and J. K. Lin, "Suppression of inducible cyclooxygenase and inducible nitric oxide synthase by apigenin and related flavonoids in mouse macrophages," *Carcinogenesis*, vol. 20, no. 10, pp. 1945–1952, 1999.

[67] K. Imada and W. J. Leonard, "The Jak-STAT pathway," *Molecular Immunology*, vol. 37, no. 1-2, pp. 1–11, 2000.

[68] P. Kovarik, M. Mangold, K. Ramsauer et al., "Specificity of signaling by STAT1 depends on SH2 and C-terminal domains that regulate Ser727 phosphorylation, differentially affecting specific target gene expression," *EMBO Journal*, vol. 20, no. 1-2, pp. 91–100, 2001.

[69] R. W. Ganster, B. S. Taylor, L. Shao, and D. A. Geller, "Complex regulation of human inducible nitric oxide synthase gene transcription by Stat 1 and NF-κB," *Proceedings of the National Academy of Sciences of the United States of America*, vol. 98, no. 15, pp. 8638–8643, 2001.

[70] Z. Wen, Z. Zhong, and J. E. Darnell Jr., "Maximal activation of transcription by Stat1 and Stat3 requires both tyrosine and serine phosphorylation," *Cell*, vol. 82, no. 2, pp. 241–250, 1995.

[71] Y. Zhang, P. Talalay, C. G. Cho, and G. H. Posner, "A major inducer of anticarcinogenic protective enzymes from broccoli: isolation and elucidation of structure," *Proceedings of the National Academy of Sciences of the United States of America*, vol. 89, no. 6, pp. 2399–2403, 1992.

[72] T. Nomura, S. Shinoda, T. Yamori et al., "Selective sensitivity to wasabi-derived 6-(methylsulfinyl)hexyl isothiocyanate of human breast cancer and melanoma cell lines studied in vitro," *Cancer Detection and Prevention*, vol. 29, no. 2, pp. 155–160, 2005.

[73] S. Löhr, C. Jacobi, A. Johann, G. Gottschalk, and A. De Meijere, "Cyclopropyl building blocks in organic synthesis, 57—convenient syntheses and biological activity of novel ω-trans-(bicyclopropyl)-and ω-(bicyclopropylidenyl)-substituted fatty acids and their derivatives," *European Journal of Organic Chemistry*, no. 17, pp. 2979–2989, 2000.

[74] T. J. Ding, L. Zhou, and X. P. Cao, "A facile and green synthesis of sulforaphane," *Chinese Chemical Letters*, vol. 17, no. 9, pp. 1152–1154, 2006.

[75] Y. Zhang and P. Talalay, "Mechanism of differential potencies of isothiocyanates as inducers of anticarcinogenic Phase 2 enzymes," *Cancer Research*, vol. 58, no. 20, pp. 4632–4639, 1998.

[76] Y. Zhang, "Role of glutathione in the accumulation of anti-carcinogenic isothiocyanates and their glutathione conjugates by murine hepatoma cells," *Carcinogenesis*, vol. 21, no. 6, pp. 1175–1182, 2000.

[77] L. Mi, A. J. Di Pasqua, and F. L. Chung, "Proteins as binding targets of isothiocyanates in cancer prevention," *Carcinogenesis*, vol. 32, no. 10, pp. 1405–1413, 2011.

[78] S. M. Deneke and B. L. Fanburg, "Regulation of cellular glutathione," *American Journal of Physiology*, vol. 257, no. 4, pp. L163–L173, 1989.

[79] I. A. Cotgreave and R. G. Gerdes, "Recent trends in glutathione biochemistry-glutathione-protein interactions: a molecular link between oxidative stress and cell proliferation?" *Biochemical and Biophysical Research Communications*, vol. 242, no. 1, pp. 1–9, 1998.

[80] I. Rahman and W. MacNee, "Regulation of redox glutathione levels and gene transcription in lung inflammation: therapeutic approaches," *Free Radical Biology and Medicine*, vol. 28, no. 9, pp. 1405–1420, 2000.

11

Polysaccharides of St. John's Wort Herb Stimulate NHDF Proliferation and NEHK Differentiation via Influence on Extracellular Structures and Signal Pathways

S. Abakuks and A. M. Deters

Institute for Pharmaceutical Biology and Phytochemistry, Westphalian Wilhelms University of Münster, Hittorfstra Be 56, 48149 Münster, Germany

Correspondence should be addressed to A. M. Deters, adeters@uni-muenster.de

Academic Editor: Abdelwahab Omri

St. John's Wort herb extracts often contain undesirable or volitional polysaccharides. As polysaccharides exhibit structure-dependent biological functions in the present study water-soluble polysaccharides were extracted from herb material, fractionated by anion exchange chromatography into four main polysaccharide fractions (denominated as Hp1, Hp2, Hp3 and Hp4) and characterized by HPAEC-PAD, CE, IR and GC-MS. Biological activity on human skin keratinocytes and fibroblasts was assessed by investigation of their effect on proliferation, metabolism, cytotoxicity, apoptosis and differentiation. The underlying mechanisms were investigated in gene expression studies. Polysaccharide fraction Hp1 was mainly composed of β-D-glucose. Hp2, Hp3 and Hp4 contained pectic structures and arabinogalactan proteins varying in composition and quantity. Polysaccharides of Hp1 induced the keratinocyte differentiation by inhibiting the gene expression of the epidermal growth factor and insulin receptor. While the collagen secretion of fibroblasts was stimulated by each polysaccharide fraction only Hp1 stimulated the synthesis. The fibroblast proliferation was reduced by Hp1 and increased by Hp4. This effect was related to the influence on genes that referred to oxidative stress, metabolism, transcription processes and extracellular proteins. In conclusion polysaccharides have been shown as biologically active ingredients of aqueous St. John's Wort extracts with a relation between their structural characteristics and function.

1. Introduction

Extracts of St. John's Wort (*Hypericum perforatum* L., Hypericaceae) are well investigated and widely used in regard to their effectiveness against moderate depressions. The responsible naphthodianthrones, phloroglucinol derivates, and flavonoids were extensively investigated [1]. Concerning biological activity on the skin the investigations focused on the phototoxicity of lipophilic and aqueous-ethanolic extracts for many years. Beside the ongoing discussion concerning the phototoxicity of St. John's Wort extracts [2, 3], it has been reported that hyperforin induced keratinocyte differentiation *in vitro* and the skin hydration *in vivo* [4, 5]. Nevertheless more information is needed concerning the less investigated side products of extraction. Especially the carbohydrates that conflict with formulation, development,

and production of solid dosage forms [6] were mostly seen as nonactive byproducts. There are some reasons for investigation of St. John's Wort polysaccharides. First of all no information is available concerning composition and structure of polysaccharides in *Hypericum* species and cognate plants. Again aqueous-ethanolic extracts of St. John's Wort possess high viscosity indicating coextraction of plant polysaccharides. According to their structural characteristics, herbal polysaccharides are able to influence the immunologic response [7], bacterial adhesion [8], and tumor inhibition [9]. Furthermore they promote the tissue regeneration [10], protect against tissue injury [11], or reduce skin aging [12]. With respect to the multifunctional bioactivities of polysaccharides, it is likely that the effect of St. John's Wort extracts is not only related to the main components. As the bioactivity of polysaccharides is closely related to their composition, water-soluble polysaccharides of St John's Wort were fractionized according to their acidity and analyzed concerning composition and linkage prior to the investigation of their activity on skin cells. Normal human dermal fibroblasts (NHDF), HaCaT, and normal human epidermal keratinocytes (NHEK) are useful tools to investigate different aspects of cell physiology in *in vitro* studies and allow the examination of underlying mechanisms. The investigations of the present study focused on the proliferation (BrdU-incorporation), the reductive enzyme activity (MTT and WST-1), involucrin and collagen expression and necrotic (extracellular lactate dehydrogenase activity) and apoptotic (Annexin V) effects of human skin cells. Mechanistical studies were carried out using real-time PCR and gene microarrays. As representative factors for RT-PCR, the fibroblast growth factor 7 (FGF-7), epidermal growth factor receptor (EGFR), insulin receptor, and the signal transducer and activator of transcription 6 (STAT6) were chosen as representative for proliferation related processes [13]. Regulation of differentiation on the gene level was assessed by phospholipase α (PLA2) [14] and involucrin [15]. An overlook over the affected signal pathways was obtained by gene microarray analysis of 1308 genes that refer to human skin.

2. Materials and Methods

2.1. Isolation and Characterization of Polysaccharides. 250 g of powdered St. John's Wort herb from Caesar and Loretz GmbH, Bonn, Germany, was exhaustively extracted for 24 h in a Soxhlet extractor with acetone and methanol. The drug was identified by microscopic characterization, and a voucher specimen is deposited in the archive of the Institute for Pharmaceutical Biology and Phytochemistry (no. HP561/D). The residue was dried at room temperature and extracted 3 times each with 2 L Aqua Millipore under permanent stirring. The combined water extracts were concentrated using a rotary evaporator at 35°C and precipitated with ethanol 96% (V/V) to a final concentration of 80%. The entire precipitated polysaccharides (RPSs) were isolated by centrifugation at 3600 x g, dialyzed against Aqua Millipore using cellulose membranes (MWCO 3.5 kDa) for 5 days at 4°C, and lyophilized. Fractionation of RPS was performed according to the polysaccharides acidity by anion exchange chromatography on DEAE-Sephadex. Stepwise elution of polysaccharides was done with water and sodium phosphate buffers of increasing ionic strength (NaPB) according to Deters et al., 2005 [16]. For determination of the total carbohydrate, uronic acid and protein amounts polysaccharides were hydrolyzed with trifluoroacetic acid 2 mol/L at 121°C for 60 min and analyzed by TLC on silica gel F_{254} glass plates using acetonitrile-water 80 : 20 (V/V) as a mobile phase. After threefold development the monosaccharides were detected using 2-isopropyl-5-methylphenol/sulphuric acid spray reagent and heating at 120°C for 5 min. Reference standards for detection of neutral carbohydrates [17] and uronic acids [18] were prepared according to the monosaccharide and uronic acid composition determined via TLC. The protein contents were determined against reference concentrations of BSA (PAA, Laboratories, Coelbe) with Coomassie brilliant blue G250 [19]. Each of these tests was modified for use in 96-well-microtiter plates. A radial gel diffusion experiment using β-D-glucosyl-Yariv reagent [20] against gum arabic as reference (0.25 mg/mL, 0.5 mg/mL, 1 mg/mL, 2.5 mg/mL, 5 mg/mL, 10 mg/mL) was used to test the polysaccharide fractions for the occurrence of arabinogalactan proteins (AGP). Starch was assayed using Lugol's solution.

2.2. Linkage Analysis of Polysaccharides. Uronic acid was identified by ion-exchange HPLC with pulsed-amperometric detection (Bio-LC, Dionex, Idstein, Germany) with an AS50 autosampler, GS50 gradient pump, AS50 oven, and ED50 electrochemical detector on a CarboPacTM PA1 analytical column, 2 mm × 250 mm, CarboPacTM PA1, guard column 2 mm × 50 mm, and BorateTrapTM, 4 mm × 50 mm using a ternary gradient of water, 0.1 mM sodium hydroxide, and 0.5 mM sodium acetate. Neutral sugars were quantified by preparing trimethylsilyl derivatives: 10 mg of hydrolyzed polysaccharide was mixed with 1 mL TriSil-Z (Pierce, Bonn, Germany) and heated for two hours at 80°C. The separation and detection were done on a AGILENT Technologies 6890 system using an HP-PAS 1701 column (0.32 μm × 25 m × 0.25 μm) with helium as carrier gas and a temperature program from 160°C to 220°C with a heating-up rate of 10°C/min (injector: 275°C). Detection took place with a mass selective detector (70 eV ionization energy; 8 kV acceleration voltage), AGILENT Technologies, Santa Clara, USA). Structures of polysaccharides were analyzed according to the permethylation method of [21, 22], and the reduction of uronic acids with sodium borodeuteride was performed as described by [23]. Permethylated alditol acetates were injected at 220°C, gas chromatographed with a AGILENT Technologies 6890 N system on an HP-5MS column (0.25 mm × 30 m × 0.25 μm) with helium as carrier gas and a temperature program from 170°C to 220°C with a temperature slope of 1°C/min. Mass fragments were detected with a mass selective detector (AGILENT Technologies, Santa Clara, USA) using 70 eV ionization energy and 8 kV acceleration voltage. The configuration of monosaccharides was determined by capillary electrophoresis versus D and L references using a P/ACE 5010 Instrument (Beckman Coulter, Krefeld, Germany) with an uncoated silica capillary (77 cm × 50 μm) and DAD UV detector at 200 nm according to the method of Noe and Freissmuth, 1995 [24]. Polysaccharides were investigated in regard to esterification with IR-spectroscopy (mid-infrared) on a FT/IR-4100 type A (Jasco, Tokio, Japan) and a pectin C, which contained 70% ester bounds as reference.

2.3. Cell Culture. Confined cell lines were obtained after isolation of normal human dermal fibroblasts (NHDFs) and normal human epidermal keratinocytes (NHEKs) from human skin grafts (University Clinical Centre of Münster, Germany, Department of Dermatology, Department of Pediatrics) of various Caucasian subjects. The studies were approved by the local ethical committee of the University of Münster (acceptance no. 2006-117-f-S). Subculture of cells was done as described earlier [16, 25]. HaCaT keratinocytes, a friendly gift of Professor Fusenig, DKFZ, Heidelberg, were used for apoptosis-related experiments.

2.4. Cell Viability, Proliferation, and Differentiation. For investigation, polysaccharides were solved in Aqua Millipore to a concentration of 1 mg/mL, sterile filtered through a $0.2\,\mu$m regenerated cellulose acetate membrane, and solved in the recommended serum-free media to a final concentration of $10\,\mu$g/mL. As positive control, 10% FCS was added to test medium. All tests were realized in 96-well plates (Sarstedt, Nuembrecht, Germany) at starting cell densities of 5×10^3 NHEK and 3×10^3 NHDF in each well. Incubation with polysaccharides started 24 h after seeding when the cells had reached a confluence of 50% and ended 48 h later by adding BrdU and WST-1 reagents. BrdU incorporation assay and WST-1 and LDH assays were performed according to the manufacturer instructions (Roche Diagnostics, Penzberg, Germany). Activity of intracellular reducing enzymes was measured with MTT [26]. Apoptosis was measured after incubation of NHDF and NHEK with $10\,\mu$g/mL polysaccharide by treating with Annexin V-PE and counterstaining with 7-aminoactinomycin (7-AAD) on a FACSCalibur flow cytometer (Becton Dickinson GmbH, Heidelberg, Germany). Cells were harvested by scraping in ice-cold Annexin V binding buffer, further proceeding following manufacture description. Differentiation of NHEK was elucidated by semiquantitative determination of involucrin amounts using the dot blot technique as described earlier [25].

2.5. Protein Expression of Cells. The collagen expression of fibroblasts was analyzed by a colorimetric method based upon Sirius Red. Therefore, NHDFs were seeded in 24-well cell culture plates (Greiner, Frickenhausen, Germany) with 7×10^4 cells/well. At 70% confluence the cells were incubated with $10\,\mu$g/mL polysaccharides solved in test medium, 100 mM L-ascorbic acid was used as positive control [27]. After 48 h, the culture supernatant (0.5 mL) was transferred to an Eppendorf cup and mixed with protease inhibitor mix (Roche Diagnostics, Penzberg, Germany). NHDFs were lysed by a fivefold freeze-thaw-cycle in $200\,\mu$L 0.5 M acetic acid containing protease inhibitor mix and scraped from the plate. The resulting cell suspension was conveyed in a new Eppendorf cup. Solutions of cells and culture supernatants were stirred overnight at 4°C and afterwards centrifuged for 10 min at 14,000 x g to remove the cell debris. $50\,\mu$L of the resulting solution was mixed with $450\,\mu$L Sirius Red ($69\,\mu$g/mL, 0.5 M acetic acid), agitated for 30 min, and again centrifuged (10 min, 14 000 x g). Subsequently, the resulting pellet was solved in $50\,\mu$L 0.1 M potassium hydroxide, and the intensity of color was determined at 540 nm with a reference wavelength of 690 nm.

2.6. Gene Expression Analysis of Keratinocytes and Fibroblasts by Real-Time PCR. Analysis of cellular signal transduction effected by St. John's Wort polysaccharides was done by gene expression analysis with real-time PCR after reverse transcription of total RNA. To exclude effects of FCS

the fibroblasts were adapted to minimal MEM containing glucose (4.5 g/L) and L-glutamine (1%) but no other supplements for 12 h. $10\,\mu$g/mL polysaccharides and 10% FCS as positive control were solved in the minimal MEM prior to the incubation with NHDF for 6 h, 12 h, and 24 h. For untreated control cells fresh minimal MEM was used. After trypsinization of cells, the total RNA was isolated with the innuPREP RNA Mini Kit (Analytik Jena, Jena, Germany). After qualitative and quantitative analysis of obtained RNA with the biophotometer (Eppendorf, Hamburg, Germany) it was reverse-transcribed using the High-Capacity cDNA Reverse Transcription Kit. cDNA was diluted with RNAse-free water to 20 ng cDNA, and real-time-PCR was performed with TaqMan gene expression assays (Table 1) and the TaqMan Universal MasterMix, without AmpErase on a 7300 Real Time PCR System (all Applied Biosystems, Foster City, USA). The gene expression was calculated with the comparative Ct method.

2.7. Microarray Analysis of Gene Expression. For gene microarray analysis, NHDFs were seeded at a cell density of 5×10^5 cells/75 cm² cell culture flask (Sarstedt, Nuembrecht, Germany). At a confluence of 70% the medium was changed against minimal MEM, containing 4.5 g/L glucose as well as 1% L-glutamine and kept for 12 h to adapt cells to minimal culture conditions. For 24 h the cells were incubated with polysaccharides, solved in minimal MEM ($10\,\mu$g/mL), or only with fresh minimal MEM (control sample). After trypsinization the cells were washed with PBS and frozen in liquid nitrogen. Isolation and amplification of the RNA as well as the analysis of the gene expression via PIQOR Skin Microarray was performed by Miltenyi Biotech, Bergisch-Gladbach, Germany. For quality control the RNA integrity number (RIN) was determined with 8.2 (must be >6), indicating sufficient quality for gene expression experiments.

2.8. Statistical Analysis. Statistical evaluation was performed by Dunnett's post hoc test for comparison of three to four treatment groups after variance calculation by Levene. The results of three independent biological repeats were considered significant when the P value was less than 0.05. All data presented are the means of 24 random samples (errors bars: $\pm$SE) or representative with $n = 8$.

3. Results

3.1. Isolation and Characterization of St. John's Wort Herb Polysaccharides. Carbohydrates were isolated from defatted St. John's Wort herb in a yield of 1.3% related to the starting material. The ochre brown product was assessed to be a polysaccharide with neutral sugar content of 78%, 16% of uronic acids, and a residual protein content of 6%. According to the ionic strength of the respective elution buffer and the acidity of polysaccharides, the AEC resulted in four polysaccharide fractions further referred to as Hp1, Hp2, Hp3, and Hp4. Main amounts of polysaccharides were eluted using 0.25 M NaPB (Hp3, 47%). High acidic (0.5 M NaPB; Hp4) and low acidic polysaccharides (0.1 M NaPB; Hp2) reached values of almost 23% each. 7% of

TABLE 1: TaqMan Assay IDs (Applied Biosystems, Foster City, USA) of specific proteins and representatives of signal pathways expressed in normal human fibroblasts (NHDFs) and normal human keratinocytes (NHEKs) investigated by real-time PCR after treatment with 10 μg/mL St. John's Wort herb polysaccharide fractions.

Gene	Function	TaqMan Assay ID
Epidermal growth factor receptor (EGFR)	Proliferation	Hs01076068m1
Fibroblast growth factor 7 (FGF7)	Proliferation	Hs00384281_m1
Insulin receptor (InsR)	Survival/proliferation	Hs00169631m1
Involucrin (Inv)	Differentiation-specific protein	Hs00846307s1
Signal transducer and activator of transcription 6 (STAT6)	IL-4 signal transduction	Hs00598618_m1
Phospholipase α (PLA2)	Ca^{2+} signaling	Hs00179898_m1
Human 18s rRNA (18s)	Endogenous control	Hs99999901s1

polysaccharides were received by water elution (Hp1). The proportion of neutral sugars in the particular AEC fractions was determined as 93% (Hp1), 69% (Hp2), 63% (Hp3), and 47% (Hp4). By HPEAC-PAD uronic acids were identified and quantified as galacturonic acid and glucuronic acid. Protein analysis revealed protein amounts of 4% (Hp1), 6% (Hp2), 5% (Hp3), and 8% (Hp4). The reaction with Yarif-reagent showed that the protein amounts originate from arabinogalactan proteins (AGP) in fractions Hp2 (75%), Hp3 (3%), and Hp4 (3%) but not in fraction Hp1. Structural analysis was done after derivatization of hydrolyzed polysaccharides to silylated (TMS) derivates and permethylated alditol acetates (PMAA) followed by gas chromatographic separation and mass spectrometric detection. TMS derivatives were identified as arabinose, galactose, and glucose as well as rhamnose, xylose and mannose. Arabinose and galactose were present in a ratio of 1 : 1 in all fractions being the main monosaccharides in AGP containing fractions whereas Hp1 mainly contained glucose. Rhamnose was only present in amounts more than 10% in Hp2 and Hp4. Xylose and mannose were detected in minor amounts. In all fractions arabinose was found as terminal, $(1 \rightarrow 5)$, and 1,3,5 linked. The acidic fractions Hp2, Hp3, and Hp4 contained rhamnose linked in terminal, $(1 \rightarrow 2)$, and 1,2,3-linked forms. Xylose was linked in $(1 \rightarrow 2)$ position and terminal in Hp1. All fractions contained $(1 \rightarrow 4)$-linked mannose and $(1 \rightarrow 4)$-linked glucose but the test for starch was negative. Especially in Hp1 glucose was also linked in positions $(1 \rightarrow 6)$, terminal, $(1 \rightarrow 2)$, and 1,4,6. $(1 \rightarrow 3)$-, $(1 \rightarrow 6)$-, and 1,3,6-linked galactose was detected in all fractions as well as $(1 \rightarrow 4)$ linked glucuronic acid. Galacturonic acid was found as $(1 \rightarrow 3)$, $(3 \rightarrow 6)$, or 1,4,6 linked (Table 2). Capillary electrophoresis revealed an L-configuration of arabinose and D-configuration of xylose, galactose, and glucose. Infrared spectrometry revealed that the galacturonic containing fractions exhibited absorptions at wavenumbers 1233 cm^{-1} and 1733 cm^{-1} in consequence of a partial esterification of the galacturonic acid residues.

3.2. Influence of St. John's Wort Herb Polysaccharides on Cell Physiology of Human Keratinocytes.
The proliferation of NHEK was marginally influenced by each polysaccharide fraction with less than 20%. Contrary to the polysaccharides of fractions Hp1, Hp2, and Hp4, the polysaccharides of Hp3

reduced the proliferation rates. MTT test revealed a slight but not significant increase of intracellular reducing enzymes activity after treatment of NHEK with all polysaccharide fractions. Necrotic effects of St. John's Wort herb polysaccharides were not observed on keratinocytes. Just weak apoptotic effects were observed with exception of HaCaT keratinocytes that were incubated with polysaccharides of fraction Hp3 (Table 3) whereas this effect was not significant.

After prolonged incubation time, NHEKs showed morphological changes in consequence of an incipient differentiation. For that after nine days the cellular proteins were extracted followed by a semi-quantitative determination of the differentiation-specific protein involucrin using dot blot technique.

As shown in Figure 1 the involucrin expression was significantly enhanced by polysaccharides of Hp1 whereas the other polysaccharide fractions had no significant influence.

The large variations resulted from the different behavior of normal cells due to their diverse sources. First investigation of gene expression of differentiation-specific proteins and proliferation-related pathways indicated that after short incubation time of 6 h the involucrin gene expression is not altered independent of the used polysaccharide fraction for treatment. But in case of Hp1, which showed the most impact on the differentiation, the gene expression of proliferation-related genes like EGFR and InsR was inhibited. The decrease in PLA2 expression that is part of the Ca^{2+} signaling and for that involved in the differentiation process revealed that the differentiation of NHEK is induced in a different way (Table 4).

3.3. Reactivity of Normal Human Dermal Fibroblasts to Polysaccharides of St. John's Wort Herb.
Polysaccharide fractions of St. John's Wort herb did not influence the activity of reducing enzymes in the cells as measured by MTT reduction assay. But as shown in Figure 2 the extracellular enzymes of Hp1-, Hp3-, and Hp4-treated NHDF reduced significantly more WST-1 than the untreated cells. The proliferation of NHDF was significantly stimulated by polysaccharide fraction Hp4 and reduced by high glucose amount containing fraction Hp1. Fractions Hp2, and Hp3 had no influence on the proliferation. Cytotoxic activity was not observed. Even the amount of necrotic cells was reduced compared to the untreated cells (0%): −2% in case of Hp2, Hp3 and Hp4

TABLE 2: Results of methylation analysis and AGP determination of St. John's Wort polysaccharides. Data indicate the respective molar composition [%], calculated from results of HPAEC-PAD and silylation analysis. AGP amounts were detected by the agar diffusion test according to van Holst and Clarke, 1985 [20].

	Hp1	Hp2	Hp3	Hp4
1-Ara	6	23	6	1
1,2-Ara		1		1
1,3-Ara	3		2	
1,5-Ara	6	5	12	10
1,3,5-Ara	2	3	1	2
1,2,3-Ara			2	3
1,2,5-Ara	2		1	7
1,3,4,5-Ara			1	
Arapent			1	
1-Rha		1	3	4
1,2 Rha		1	2	2
3,4/1,4-Rha		9		2
1,2,3-Rha		1	2	6
1-Xyl	1			
1,2-Xyl	1	1		1
1,3,5-Xyl			1	
1-Man				1
1,4-Man	2	2	3	3
1,4,6-Man	1		1	
1-Glc	7			1
1,3-Glc	5			2
1,4-Glc	11	1	1	3
1,6-Glc	26		2	1
1,2,4-Glc	2			
1,4,6-Glc	3			1
1-Gal	1	1	1	
1,3-Gal	2	1	3	3
1,6-Gal	5	5	5	3
3,6-Gal	1		1	1
1,2,4-Gal			1	1
1,4,6-Gal	3	2		1
1,3,6-Gal	6	23	21	5
1,3,4,6-Gal	1		2	1
1,4-GlcAc	3	18	8	6
1,3-GalAc			17	
3,6-GalAc				15
1,3,6-GalAc		2		
1,2,4-GalAc				13
AGP amount [%]	0	75	3	3

and −12% if NHDF. Apoptotic processes in NHDF were not affected by St. John's Wort polysaccharides. In Hp1-treated NHDF −12% ± 10 of apoptotic cells were detected, NHDF incubated with Hp2, and Hp3 exhibited −8% ± 6 respective −8% ± 8 of apoptotic cells while Hp4 had no influence (1% ± 24).

Collagen synthesis and release as parameter of fibroblast activity was measured indirectly by determination of hydroxyproline amounts with Direct Red 80 in cells and cell culture supernatant. Compared to untreated control fibroblasts the collagen release was significantly stimulated if NHDFs were incubated with each polysaccharide fraction but in

TABLE 3: Influence of St. John's Wort polysaccharides on cell physiology of keratinocytes (NEHK and HaCaT). Results were normalized to the untreated cells calculated as 0%. Proliferation was determined by BrdU incorporation ELISA. MTT reduction assay was performed to investigate the intracellular enzyme activity. The cytotoxicity was determined by calculating the extracellular LDH activity compared to total LDH activity according to the manufacturer instructions. Apoptosis was measured by flow cytometry using Annexin V and 7-AAD.

Polysaccharide fraction	Proliferation rate (NHEK)	Intracellular enzyme activity (NHEK)	Amount of necrotic cells (NHEK)	Amount of apoptotic cells (HaCaT)
Hp1	16% ± 8	17% ± 7	0%	13% ± 11
Hp2	16% ± 9	23% ± 7	4%	15% ± 10
Hp3	−17% ± 8	21% ± 10	8%	21% ± 9
Hp4	10% ± 7	13% ± 6	5%	6% ± 3

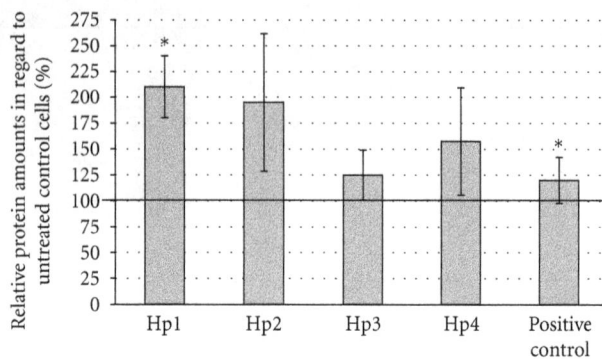

FIGURE 1: Expression of differentiation-specific protein involucrin of NHEK after treatment with 10 μg/mL St. John's Wort polysaccharide fractions for nine days. Protein amounts were determined by semiquantitative dot blot technique. Obtained values with n = 8 were normalized to untreated NHEK (—: untreated NHEK = 100%). To induce the differentiation, the serum-starved MCDB 153 complete media were supplemented with 13 μg/mL A23187 and 2 mM Ca^{2+} (positive control).

TABLE 4: Gene expression of NHEK after 6 h of incubation with 10 μg/mL St. John's Wort polysaccharides in serum-starved media. Results of RT-PCR with TaqMan Assays were normalized to endogenous control 18srRNA and to respective target gene expression of untreated control cells. Regulation was defined as significant with >2 (+) and <0.5 (−). No change in gene expression is shown as "o".

	Involucrin	PLA2	EGFR	InsR
Hp1	o	−	−	−
Hp2	o	o	o	o
Hp3	o	o	o	o
Hp4	o	+	o	o

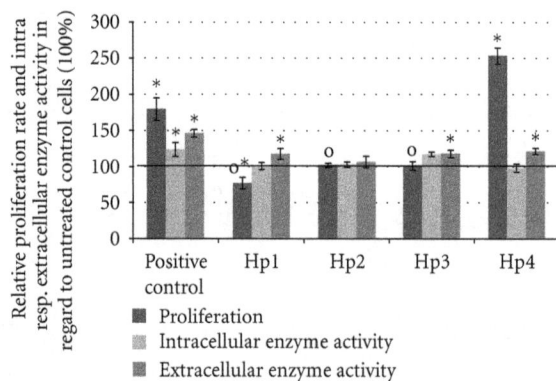

FIGURE 2: Results of relative proliferation (BrdU incorporation, representative with n = 8) and intracellular (MTT-reduction) and extracellular enzyme activity (WST-1 reduction) of NHDF treated with 10 μg/mL St. John's Wort polysaccharides for 48 h. As positive control, 10% FCS was used. Values were normalized to untreated cells (—: untreated control = 100%). n = 24. Error bars = SE; *P < 0.05 compared to untreated cells and o: P < 0.05 to Hp4.

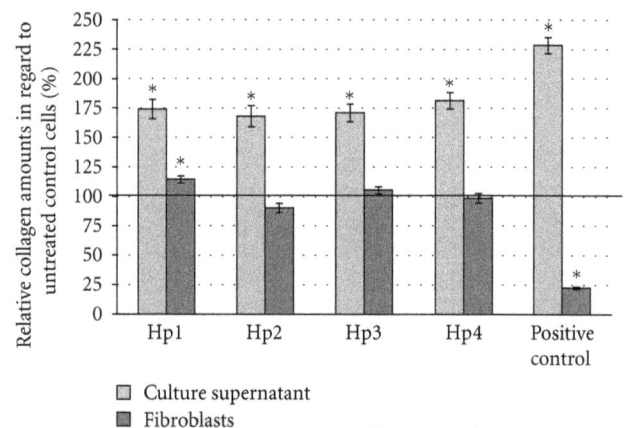

FIGURE 3: Relative amounts of acid soluble collagen of fibroblast culture supernatants and fibroblasts after incubation with 100 mM L-ascorbic acid as positive control and polysaccharide fractions (10 μg/mL). Results were indirectly calculated by determination of hydroxyproline with Direct Red 80. Values shown are normalized to collagen amounts in supernatants and cells of untreated control (—: untreated control = 100%). *P < 0.05 compared to untreated cells; n = 4. Error bars = SE.

less amounts compared to L-ascorbic-acid-treated NHDF (positive control). The amount of remaining intracellular collagen soluble within acetic acid was significantly increased if NHDFs were incubated with Hp1 but was not altered after incubation with polysaccharide fractions Hp3 and Hp4. Polysaccharides of Hp2 slightly reduced the intracellular acidic collagen amounts (Figure 3).

TABLE 5: Gene expression of NHDF after incubation with 10 μg/mL St. John's Wort polysaccharide fractions in minimal MEM for 6 h, 12 h, and 24 h. Results of RT-PCR with TaqMan assays were normalized to endogenous control 18 srRNA and to the respected expression of target genes in untreated control cells. Regulation was defined as significant with >2 (+) and <0.5 (−). No change in gene expression is shown as "o".

Polysaccharide fraction	EGFR	STAT6	FGF7	Incubation time
Hp1	−	−	−	
Hp2	o	o	o	
Hp3	o	o	o	6 h
Hp4	o	o	o	
Hp1	o	o	o	
Hp2	+	o	o	
Hp3	o	o	+	12 h
Hp4	o	o	+	
Hp1	−	o	−	
Hp2	+	o	−	
Hp3	o	o	−	24 h
Hp4	o	o	o	

3.4. Influence on the Gene Expression of NHDF. NHDF were incubated for 6 h, 12 h, and 24 h with St. John's Wort herb polysaccharide fractions. The epidermal growth factor receptor (EGFR) was not affected by Hp3 and Hp4 independent of the incubation time while an increase in gene expression was observed after 12 h of incubation with Hp2. Hp1 repressed the EGFR gene expression after 6 h and 24 h of incubation. The gene expression of the fibroblast growth factor 7 (FGF7) depended on incubation time and used polysaccharide fraction. At 6 h of incubation the gene expression was reduced by Hp1 and not changed by the other fractions. If the incubation was prolonged for 6 h an upregulation occurred if the NHDFs were treated with Hp3 and Hp4 but after 24 h this effect inverted. Incubation of Hp2 resulted in a downregulation of FGF7 gene expression but only after 24 h. The gene expression of the signal transducer and activator of transcription 6 (STAT6) involved in the signaling of IL-4 was not changed by Hp2, Hp3, and Hp4 independent of incubation time. During the first 6 h of incubation Hp1 reduced the STAT6 gene expression but this effect was reverted if the incubation time was prolonged (Table 5).

Gene expression analysis by RT-PCR did not explain the activity of St. John's Wort polysaccharide fractions on NHDF. To get an idea which signal pathways were altered a microarray analysis was carried out. For the microarray analysis polysaccharides of AEC fraction Hp4 were chosen exemplarily because of their prominent effect on NHDF proliferation. DNA microarray indicated that the expression of 142 of 1308 genes in total changed after incubation for 24 h. But a significant regulation (>2 and <0.5 compared to untreated cells) was only found in case of 44 genes (Table 6). These genes were part of cellular processes like inflammation/stress response, transcription, metabolism, cell adhesion/extracellular matrix, and receptor

signaling. Mostly an increase in gene expression occurred but the genes related to receptor signaling were predominantly downregulated. This coincides with the results of RT-PCR analysis concerning the gene expression of EGFR and KGF. Furthermore, the microarray revealed no influence on the cytokine signaling as it had been shown by RT-PCR with STAT6. In more detail prominent changes (>2) in gene expression were observed in case of genes that referred to cellular processes like inflammation (IKBE, FEN1, CXCL1), response to toxins (CMTM7, BGLAP), oxidative stress (SOD2, MUTYH), metabolism (NNMT), extracellular matrix (HSPG2), transcription (HOXD10, EXOSC10), cell motility (ACTG2) and of unknown function (LOC387763, C9ORF16). To a less extent but still significant was the up-regulation of genes referring to metabolism and transcription as well as cell adhesion and extracellular matrix as shown in Table 6. Additionally to genes related to receptor signalling (INHBC, CD16, GJB6, ZAP70) the gene expression of IL17A, C-FOS, AFM, CYP3A7, MMP7, and SPARCL1 was significantly decreased. No influence was observed concerning apoptosis, MAPK pathways, TNF signalling, mitochondria-associated metabolism, calcium signalling, cytoskeleton and translation-related processes.

4. Discussion

The presented results show that polysaccharide fractions denominated as Hp1, Hp2, Hp3, and Hp4 differ in acidity, monosaccharide composition, monosaccharide linkage, and their influence on human skin cells.

The polysaccharides belong to water-soluble hemicelluloses, nonswelling pectin, and arabinogalactan proteins (AGPs). In detail the most obvious difference was seen in fraction Hp1 that was composed of a high amount of glucose. Since the test with Lugol solution that only reacts with helical linked α-D-glucose, was negative, the glucose must be part of a β-D-glucan [28]. In regard to 1 : 1 ratio and linkage of galactose and arabinose a coexistence of an arabinogalactan is likely a result of the limited separation according to the polysaccharide acidity. For the same reason the acidic polysaccharide fractions Hp2, Hp3, and Hp4 would contain more than one polysaccharide. According to the positive reaction with the Yarif reagent, linkage of arabinose and galactose residues and their proportion pointed to the occurrence of arabinogalactan proteins (AGPs). Furthermore the ratio and linkage of arabinose, rhamnose, galactose, and galacturonic acid as well as the esterification of galacturonic acid indicates the presence of pectic structures. The increasing amounts of galacturonic acid and the different linkage types point to structural differences [29, 30]. To confirm these data the fractions must be purified and structurally characterized by NMR within future investigations.

Nevertheless the cell-based investigations showed that the polysaccharide fractions affect the skin cells corresponding to their composition and linkage of monosaccharide residues. Obvious was that polysaccharides of fraction Hp1 had the most efficient activity on NHEK differentiation and collagen synthesis of NHDF compared to the other polysaccharide fractions. According to previous investigations it is

TABLE 6: Summary of genes with significantly changed expression (>1.7, <0.5) from 1308 genes in total within gene expression analysis using topic-defined PIQOR skin microarray (Miltenyi Biotech, Cologne, Germany) from NHDF after treatment with polysaccharides of Hp4 (10 μg/mL) compared to an untreated control (=1) for 24 h.

Gene	Description and function according to NCBI gene database	Relative regulation (SD %)
Miscellaneous		
LOC387763	LOC387763 protein (unknown)	2.70/9%
C9ORF16	C9ORF16 (unknown)	2.37/21%
ACTG2	Gamma-2-actin (cell motility)	2.01/29%
GJB6	Connexin 30 (hyperproliferation)	0.48/32%
Cell adhesion and extracellular matrix		
HSPG2	Perlecan	3.05/33%
L1CAM	L1 cell adhesion molecule	1.93/13%
FGF11	Fibroblast growth factor 11	1.93/13%
PTK7	Protein-tyrosine kinase 7	1.78/19%
FAT	Cadherin-related tumor suppressor	1.73/13%
SPARCL1	SPARC-like protein 1	0.48/22%
MMP7	Matrilysin	0.42/14%
Metabolism		
NNMT	Nicotinamide N-methyltransferase	2.83/17%
CA12_2	Carbonic anhydrase XII	1.98/11%
SLC20A1	Member of solute carrier family 20 (phosphate transporter)	1.89/10%
MDH1	Cytoplasmic malate dehydrogenase	1.84/21%
CFTR	cAMP-dependent chloride channel	1.80/4%
GLUT1	Solute carrier family 2 member 1 (facilitated glucose transporter)	1.78/29%
PEG1-MEST	Mesoderm-specific transcript homolog (mouse)	1.71/17%
CYP3A7	Cytochrome P450 3A7	0.47/23%
AFM	Afamin (α-albumin)	0.33/15%
Receptor signaling		
NRP1	Neuropilin-1 (CD304 Antigen)	1.79/26%
INHBC	Inhibin βC	0.46/19%
CD16	IGG FC receptor III-2	0.43/21%
ZAP70	Zeta-chain (TCR) associated protein kinase 70 kDa	0.41/24%
Transcription		
EXOSC10	Exosome component 10	2.96/37%
HOXD10	Homeobox D10	2.04/20%
SRRM2	Serine/arginine-rich splicing factor-related nuclear matrix protein of 300 kDa	1.92/33%
MAZ	MYC-associated zinc finger protein (purine-binding transcription factor)	1.91/17%
ANKRD11	Ankyrin repeat domain 11	1.81/23%
MRPL28	Mitochondrial ribosomal protein L28	1.74/15%
C-FOS	G0/G1 switch regulatory protein 7	0.21/1%

TABLE 6: Continued.

Gene	Description and function according to NCBI gene database	Relative regulation (SD %)
Inflammation, stress, and DNA repair		
SOD2	Mitochondrial superoxide dismutase 2	4.78/22%
CMTM7	CKLF-like MARVEL transmembrane domain-containing protein 7	3.86/38%
CXCL1	Chemokine (C-X-C motif) ligand 1	3.33/18%
IKBE	Nuclear factor of kappa light polypeptide gene enhancer in B-cells inhibitor, epsilon	3.18/38%
FEN1	Flap structure-specific endonuclease 1	2.34/11%
BGLAP	Bone gamma-carboxyglutamate (gla) protein	2.07/10%
MUTYH	A/G-specific adenine DNA glycosylase	2.05/20%
BTF2P44	Basic transcription factor 2 44 kDa subunit	1.99/18%
IKBA	Nuclear factor of kappa light polypeptide gene enhancer in B-cells inhibitor, alpha	1.89/5%
SERPIN 1	Serine proteinase inhibitor	1.83/6%
XBP1	X-box binding protein 1	1.73/12%
HSP90B1	Endoplasmin (heat shock protein 90 b1)	1.73/21%
POLH	Polymerase eta (DNA directed)	1.70/20%
IL17A	Interleukin 17	0.45/20%

SD: standard deviations from $n = 4$ replicates of three biologic repeats.

more likely that the β-D-glucan is responsible for this effect than the arabinogalactan. Arabinogalactans as well as AGPs have mostly shown to influence the proliferation of different cell types [7, 16, 30–32] while a similar β-D-glucan has proven to induce the differentiation of NHEK differentiation. We previously observed this effect in a study about Reed mace fruit polysaccharides [25]. Gene expression studies with keratinocytes and fibroblasts pointed to an influence of Hp1 on differentiation and proliferation processes by down-regulation of genes for growth factors (FGF7), growth factor receptors (EGFRs), and insulin receptor (InsR), which are involved in promotion of proliferation and migration [13]. Especially a decreased EGFR signaling promotes epidermal differentiation [33]. Interestingly the differentiation was not influenced via PLA2 known to regulate the differentiation of keratinocytes [14]. Polysaccharide fractions Hp2, Hp3, and Hp4 were composed of AGP and pectic structures of different composition and linkage. AGPs as well as pectins are known to be biologically active in regard to their specific structure [30, 34]. The data of the present study does not allow to allocate the biologic activities neither to a specific AGP nor to a distinct pectic structure. However, it appeared that minor differences concerning linkage and amounts of monosaccharides are responsible for the different activity of these three polysaccharide fractions. Since differences in monosaccharide linkage will alter the structure of the whole polymer the polysaccharides of Hp4 differed from the polysaccharides of fractions Hp2 and Hp3. Treatment of fibroblasts with these three acidic fractions caused a stimulation of the proliferation rates only in case of fraction Hp4. Additionally, ANOVA analysis revealed that this effect

was significant not only to untreated control cells but also to the effect of the other polysaccharide fractions. Gene expression analysis by RT-PCR revealed additional difference in their activity on cellular gene level. The effect of Hp4 polysaccharides on the fibroblast proliferation was not based on an influence on the gene expression of growth factors or their receptors as RT-PCR and microarray analysis revealed. At the investigated time point the predominant upregulation pertained to genes that refer to processes involved in oxidative stress (SOD2), response to toxins (CMTM7), and DNA repair (BGLAP). For that it is possible that the increased proliferation is due to a hyperproliferation as stress response. But the down regulation of connexin 30 (GJB6), a marker for hyperproliferation [35], and C-FOS, the lack of induction of inflammation-specific proteins like hypoxia inducible factor 1α (HIF1A), catalase (CAT), LPS binding protein (LPB), soluble epoxide hydrolase (EPHX2), chaperons and proinflammatory cytokines that are additionally part of the microarray contradict this hypothesis. Additionally the unaltered activity of reducing or antioxidative enzymes in the cells as determined with MTT test disagrees with a cellular response to oxidative stress.

The upregulation of the cytoplasmic malate dehydrogenase (MDH1) is interesting for its involvement in the carbohydrate metabolism. This and the fact that the other regulated genes are involved in transport mechanisms (CFTR, GLUT1, and AFM), drug metabolism (CYP3A7, PEG1-MEST, and NNMT) transcription processes (EXOSC10, HOXD10, SRRM2, ANKRD11, and MAZ) led to the hypothesis that the polysaccharides were internalized and catabolized by the cells and that the influence on the cells derives from inside and not outside the cell. According to the significant increase in extracellular enzyme activity the catabolism of polysaccharides may already start outside the cell followed by internalization. An internalization of an arabinogalactan with similar activity on cellular processes on gene level has been shown recently [32]. For that future studies must show if the polysaccharides were internalized or if they were degraded on the cell surface. Anyway the proliferation process is also influenced from outside the cell. The significantly upregulated genes of neuropilin (NRP1) and fibroblast growth factor 11 (FGF11) point to an influence of Hp4 polysaccharides on the FGF signaling [36]. Moreover, the proliferation process is influenced by other signal pathways as indicated by the regulation of perlecan (HSPG2), matrilysin (MMP7), and SPARC-like protein1 (SPARCL1). Another way to support the cell proliferation is to maintain cell adhesion and migration. So it is not surprising that the L1 adhesion molecule (L1CAM) and the cadherin-related tumor suppressor homolog (FAT) gene expression was affected by Hp4 polysaccharides. The regulation of gene expression may vary over the incubation time as mostly late signal pathway steps were affected. So shortening of incubation time for gene expression studies will show a different pattern of gene expression shifted towards earlier signaling processes and extracellular proteins [37]. The lacking influence on collagen expression coincides with unchanged intracellular collagen amounts indicating no increased or induced collagen synthesis.

Present results show that polysaccharides of different composition and linkage influence human skin cells in different ways. Gene expression studies support the physiologic data and reveal a foundation for the underlying mechanisms of polysaccharide activity.

5. Conclusion

Concluding, the water-soluble polysaccharides isolated and characterized from St. John's Wort herb are similar to already described water-soluble plant polysaccharides. Anyway the high β-D-glucose content and linkage of neutral AEC fraction Hp1 are characteristic for St. John's Wort herb and uncommon for already described polysaccharides of dicotyledons. Cell physiological investigations showed that the polysaccharides of Hp1 differ not only in their structure but also in their biological activity from the other extracted polysaccharides. Furthermore, the results obtained with acidic polysaccharides illustrate that slight structural differences lead to obvious differences in the biologic activity. However, future studies are necessary to determine the effective polysaccharide structure. Nevertheless, the presented data demonstrate that polysaccharides play a role in the effect of St. John's Wort extracts on skin cells.

Acknowledgments

The authors thank Dr. Lohse, Department of Paediatric Surgery, University of Münster, for support with dermal resectates and Mrs. Possemeyer for technical assistance (Institute for Pharmaceutical Biology and Phytochemistry, University of Münster). The study was financially supported by Professor Hensel, Institute for Pharmaceutical Biology and Phytochemistry, University of Münster.

References

[1] V. Butterweck and A. Nahrstedt, "What is known about St John's wort? Phytochemistry and pharmacology," *Pharmazie in Unserer Zeit*, vol. 32, no. 3, pp. 212–219, 2003.

[2] S. Onoue, Y. Seto, M. Ochi et al., "*In vitro* photochemical and phototoxicological characterization of major constituents in St. John's Wort (*Hypericum perforatum*) extracts," *Phytochemistry*, vol. 72, pp. 1814–1820, 2011.

[3] M. C. Meinke, S. Schanzer, S. F. Haag et al., "*In vivo* photoprotective and anti-inflammatory effect of hyperforin is associated with high antioxidant activity *in vitro* and *ex vivo*," *European Journal of Pharmaceutics and Biopharmaceutics*, vol. 81, no. 2, pp. 346–350, 2012.

[4] M. Müller, K. Essin, K. Hill et al., "Specific TRPC6 channel activation, a novel approach to stimulate keratinocyte differentiation," *The Journal of Biological Chemistry*, vol. 283, no. 49, pp. 33942–33954, 2008.

[5] C. M. Schempp, T. Windeck, S. Hezel, and J. C. Simon, "Topical treatment of atopic dermatitis with St. John's wort cream—a randomized, placebo controlled, double blind half-side comparison," *Phytomedicine*, vol. 10, no. 4, pp. 31–37, 2003.

[6] S. G. von Eggelkraut-Gottanka, S. Abu Abed, W. Müller, and P. C. Schmidt, "Quantitative analysis of the active components and the by-products of eight dry extracts of *Hypericum perforatum* L. (St John's Wort)," *Phytochemical Analysis*, vol. 13, no. 3, pp. 170–176, 2002.

[7] C. S. Nergard, T. Matsumoto, M. Inngjerdingen et al., "Structural and immunological studies of a pectin and a pectic arabinogalactan from *Vernonia kotschyana* Sch. Bip. ex Walp. (Asteraceae)," *Carbohydrate Research*, vol. 340, no. 1, pp. 115–130, 2005.

[8] C. Lengsfeld, F. Titgemeyer, G. Faller, and A. Hensel, "Glycosylated compounds from okra inhibit adhesion of *Helicobacter pylori* to human gastric mucosa," *Journal of Agricultural and Food Chemistry*, vol. 52, no. 6, pp. 1495–1503, 2004.

[9] X. Shu, X. Liu, C. Fu, and Q. Liang, "Extraction, characterization and antitumor effect of the polysaccharides from star anise (*Illicium verum* Hook. f.)," *Journal of Medicinal Plant Research*, vol. 4, no. 24, pp. 2666–2673, 2010.

[10] G. Biagini, A. Bertani, R. Muzzarelli et al., "Wound management with N-carboxybutyl chitosan," *Biomaterials*, vol. 12, no. 3, pp. 281–286, 1991.

[11] S. P. Liu, W. G. Dong, D. F. Wu, H. S. Luo, and J. P. Yu, "Protective effect of *Angelica sinensis* polysaccharide on experimental immunological colon injury in rats," *World Journal of Gastroenterology*, vol. 9, no. 12, pp. 2786–2790, 2003.

[12] G. Peterszegi, N. Isnard, A. M. Robert, and L. Robert, "Studies on skin aging. Preparation and properties of fucose-rich oligo- and polysaccharides. Effect on fibroblast proliferation and survival," *Biomedicine and Pharmacotherapy*, vol. 57, no. 5-6, pp. 187–194, 2003.

[13] V. Mitev and L. Miteva, "Signal transduction in keratinocytes," *Experimental Dermatology*, vol. 8, no. 2, pp. 96–108, 1999.

[14] J. Zhou, J. G. Haggerty, and L. M. Milstone, "Growth and differentiation regulate CD44 expression on human keratinocytes," *In vitro Cellular and Developmental Biology*, vol. 35, no. 4, pp. 228–235, 1999.

[15] M. B. Yaffe, H. Beegen, and R. L. Eckert, "Biophysical characterization of involucrin reveals a molecule ideally suited to function as an intermolecular cross-bridge of the keratinocyte cornified envelope," *The Journal of Biological Chemistry*, vol. 267, no. 17, pp. 12233–12238, 1992.

[16] A. M. Deters, K. R. Schröder, and A. Hensel, "Kiwi fruit (*Actinidia chinensis* L.) polysaccharides exert stimulating effects on cell proliferation via enhanced growth factor receptors, energy production, and collagen synthesis of human keratinocytes, fibroblasts, and skin equivalents," *Journal of Cellular Physiology*, vol. 202, no. 3, pp. 717–722, 2005.

[17] M. Monsigny, C. Petit, and A. C. Roche, "Colorimetric determination of neutral sugars by a resorcinol sulfuric acid micromethod," *Analytical Biochemistry*, vol. 175, no. 2, pp. 525–530, 1988.

[18] N. Blumenkrantz and G. Asboe Hansen, "New method for quantitative determination of uronic acids," *Analytical Biochemistry*, vol. 54, no. 2, pp. 484–489, 1973.

[19] M. M. Bradford, "A rapid and sensitive method for the quantitation of microgram quantities of protein utilizing the principle of protein dye binding," *Analytical Biochemistry*, vol. 72, no. 1-2, pp. 248–254, 1976.

[20] G. J. Van Holst and A. E. Clarke, "Quantification of arabinogalactan-protein in plant extracts by single radial gel diffusion," *Analytical Biochemistry*, vol. 148, no. 2, pp. 446–450, 1985.

[21] S. I. Hakomori, "A rapid permethylation of glycolipid, and polysaccharide catalyzed by methylsulfinyl carbanion in dimethyl sulfoxide," *Journal of Biochemistry*, vol. 55, no. 2, pp. 205–208, 1964.

[22] P. J. Harris, R. J. Henry, A. B. Blakeney, and B. A. Stone, "An improved procedure for the methylation analysis of oligosaccharides and polysaccharides," *Carbohydrate Research*, vol. 127, no. 1, pp. 59–73, 1984.

[23] R. L. Taylor and H. E. Conrad, "Stoichiometric depolymerization of polyuronides and glycosaminoglycuronans to monosaccharides following reduction of their carbodiimide-activated carboxyl groups," *Biochemistry*, vol. 11, no. 8, pp. 1383–1388, 1972.

[24] C. R. Noe and J. Freissmuth, "Capillary zone electrophoresis of aldose enantiomers: separation after derivatization with S-(−)-1-phenylethylamine," *Journal of Chromatography A*, vol. 704, no. 2, pp. 503–512, 1995.

[25] K. Gescher and A. M. Deters, "*Typha latifolia* L. fruit polysaccharides induce the differentiation and stimulate the proliferation of human keratinocytes *in vitro*," *Journal of Ethnopharmacology*, vol. 137, pp. 352–358, 2011.

[26] T. Mosmann, "Rapid colorimetric assay for cellular growth and survival: application to proliferation and cytotoxicity assays," *Journal of Immunological Methods*, vol. 65, no. 1-2, pp. 55–63, 1983.

[27] J. M. Davidson, P. A. LuValle, O. Zoia, D. Quaglino Jr., and M. Giro, "Ascorbate differentially regulates elastin and collagen biosynthesis in vascular smooth muscle cells and skin fibroblasts by pretranslational mechanisms," *The Journal of Biological Chemistry*, vol. 272, no. 1, pp. 345–352, 1997.

[28] D. Reis, B. Vian, D. Darzens, and J. C. Roland, "Sequential patterns of intramural digestion of galactoxyloglucan in tamarind seedlings," *Planta*, vol. 170, no. 1, pp. 60–73, 1987.

[29] D. Mohnen, "Pectin structure and biosynthesis," *Current Opinion in Plant Biology*, vol. 11, no. 3, pp. 266–277, 2008.

[30] B. S. Paulsen and H. Barsett, "Bioactive pectic polysaccharides," *Advances in Polymer Science*, vol. 186, pp. 69–101, 2005.

[31] G. J. Seifert and K. Roberts, "The biology of arabinogalactan proteins," *Annual Review of Plant Biology*, vol. 58, pp. 137–161, 2007.

[32] J. Zippel, A. Deters, D. Pappai, and A. Hensel, "A high molecular arabinogalactan from *Ribes nigrum* L.: influence on cell physiology of human skin fibroblasts and keratinocytes and internalization into cells via endosomal transport," *Carbohydrate Research*, vol. 344, no. 8, pp. 1001–1008, 2009.

[33] S. Getsios, C. L. Simpson, S. I. Kojima et al., "Desmoglein 1-dependent suppression of EGFR signaling promotes epidermal differentiation and morphogenesis," *Journal of Cell Biology*, vol. 185, no. 7, pp. 1243–1258, 2009.

[34] B. Westereng, T. E. Michaelsen, A. B. Samuelsen, and S. H. Knutsen, "Effects of extraction conditions on the chemical structure and biological activity of white cabbage pectin," *Carbohydrate Polymers*, vol. 72, no. 1, pp. 32–42, 2008.

[35] G. Lemaître, V. Sivan, J. Lamartine et al., "Connexin 30, a new marker of hyperproliferative epidermis," *British Journal of Dermatology*, vol. 155, no. 4, pp. 844–846, 2006.

[36] T. P. Yamaguchi and J. Rossant, "Fibroblast growth factors in mammalian development," *Current Opinion in Genetics and Development*, vol. 5, no. 4, pp. 485–491, 1995.

[37] A. Balsalobre, F. Damiola, and U. Schibler, "A serum shock induces circadian gene expression in mammalian tissue culture cells," *Cell*, vol. 93, no. 6, pp. 929–937, 1998.

12

Anxiolytic and Antidepressant-Like Effects of the Aqueous Extract of *Alafia multiflora* Stem Barks in Rodents

Harquin Simplice Foyet,[1] David Emery Tsala,[2] Armand Abdou Bouba,[1] and Lucian Hritcu[3]

[1] *Department of Agriculture, Livestock and By-Products, The Higher Institute of the Sahel, University of Maroua,*
P.O. Box 46, Maroua, Cameroon
[2] *Department of Life and Earth Sciences, Higher Teachers' Training College, University of Maroua, P.O. Box 55, Maroua, Cameroon*
[3] *Department of Biology, Alexandru Ioan Cuza University, Bou/evard Carol I 11, 700506 Iasi, Romania*

Correspondence should be addressed to Harquin Simplice Foyet, fharquins@yahoo.fr

Academic Editor: Alison Oliveto

The present study examined the anxiolytic and antidepressant effects of the aqueous extract of *Alafia multiflora Stapf* (AM) stem barks (150 and 300 mg/kg, 7 days administration) on rats and mice, using experimental paradigms of anxiety and depression. In the open field, the aqueous extract increased significantly the number of center square crossed and the time spent at the center of the field as well as the rearing time, while the grooming time was reduced significantly. In the elevated plus maze, the aqueous extract increased the time spent and the number of entries in the open arms. All these effects were also completely reversed by flumazenil, an antagonist of benzodiazepine receptors and pindolol a β-adrenoceptors blocker/5-HT 1A/1B receptor antagonist. The time spent in the light compartment, the latency time, and the number of the light-dark transitions increased significantly in the light/dark exploration test after the treatment with AM. The extract was able to reduce significantly the immobility time and increase swimming as well as climbing duration. Taken together, the present work evidenced anxiolytic effects of the aqueous extract of AM that might involve an action on benzodiazepine-type receptors and an antidepressant effect where noradrenergic mechanisms will probably play a role.

1. Introduction

Anxiety and depressive disorders are frequent psychiatric conditions identified as the most common stress-related mood disorders causing disability and premature death. More than 20% of the adult population suffer from these conditions at some time during their life [1]. The World Health Organization envisaged that depression will become the second leading cause of premature death or disability worldwide by the year 2020 [2]. The complexity of daily life in modern society leads to various degrees of anxiety and depression. Mood, depression, and anxiety disorders have been found to be associated with chronic pain among medical patients in both developed and developing countries [3]. For many years, they were considered as two different mental diseases, with the benzodiazepines used as the drugs of choice for acute anxiety states and the amine uptake inhibitors and monoamine oxidase inhibitors to treat depression. However, in the clinical practices of the treatment of anxiety disorders, benzodiazepines are now slowly replaced by antidepressants, which are not only efficacious in depression but also in the acute and chronic treatment anxiety disorders [1].

The GABAergic system and the serotoninergic neurotransmission are involved in anxiety. In addition, selective serotonin reuptake inhibitors (SSRIs) are effective in anxiety disorders and are known to have strong antidepressant effects [4, 5]. Depression is related to monoamines in the brain, especially to 5-HT and noradrenaline. Although benzodiazepines have well-known benefits, their side effects are prominent, including muscle relaxation, sedation, physical dependence, memory disturbance, and interaction with other drugs [6]. In these conditions, the efficacy of such drugs is very limited so the need for newer, better-tolerated, and more efficacious treatments remains high.

Herbal therapies could be considered as alternative or complementary medicines. In the search for new molecules useful for the treatment of neurological disorders, worldwide medicinal plant research has continued to progress, demonstrating the pharmacological effectiveness of different plant species in a variety of animal's models [7]. This is reflected in the large number of herbal medicines whose psychotherapeutic potential has been assessed in a variety of animal models. These studies have provided useful information for the development of new pharmacotherapies from medicinal plants and for new isolated active phytoconstituents.

Alafia multiflora (Apocynaceae) is a medicinal plant widely distributed in the tropical region of Africa, traditionally used for ulcerous wounds and occasionally used for abdominal pain. Previously, we showed the protective effect of the methanol/methylene chloride extract of this plant on carbon tetrachloride- (CCl_4-) induced oxidative stress in rats. Furthermore, antibacterial and antiradical activities of different extracts of this plant have been demonstrated along with a high LD_{50} (>5 g/kg) in rats. Recently both biochemical and histopathological studies in rats demonstrated that the methanolic extract of *A. multiflora* at doses of 125 and 250 mg/kg has hepatoprotective activity due to its antioxidant potential [8]. Phytochemical screening of the stem bark showed the presence of phenols, tannins, flavonoids, anthraquinones, and alkaloids [9].

A wide range of plant-derived flavonoids, terpenes, can cross the blood-brain barrier and are able to influence brain function [10] such as the modulation of the function of ionotropic GABA receptors. Due to the presence of flavonoids in the extract of *A. multiflora* and its higher antioxidant activities, it is presumed that this plant might have benefic pharmacological effects at the level of the central nervous system.

Therefore, the objective of the present work was to analyse the possible anxiolytic and antidepressant-like effects of the aqueous extract of *A. multiflora* stem bark in rats and mice using the open field, elevated plus-maze and light-dark box tests as animal models of anxiety, and forced swimming test as an animal model of depression, respectively.

2. Materials and Methods

2.1. Plant Material and Extraction. Plant material (stem bark) was collected in the centre region of Cameroon in May and authenticated at the National Herbarium-Yaoundé, where the voucher specimen was conserved under the reference number 43196/HNC. Aqueous extract was prepared as follows: after drying fresh stem bark and powdering it, 900 g of the powder were dissolved in boiled distilled water (1 litre) for 24 hours. This was followed by filtration and elimination of the solvent under air-dried oven at 50°C. The given powder yielded 3.24% of a dark brown extract.

2.2. Experimental Animals. Wistar albino rats (weighing 160–180 g) and Swiss albino mice (weighing 20–25 g) of both sexes were obtained from the veterinary national laboratory (LANAVET) of Garoua, Cameroun. The animals were

housed in polyacrylic cages (6 animals/cage) and maintained in a temperature and light-controlled room (25 ± 2°C, a 12 h cycle). The animals were acclimatized to laboratory condition for 10 days before the start of experiment. Prior to and after treatment, the animals were fasted for 12 and 7 h, respectively. However, all animals were allowed to drink water *ad libitum*. The authorization for the use of laboratory animals in this study was obtained from the Cameroun National Ethical Committee (Registration number: FWA-IRB00001954).

2.3. Chemicals. Diazepam hydrochloride, pindolol, flumazenil, and fluoxetine were purchased from Sigma-Aldrich Co., USA, and used as a reference drugs. All drugs and extracts were freshly prepared in saline on the day of the experiments and administered intraperitoneally (i.p.). Control animals received 10 mL/kg body of the vehicle in the same route of administration.

3. Behavioral Evaluation

3.1. Open Field Activity Test (OFT). The open field apparatus was constructed of white polywood and measured 72×72 cm with 36 cm walls. Red lines were drawn on the floor with a marker and were clearly visible through the clear Plexiglas floor. Mice were injected (i.p) with the aqueous extract of *A. multiflora* stem bark once per day for 7 days. The test was performed 30 min after the last administration of the aqueous extract of *A. multiflora* stem bark (150 and 300 mg/kg, i.p.) or saline (10 mL/kg). The standard drug diazepam (1 mg/kg, i.p.) was given once 30 min before the test. The mice were placed in the open field box for 6 min, and their behaviors were recorded. The behaviors scored included time spent at the center square, number of the lines crossed in the floor of the maze, rearing frequency (number of times the animal stood on its hind legs), and grooming (duration of time the animal spent licking or scratching itself while stationary) [11].

3.2. Elevated Plus-Maze Test (EPM). Behavior in the elevated plus maze (EPM) is used to assess exploration, anxiety, and motor behavior. The possible anxiolytic effects of the aqueous extract of *A. multiflora* stem bark were assessed, basically using the same method described by Foyet et al. [12]. The EPM consists of four arms, 49 cm long and 10 cm wide, arranged in such a way that the two arms of each type were opposite to each other. The maze was elevated 50 cm above the floor. Two arms were enclosed by walls 30 cm high and the other two arms were exposed. Rats were injected i.p. with the aqueous extract of *A. multiflora* stem bark (150 and 300 mg/kg, i.p) or saline (10 mL/kg, i.p) once per day for 7 days. The positive control diazepam (1 mg/kg, i.p) was given once 30 min before the test. Thirty minutes after the i.p. injection of the last dose of extract or saline, each animal was placed at the center of the maze facing one of the enclosed arms. During a 5 min test period, the number of open and enclosed arms entries, as well as the time spent in open and enclosed arms, was recorded as previously described [12, 13].

Entry into an arm was defined as the point when the animal places all four paws into the arm. After the test, the maze was carefully cleaned with 10% ethanol solution and allowed to dry before the next animal.

In another set of experiments, rats were subjected to the coadministration of the aqueous extract of *A. multiflora* leaves and pindolol or flumazenil. Thirty minutes before the oral administration, the plant extract (150 and 300 mg/kg), pindolol (10 mg/kg), flumazenil (10 mg/kg), or vehicle (10 mL/kg) were administered intraperitoneally. Two other groups of rats were treated with pindolol or flumazenil during the same period [14].

3.3. Light-Dark Transition Test (LDB). The LDB test was performed according to the method of Gong et al. [15], with minor modifications. Our light/dark box (45 × 27 × 27 cm) was made of polywood and consisted of two chambers connected by an opening (7.5 × 7.5 cm) located at the floor level in the center of the dividing wall. The floor was divided into 9 × 9 cm squares and was covered with Plexiglas. The small chamber (18 × 27 cm) was painted black and the larger chamber (27 × 27 cm) was painted white. Bright illumination was provided by a 60 watt table lamp located 40 cm above the center of the white chamber. Mice were injected (i.p) with the aqueous extract of *A. multiflora* stem bark once per day for 7 days. The test was performed 1 h after the last extract administration. Standard drug diazepam (i.p.) was given once 30 min before the test. During the test, the mice were placed at the center of the light compartment with their back to the dark compartment, and then transition behavior over 10 min was observed, including the latency time (latency before entering the dark compartment), the transition number (the number of dark compartment to light compartment transitions), and the total time spent visiting the light compartment [16, 17]. After 5 min, mice were removed from the box by the base of their tails and returned to their home cage. The maze was then cleaned with a solution of 10% ethanol and permitted to dry between tests.

3.4. Forced Swimming Test (FST). The FST is the most widely used pharmacological model for assessing antidepressant activity [18]. The development of immobility when the rodents are placed in an inescapable cylinder of water reflects the cessation of persistent escape-directed behavior [19]. The possible antidepressant effects of the aqueous extract of *A. multiflora* stem bark were assessed, basically using the same method described by Foyet et al. [12] with minor modifications. Rats were administered with aqueous extract of *A. multiflora* stem bark (150 and 300 mg/kg, i.p) or saline (10 mL/kg, i.p) once per day for 7 days. The standard drug fluoxetine (10 mg/kg, i.p) was given once 30 min before the test. On the first day of the experiments (pretest session), rats were individually placed into transparent Plexiglas cylinder (50 cm high and 20 cm wide) filled to a 30 cm depth with water at 26 ± 1°C. The animals were left to swim for 15 min before being removed, dried, and returned to their cages.

The procedure was repeated 24 h later, in a 6 min swim session (test session) 30 min after the last dose of the extract of *A. multiflora* stem bark, fluoxetine, or saline. During the test session, the following behavioral responses were recorded: immobility time (time spent floating with the minimal movements to keep the head above the water), swimming time (time spent with active swimming movements), and climbing time (time spent with upward movements of the forepaws directed to the cylinder wall). Increases in active responses, such as climbing or swimming and reduction in immobility, were reconsidered as behavioral profiles consistent with an antidepressant-like action [18].

3.5. Statistical Analysis. Data were presented as mean ± SEM values. One-way ANOVA with Dunnett's posttest was performed using Graph Pad Prism version 5.00 for Windows, Graph Pad Software, San Diego, CA, USA, http://www.graphpad.com. A probability level of 0.05 or less was accepted as significant.

4. Results

4.1. Effects of the Extract in the OFT. The open field test was performed for 30 min after the administration of the last dose of the extract or 30 min after single dose of diazepam. The extract did not significantly increase the number of lines crossed by the mice at any dose tested, but did significantly increase rearing time at the 300 mg/kg dose. In contrast, diazepam significantly decreased both the number of lines crossed and rearing time. The grooming time was significantly reduced by the extract and the standard drug, compared with the control group. Diazepam significantly increased the time mice spent at the center of the field. Moreover, this parameter was also significantly increased by the chronic administration of the extract (Table 1).

4.2. Effects of the Extract in the EPM. The extract at doses of 150 and 300 mg/kg i.p. produced anxiolytic-like effects as determined by the increase of the time spent in the open arms compared to control animals ($P < 0.001$, Figure 1(a)). Consequently, the plant extract significantly ($P < 0.05$, Figure 1(b)) increased the number of entries in the open arms of the plus maze. Conversely, the time spent and the numbers of entries in the enclosed arms were reduced by the extract treatment compared to control animals (Figures 1(a) and 1(b)).

4.3. Effect of Pindolol and Flumazenil Antagonism on the Anxiolytic Effect of the Extract. As shown in Figures 2 and 3, the behavioral effects of the aqueous extract of *A. multiflora* stem bark were completely antagonized by pindolol (10 mg/kg) and flumazenil (3 mg/kg).

4.4. Effects of the Extract in the LDB. The extract at 150 mg/kg significantly increased the latency time, the number of the light-dark transitions, and the time spent in the light compartment. Diazepam (1 mg/kg, i.p) significantly increased the number of transitions and the time spent in the light compartment while the latency time significantly decreased (Table 2).

TABLE 1: Effects of the aqueous extract of A. multiflora stem bark and diazepam in the open field test in mice.

Groups	Dose (mg/kg)	Number of line traversed	Rearing time (s)	Grooming time (s)	Time spent at the center (s)
Control	—	35 ± 5.2	23.54 ± 5.14	87.54 ± 12.62	5.70 ± 1.36
AM	150	49.12 ± 2.24	29.25 ± 3.46	57.32 ± 13.17	$41.22 \pm 5.61^*$
AM	300	48.21 ± 3.56	$35.42 \pm 2.20^*$	$34.20 \pm 6.16^{**}$	$56.50 \pm 4.04^*$
Diazepam	1	$5.40 \pm 4.32^{***}$	$9.10 \pm 3.10^{***}$	$10.70 \pm 8.56^{***}$	$123.00 \pm 18.120^{**}$

Mice activity was measured 30 min after the last chronic administration of the aqueous extract of A. multiflora or 30 min after the single dose of diazepam administration. Data are expressed as mean $\pm$ SEM of 6 animals. $*P < 0.05$, $**P < 0.01$, and $**P < 0.001$, compared to the vehicle-treated control group.

TABLE 2: Effects of repeated administration of the aqueous extract of A. multiflora (i.p.) on the light-dark transition test with mice.

Groups	Dose (mg/kg)	Latency time (s)	Transition number	Time spent in light compartment (s)
Control	—	116.2 ± 12.16	3.4 ± 0.73	38.60 ± 2.26
AM	150	$196.60 \pm 8.90^{***}$	$7.2 \pm 0.86^{**}$	$53.80 \pm 3.13^*$
AM	300	$181.20 \pm 11.20^{***}$	$8.8 \pm 0.86^{***}$	$83.60 \pm 4.06^{***}$
Diazepam	1	$57.40 \pm 3.73^{***}$	$15.40 \pm 1.20^{***}$	$105.00 \pm 3.33^{***}$

Aqueous extract of A. multiflora stem bark was given (i.p) once per day for 7 days. Diazepam was given (i.p.) only once 30 min prior to the test. Data are expressed as means $\pm$ SEM. $n = 6$ animals per group. $*P < 0.05$; $**P < 0.01$; $***P < 0.001$ versus control.

4.5. Effects of the Extract in the FST. The impact of the extract on immobility time in the forced swimming test in rats is shown in Figure 4. After 7 days i.p. administration of this extract, the immobility time was significantly reduced in rats that received a daily dose of 300 mg/kg but not 150 mg/kg. This activity was similar to that of fluoxetine at 10 mg/kg. Conversely, the swimming and the climbing time (Figure 4) were significantly ($P < 0.01$ and $P < 0.05$, resp.) increased by the aqueous extract of A. *multiflora* stem bark. Fluoxetine had no significant effect on climbing time, but did increase swimming time.

5. Discussion

In the present study, the anxiolytic and antidepressant-like effects of the chronic administration of the aqueous extract of *Alafia multiflora* stem bark were studied in different animal models of anxiety and depression. The *Alafia multiflora* stem bark extract was first studied using the open field which gives a better indication of the animal's emotional state. The administration of the plant extract and diazepam produced a significant reduction of the grooming time and an increase in the time spent at the centre of the field. Grooming behavior following exposure to stress and the increase of the time at the center of the field clearly indicate that the plant extract has anxiolytic activity. The *Alafia multiflora* spontaneous activities were studied by rearing and the number of line crossed. The rearing (vertical movement) is an index of the locomotor activity [20] while the increased number of line crossed (horizontal movement) is an indication of the central nervous system stimulant properties. The chronic administration of the aqueous extract of the *Alafia multiflora* stem bark significantly increased the rearing time and the number of crossings. These results taking together indicate that, in contrast to diazepam, the aqueous extract of *Alafia multiflora* showed anxiolytic-like effects without affecting locomotor activity or without producing central nervous depression. However, the significant decrease in the number

of line crossed by animals treated with diazepam suggests a sedative effect of this drug at the dose used.

One of the most widely used animal models for screening putative anxiolytics is the elevated plus maze, in which rodents display an avoidance of exposed open areas of the maze, which are presumed to be the most aversive, and a preference for sections enclosed by protective walls [21]. The anxiolytic effectiveness of a drug can be demonstrated by a statistically significant increase in rodent activity in the open arms. In the elevated plus maze test, the aqueous extract of *Alafia multiflora* increased but not in a dose-dependant manner, the time spent, and the numbers of entries in the open arms ($P < 0.001$). This anxiolytic effect of *Alafia multiflora* is similar to the one observed with diazepam, a typical benzodiazepine drug which induced significant increase in open arm time and in number of entries into the open arm. The effect of anxiolytic agents is to enhance the response to GABA, by facilitating the opening the GABAA-activated chloride channels. It can therefore be hypothesized that *Alafia multiflora* may be acting like a benzodiazepine-like substance. Supporting this view, the treatment with flumazenil, a specific antagonist of the benzodiazepine site in the GABA-BDZ receptor complex, at the dose of 10 mg/kg, was able to block significantly the anxiolytic effect induced by the *Alafia multiflora* extract and the diazepam. The benzodiazepines receptor agonists are commonly prescribed for the treatment of anxiety, sleep, and seizure disorders for over 40 years. Based on this antagonism study, it could be concluded that the aqueous extract of *Alafia multiflora* may probably work via the activation of the benzodiazepine site of the GABA receptors in the central nervous system. Similar results were obtained by Yu et al. [22], testing the anxiolytic-like effects of *Cinnamomum cassia* in mice. In the other hand, the anxiolytic effect of the aqueous extract of *Alafia multiflora* stem bark was significantly reversed by pindolol. Pindolol blocks 5-HT$_{1A}$ autoreceptors, thus inhibiting the negative feedback produced by the rapid increase of 5-HT resulting from the blockade of 5-HT transporters [23]. Therefore, we

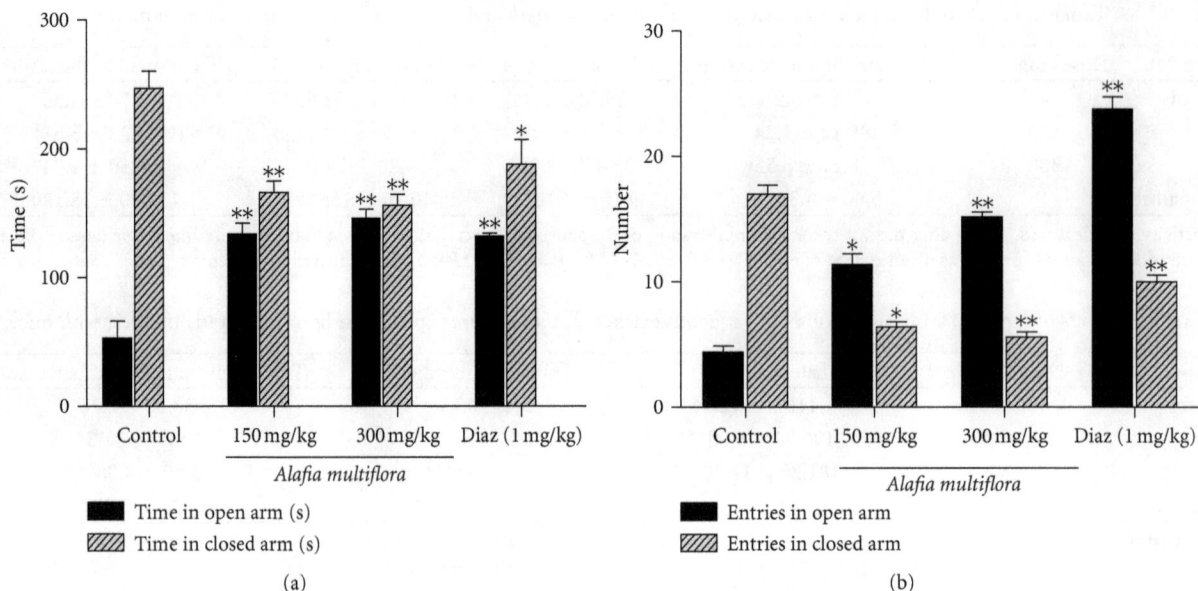

FIGURE 1: Effect of the aqueous extract of *A. multiflora* stem bark on the time spent in open and closed arms (a) and the numbers of entries in open and closed arms (b) in the elevated maze test. Experiments were performed 30 min after the last chronic administration of the aqueous extract *of A. multiflora* or 30 min after the single dose of diazepam (Diaz) administration. Data are expressed as mean ± SEM of 6 animals. *$P < 0.05$, **$P < 0.01$, compared to the vehicle-treated control group.

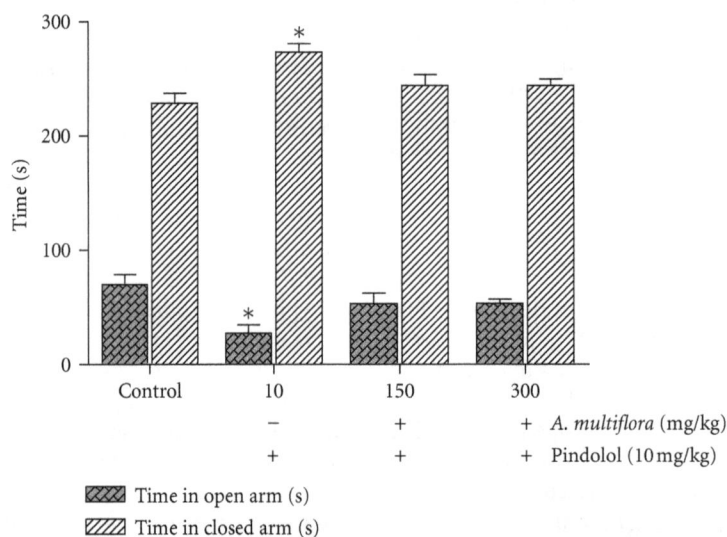

FIGURE 2: Antagonistic effect of pindolol on the anxiolytic-like effect of the aqueous extract of *A. multiflora* stem bark. Pindolol (10 mg/kg) was given 30 min before the extract and during the same period. Data are expressed as mean ± SEM of the time spent in the closed and open arms in rats given 5 min test 30 min after the last administration of the extract. *$P < 0.05$, compared to the vehicle-treated control group, $n = 6$ rats per group.

think that the anxiolytic-like effect of *Alafia multiflora* is also mediated by the 5-HT$_{1A}$ receptor. However, it is known that one of the pharmacological actions of pindolol include the blockade of the β-adrenergic receptor activity. Thus, a definitive conclusion that the anxiolytic activity of the plant extract is mediated through 5-HT$_{1A}$, in addition to GABA, receptors cannot be made at this time.

The present study also characterized the effects of the aqueous extract of *A. multiflora* stem bark, on rat's perform-

ance in forced swimming test (FST) following short-term (7 days) treatment. In this experiment, the immobility displayed by rodents when subjected to unavoidable stress such as forced swimming is thought to reflect a state of despair or lowered mood, which is thought to reflect depressive disorders in humans [12]. The immobility time has been shown to be reduced by treatment with antidepressant drugs [24]. Because the pharmacotherapy of depression typically requires chronic drug treatment to obtain a full response

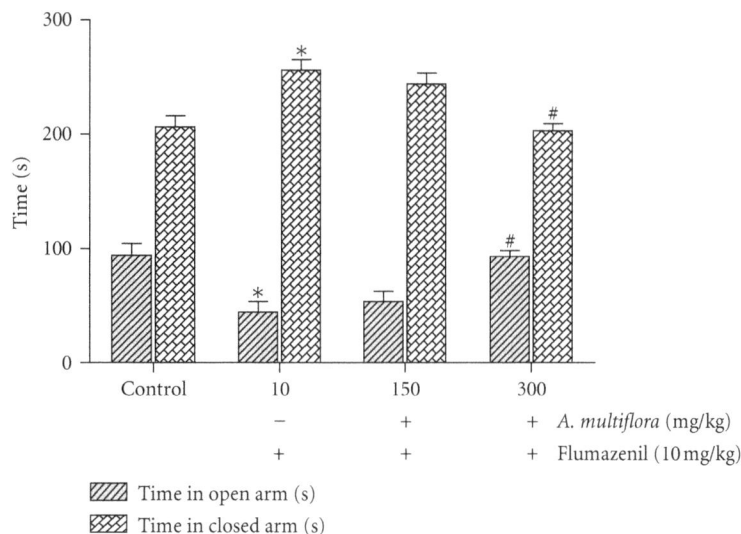

FIGURE 3: Antagonistic effect of flumazenil on the anxiolytic-like effect of the aqueous extract of *A. multiflora* stem bark in rats. Flumazenil (10 mg/kg) or vehicle was administered intraperitoneally. The data is expressed as the mean ± SEM of the percentage of the time spent and the number of entries into the open arms of the elevated plus maze over 5 min test period. $*P < 0.05$ compared to the vehicle-treated control group; $\#P < 0.05$ versus the flumazenil treated group, $n = 6$ rats per group.

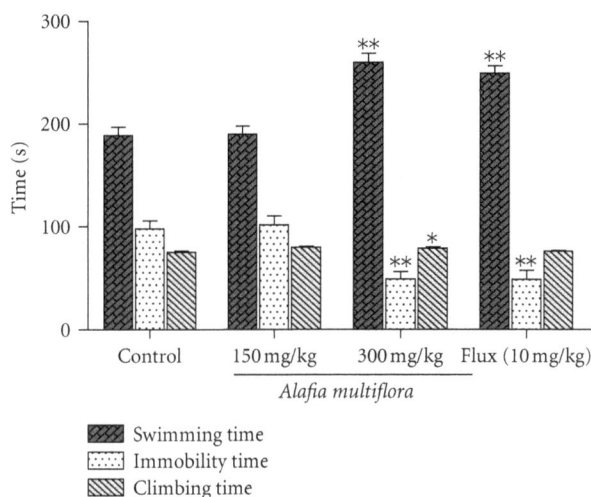

FIGURE 4: Effects of the aqueous extract of *A. multiflora* stem bark or fluoxetine on the forced swimming test in rats. Animals were treated with the extract (150 mg/kg or 300 mg/kg, i.p.) or distilled water once a day for 7 days. In the positive control, fluoxetine (Flux) was given only once (10 mg/kg, i.p.) 30 min prior to the test. Each column represents the mean ± SEM of 6 animals. Data analysis was performed using Dunnett's t-test, $*P < 0.05$; $**P < 0.01$ significantly different from saline-treated animals.

in terms of antidepressant effect, it is critical to perform repeated treatments in the FST rat model [25].

Reduction of immobility was comparable to that observed after i.p. administration of fluoxetine (10 mg/kg), the reference antidepressant drug. The decrease in immobility induced by fluoxetine is generally accompanied by an increase in swimming, whereas climbing duration was not affected by this drug [26]. It is widely known that

swimming is sensitive to serotoninergic compounds, such as the selective serotonin reuptake inhibitor fluoxetine while the climbing behavior is sensitive to tricyclic antidepressants and drugs with selective effects on catecholamine transmission [27]. Taken this into account, the results obtained in this study strongly suggested the implication of the serotoninergic and catecholaminergic pathway in the antidepressant effect of the aqueous extract of *A. multiflora*.

The biological effects of the aqueous extract of *A. multiflora* observed in this study might be attributed to phytoconstituents in the plant. Our preliminary phytochemical screening revealed the presence of flavonoids and polyphenols in the extract of this plant [9]. It has been reported that some flavonoids bind with high affinity to the benzodiazepine site of the GABA receptor [28, 29]. Their general bioavailability and particularly their presence in the brain *in vivo* appear to play an important role in the expression of their effects on the CNS [12]. It is possible that the presence in the aqueous extract of the stem bark of *A. multiflora* of flavonoids could account for its effects on CNS [30, 31].

The use of two types of animal species was simply due to lack of animals at the time in our institution. The behavioral field has adapted tests developed in the rat to the mouse with success and some tests like OFT and LDB have been easily retooled and validated for the mouse [32, 33]. Thus, we believe that the use of mice instead of rats does not fundamentally alter the trends of the results obtained in this study.

In conclusion, our results provide evidence that the aqueous extract of the stem bark of *Alafia multiflora* possesses anxiolytic and antidepressant properties in rodents with no significant decrease in locomotor activity. Further neurochemical studies are necessary to elucidate the influence of this extract on the monoamine systems (5-HT, NA, and DA), which are critically involved in the development of clinical depression.

References

[1] H. Dang, L. Sun, X. Liu et al., "Preventive action of Kai Xin San aqueous extract on depressive-like symptoms and cognition deficit induced by chronic mild stress," *Experimental Biology and Medicine*, vol. 234, no. 7, pp. 785–793, 2009.

[2] S. A. Onasanwo, M. Chatterjee, and G. Palit, "Antidepressant and anxiolytic potentials of dichloromethane fraction from *Hedranthera barteri*," *African Journal of Biomedical Research*, vol. 13, no. 1, pp. 76–81, 2010.

[3] D. L. Evans, D. S. Charney, L. Lewis et al., "Mood disorders in the medically ill: scientific review and recommendations," *Biological Psychiatry*, vol. 58, no. 3, pp. 175–189, 2005.

[4] D. P. Figgitt and K. J. McClellan, "Fluvoxamine: an updated review of its use in the management of adults with anxiety disorders," *Drugs*, vol. 60, no. 4, pp. 925–954, 2000.

[5] Y. Sugimoto, S. Furutani, K. Nishimura et al., "Antidepressant-like effects of neferine in the forced swimming test involve the serotonin1A (5-HT1A) receptor in mice," *European Journal of Pharmacology*, vol. 634, no. 1–3, pp. 62–67, 2010.

[6] C. C. Barua, J. D. Roy, B. Buragohain, A. G. Barua, P. Borah, and M. Lahkar, "Anxiolytic effect of hydroethanolic extract of *Drymaria cordata* L Willd," *Indian Journal of Experimental Biology*, vol. 47, no. 12, pp. 969–973, 2009.

[7] P. M. Galdino, M. V. M. Nascimento, B. L. Sampaio, R. N. Ferreira, J. R. Paula, and E. A. Costa, "Antidepressant-like effect of *Lafoensia pacari* A. St.-Hil. ethanolic extract and fractions in mice," *Journal of Ethnopharmacology*, vol. 124, no. 3, pp. 581–585, 2009.

[8] D. E. Tsala, B. V. Penlab, N. Nga, N. J. Mendimi, K. Jonas, and D. Théophile, "Protective activity of the stem bark methanol extract of *Alafia multiflora* against Carbon tetrachloride-induced hepatotoxicity in rats," *International Journal of Pharmaceutical Sciences Review and Research*, vol. 3, no. 2, pp. 157–163, 2010.

[9] D. E. Tsala, D. Theophile, N. Judith et al., "Screening of *Alafia multiflora* for antibacterial, antiradical activity and LD50 investigation," *International Journal of Pharmacology*, vol. 3, no. 4, pp. 327–333, 2007.

[10] G. A. R. Johnston, J. R. Hanrahan, M. Chebib, R. K. Duke, and K. N. Mewett, "Modulation of ionotropic GABA receptors by natural products of plant origin," *Advances in Pharmacology*, vol. 54, pp. 285–316, 2006.

[11] N. Carrey, M. P. McFadyen, and R. E. Brown, "Effects of subchronic methylphenidate hydrochloride administration on the locomotor and exploratory behavior of prepubertal mice," *Journal of Child and Adolescent Psychopharmacology*, vol. 10, no. 4, pp. 277–286, 2000.

[12] H. S. Foyet, L. Hritcu, A. Ciobica, M. Stefan, P. Kamtchouing, and D. Cojocaru, "Methanolic extract of *Hibiscus asper* leaves improves spatial memory deficits in the 6-hydroxydopamine-lesion rodent model of Parkinson's disease," *Journal of Ethnopharmacology*, vol. 133, no. 2, pp. 773–779, 2011.

[13] O. O. Adeyemi, A. J. Akindele, O. K. Yemitan, F. R. Aigbe, and F. I. Fagbo, "Anticonvulsant, anxiolytic and sedative activities of the aqueous root extract of *Securidaca longepedunculata*

Fresen," *Journal of Ethnopharmacology*, vol. 130, no. 2, pp. 191–195, 2010.

[14] P. Van Meer and J. Raber, "Mouse behavioural analysis in systems biology," *Biochemical Journal*, vol. 389, no. 3, pp. 593–610, 2005.

[15] Z. H. Gong, Y. F. Li, N. Zhao et al., "Anxiolytic effect of agmatine in rats and mice," *European Journal of Pharmacology*, vol. 550, no. 1–3, pp. 112–116, 2006.

[16] J. A. Bouwknecht and R. Paylor, "Behavioral and physiological mouse assays for anxiety: a survey in nine mouse strains," *Behavioural Brain Research*, vol. 136, no. 2, pp. 489–501, 2002.

[17] M. Bourin and M. Hascoët, "The mouse light/dark box test," *European Journal of Pharmacology*, vol. 463, no. 1–3, pp. 55–65, 2003.

[18] J. F. Cryan, A. Markou, and I. Lucki, "Assessing antidepressant activity in rodents: recent developments and future needs," *Trends in Pharmacological Sciences*, vol. 23, no. 5, pp. 238–245, 2002.

[19] G. Ulak, O. Mutlu, F. Y. Akar, F. I. Komsuoğlu, P. Tanyeri, and B. F. Erden, "Neuronal NOS inhibitor 1-(2-trifluoromethylphenyl)-imidazole augment the effects of antidepressants acting via serotonergic system in the forced swimming test in rats," *Pharmacology Biochemistry and Behavior*, vol. 90, no. 4, pp. 563–568, 2008.

[20] G. H. Vogel, *Drug Discovery and Evaluation, Pharmacological Assays*, Springer, Berlin, Germany, 2nd edition, 2002.

[21] X. Y. Wei, J. Y. Yang, J. H. Wang, and C. F. Wu, "Anxiolytic effect of saponins from *Panax quinquefolium* in mice," *Journal of Ethnopharmacology*, vol. 111, no. 3, pp. 613–618, 2007.

[22] H. S. Yu, S. Y. Lee, and C. G. Jang, "Involvement of 5-HT1A and GABAA receptors in the anxiolytic-like effects of *Cinnamomum cassia* in mice," *Pharmacology Biochemistry and Behavior*, vol. 87, no. 1, pp. 164–170, 2007.

[23] G. Gobbi and P. Blier, "Effect of neurokinin-1 receptor antagonists on serotoninergic, noradrenergic and hippocampal neurons: comparison with antidepressant drugs," *Peptides*, vol. 26, no. 8, pp. 1383–1393, 2005.

[24] V. K. Sharma, N. S. Chauhan, S. Lodhi, and A. K. Singhai, "Anti-depressant activity of *Zizyphus xylopyrus*," *International Journal of Phytomedicine*, vol. 1, no. 1, pp. 12–17, 2009.

[25] M. C. Hellión-Ibarrola, D. A. Ibarrola, Y. Montalbetti et al., "The antidepressant-like effects of *Aloysia polystachya* (Griseb.) Moldenke (Verbenaceae) in mice," *Phytomedicine*, vol. 15, no. 6-7, pp. 478–483, 2008.

[26] S. Mora, G. Diaz-Veliz, H. Lungenstrass et al., "Central nervous system activity of the hydroalcoholic extract of *Casimiroa edulis* in rats and mice," *Journal of Ethnopharmacology*, vol. 97, no. 2, pp. 191–197, 2005.

[27] J. F. Cryan and I. Lucki, "Antidepressant-like behavioral effects mediated by 5-hydroxytryptamine(2C) receptors," *Journal of Pharmacology and Experimental Therapeutics*, vol. 295, no. 3, pp. 1120–1126, 2000.

[28] P. Kahnberg, E. Lager, C. Rosenberg et al., "Refinement and evaluation of a pharmacophore model for flavone derivatives binding to the benzodiazepine site of the GABAA receptor," *Journal of Medicinal Chemistry*, vol. 45, no. 19, pp. 4188–4201, 2002.

[29] C. Wasowski, L. Gavernet, I. A. Barrios et al., "N, N-dicyclohexylsulfamide and N, N-diphenethylsulfamide are anticonvulsant sulfamides with affinity for the benzodiazepine binding site of the GABAA receptor and anxiolytic activity in

mice," *Biochemistry and Pharmacology*, vol. 83, no. 2, pp. 253–259, 2012.

[30] R. Estrada-Reyes, M. Martínez-Vázquez, A. Gallegos-Solís, G. Heinze, and J. Moreno, "Depressant effects of *Clinopodium mexicanum* Benth. Govaerts (Lamiaceae) on the central nervous system," *Journal of Ethnopharmacology*, vol. 130, no. 1, pp. 1–8, 2010.

[31] K. E. Heim, A. R. Tagliaferro, and D. J. Bobilya, "Flavonoid antioxidants: chemistry, metabolism and structure-activity relationships," *Journal of Nutritional Biochemistry*, vol. 13, no. 10, pp. 572–584, 2002.

[32] J. F. Cryan, R. J. Valentino, and I. Lucki, "Assessing substrates underlying the behavioral effects of antidepressants using the modified rat forced swimming test," *Neuroscience and Biobehavioral Reviews*, vol. 29, no. 4-5, pp. 547–569, 2005.

[33] M. Bourin, B. Petit-Demoulière, B. Nic Dhonnchadha, and M. Hascöet, "Animal models of anxiety in mice," *Fundamental and Clinical Pharmacology*, vol. 21, no. 6, pp. 567–574, 2007.

13

Trends in Ambulatory Prescribing of Antiplatelet Therapy among US Ischemic Stroke Patients: 2000–2007

Sudeep Karve,[1,2] Deborah Levine,[3,4,5] Eric Seiber,[6] Milap Nahata,[1] and Rajesh Balkrishnan[7,8]

[1] College of Pharmacy, The Ohio State University, Columbus, OH 43210, USA
[2] RTI Health Solutions, Research Triangle Park, Durham, NC 27709, USA
[3] Department of Internal Medicine, College of Medicine, The Ohio State University, Columbus, OH, USA
[4] Division of Health Services Management and Policy, College of Public Health, The Ohio State University, Columbus, OH 43210, USA
[5] Ann Arbor VA Healthcare System and Departments of Medicine and Neurology, The University of Michigan, Ann Arbor, MI 48109, USA
[6] Health Services Management and Policy, The Ohio State University, Columbus, OH 43210, USA
[7] Department of Clinical, Social and Administrative Sciences, University of Michigan, Ann Arbor, MI 48109, USA
[8] Clinical, Social and Administrative Sciences, College of Pharmacy, University of Michigan, 428 Church Street, Ann Arbor, MI 48109, USA

Correspondence should be addressed to Rajesh Balkrishnan, rbalkris@umich.edu

Academic Editor: Paola Patrignani

Objective. Study objectives were to assess temporal trends and identify patient- and practice-level predictors of the prescription of antiplatelet medications in a national sample of ischemic stroke (IS) patients seeking ambulatory care. *Methods*. IS-related outpatient visits by adults were identified using the National Ambulatory Medical Care Survey and National Hospital Ambulatory Medical Care Survey for the years 2000–2007. We assessed prescribing of antiplatelet medications using the generic drug code and drug entry codes in these data. Temporal trends in antiplatelet prescribing were assessed using the Cochran-Mantel-Haenszel test for trend. *Results*. We identified 9.5 million IS-related ambulatory visits. Antiplatelet medications were prescribed at 35.5% of visits. Physician office prescribing of the clopidogrel-aspirin combination increased significantly from 0.5% in 2000 to 22.0% in 2007 ($P = 0.05$), whereas prescribing of aspirin decreased from 17.9% to 7.0% ($P = 0.50$) during the same period. *Conclusion*. We observed a continued increase in prescription of the aspirin-clopidogrel combination from 2000 to 2007. Clinical trial evidence suggests that the aspirin-clopidogrel combination does not provide any additional benefit compared with clopidogrel alone; however, our study findings indicate that even with lack of adequate clinical evidence physician prescribing of this combination has increased in real-world community settings.

1. Introduction

In 2008, approximately 7 million individuals were reported to have a history of stroke [1]. Stroke survivors have a 4 to 14% annual risk of recurrent stroke and a 1–5% annual risk of myocardial infarction (MI). To reduce the recurrence of ischemic stroke (IS), the major stroke type accounting for 85% of strokes, modification of vascular risk factors [2–4], and antithrombotic therapy are recommended for stroke survivors [5, 6]. Antithrombotic therapy may include vitamin K antagonist therapy if atrial fibrillation is present (cardioembolic strokes) or antiplatelet therapy

(noncardioembolic strokes). Antiplatelet therapy can reduce the relative risk of IS by approximately 15% [7]. Four antiplatelet agents (aspirin, clopidogrel, ticlopidine, and dipyridamole) are used alone or in combination to treat IS patients. However, few clinical trials of IS patients provide direct comparisons among antiplatelet alternatives. As a result, clinicians have uncertainty regarding the selection of antiplatelet therapy for secondary stroke prevention among patients with noncardioembolic IS [8–17].

Between 2001 and 2006, several clinical trials were published that may influence clinicians' prescribing of anti-platelet therapy to IS patients: CURE (Clopidogrel in Unstable Angina to Prevent Recurrent Events) [18], CREDO (Clopidogrel for the Reduction of Events During Observation trial) [19], and MATCH (Management of ATherothrombosis with Clopidogrel in High-risk patients with Recent Transient Ischemic Attacks or Ischemic Stroke) [20]. The CURE trial which showed that the combination of clopidogrel and aspirin was more effective than aspirin in reducing cardiovascular events in patients with coronary heart disease (absolute risk reduction 2%) may have led to increases in prescription of the clopidogrel-aspirin combination to patients with other types of vascular disease such as IS. Subsequently, this enthusiasm may have dampened when later trials (MATCH and CHARISMA) showed that dual antiplatelet therapy with aspirin and clopidogrel was no more effective than clopidogrel therapy alone and, in fact, the combination may be harmful. Alternatively, the European/Australasian Stroke Prevention in Reversible Ischaemia trial (ESPRIT) showed that, in patients with nonembolic recent minor cerebral ischemia, aspirin plus dipyridamole was more effective than aspirin alone in preventing vascular events, findings consistent with other studies. In 2006, updated clinical practice guidelines for secondary stroke prevention were published that generated much of these trial data and also discouraged the routine use of the aspirin and clopidogrel combination in IS patients.

Despite these major changes in the evidence and recommendations for antiplatelet therapy in vascular patients, few studies have examined temporal trends in physicians' prescribing of antiplatelet therapy to IS stroke patients in the ambulatory setting or in a population-based fashion [12]. As a result, little is known about temporal changes in ambulatory prescribing practices of antiplatelet agents to the US population of stroke survivors. In addition, the patient and physician predictors of antiplatelet therapy selection are unknown. Therefore, we assessed the temporal trends in prescribing of the various antiplatelet agents, alone or in combination, among patients with IS seeking ambulatory care using a nationally representative population-based survey. We also explored patient-level and physician-level characteristics associated with prescription of specific antiplatelet therapies.

2. Materials and Methods

2.1. Data Source. This study was a retrospective analysis of two national surveys: (1) National Ambulatory Medical Care Survey (NAMCS) [21] and (2) National Hospital Ambulatory Medical Care Survey (NHAMCS) [22] for the years 2000 through 2007. The NAMCS is a national survey on the utilization of ambulatory medical care services provided by nonfederally employed physicians. The NHAMCS is a national survey on ambulatory care services provided in general and short stay (average length of stay < 30) hospital outpatient departments (OPD) and emergency departments (ED). Federal, military, and veterans administration hospitals are excluded from this survey. Both NAMCS and NHAMCS are conducted annually and they utilize a multistage probability sampling with counties, groups of counties, county equivalents or towns, and townships within the

US and the District of Columbia as the primary sampling unit. Both surveys provide information related to patient demographic characteristics, patient described reason for visit, physician diagnosis, payment source for the visit, and physician office/hospital location. Additionally, information on medication provided/prescribed (2000–2002: up to 6 medications are recorded; 2003–2007: up to 8 medications are recorded) during the visit is available. Each record in the data represents a patient visit. Patient visit weights provided in these data were used to obtain national estimates on ambulatory utilization at the physician office, hospital OPD, and hospital ED.

2.2. Patient Population. We identified all patients age 18 years or older who had an ambulatory visit with a primary physician diagnosis of ischemic stroke (IS) using valid ICD-9-CM codes (433.x1, 434.xx, 436.xx) [23–26] and recorded in the NAMCS and NHAMCS data from January 2000 through December 2007. Patients with a diagnosis for atrial fibrillation (ICD-9-CM code = 427.3x) or prescription for warfarin (generic drug code: 56205, drug entry codes: 34775, 07930; multum code: d00022) were excluded because these patients are likely to have cardioembolic stroke. The antiplatelet agents are primarily recommended for patients with noncardioembolic stroke and thus we excluded IS patients with diagnosis of atrial fibrillation or drug mention of warfarin.

2.3. Outcome Measure. The primary outcome was an ambulatory IS visit with medication mention for antiplatelet agents. The antiplatelet agents considered for this study were aspirin, clopidogrel, dipyridamole, and ticlopidine as these agents were available during 2000 to 2007. We then categorized the antiplatelet agents into the following mutually exclusive categories: (1) aspirin only, (2) clopidogrel only, (3) aspirin and clopidogrel, (4) aspirin and dipyridamole, (5) dipyridamole only, and (6) ticlopidine.

The NAMCS [21] and NHAMCS [22] collect data on medications ordered or supplied at the physician office or ED/OPD visit. The medication data is then classified and coded using the drug coding system developed by the National Center for Health Statistics (NCHS) and is made available in the NAMCS and NHAMCS dataset. To assess the proportion of IS visits resulting in an antiplatelet medication documentation we used antiplatelet drug codes provided in the NAMCS and NHAMCS data.

2.4. Covariates. The various patient characteristics considered in the analysis included race (white, black, and other), age (18–44 years, 45–64 years, and ≥65 years), gender (male and female), and primary payment source for the visit (private, Medicare, Medicaid and other). The various physician office/hospital characteristics in the analysis included region of the physician office or the hospital as defined by the US census bureau (Northeast, Midwest, South, West), location (urban: Metropolitan Statistical Area (MSA), rural: non-MSA), and visit setting (physician office, hospital OPD, and hospital ED).

3. Statistical Analysis

Patient visit weights were used to assess the national estimate on annual IS visits with and without a mention of antiplatelet agents. Temporal changes in the proportion of IS visits resulting in mention of antiplatelet agents were assessed during the 8-year study period, that is, 2000 to 2007, using the Cochran-Mantel-Haenszel test for trend. We further stratified the utilization trends by visit setting, that is, physician office, hospital ED, and hospital OPD, using indicator variable for visit setting available in the dataset. Associations between antiplatelet prescribing and patient and physician office/hospital characteristics were tested using the Chi-square test. All the statistical analyses were performed in SAS-callable SUDAAN (version 10.0.1 hosted on the Windows platform) to account for the complex survey design of the NAMCS and NHAMCS and to provide weighted results that reflect population estimates. This study was approved by the Institutional Review Board at the Ohio State University.

4. Results and Discussion

4.1. Results

4.1.1. Patient Characteristics. During the 8 year period, there were 9.5 million ischemic stroke-related ambulatory visits of which 6.8 million (71.1%) occurred in a physician office, 0.3 million (3.4%) in a hospital OPD, and 2.4 million (25.5%) in a hospital ED (Table 1). Over 77% of the visits were by whites and approximately 50.1% were by females; 67.5% were by patients aged over 65 years. Among persons aged <65 years the proportion of visits increased from 26.8% in 2000-01 to 36.7% in 2006-07, whereas, the proportion of visits in the MSA region increased from 71.1% in 2000-01 to 92.4% in 2006-07.

4.1.2. Associations between Patient and Physician Office/ Hospital Characteristics and Antiplatelet Medications Prescribed. Table 2 represents the univariate association between patient and physician office/hospital characteristics and antiplatelet drugs prescribed. No significant differences in prescribing of aspirin or clopidogrel monotherapy or aspirin-clopidogrel combination were observed by race or region. Older adults were more likely to receive clopidogrel monotherapy compared with younger adults ($P = 0.03$). The aspirin-clopidogrel combination was significantly more likely to be prescribed among men compared with women (80.3% versus 19.7%; $P < 0.01$). Clopidogrel monotherapy (88.7%, $P < 0.01$) or in combination with aspirin (89.0%, $P = 0.01$) was more likely to be prescribed in a physician office compared with a hospital ED or a OPD. Overall, 0.98 million visits resulted in prescribing of aspirin-clopidogrel combination, for which the proportion increased significantly from 2.4% (0.02 million) in 2000-01 to 31.2% (0.30 million) in 2006-07 ($P < 0.01$).

4.1.3. Antiplatelet Prescribing Trend. Among the IS patients, the proportion of patients receiving antiplatelet drugs

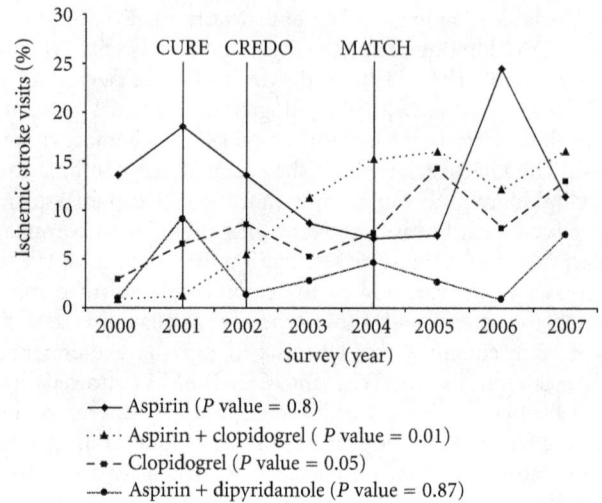

FIGURE 1: Antiplatelet prescribing trends among patients with ischemic stroke: NAMCS, NHAMCS, 2000–2007. NAMCS: National Ambulatory Medical Care Survey; NHAMCS: National Hospital Ambulatory Medical Care Survey; P values based on Cochran-Mantel-Haenszel test for trend. Years of publication of the 3 clinical trials shown in the figure above: 2001—CURE (Clopidogrel in Unstable Angina to Prevent Recurrent Events trial); 2002—CREDO (Clopidogrel for the Reduction of Events During Observation); 2004—MATCH (Management of ATherothrombosis with Clopidogrel in High-risk patients).

increased from 28.1% in 2000-01 to 47.1% in 2006-07 ($P_{trend} = 0.02$) (Table 1). In 2000, the proportion of visits resulting in clopidogrel-aspirin combination was 0.8% which significantly increased to 16.1% in 2007 ($P_{trend} = 0.01$) (Figure 1).

No significant changes in prescribing of dipyridamole-aspirin combination were seen ($P_{trend} = 0.87$) in this study. During the same period, the proportion of patients receiving aspirin monotherapy declined from 13.6% in 2000 to 11.4% in 2007 ($P_{trend} = 0.80$), while prescribing for clopidogrel monotherapy increased significantly from 2.9% in 2000 to 13.0% in 2007 ($P_{trend} = 0.05$).

Prescribing trends varied significantly by the physician practice setting (Figure 2). Proportion of IS patients receiving clopidogrel-aspirin combination significantly increased in the physician office setting (2000: 0.5%–2007: 22.0%; $P_{trend} = 0.02$) whereas no significant changes in prescribing were observed in the hospital OPD/ED (2000: 1.4%–2007: 3.2%; $P_{trend} = 0.81$) (Figure 2). In contrast, the proportion of IS patients receiving aspirin decreased considerably in the physician office setting (2000: 17.9%–2007: 7.0%; $P_{trend} = 0.50$), while it increased significantly in the hospital OPD/ED setting (2000: 6.5%–2007: 20.9%; $P_{trend} = 0.06$) (Figure 2). No significant differences in prescribing of clopidogrel monotherapy and dipyridamole-aspirin combination in either setting were observed.

5. Discussion

To the authors knowledge this is the first comprehensive study evaluating the ambulatory (physician office, hospital

TABLE 1: Ischemic stroke patient characteristics and antiplatelet agents prescribed: NAMCS, NAMCS 2000–2007[a,b].

	2000-01 (N = 285)		2002-03 (N = 330)		2004-05 (N = 352)		2006-07 (N = 304)	
Characteristic	Population estimate	%	Population estimate	%	Population estimate	%	Population estimate	%
Total ischemic stroke visits	2,221,277	100%	2,238,540	100%	2,917,650	100%	2,150,851	100%
Race								
White	1,605,408	72.3%	1,760,410	78.6%	2,266,603	77.7%	1,716,210	79.8%
Black	448,739	20.2%	184,064	8.2%	551,036	18.9%	392,536	18.3%
Other	167,130	7.5%	294,066	13.1%	100,011	3.4%	42,105	2.0%
Region								
Northeast	340,302	15.3%	509,922	22.8%	393,472	13.5%	339,938	15.8%
Midwest	491,280	22.1%	366,347	16.4%	1,058,706	36.3%	536,408	24.9%
South	703,364	31.7%	579,150	25.9%	1,119,719	38.4%	928,226	43.2%
West	686,331	30.9%	783,121	35.0%	345,753	11.9%	346,279	16.1%
Age								
18–44 years	46,907	2.1%	141,937	6.3%	137,665	4.7%	116,652	5.4%
45–64 years	549,189	24.7%	536,338	24.0%	885,617	30.4%	673,635	31.3%
≥65 years	1,625,181	73.2%	1,560,265	69.7%	1,894,368	64.9%	1,360,564	63.3%
Gender								
Female	1,177,727	53.0%	1,196,813	53.5%	1,572,905	53.9%	834,076	38.8%
Male	1,043,550	47.0%	1,041,727	46.5%	1,344,745	46.1%	1,316,775	61.2%
Insurance[c]								
Private insurance	523,035	23.5%	553,314	24.7%	860,712	29.5%	633,122	29.4%
Medicare	1,488,002	67.0%	1,364,738	61.0%	1,538,343	52.7%	1,224,087	56.9%
Medicaid	76,721	3.5%	61,621	2.8%	106,824	3.7%	128,987	6.0%
Other	90,939	4.1%	206,476	9.2%	145,752	5.0%	75,490	3.5%
Location								
MSA[d]	1,580,138	71.1%	2,003,578	89.5%	2,546,768	87.3%	1,986,970	92.4%
Non-MSA	641,139	28.9%	234,962	10.5%	370,882	12.7%	163,881	7.6%
Antiplatelet prescribing								
Overall antiplatelet agents	623,998	28.1%	641,900	28.7%	1,101,786	37.8%	1,010,462	47.0%
Aspirin only	360,067	16.2%	244,855	10.9%	213,034	7.3%	377,002	17.5%
Clopidogrel only	107,873	4.9%	151,764	6.8%	327,148	11.2%	231,652	10.8%
Aspirin and clopidogrel	23,542	1.1%	192,779	8.6%	456,787	15.7%	305,702	14.2%
Aspirin and dipyridamole	118,183	5.3%	47,861	2.1%	104,817	3.6%	96,106	4.5%
Dipyridamole only	3,148	0.1%	0	0.0%	0	0.0%	0	0.0%
Ticlopidine only	11,185	0.5%	4,641	0.2%	0	0.0%	0	0.0%
Setting								
Physician office	1,502,370	67.6%	1,550,687	69.3%	2,231,054	76.5%	1,493,699	69.4%
Hospital OPD	65,065	2.9%	102,196	4.6%	62,847	2.2%	92,825	4.3%
Hospital ED	653,842	29.4%	585,657	26.2%	623,749	21.4%	564,327	26.2%

a NAMCS: National Ambulatory Medical Care Survey; NHAMCS: National Hospital Ambulatory Medical Care Survey.
b Population estimates were calculated using SAS-callable SUDAAN software, version 10.0.1 (Research Triangle Institute) to obtain proper variance estimations that accounted for the complex sampling design of the National Ambulatory Medical Care Survey and National Hospital Ambulatory Medical Care Survey and results that were weighted to reflect national population estimates.
c Insurance (payment source) does not sum to 100% because of missing data. d MSA: Metropolitan Statistical Area.

TABLE 2: Association between patient demographic and physician office/hospital characteristics and antiplatelet agent prescribed: NAMCS, NHAMCS 2000–2007[a,b].

| | Antiplatelet medication | | | | | | | | | | | |
| | Aspirin only (N = 233) | | | Clopidogrel only (N = 95) | | | Aspirin and clopidogrel (N = 63) | | | Aspirin and dipyridamole (N = 39) | | |
Characteristic	Population estimate	%	P value	Population estimate	%	P value	Population estimate	%	P value	Population estimate	%	P value
Total	1,194,958	—		818,437	—		978,810	—		366,967	—	
Race												
White	958,151	80.2%		581,489	71.0%		708,008	72.3%		341,339	93.0%	
Black	201,745	16.9%	0.40	150,228	18.4%	0.68	203,509	20.8%	0.91	22,867	6.2%	0.11
Other	35,062	2.9%		86,720	10.6%		67,293	6.9%		2761	0.8%	
Region												
Northeast	304,874	25.5%		82,604	10.1%		111,832	11.4%		62,510	17.0%	
Midwest	217,812	18.2%	0.38	287,327	35.1%	0.52	161,843	16.5%	0.47	108,731	29.6%	0.75
South	433,594	36.3%		259,449	31.7%		466,195	47.6%		84,482	23.0%	
West	238,678	20.0%		189,057	23.1%		238,940	24.4%		111,244	30.3%	
Age												
18–44 years	65,453	5.5%		10,958	1.3%		17,561	1.8%		12364	3.4%	
45–64 years	436,552	36.5%	0.39	116,735	14.3%	**0.03**	404,818	41.4%	0.20	95,313	26.0%	0.90
≥65 years	692,953	58.0%		690,744	84.4%		556,431	56.8%		259,290	70.7%	
Gender												
Female	632,517	52.9%		522,671	63.9%		192,540	19.7%		113,778	31.0%	
Male	562,441	47.1%	0.71	295,766	36.1%	0.15	786,270	80.3%	**<0.01**	253,189	69.0%	0.22
Insurance[c]												
Private insurance	355,686	29.8%		187,508	22.9%		405,119	41.4%		64,802	17.7%	
Medicare	656,260	54.9%	0.31	572,429	69.9%	0.47	461,148	47.1%	0.21	267,898	73.0%	0.73
Medicaid	71,523	6.0%		26,884	3.3%		53,025	5.4%		10,678	2.9%	
Other	55,345	4.6%		21,151	2.6%		14,927	1.5%		10,620	2.9%	
Location												
MSA[d]	994,903	83.3%		646,403	79.0%		852,053	87.0%		224,322	61.1%	
Non-MSA	200,055	16.7%	0.82	172,034	21.0%	0.58	126,757	13.0%	0.72	142,645	38.9%	0.30
Setting												
Physician office	711,071	59.5%		726,058	88.7%		870,856	89.0%		317,518	86.5%	
Hospital OPD[e]	56,218	4.7%	**0.05**	49,195	6.0%	**<0.01**	5,305	0.5%	**0.01**	8,951	2.4%	0.21
Hospital ED	427,669	35.8%		43,184	5.3%		102,649	10.5%		40,498	11.0%	
Year												
2000-01	360,067	30.1%		107,873	13.2%		23,542	2.4%		118,183	32.2%	
2002-03	244,855	20.5%	0.13	151,764	18.5%	0.22	192,779	19.7%	**<0.01**	47,861	13.0%	0.62
2004-05	213,034	17.8%		327,148	40.0%		456,787	46.7%		104,817	28.6%	
2006-07	377,002	31.5%		231,652	28.3%		305,702	31.2%		96,106	26.2%	

[a] NAMCS: National Ambulatory Medical Care Survey, NHAMCS: National Hospital Ambulatory Medical Care Survey.
[b] Population estimates were calculated using SAS-callable SUDAAN software, version 9.0.1 (Research Triangle Institute) to obtain proper variance estimations that accounted for the complex sampling design of the National Ambulatory Medical Care Survey and National Hospital Ambulatory Medical Care Survey and results that were weighted to reflect national population estimates.
[c] Insurance (payment source) does not sum to 100% because of missing data, [d] MSA: Metropolitan Statistical Area.
[e] OPD: Outpatient Department.

Physician office visits

(a)

Hospital OPD/ED

(b)

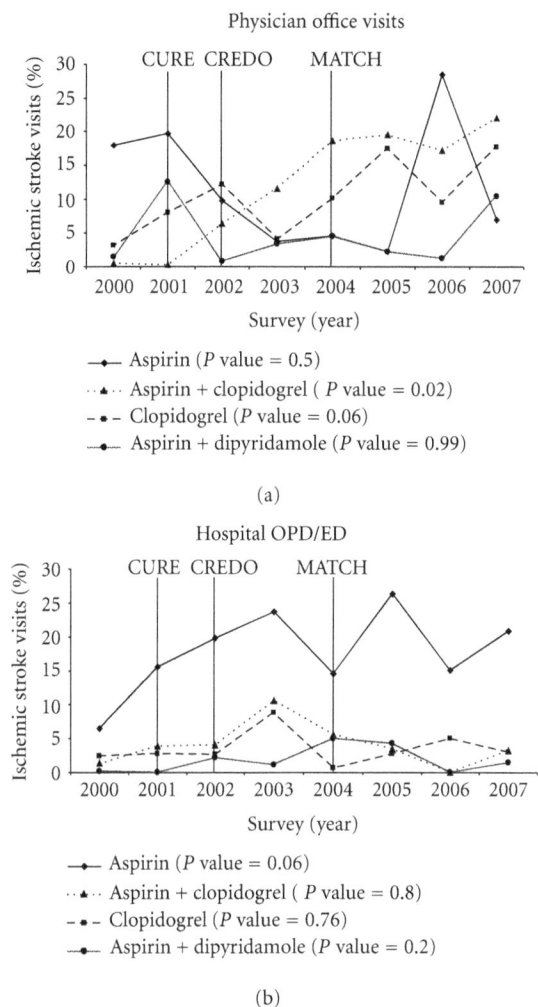

FIGURE 2: Antiplatelet prescribing trends among patients with ischemic stroke, by visit setting: 2000–2007. Physician office visits based on National Ambulatory Medical Care Survey data; Hospital ED/OPD visits based on National Hospital Ambulatory Medical Care Survey data; OPD: Outpatient Department; ED: Emergency Department; P values based on Cochran-Mantel-Haenszel test for trend. Years of publication of the 3 clinical trials shown in the figure above: 2001—CURE (Clopidogrel in Unstable Angina to Prevent Recurrent Events trial); 2002—CREDO (Clopidogrel for the Reduction of Events During Observation); 2004—MATCH (Management of ATherothrombosis with Clopidogrel in High-risk patients).

ED, and hospital OPD) prescribing trends for antiplatelet agents among community dwelling IS patients. We have identified significant changes in utilization pattern of antiplatelet agents among IS patients. During the 8 year study period (2000–2007), clopidogrel-aspirin prescribing increased significantly in the physician office setting. In contrast, the prescribing of clopidogrel-aspirin combination remained relatively low and stable in the hospital OPD and ED during the same period. However, the prescription of aspirin monotherapy increased dramatically in the hospital OPD and ED settings while it declined significantly in the physician office setting. We found that prescribing of

clopidogrel alone was considerably higher among elderly compared with younger IS patients. Prior study findings suggest that the risk of bleeding is higher among elderly patients using aspirin plus clopidogrel combination compared with patients only using clopidogrel [27]. Additionally, a study assessing risk factors associated with bleeding reported that compared with aspirin only users, patients using aspirin in combination with ticlopidine or clopidogrel had a 68% higher risk of bleeding (odds ratio: 1.68; 95% confidence interval: 1.02–1.77) [20]. We also found a higher use of clopidogrel plus aspirin combination among males compared with females. Findings of a recent meta-analysis suggest that the use of clopidogrel plus aspirin was associated with lower risk of CVD events among both men and women; however, the addition of clopidogrel to aspirin therapy was associated with a 43% and 21% increased risk of bleeding among females and males, respectively [28].

Our findings suggest that physician prescribing of clopidogrel-aspirin combination may have been influenced by the publication of three major clinical trials. Findings from both CURE (08/01) [18] and CREDO (11/02) [19] suggest that the use of clopidogrel-aspirin combination can significantly reduce the relative risk for the primary outcome measure (death from cardiovascular causes, nonfatal myocardial infarction, or IS). Publication of these trials along with aggressive marketing and promotion by the drug manufacturers [12] may have resulted in the increased prescribing of the clopidogrel-aspirin combination during the study period.

During the period under consideration for this study, MATCH [20] was the third major published trial evaluating clopidogrel-aspirin combination versus aspirin monotherapy for the primary composite endpoint; that is, ischemic stroke, myocardial infarction, vascular death, or rehospitalization for acute ischemia. The findings of this study did not indicate any benefit of adding aspirin to clopidogrel treatment in reducing the risk of the primary outcome but in contrast increased the risk of bleeding. Hill and Johnston reported a decline in hospital use of this combination following the publication of MATCH [12, 20], in contrast we found that the use of this combination continued to increase especially in the physician office setting after publication of MATCH. However, we did observe an increase in the prescribing of clopidogrel monotherapy in physician office setting following the publication of MATCH. Similarly, the American Heart Association/American Stroke Association guidelines published in 2006 that cautioned on the use of aspirin-clopidogrel combination did not seem to have an effect on physician office prescribing of this combination [6].

We found a significant increase in prescribing of aspirin monotherapy in the hospital OPD and ED settings from 2000 to 2007. One of the reasons for this increased use may be the publication of the Chinese Acute Stroke Trial [29] and International Stroke Trial [30] and subsequent publication of the American Stroke Association guidelines (07/02) [31], recommending the use of aspirin among patients suspected with acute stroke. Moreover since patients visiting hospital ED were more likely to present with acute IS it may explain the increased use of aspirin monotherapy in hospital ED setting.

Surprisingly, during the entire study period the prescribing of dipyridamole-aspirin combination remained low even though this combination was shown to be effective in reducing the risk of recurrent IS or death as compared to aspirin monotherapy in the European Stroke Prevention Study 2 (ESPS-2) published in 1996 [32]. However, we did observe a considerable increase in prescribing of this combination in 2007. This increase may be due to the publication of ESPRIT trial in 2006, which highlighted the relative risk reduction in the primary outcome measure (i.e., composite of death from all vascular causes, nonfatal stroke, nonfatal myocardial infarction, or major bleeding complication) among patients using dipyridamole-aspirin combination compared with patients using aspirin monotherapy [33].

In the wake of the above findings, there is a need to recognize certain limitations of this study. In this study the proportion of patients receiving antiplatelet medications ranged from 28% to 47% compared to 89% reported by Hill and Johnston [12]. This may be due to several reasons; firstly, both the NAMCS and NHAMCS data do not provide information on several important factors such as stroke severity, stroke type (first versus recurrent, acute versus nonacute), and contraindication to antiplatelet therapy. Secondly, antiplatelet agents are primarily recommended for patients with noncardioembolic IS; the data we used does not permit distinction between patients with cardioembolic or noncardioembolic stroke. However, we excluded patients with atrial fibrillation and those using warfarin considering this as a proxy for patients with cardioembolic stroke. Moreover, the important distinction between these two studies is the setting; our study focused on the ambulatory prescribing trends which may vary significantly from inpatient prescribing. Additionally, our analysis was restricted to patients with primary IS diagnosis selected using previously validated high sensitivity and specificity ICD-9-CM codes (433.x1, 434.xx, and 436.xx). Expanding the analysis to patients with secondary IS diagnosis or the use of other low sensitivity ICD-9-CM code(s) (e.g., 433.xx—without the 5th digit modifier) may affect the national estimates on IS-related outpatient visits and anti-platelet prescribing trends. In sensitivity analyses using a low-specificity algorithm (433.xx, 434.xx, and 436.xx) [34, 35], estimates on the number of IS-related ambulatory visits varied; however the proportion of patients receiving antiplatelet therapy remained relatively similar (data available upon request). The cross-sectional nature of the survey does not permit the evaluation of a patient's prior IS treatment. Even though the data provide information on both prescription and over the counter (OTC) medications prescribed or provided at the visit, the OTC availability of aspirin may underestimate the actual reporting of the aspirin use. Moreover, for both NAMCS and NHAMCS data the information on maximum number of medications provided has changed over the years; information on 6 medications was available during 2000 to 2002 which increased to 8 medications in 2003 to 2007. Finally, NHAMCS data do not contain information

on physician specialty and thus we could not assess the association between physician specialty and antiplatelet use.

6. Conclusions

Our study highlights important changes in the prescribing patterns of antiplatelet therapy among IS patients. Our findings suggest that even with the lack of adequate efficacy evidence, safety concerns, and higher cost, the prescribing of clopidogrel-aspirin combination increased substantially during the study period. Quality improvement measures are warranted to educate physicians of the evidence regarding antiplatelet drugs for secondary stroke prevention and improve prescribing of safe antiplatelet drugs among IS patients.

References

[1] V. L. Roger, A. S. Go, D. M. Lloyd-Jones et al., "Heart disease and stroke statistics—2011 update: a report from the American Heart Association," *Circulation*, vol. 123, no. 4, pp. e18–e209, 2011.

[2] K. Hardie, G. J. Hankey, K. Jamrozik, R. J. Broadhurst, and C. Anderson, "Ten-year risk of first recurrent stroke and disability after first-ever stroke in the perth community stroke study," *Stroke*, vol. 35, no. 3, pp. 731–735, 2004.

[3] T. Thom, N. Haase, and W. Rosamond, "American Heart Association Statistics Committee and Stroke Statistics Subcommittee. Heart disease and stroke statistics—2006 update: a report from the American Heart Association Statistics Committee and Stroke Statistics Subcommittee," *Etal Circulation*, vol. 14113, no. 6, pp. e85–e151, 2006.

[4] K. S. Wong and H. Li, "Long-term mortality and recurrent stroke risk among Chinese stroke patients with predominant intracranial atherosclerosis," *Stroke*, vol. 34, no. 10, pp. 2361–2366, 2003.

[5] G. W. Albers, P. Amarenco, J. D. Easton, R. L. Sacco, and P. Teal, "Antithrombotic and thrombolytic therapy for ischemic stroke: American College of Chest Physicians evidence-based clinical practice guidelines (8th edition)," *Chest*, vol. 133, supplement 6, pp. 630S–669S, 2008.

[6] R. L. Sacco, R. Adams, G. Albers et al., "Guidelines for prevention of stroke in patients with ischemic stroke or transient ischemic attack: a statement for healthcare professionals from the American Heart Association/American Stroke Association council on stroke: co-sponsored by the council on cardiovascular radiology and intervention. The American Academy of Neurology affirms the value of this guideline," *Stroke*, vol. 37, no. 2, pp. 577–617, 2006.

[7] G. J. Hankey and C. P. Warlow, "Treatment and secondary prevention of stroke: evidence, costs, and effects on individuals and populations," *The Lancet*, vol. 354, no. 9188, pp. 1457–1463, 1999.

[8] G. W. Albers, P. Amarenco, J. D. Easton, R. L. Sacco, and P. Teal, "Antithrombotic and thrombolytic therapy for ischemic stroke," *Chest*, vol. 119, supplement 1, pp. 300S–320S, 2001.

[9] J. Biller, "Antiplatelet therapy in ischemic stroke: variability in clinical trials and its impact on choosing the appropriate therapy," *Journal of the Neurological Sciences*, vol. 284, no. 1-2, pp. 1–9, 2009.

[10] G. Howard, L. A. McClure, J. W. Krakauer, and C. S. Coffey, "Stroke and the statistics of the aspirin/clopidogrel secondary

prevention trials," *Current Opinion in Neurology*, vol. 20, no. 1, pp. 71–77, 2007.

[11] P. A. Wolf, G. P. Clagett, J. D. Easton et al., "Preventing ischemic stroke in patients with prior stroke and transient ischemic attack : a statement for healthcare professionals from the Stroke Council of the American Heart Association," *Stroke*, vol. 30, no. 9, pp. 1991–1994, 1999.

[12] N. K. Hills and S. C. Johnston, "Trends in usage of alternative antiplatelet therapy after stroke and transient ischemic attack," *Stroke*, vol. 39, no. 4, pp. 1228–1232, 2008.

[13] G. W. Albers, "Choice of endpoints in antiplatelet trials. Which outcomes are most relevant to stroke patients?" *Neurology*, vol. 54, no. 5, pp. 1022–1028, 2000.

[14] N. E. Schwartz and G. W. Albers, "Use of antiplatelet agents to prevent stroke: What is the role for combinations of medications?" *Current Neurology and Neuroscience Reports*, vol. 8, no. 1, pp. 29–34, 2008.

[15] A. Kumar, G. C. Fonarow, K. A. Eagle et al., "Regional and practice variation in adherence to guideline recommendations for secondary and primary prevention among outpatients with atherothrombosis or risk factors in the United States: a report from the REACH registry," *Critical Pathways in Cardiology*, vol. 8, no. 3, pp. 104–111, 2009.

[16] L. B. Goldstein, A. J. Bonito, D. B. Matchar, P. W. Duncan, and G. P. Samsa, "US national survey of physician practices for the secondary and tertiary prevention of ischemic stroke: medical therapy in patients with carotid artery stenosis," *Stroke*, vol. 27, no. 9, pp. 1473–1478, 1996.

[17] L. B. Goldstein, A. J. Bonito, D. B. Matchar et al., "US national survey of physician practices for the secondary and tertiary prevention of ischemic stroke: design, service availability, and common practices," *Stroke*, vol. 26, no. 9, pp. 1607–1615, 1995.

[18] S. Yusuf, F. Zhao, S. R. Mehta, S. Chrolavicius, G. Tognoni, and K. K. Fox, "Effects of clopidogrel in addition to aspirin in patients with acute coronary syndromes without ST-segment elevation," *New England Journal of Medicine*, vol. 345, no. 7, pp. 494–502, 2001.

[19] S. R. Steinhubl, P. B. Berger, J. T. Mann III et al., "Early and sustained dual oral antiplatelet therapy following percutaneous coronary intervention: a randomized controlled trial," *Journal of the American Medical Association*, vol. 288, no. 19, pp. 2411–2420, 2002.

[20] P. H. C. Diener, P. J. Bogousslavsky, P. L. M. Brass et al., "Aspirin and clopidogrel compared with clopidogrel alone after recent ischaemic stroke or transient ischaemic attack in high-risk patients (MATCH): randomised, double-blind, placebo-controlled trial," *The Lancet*, vol. 364, no. 9431, pp. 331–337, 2004.

[21] National Center for Health Statistics, "National Ambulatory Medical Care Survey (NAMCS)-Micro-Data File Documentation," ftp://ftp.cdc.gov/pub/Health_Statistics/NCHS/namcs_public_use_files/.

[22] National Center for Health Statistics, "National Hospital Ambulatory Medical Care Survey (NHAMCS)-Micro-Data File Documentation," ftp://ftp.cdc.gov/pub/Health_Statistics/Statistics/NCHS/Dataset_Documentation/NHAMCS/.

[23] C. L. Roumie, E. Mitchel, P. S. Gideon, C. Varas-Lorenzo, J. Castellsague, and M. R. Griffin, "Validation of ICD-9 codes with a high positive predictive value for incident strokes resulting in hospitalization using Medicaid health data," *Pharmacoepidemiology and Drug Safety*, vol. 17, no. 1, pp. 20–26, 2008.

[24] L. B. Goldstein, "Accuracy of ICD-9-CM coding for the identification of patients with acute ischemic stroke: effect of modifier codes," *Stroke*, vol. 29, no. 8, pp. 1602–1604, 1998.

[25] D. L. Tirschwell and W. T. Longstreth, "Validating administrative data in stroke research," *Stroke*, vol. 33, no. 10, pp. 2465–2470, 2002.

[26] D. M. Reker, A. K. Rosen, H. Hoenig et al., "The hazards of stroke case selection using administrative data," *Medical Care*, vol. 40, no. 2, pp. 96–104, 2002.

[27] K. Buresly, M. J. Eisenberg, X. Zhang, and L. Pilote, "Bleeding complications associated with combinations of aspirin, thienopyridine derivatives, and warfarin in elderly patients following acute myocardial infarction," *Archives of Internal Medicine*, vol. 165, no. 7, pp. 784–789, 2005.

[28] J. S. Berger, D. L. Bhatt, C. P. Cannon et al., "The relative efficacy and safety of clopidogrel in women and men. A sex-specific collaborative meta-analysis," *Journal of the American College of Cardiology*, vol. 54, no. 21, pp. 1935–1945, 2009.

[29] Z. Chen, "CAST: randomised placebo-controlled trial of early aspirin use in 20,000 patients with acute ischaemic stroke," *The Lancet*, vol. 349, no. 9066, pp. 1641–1649, 1997.

[30] International Stroke Trial Collaborative Group, "The International Stroke Trial (IST): a randomised trial of aspirin, subcutaneous heparin, both, or neither among 19 435 patients with acute ischaemic stroke," *The Lancet*, vol. 349, no. 9065, pp. 1569–1581, 1997.

[31] T. A. Pearson, S. N. Blair, S. R. Daniels et al., "AHA guidelines for primary prevention of cardiovascular disease and stroke: 2002 update: consensus panel guide to comprehensive risk reduction for adult patients without coronary or other atherosclerotic vascular diseases," *Circulation*, vol. 106, no. 3, pp. 388–391, 2002.

[32] H. C. Diener, L. Cunha, C. Forbes, J. Sivenius, P. Smets, and A. Lowenthal, "European stroke prevention study 2. Dipyridamole and acetylsalicylic acid in the secondary prevention of stroke," *Journal of the Neurological Sciences*, vol. 143, no. 1-2, pp. 1–13, 1996.

[33] ESPRIT Study Group, P. H. Halkes, J. van Gijn, L. J. Kappelle, P. J. Koudstaal, and A. Algra, "Aspirin plus dipyridamole versus aspirin alone after cerebral ischaemia of arterial origin (ESPRIT): randomised controlled trial," *The Lancet*, vol. 367, no. 9523, pp. 1665–1673, 2006.

[34] J. Fang, M. H. Alderman, N. L. Keenan, and J. B. Croft, "Declining US stroke hospitalization since 1997: national hospital discharge survey, 1988–2004," *Neuroepidemiology*, vol. 29, no. 3-4, pp. 243–249, 2008.

[35] J. Fang and M. H. Alderman, "Trend of stroke hospitalization, United States, 1988–1997," *Stroke*, vol. 32, no. 10, pp. 2221–2225, 2001.

14

Chronic Administration of a Combination of Six Herbs Inhibits the Progression of Hyperglycemia and Decreases Serum Lipids and Aspartate Amino Transferase Activity in Diabetic Rats

Reza Shafiee-Nick,[1,2] Ahmad Ghorbani,[1]
Farzaneh Vafaee Bagheri,[1] and Hassan Rakhshandeh[1,2]

[1] *Pharmacological Research Center of Medicinal Plants, School of Medicine, Mashhad University of Medical Sciences, Mashhad 9177948564, Iran*
[2] *Department of Pharmacology, School of Medicine, Mashhad University of Medical Sciences, Mashhad 9177948564, Iran*

Correspondence should be addressed to Ahmad Ghorbani, ghorbania@mums.ac.ir

Academic Editor: Owen L. Woodman

The effects of a polyherbal compound, containing six plants (Allium sativum, Cinnamomum zeylanicum, Nigella sativa, Punica granatum, Salvia officinalis and Teucrium polium) were tested on biochemical parameters in streptozotocin-induced diabetic rats. Streptozotocin caused an approximately 3-fold increase in fasting blood sugar level after 2 days. The diabetic control rats showed further increase in blood glucose after 30 days (384 ± 25 mg/dl in day 30 versus 280 ± 12 mg/dl in day 2, $P < 0.001$). Administration of the compound blocked the increase of blood glucose (272 ± 7 and 269 ± 48 mg/dl at day 2 and day 30, respectively). Also, there was significant difference in the level of triglyceride (60 ± 9 versus 158 ± 37 mg/dl, $P < 0.01$), total cholesterol (55 ± 2 versus 97 ± 11 mg/dl, $P < 0.01$) and aspartate amino transferase activity (75 ± 12 versus 129 ± 18 U/L, $P < 0.05$) between treated rats and diabetic control group. In conclusion, the MSEC inhibited the progression of hyperglycemia and decreased serum lipids and hepatic enzyme activity in diabetic rats. Therefore, it has the potential to be used as a natural product for the management of diabetes.

1. Introduction

Diabetes mellitus, a metabolic disease with manifestation of hyperglycemia, is a fast growing health problem through out the world. The World Health Organization estimates that 346 million people suffer from diabetes worldwide. Without urgent action, this number is likely to double by 2030. Generally, diabetes is classified into two main types: type-1 diabetes, a state of insulin deficiency because of defect in islet β-cell function and type-2 diabetes which mainly characterized by resistance to the actions of insulin. Over time, diabetes leads to serious microvascular and macrovascular complications such as nephropathy, retinopathy, neuropathy, and cardiovascular disease [1]. Although early onset manifestations of diabetes can be controlled by current oral hypoglycemic drugs or insulin treatment, serious late onset complications appear in many patients [2]. Moreover, the hypoglycemic drugs lead to some unpleasant side effects such as lactic acidosis, peripheral edema, severe hypoglycemia, and abdominal discomfort [3]. Therefore, the search for new antidiabetic agents has continued.

Plants have always been a good source for finding new therapeutic agents for human diseases. Antidiabetic effects of several plants have been supported by results from animal models and clinical trials [4, 5]. Among them, *Allium sativum, Cinnamomum zeylanicum, Nigella sativa, Punica granatum, Salvia officinalis,* and *Teucrium polium* are widely used as medicinal plants for management of diabetes in Middle East [6, 7]. Recently, several studies have shown that each one of the six plants is effective in decrease of plasma glucose and serum lipids in diabetes [8–18]. We hypothesized that a combination of their extracts may have more effect

TABLE 1: Composition of polyherbal compounds.

Herbs	Quantity (g/100 g of compound)		
	MEC	SEC	MSEC (MEC + SEC)
Allium sativum	16	16	8 + 8
Cinnamomum zeylanicum	14	14	7 + 7
Nigella sativa	28	28	14 + 14
Punica granatum	14	14	7 + 7
Salvia officinalis	14	14	7 + 7
Teucrium polium	14	14	7 + 7

MEC: macerated extracts compound; SEC: Soxhlet extracts compound; MSEC: combination of both MEC and SEC.

on improving metabolic indexes in diabetes. Therefore, the present work was carried out to investigate antidiabetic activity of a polyherbal compound containing these six plant species.

2. Materials and Methods

2.1. Preparation of Extracts. The air-dried *A. sativum* (cloves), *C. zeylanicum* (bark), *N. sativa* (seeds), *P. granatum* (fruits), *S. officinalis* (areal parts), and *T. polium* (areal parts) were powdered and used for extraction. For each plant two types of hydroalcoholic extract were prepared: macerated extract (ME) and Soxhlet extract (SE). The ME was prepared by suspension of each powdered plant material in 70% ethanol and incubated for 72 h at 37°C. The SE was made in a Soxhlet apparatus with 70% ethanol for 24 h [19, 20]. The ME and SE of each plant were evaporated to dryness and then mixed as indicated in Table 1 to make three test compounds: MEs compound (MEC), SEs compound (SEC) and a combination of both MEC and SEC (MSEC).

2.2. Animals. Male albino Wistar rats (280–330 g) were used for each experiment. They were housed in a room with controlled lighting (12 h light/12 h darkness) and temperature (22 ± 2°C). The animals were given standard pellets diet and water *ad libitum*. The study protocol using laboratory animals complied with the guidelines of the animal care of the Mashhad University of Medical Sciences, Mashhad, Iran.

2.3. Induction of Diabetes. The animals were given a single dose (55 mg/kg, ip) of streptozotocin (STZ) (Enzo Life, USA). Development of diabetes was confirmed by measuring fasting blood sugar (FBS) two days after STZ injection [21, 22]. Rats with FBS level of 250 mg/kg or higher were considered to be diabetic.

2.4. Glucose Tolerance Test. Oral glucose tolerance test (GTT) was performed on normal rats that were fasted 16 h. The animals were divided into 4 groups comprising of 8 animals in each groups. The rats in group 1, 2, 3, and 4 were received vehicle, MEC (1 g/kg), SEC (1 g/kg), and glibenclamide (1 mg/kg), respectively. The vehicle or test compounds were given orally thirty minutes before administration of glucose (2 g/kg). A fasting blood sample was first collected from

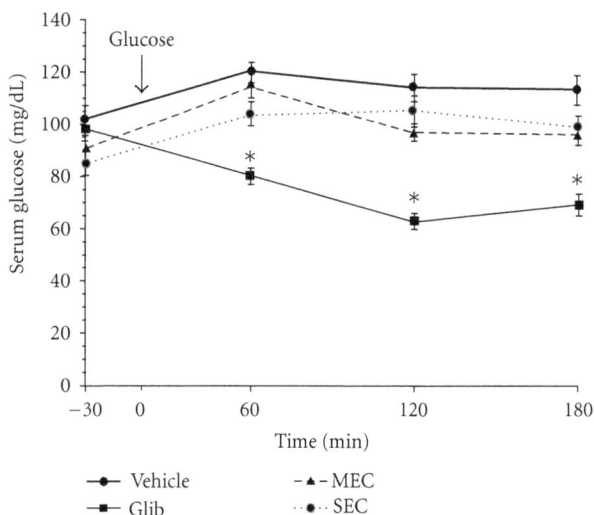

FIGURE 1: Effect of test compounds on glucose tolerance test (GTT) in normal rats. After 16 h fasting, the animals were received water as vehicle, glibenclamide (1 mg/kg), or test compounds (1 g/kg) orally thirty minutes before administration of glucose (2 g/kg). The data are expressed as mean ± SEM ($n = 8$). *$P < 0.01$ compared with the corresponding values at all other groups. Glib: glibenclamide-MEC: macerated extracts compound; SEC: Soxhlet extracts compound.

retroorbital sinus, and then three more samples were taken at the 60, 120, and 180 min intervals following glucose administration.

2.5. Long-Term Administration of Test Compounds. Diabetic rats were randomized into two groups, 7 animals each: (1) diabetic control rats which were fed standard pellets diet, and (2) diabetic rats which were received diet containing 4% (w/w) of MSEC. The treatment was initiated two days after STZ injection and continued for 4 weeks. At the end of the 30th day, the rats were fasted 16 h and blood samples were collected from retroorbital sinus for biochemical measurements. Also, a 2 h glucose tolerance assay was conducted in the 30th day.

2.6. Biochemical Assays. Blood glucose was measured using glucose oxidase reagent (Ziest Chem Diagnostics, Iran). Total cholesterol and high-density lipoprotein (HDL) were evaluated with standard enzymatic colorimetric kits from Pars Azmun (Iran). Serum triglyceride was measured using an enzymatic colorimetric test (Ziest Chem Diagnostics, Iran). Serum alanine aminotransferase (ALT) and aspartate aminotransferase (AST) activities were measured colorimetrically by commercially available kits (Pars Azmun, Iran).

2.7. Statistical Analysis. Statistical analysis of changes from baseline was performed by paired *t*-test within groups. Intergroup comparison was done by one-way ANOVA with Turkey's post-hoc test. Results showing *P* values less than 0.05 were considered significant.

TABLE 2: Effect of long-term administration of MSEC on blood glucose level in diabetic rats.

Animal groups	Blood glucose (mg/dL)			
	Day 0 (FBS)	Day 2 (FBS)	Day 30 (FBS)	Day 30 (2 h GTT)
Normal control	85 ± 5	82 ± 6	86 ± 8	115 ± 6#
Diabetic control	91 ± 5	280 ± 12*	384 ± 25*†	451 ± 26*
Diabetic + MSEC	96 ± 4	272 ± 7*	269 ± 48*	347 ± 29*

The data are expressed as mean ± SEM ($n = 7$). *$P < 0.001$ compared with the corresponding values at day 0 in each group. #$P < 0.05$ compared with FBS value at day 30 for normal control group. †$P < 0.05$ compared with the corresponding values at day 2 for Diabetic control group. FBS: fasting blood sugar; MSEC: combination of both macerated and Soxhlet extracts (see Table 1); GTT: glucose tolerance test.

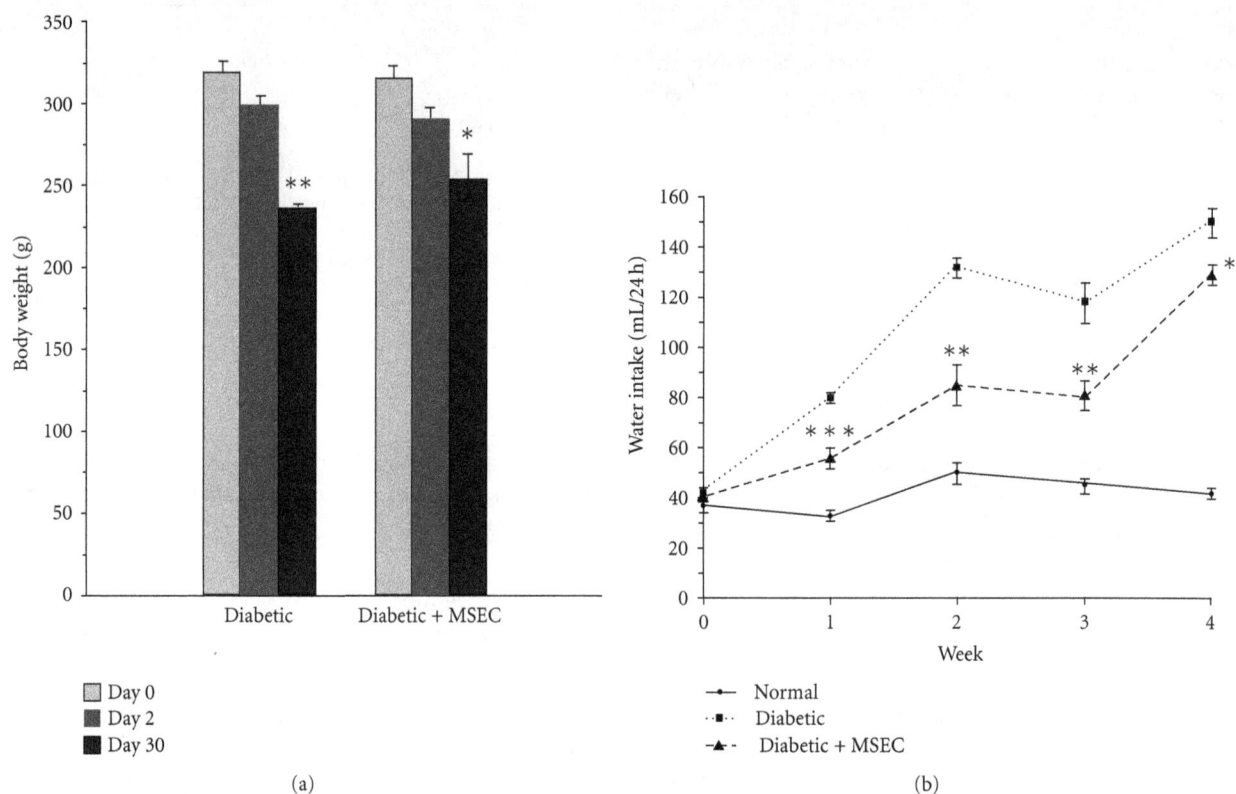

FIGURE 2: Effect of long-term administration of MSEC on body weight and water intake in diabetic rats. The animals in group of diabetic + MSEC received diet containing 4% (w/w) of MSEC for 1 month. (a): *$P < 0.01$ compared with the corresponding values at day 2 and day 0. **$P < 0.001$ compared with the corresponding values at day 2 or day 0. (b): *$P < 0.001$ and $P < 0.05$ compared with the corresponding values of normal and diabetic + MSEC group, respectively. **$P < 0.01$ compared with the corresponding values of normal or diabetic + MSEC group. ***$P < 0.001$ compared with the corresponding values of normal or diabetic + MSEC group. The data are expressed as mean ± SEM for seven (body weight) or six (water intake) rats. MSEC: combination of both macerated and Soxhlet extracts (see Table 1).

3. Results

3.1. Effect of Test Compounds on Glucose Tolerance.
Results of GTT conducted on normal rats are shown in Figure 1. The plasma glucose levels of the control rats reached a peak at 60 min after administration of glucose and gradually decreased. The glibenclamide produced plasma glucose levels significantly ($P < 0.001$) lower than those of the control group at 60–120 min after the glucose administration. When the basal glucose levels were adjusted to 100%, neither the MEC nor the SEC showed significant effect on serum glucose

at 60, 120, or 180 min as compared to those of the control group.

3.2. Effect of MSEC on Blood Glucose.
As shown in Table 2, prior to STZ injection, FBS levels of all the groups were not statistically different from each other. At day 2, administration of STZ to rats caused an approximately 3-fold increase in FBS level compared to normal controls. The diabetic control rats showed further increase in FBS level after 30 days (384 ± 25 mg/dL in day 30 versus 280 ± 12 mg/dL in day 2,

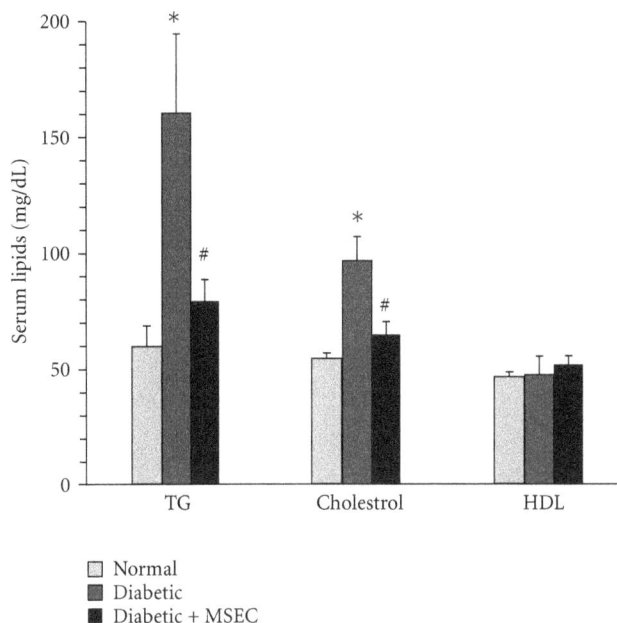

FIGURE 3: Effect of long-term administration of MSEC on the levels of plasma lipids in diabetic rats. The animals in group of diabetic + MSEC received diet containing 4% (w/w) of MSEC for 1 month. *$P < 0.01$ versus normal rats. #$P < 0.05$ versus diabetic group. The data are expressed as mean ± SEM for eight (normal and diabetic + MSEC groups) or six (diabetic groups) rats. MSEC: combination of both macerated and Soxhlet extracts; TG: triglycerides; TC: total cholesterol; HDL: high-density lipoprotein.

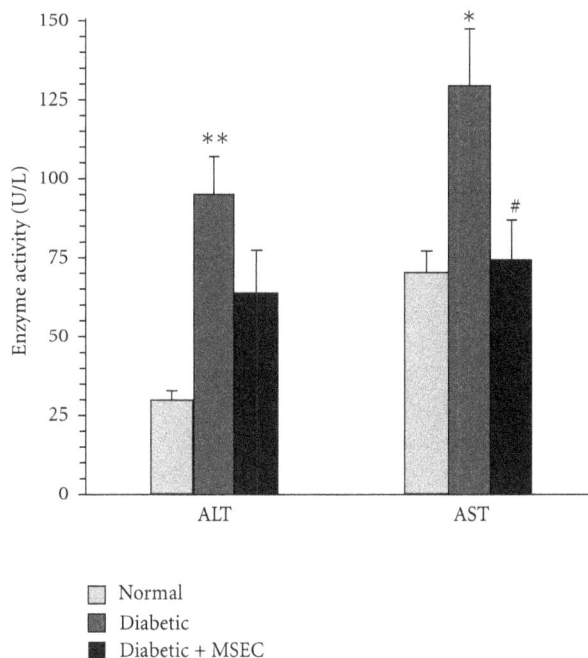

FIGURE 4: Effect of MSEC on serum alanine aminotransferase (ALT) and aspartate aminotransferase (AST) activities in diabetic rats. The animals in group of diabetic + MSEC received diet containing 4% (w/w) of MSEC for 1 month. *$P < 0.05$ versus normal and diabetic + MSEC groups. **$P < 0.01$ versus normal rats. #$P < 0.05$ versus diabetic group. The data are expressed as mean ± SEM for eight (normal and diabetic + MSEC groups) or six (diabetic groups) rats. MSEC: combination of both macerated and Soxhlet extracts.

$P < 0.001$). However, administration of MSEC to diabetic rats blocked the increase of blood glucose. The level of FBS in this group was 272 ± 7 and 269 ± 48 mg/dL at day 2 and day 30, respectively.

Two hours after feeding of glucose, the blood sugar rose to 451 ± 26 mg/dL from 384 ± 25 mg/dL and to 347 ± 29 mg/dL from 269 ± 48 mg/dL in the case of diabetic controls and MSEC-treated rats, respectively.

3.3. Effect of MSEC on Body Weight and Water Intake. After two days of STZ injection, the diabetic rats in control and MSEC-treated groups showed a significant reduction in their original body weight from 320 ± 6 to 300 ± 5 g ($P < 0.01$) and from 315 ± 7 to 292 ± 6 g ($P < 0.01$), respectively. The weight reduction was continued for both groups and at 30th day reached to 236 ± 4 g ($P < 0.01$ versus day 2) and 254 ± 16 g ($P < 0.05$ versus day 2) for control and MSEC-treated animals, respectively (Figure 2(a)).

In all groups prior to diabetes induction, the levels of water intake were not significantly different. However, there was a significant increase in the levels of water intake in both groups of diabetic rats after STZ administration (Figure 2(b)). Although the polydipsia condition was evident from the first week to the end of the experiment period, the level of water intake in MSEC-treated rats was significantly lower than that of control diabetic group.

3.4. Effect of MSEC on the Levels of Serum Lipids. Figure 3 shows the effect of MSEC on serum lipids in diabetic rats. There was a significant elevation in the level of triglyceride (60 ± 9 mg/dL versus 158 ± 37 mg/dL, $P < 0.01$) and total cholesterol (55 ± 2 mg/dL versus 97 ± 11 mg/dL, $P < 0.01$) in diabetic rats as compared with normal rats. The MSEC was found to be effective in decreasing the serum lipids. The levels of triglyceride and total cholesterol in MSEC-treated group were 80 ± 9 mg/dL ($P < 0.01$ versus the corresponding value of diabetic rats) and 65 ± 6 mg/dL ($P < 0.01$ versus the corresponding value of diabetic rats), respectively. There was no significant difference between the groups in serum HDL level.

3.5. Effect of MSEC on the Serum Enzyme Activity. After 30 days of diabetes induction, the activity of serum ALT was more than three times relative to the normal animals (95 ± 12 versus 30 ± 3 U/L, $P < 0.01$). Similarly, diabetic rats showed higher AST activity than normal group (129 ± 18 versus 70 ± 7 U/L, $P < 0.05$). Treatment with MSEC decreased the ALT activity (64 ± 13 U/L); however, the effect was statistically insignificant (Figure 4). On the other hand, there was significant difference in the AST activity between MSEC-treated rats (75 ± 12 U/L, $P < 0.05$) and diabetic control group (129 ± 18 U/L).

4. Discussion

In the present study, we tested the possible beneficial effects of a polyherbal compound, containing six plants (*A. sativum*, *C. zeylanicum*, *N. sativa*, *P. granatum*, *S. officinalis*, and *T. polium*) on biochemical parameters of diabetic rats. Although this compound (MSEC) failed to completely restore STZ-induced hyperglycemia and had no remarkable effect on weight reduction; however, it significantly prevented further elevation of blood sugar and improved the polydipsia state. Therefore, it seems that administration of MSEC can only inhibit progression and deterioration of hyperglycemia. Additionally, normal rats treated with MEC or SEC did not change significantly the glycaemia values on GTT, which indicates an antihyperglycemic effect rather than a hypoglycaemic one for the constituents of MSEC. This effect is expected to happen as antihyperglycemic property of its herbal constituents (i.e., the six plants) has been confirmed with repeated studies [8–18].

Antihyperglycemic effect of plants is achieved by enhancing insulin secretion from beta cells, increasing glucose uptake by tissues, decreasing glucose absorption from intestine, inhibiting glucose production in liver, increasing pancreatic tissue regeneration [23], and/or presence of insulin-like agents in plants [4, 23, 24]. Recent studies have shown that *P. granatum* inhibits α-glucosidase, rate-limiting enzymes for digestion of oligosaccharides which are necessary for intestinal absorption of glucose. Also, it has been demonstrated that *N. sativa* and *S. officinalis* decrease hepatic glucose production through inhibition of gluconeogenic enzymes. Moreover, beneficial effect of *T. polium* on regeneration of pancreatic islets was reported [25–28].

The levels of serum triglyceride and cholesterol are usually elevated in diabetic patients [29]. The hyperlipidemia mainly occurs as a result of insulin deficiency and thereby dysregulation of metabolic processes like lipolysis and lipogenesis [30]. In the present study also, the diabetic animals showed hypertriglyceridemia, and hypercholesterolemia and the treatment with MSEC significantly decreased the hyperlipidemia. Therefore, the product most probably can prevent dyslipidemia-related complications of diabetic patients. The hypolipidemic action of MSEC is in agreement with earlier studies that reported that *A. sativum*, *C. zeylanicum*, *N. sativa*, *S. officinalis*, and *T. polium* decrease the levels of serum triglyceride and cholesterol in diabetic animals [8, 11, 12, 16, 18].

Measurements of serum ALT and AST are used in the evaluation of liver damage. Elevation of these enzyme activities is considered as evidence for hepatic damage. An increase of these enzyme activities is also associated with fatty liver disease and decreased hepatic insulin sensitivity in type-2 diabetes [31, 32]. Recently, it has shown that fatty liver disease is associated with an increased risk of death among diabetic patients [33]. In our study, recovery of serum ALT and AST activities of diabetic rats towards normal level shows that the MSEC has protective effect against liver damage and therefore can improve prognosis of diabetic patients. According to the results of previous studies, the main components responsible for this protective effect are most likely found in *A. sativum*, *S. officinalis*, and *T. polium* [8, 16, 34].

In conclusion, the present study demonstrated that MSEC has antidiabetic actions mainly through its hypolipidemic and hepatoprotective effects as well as through inhibition of progression and deterioration of glycemia. Therefore, it has the potential to be used as a new natural product for the management of diabetes.

Conflict of Interests

The authors declare that they have no conflict of interests.

Acknowledgments

This work was supported by a grant from Research Council of Mashhad University of Medical Sciences, Mashhad, Iran.

References

[1] A. D. Deshpande, M. Harris-Hayes, and M. Schootman, "Epidemiology of diabetes and diabetes-related complications," *Physical Therapy*, vol. 88, no. 11, pp. 1254–1264, 2008.

[2] I. Tzoulaki, M. Molokhia, V. Curcin et al., "Risk of cardiovascular disease and all cause mortality among patients with type 2 diabetes prescribed oral antidiabetes drugs: retrospective cohort study using UK general practice research database," *British Medical Journal*, vol. 339, p. b4731, 2009.

[3] B. Lorenzati, C. Zucco, S. Miglietta, F. Lamberti, and G. Bruno, "Oral hypoglycemic drugs: pathophysiological basis of their mechanism of action," *Pharmaceuticals*, vol. 3, no. 9, pp. 3005–3020, 2010.

[4] H. Hui, G. Tang, and V. L. W. Go, "Hypoglycemic herbs and their action mechanisms," *Chinese Medicine*, vol. 4, no. 1, article 11, 2009.

[5] M. Modak, P. Dixit, J. Londhe, S. Ghaskadbi, and T. P. A. Devasagayam, "Indian herbs and herbal drugs used for the treatment of diabetes," *Journal of Clinical Biochemistry and Nutrition*, vol. 40, no. 3, pp. 163–173, 2007.

[6] A. Ghorbani and H. Rakhshandeh, *The Most Effective Herbs for Diabetes*, Mashhad University of Medical Sciences, Mashhad, Iran, 2012.

[7] S. Hasani-Ranjbar, B. Larijani, and M. Abdollah, "A systematic review of iranian medicinal plants useful in diabetes mellitus," *Archives of Medical Science*, vol. 4, no. 3, pp. 285–292, 2008.

[8] A. Eidi, M. Eidi, and E. Esmaeili, "Antidiabetic effect of garlic (*Allium sativum* L.) in normal and streptozotocin-induced diabetic rats," *Phytomedicine*, vol. 13, no. 9-10, pp. 624–629, 2006.

[9] F. M. El-Demerdash, M. I. Yousef, and N. I. Abou El-Naga, "Biochemical study on the hypoglycemic effects of onion and garlic in alloxan-induced diabetic rats," *Food and Chemical Toxicology*, vol. 43, no. 1, pp. 57–63, 2005.

[10] B. Mang, M. Wolters, B. Schmitt et al., "Effects of a cinnamon extract on plasma glucose, HbA$_{1c}$, and serum lipids in diabetes mellitus type 2," *European Journal of Clinical Investigation*, vol. 36, no. 5, pp. 340–344, 2006.

[11] S. A. Hassan, R. Barthwal, M. S. Nair, and S. S. Haque, "Aqueous bark extract of *Cinnamomum Zeylanicum*: a potential therapeutic agent for streptozotocin-induced type 1 diabetes

mellitus (T1DM) rats," *Tropical Journal of Pharmaceutical Research*, vol. 13, no. 3, pp. 429–435, 2012.

[12] M. Kaleem, D. Kirmani, M. Asif, Q. Ahmed, and B. Bano, "Biochemical effects of *Nigella sativa* L seeds in diabetic rats," *Indian Journal of Experimental Biology*, vol. 44, no. 9, pp. 745–748, 2006.

[13] I. Meral, Z. Yener, T. Kahraman, and N. Mert, "Effect of *Nigella sativa* on glucose concentration, lipid peroxidation, antioxidant defence system and liver damage in experimentally-induced diabetic rabbits," *Journal of Veterinary Medicine A*, vol. 48, no. 10, pp. 593–599, 2001.

[14] A. Esmaillzadeh, F. Tahbaz, I. Gaieni, H. Alavi-Majd, and L. Azadbakht, "Cholesterol-lowering effect of concentrated pomegranate juice consumption in type II diabetic patients with hyperlipidemia," *International Journal for Vitamin and Nutrition Research*, vol. 76, no. 3, pp. 147–151, 2006.

[15] M. A. Jafri, M. Aslam, K. Javed, and S. Singh, "Effect of *Punica granatum* Linn. (flowers) on blood glucose level in normal and alloxan-induced diabetic rats," *Journal of Ethnopharmacology*, vol. 70, no. 3, pp. 309–314, 2000.

[16] A. Eidi and M. Eidi, "Antidiabetic effects of sage (*Salvia officinalis* L.) leaves in normal and streptozotocin-induced diabetic rats," *Diabetes & Metabolic Syndrome*, vol. 3, no. 1, pp. 40–44, 2009.

[17] M. R. Shahraki, M. R. Arab, E. Mirimokaddam, and M. J. Palan, "The effect of *Teucrium polium* (Calpoureh) on liver function, serum lipids and glucose in diabetic male rats," *Iranian Biomedical Journal*, vol. 11, no. 1, pp. 65–68, 2007.

[18] F. Karimi, S. Abbasi, and A. R. Bateni, "The effect of *Teucrium polium* on blood glucose in diabetes mellitus type 2; a comparison with glibenclamide," *Iranian South Medical Journal*, vol. 2, no. 2, pp. 96–103, 2002.

[19] S. M. Mortazavian and A. Ghorbani, "Antiproliferative effect of *Viola tricolor* on neuroblastoma cells in vitro," *Australian Journal of Medicinal Herbalism*, vol. 24, no. 3, pp. 93–96, 2012.

[20] A. Ghorbani, N. J. Youssofabad, and H. Rakhshandeh, "Effect of *Viola tricolor* on pentobarbital-induced sleep in mice," *African Journal of Pharmacy and Pharmacology*, vol. 6, no. 33, pp. 2503–2509, 2012.

[21] A. Ghorbani, M. Varedi, M. A. R. Hadjzadeh, and G. H. Omrani, "Type-1 diabetes induces depot-specific alterations in adipocyte diameter and mass of adipose tissues in the rat," *Experimental and Clinical Endocrinology and Diabetes*, vol. 118, no. 7, pp. 442–448, 2010.

[22] A. Ghorbani, G. H. Omrani, M. R. Hadjzadeh, and M. Varedi, "Proinsulin C-peptide inhibits lipolysis in diabetic rat adipose tissue through phosphodiesterase-3Benzyme," *Hormone and Metabolic Research*. In press.

[23] K. R. Shanmugasundaram, C. Panneerselvam, P. Samudram, and E. R. B. Shanmugasundaram, "The insulinotropic activity of *Gymnema sylvestre*, R. Br. an Indian medical herb used in controlling diabetes mellitus," *Pharmacological Research Communications*, vol. 13, no. 5, pp. 475–486, 1981.

[24] A. M. Gray and P. R. Flatt, "Insulin-releasing and insulin-like activity of the traditional anti-diabetic plant *Coriandrum sativum* (coriander)," *British Journal of Nutrition*, vol. 81, no. 3, pp. 203–209, 1999.

[25] L. Pari and C. Sankaranarayanan, "Beneficial effects of thymoquinone on hepatic key enzymes in streptozotocin-nicotinamide induced diabetic rats," *Life Sciences*, vol. 85, no. 23–26, pp. 830–834, 2009.

[26] K. M. Fararh, Y. Atoji, Y. Shimizu, and T. Takewaki, "Isulinotropic properties of *Nigella sativa* oil in Streptozotocin plus Nicotinamide diabetic hamster," *Research in Veterinary Science*, vol. 73, no. 3, pp. 279–282, 2002.

[27] C. F. Lima, M. F. Azevedo, R. Araujo, M. Fernandes-Ferreira, and C. Pereira-Wilson, "Metformin-like effect of *Salvia officinalis* (common sage): is it useful in diabetes prevention?" *British Journal of Nutrition*, vol. 96, no. 2, pp. 326–333, 2006.

[28] M. Vessal, F. Zal, and M. Vasei, "Effects of *Teucrium polium* on oral glucose tolerance test, regeneration of pancreatic islets and activity of hepatic glucokinase in diabetic rats," *Archives of Iranian Medicine*, vol. 6, no. 1, pp. 35–39, 2003.

[29] J. Patel, "Diabetes: managing dyslipidaemia," *Clinical Evidence*, vol. 2008, p. 0610, 2008.

[30] P. Arner, "Human fat cell lipolysis: biochemistry, regulation and clinical role," *Best Practice & Research Clinical Endocrinology & Metabolism*, vol. 19, no. 4, pp. 471–482, 2005.

[31] R. K. Schindhelm, M. Diamant, J. M. Dekker, M. E. Tushuizen, T. Teerlink, and R. J. Heine, "Alanine aminotransferase as a marker of non-alcoholic fatty liver disease in relation to type 2 diabetes mellitus and cardiovascular disease," *Diabetes/Metabolism Research and Reviews*, vol. 22, no. 6, pp. 437–443, 2006.

[32] B. Vozarova, N. Stefan, R. S. Lindsay et al., "High alanine aminotransferase is associated with decreased hepatic insulin sensitivity and predicts the development of type 2 diabetes," *Diabetes*, vol. 51, no. 6, pp. 1889–1895, 2002.

[33] L. A. Adams, S. Harmsen, J. L. S. Sauver et al., "Nonalcoholic fatty liver disease increases risk of death among patients with diabetes: a community-based cohort study," *American Journal of Gastroenterology*, vol. 105, no. 7, pp. 1567–1573, 2010.

[34] S. Shtukmaster, P. Ljubuncic, and A. Bomzon, "The effect of an aqueous extract of *Teucrium polium* on glutathione homeostasis in vitro: a possible mechanism of its hepatoprotectant action," *Advances in Pharmacological Sciences*, vol. 2010, Article ID 938324, 7 pages, 2010.

15

Antinociceptive and Anti-Inflammatory Activities of Leaf Methanol Extract of *Cotyledon orbiculata* L. (Crassulaceae)

George J. Amabeoku and Joseph Kabatende

Discipline of Pharmacology, School of Pharmacy, University of the Western Cape, Private Bag X17, Bellville 7535, South Africa

Correspondence should be addressed to George J. Amabeoku, gamabeoku@uwc.ac.za

Academic Editor: Esra Küpeli Akkol

Leaf methanol extract of *C. orbiculata* L. was investigated for antinociceptive and anti-inflammatory activities using acetic acid writhing and hot-plate tests and carrageenan-induced oedema test in mice and rats, respectively. *C. orbiculata* (100–400 mg/kg, i.p.) significantly inhibited acetic acid-induced writhing and significantly delayed the reaction time of mice to the hot-plate-induced thermal stimulation. Paracetamol (300 mg/kg, i.p.) significantly inhibited the acetic acid-induced writhing in mice. Morphine (10 mg/kg, i.p.) significantly delayed the reaction time of mice to the thermal stimulation produced with hot plate. Leaf methanol extract of *C. orbiculata* (50–400 mg/kg, i.p.) significantly attenuated the carrageenan-induced rat paw oedema. Indomethacin (10 mg/kg, p.o.) also significantly attenuated the carrageenan-induced rat paw oedema. The LD_{50} value obtained for the plant species was greater than 4000 mg/kg (p.o.). The data obtained indicate that *C. orbiculata* has antinociceptive and anti-inflammatory activities, justifying the folklore use of the plant species by traditional medicine practitioners in the treatment of painful and inflammatory conditions. The relatively high LD_{50} obtained shows that *C. orbiculata* may be safe in or nontoxic to mice.

1. Introduction

Pain and inflammation are some of the most common manifestations of many diseases afflicting millions of people worldwide [1, 2]. Even though there are effective orthodox medicines used to alleviate these manifestations [3], traditional medicine practitioners in, mainly, developing countries have used herbal medicines to treat various ailments including pain and inflammation [4]. The dependence of the population especially in the rural communities in South Africa on plant medicines as well as traditional medicine practitioners for their healthcare needs is cultural. One of such plants used by traditional medicine practitioners to treat various ailments is *Cotyledon orbiculata* L. [5, 6]. It belongs to the family Crassulaceae. It is a small shrub with fleshy leaves and widely distributed in Southern Africa. It is known locally as "Seredile" in Sotho and Tswana, "Plakkie" in Afrikaans, and "Imphewula" in Xhosa [5, 6]. *C. orbiculata* is used in the treatment of various ailments in different parts of South Africa. The fleshy leaves have been used to treat corn and warts. The juice of the leaves is used as drops for earache and toothache and as hot poultice for boils and inflammation [5–7]. Infusion of the fleshy leaves of *C. orbiculata* has also been used by traditional medicines practitioners in South Africa for the treatment of epilepsy, inflammation, and aches (Oral communication).

According to the literature, very limited evaluation has been done on the pharmacological activities of the plant species despite the wide folklore use [8]. This study was, therefore, intended to investigate the antinociceptive and anti-inflammatory activities of *C. orbiculata* in mice and rats, respectively. The acute toxicity and HPLC studies of the plant species were also carried out.

2. Materials and Methods

2.1. Plant Material. The fleshy leaves of *C. orbiculata* were collected from Kirstenbosch National Botanical Garden, Cape Town, in September, 2010. The plant material was identified by the curator of the Gardens as well as a taxonomist in the Department of Biodiversity and Conservative Biology,

University of the Western Cape and the voucher specimen (COT 25) deposited in the University's Herbarium.

2.2. Preparation of Plant Extract. The fleshy leaves (10.5 kg) of *C. orbiculata* were washed with water, sliced into pieces, and dried in a ventilated oven at 40°C for 120 h. The dried plant material (640 g) was ground into fine powder using Waring Commercial laboratory blender and passed through 850 μm sieve. For the preparation of the methanol extract, the dried powder (120 g) was extracted in a soxhlet extractor with methanol for 72 h. The methanol filtrate was evaporated to dryness using a Buchi RE11 rotavapor and Buchi 461water bath. A yield of 55.4 g of crude methanol extract was obtained and preserved in a dessicator. Fresh solution of the crude leaf methanol extract was prepared by dissolving a given quantity of the methanol extract in a small volume of dimethylsulfoxide (DMSO) and made up to the appropriate volume with physiological saline. The methanol solution was administered intraperitoneally (i.p.) to mice and rats in a volume of 1 mL/100 g of body weight.

2.3. Animals. Male albino mice bred in the Animal House of the Discipline of Pharmacology, School of Pharmacy, University of the Western Cape, South Africa, weighing 18–30 g were used for the antinociceptive activity and acute toxicity studies. Young adult male Wistar rats, bought from the University of Cape Town, South Africa, and weighing 160–210 g were used for anti-inflammatory activity study. The animals were housed in a quiet laboratory with an ambient temperature of 22 ± 1°C and a12 h light/12 h dark cycle was maintained. They all had access to food and water *ad libitum*. All the animals were fasted for 16 h during which they had access to water prior to the commencement of the experiments. Each animal was used for one experiment only.

2.4. Drugs and Chemicals. Indomethacin (Sigma Chemical Co.) was dissolved in a minimum amount of dimethylsulfoxide (DMSO, Sigma Chemical Co.) and adjusted to the appropriate volume with physiological saline. Carrageenan (Sigma Chemical Co.) and morphine sulphate (Bodene) were dissolved in physiological saline to an appropriate volume. Acetic acid (Merck) was dissolved in physiological saline to an appropriate strength. Paracetamol (Sigma Chemical Co.) was dissolved in a minimum volume of propylene glycol 400 (BDH, UK) and adjusted to the appropriate volume with physiological saline. DMSO solution was prepared by dissolving an equal amount of DMSO used to dissolve the plant extract, in an appropriate volume of physiological saline. Indomethacin was given orally to rats by means of a bulbed steel needle. Carrageenan was injected into the subplantar surface of the right hind paws of the rats.

Morphine, acetic acid, and paracetamol were administered intraperitoneally (ip) to mice. Fresh drug solutions were prepared each morning of the experiment. All drugs were administered in a volume of 1 mL/100 g of body weight, while constant volumes of carrageenan, DMSO, physiological saline, and acetic acid were used. Control animals received equal volume injections of the appropriate vehicles.

The doses and pretreatment times of the leaf methanol extract of *C. orbiculata* and standard drugs, indomethacin, morphine, paracetamol, and the vehicles, physiological saline and DMSO, were obtained from preliminary studies in our laboratory.

3. Assessment Pharmacological Activities

3.1. Antinociceptive Activity of Cotyledon orbiculata

3.1.1. Acetic Acid Writhing Test. The methods of Koster et al. [9] and Williamson et al. [10] were used for the assessment of the antinociceptive activity of *C. orbiculata*. Mice were used in groups of 8 per dose of plant extract, standard drug, paracetamol, or DMSO. They were placed singly in a transparent perspex mouse cage and allowed to acclimatize to their environment for 30 min prior to the commencement of the experiment. In the control experiment, the animals were pretreated with 0.25 mL of physiological saline (i.p.) for 15 min and then given intraperitoneal injection of 0.20 mL of 3% acetic acid solution, an irritant, used to induce writhing (pain). The mice were then left for 5 min, and the writhes were counted for the next 20 min. A writhe is defined as contraction of the abdominal muscles accompanied by elongation of the body and the hind limbs.

In the test experiment, a group of 8 mice were pretreated for 15 min with either the plant extract (i.p.) or the standard analgesic drug, paracetamol (i.p.), after which they were injected with 0.20 mL of the 3% acetic acid intraperitoneally, allowed to stand for 5 min and then the number of writhes counted for 20 min as for the control experiment. The experiment was repeated with another group of 8 mice pretreated with 0.25 mL of DMSO solution (i.p.) for 15 min, after which they were injected with 0.20 mL of the 3% acetic acid intraperitoneally, allowed to stand for 5 min, and then the number of writhes counted for 20 min. All experiments were performed in a quite laboratory with an ambient temperature of 22 ± 1°C. The ability of the plant extract to prevent or significantly reduced the number of acetic acid-induced writhes was an indication of an antinociceptive activity.

3.1.2. Hot-Plate Test. The methods of Williamson et al. [10] and Eddy and Leimback [11] were used in the hot-plate test for the antinociceptive activity of *C. orbiculata*. Mice were used in groups of 8 per dose of plant extract, standard drug, morphine, or DMSO. Control animals were individually placed in a 21 glass beaker placed on a thermostatically controlled hot plate (model HC500, Bibby Sterilin Ltd., England) set at 50–55°C, before and 15 min after intraperitoneal injection of 0.25 mL of physiological saline. The pain threshold is considered to be reached when the animals lift and lick their paws or attempt to jump out of the beaker. The time taken for the mice to exhibit these characteristics, also known as the reaction or response time, was noted by means of a stopwatch. The animals were tested before and 15 min, 30 min, 45 min, and 60 min after intraperitoneal injection of 0.25 mL of physiological saline. The experiments were repeated using other groups of animals, which were tested before and 15 min, 30 min, 45 min, and 60 min after the intraperitoneal administration of either the plant extract, morphine, or DMSO. All experiments were performed in a quite laboratory with an ambient temperature of $22 \pm 1°C$. A cutoff time of 60 s was used to avoid harm to the mice. The ability of the plant extract to delay the reaction time was taken as an indication of an antinociceptive activity.

3.2. Anti-Inflammatory Activity of Cotyledon orbiculata

3.2.1. Rat Paw Oedema Test.
Modified method of Williamson et al. [10] and Winter et al. [12] were used to assess the anti-inflammatory activity of *C. orbiculata*. Rats were used in groups of 8 per dose of plant extract, standard drug, physiological saline, or DMSO. The rats were divided into five groups. Rats in Group I (control) were given 0.25 mL (i.p.) of physiological saline. Group II rats received plant extracts (50–400 mg/kg, i.p.). Group III rats were given the standard anti-inflammatory drug, indomethacin (10 mg/kg, p.o.), and Group IV rats received 0.25 mL (i.p.) of DMSO (vehicle). Group V rats were untreated. Oedema or acute inflammation was induced in Group I or control rats pretreated for 15 min with 0.25 mL (i.p.) of physiological saline by injecting 0.1 mL of carrageenan (1% dissolved in 0.9% saline solution) into the subplantar surface of the right hind paw. The oedema following the carrageenan injection was noticeable within 30–40 min. The volume of the right hind paw was measured before and then after the injection of carrageenan at 30 min intervals for 4 h by volume displacement method using plethysmometer (IITC Life Sciences, USA). Group II rats were pretreated for 15 min with plant extracts intraperitoneally (i.p.), Group II rats for 1 h with indomethacin orally (p.o.) and Group IV rats for 15 min with DMSO (i.p.) prior to the injection 0.1 mL of carrageenan into the subplantar surface of the right hind paws of the rats in each group. The experiments were repeated with the volumes of the rats' right hind paws measured before and then after the injection of carrageenan at 30 min intervals for 4 h using the plethysmometer. The volumes of the untreated rats' right paws were also measured at 30 min intervals for 4 h. Oedema was expressed as a mean increase in paw volume with respect to physiological saline control. Inhibition was expressed as a percentage increase or decrease in oedema volume. The ability of the plant extract to inhibit the foot oedema was taken as an indication of an anti-inflammatory activity. All experiments were performed in a quite laboratory with an ambient temperature of $22 \pm 1°C$.

3.2.2. HPLC Analysis.
Chromatographic system: Beckman HPLC system consisting of double pump Programmable Solvent Module model 126; Diode Array detector Module model 168; Samsung computer 386 with management System Gold (Gold V601) software supplied by Beckman; Column, C18 Bondapak 5 μm and dimensions (250 $\times$ 4.6 mm).

Chromatographic conditions: Mobile phase: solvent A: 1% acetic acid; solvent B: methanol; Mode: gradient; flow rate, 1 min/min; injection volume, 10 μL; detector, UV at 350 nm. The HPLC operating conditions were programmed to give the following: 0 min, solvent B: 20%; 5 min, solvent B: 40%; 15 min, solvent B: 60%; 20 min, solvent B: 80% and 27 min, solvent B: 20%. The run rate was 30 min.

3.2.3. Acute Toxicity Testing.
The method described by Lorke [13] and modified by Hilaly et al. [14] was used to determine the median lethal dose (LD_{50}) of the leaf methanol extract. Mice were fasted for 16 h and then randomly divided into groups of eight mice per cage. Graded doses of the plant extract (100, 200, 300, 400, 600, 800, 1600, 2000, 2400, 2800, 3200, 3600, and 4000 mg/kg) were separately administered orally by means of a bulbed steel needle to mice in each test group. The control group was administered with 0.25 mL (p.o.) of physiological saline by means of a bulbed steel needle. The mice in both the test and control groups were then allowed free access to food and water and observed for over 5 days for signs of acute toxicity including death. The median lethal dose (LD_{50}) of the leaf methanol extract of *C. orbiculata* would be calculated if applicable, from a plot of log dose-response curve which would be constructed for the plant species.

3.3. Statistical Analysis.
The data on the number of writhes exhibited by the mice and the effect of carrageenan on the rat's right hind paw were analysed using one way analysis of variance (ANOVA) followed by Dunnett's multiple comparison test (GraphPad Prism, version 5.0, GraphPad Software, Inc., SanDiego CA p2130, USA) and presented as mean $\pm$ standard error mean (SEM). P values of less than 5% ($P < 0.05$) were considered statistically significant.

3.4. Ethical Considerations.
The experimental protocol used in this study was approved (07/04/31) by the Ethics Committee of the University of the Western Cape, Bellville 7535, South Africa, and conforms with the University's Regulations Act concerning animal experiments.

4. Results

4.1. Pharmacological Activities: Antinociceptive Activity of Cotyledon orbiculata

4.1.1. Acetic Acid Writhing Test

Effect of Leaf Methanol Extract of Cotyledon orbiculata on Acetic Acid-Induced Writhing. 0.20 mL (i.p.) of 3% acetic acid produced a substantial number of writhes in control mice pretreated with 0.25 mL (i.p.) of physiological saline. Leaf methanol extract of *C. orbiculata* (100–400 mg/kg, i.p.) in a dose-dependent manner, significantly reduced the number of acetic acid-induced writhes. 100 mg/kg (i.p.) of the plant species reduced the writhes by 51%. 200 mg/kg (i.p.) and 400 mg/kg (i.p.) of *C. orbiculata* produced 67% and 76% reduction in writhes produced by 0.20 mL of 3% acetic acid in mice, respectively. Similarly, paracetamol (300 mg/kg, i.p.) profoundly reduced the number of writhes elicited by

0.20 mL of 3% acetic acid by 93%. DMSO (0.25 mL, i.p.) did not significantly alter the acetic acid-induced writhes in mice (Table 1).

Effect of Leaf Methanol Extract of Cotyledon orbiculata on Hot-Plate-Induced Nociception. Mice pretreated with physiological saline reacted to hot-plate thermal stimulation at 50°C–55°C either by lifting and licking their paws or attempting to jump out of the beaker. This manifestation occurred within 6.63 ± 0.60 sec in the first 15 min after intraperitoneal administration of 0.25 mL of physiological. saline and within 2.75 ± 0.31 sec, 60 min later after the injection of 0.25 mL of physiological saline. Leaf methanol extract of *C. orbiculata* (100–200 mg/kg, i.p.) significantly delayed the reaction times of the animals to hot-plate thermal stimulation 30 min after treatment. *C. orbiculata* (400 mg/kg, i.p.) significantly delayed the pain reaction time of the mice to the hot-plate-induced thermal stimulation over the 1 h period of measurement. Similarly, morphine (10 mg/kg, i.p.) significantly delayed the reaction time of the mice to the hot-plate-induced thermal stimulation over the 1 h period of measurement. DMSO (0.25 mL, i.p.) did not significantly alter the reaction time of the mice to the hot-plate-induced thermal stimulation over the 1 h period of measurement (Table 2).

Effect of Leaf Methanol Extract of C. orbiculata on Carrageenan-Induced Right Hind Paw Oedema. Carrageenan (1%) injected into the subplantar of the right hind paws of the rats pretreated with physiological saline induced oedema or acute inflammation in the paws within 30–40 min. The oedema reached its maximum intensity 3 h after injection. 50 mg/kg (i.p.) of the leaf methanol extract of *C. orbiculata* significantly reduced the carrageenan-induced oedema from 60 min up to the 4 h period of measurement. *C. orbiculata* (100–400 mg/kg, i.p.) significantly reduced the carrageenan-induced oedema over the 4 h period of measurement. Indomethacin (10 mg/kg, p.o.) profoundly reduced the carrageenan-induced oedema in the right hind paws of rats over the 4 h period of measurement (Table 3).

4.1.2. Acute Toxicity Test. There were no deaths or signs of acute toxicity observed after oral administration of 100–4000 mg/kg of the leaf methanol extract of *Cotyledon orbiculata* with the highest dose tested (4000 mg/kg, p.o.) being the no-adverse-effect-level (NOAEL). That is, the LD_{50} was probably greater than 4000 mg/kg (p.o.) in mice.

4.1.3. HPLC Analysis. The chromatographic spectrum of the leaf methanol extract of *C. orbiculata* obtained revealed major peaks at the following retention times (minutes): 6.983, 10.521, 12.088, 12.838, and 13.342 (Figure 1).

5. Discussion

In the present study, the leaf methanol extract of *C. orbiculata* significantly inhibited the acetic acid-induced writhing and significantly inhibited the nociception produced by hot

TABLE 1: Effect of leaf methanol extract of *Cotyledon orbiculata* on acetic acid-induced writhing in mice.

Treatment groups	Dose (mg/kg)	Number of writhes Mean ± SEM		Percentage reduction (%)
PS	0.25 mL	28.13	3.92	
C. orbiculata	100	13.83*	3.17	51
	200	9.20**	3.04	67
	400	6.75***	1.97	76
Paracetamol	300	2.10***	0.24	93
DMSO	0.25 mL	29.04	2.73	0

$*P < 0.025$, $**P < 0.005$, $***P < 0.001$ versus 3% acetic acid (0.20 mL, i.p.) control, ANOVA ($n = 8$). Writhes are expressed as number of counts per 20 minutes.
PS: physiological saline.
DMSO: dimethylsulfoxide.

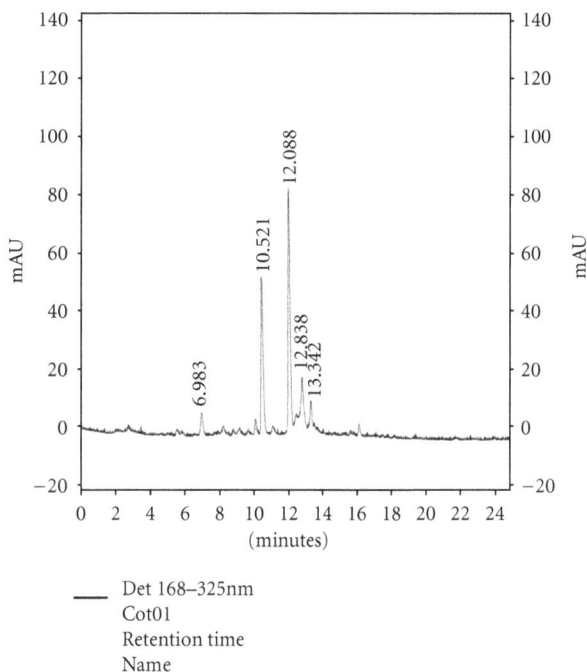

FIGURE 1: HPLC fingerprint of leaf methanol extract of *Cotyledon orbiculata*.

plate. *C. orbiculata* also significantly attenuated carrageenan-induced rat right hind paw oedema. Satyanarayana et al. [15] has shown that acetic acid produced writhing or nociception by stimulating the production of prostaglandin. Paracetamol, a standard analgesic drug [2], has been shown to inhibit prostaglandin synthesis in the brain [16]. It is, therefore, not surprising that paracetamol significantly attenuated acetic acid-induced nociception in this study. The effect of paracetamol on prostaglandin in relation to acetic-acid-induced writhes may be direct or indirect. Since *C. orbiculata* also attenuated acetic acid-induced writhing, it is probable that the plant species may be producing its antinociceptive activity by affecting the prostaglandin system. Morphine, a standard centrally acting analgesic

TABLE 2: Effect of leaf methanol extract of *Cotyledon orbiculata* on hot-plate-induced nociception in mice.

Treatment groups	Dose (mg/kg)	Response time (s)				
		0 min	15 min	30 min	45 min	60 min
PS	0.25 mL	4.13 ± 0.13	6.63 ± 0.60	4.38 ± 0.78	3.38 ± 0.68	2.75 ± 0.31
C. orbiculata	100	6.63 ± 0.92	10.25 ± 1.46	11.75** ± 1.07	7.13 ± 1.27	5.13 ± 0.08
	200	6.63 ± 0.85	7.38 ± 1.08	12.38+ ± 1.43	6.88 ± 1.57	6.25 ± 1.45
	400	5.25 ± 0.47	19.13* ± 5.01	26.63++ ± 3.35	22.63+ ± 3.41	24.5++ ± 2.55
Morphine	10	3.38 ± 0.64	26.63++ ± 4.83	36.50++ ± 6.55	22.88++ ± 2.93	16.63++ ± 2.07
DMSO	0.25 mL	5.00 ± 0.76	6.13 ± 0.99	3.88 ± 0.38	4.75 ± 0.86	4.50 ± 0.91

*$P < 0.05$, **$P < 0.025$, +$P < 0.02$, ++$P < 0.001$ versus physiological saline control, ANOVA ($n = 8$). The response time in seconds was expressed as Mean ± SEM.
PS: physiological saline.
DMSO: dimethylsulfoxide.

TABLE 3: Effect of leaf methanol extract of Cotyledon orbiculata on carrageenan-induced oedema in the right hind paw of rat.

Treatment group	Dose (mg/kg)	Paw volume (mL) (Mean ± SEM)								
		0	30	60	90	120	150	180	210	240 (min)
UR	—	0.11 ± 0.01	0.12 ± 0.08	0.10 ± 0.03	0.09 ± 0.01	0.11 ± 0.04	0.11 ± 0.05	0.09 ± 0.07	0.10 ± 0.03	0.09 ± 0.05
PS	0.25 mL	0.09 ± 0.04	0.35 ± 0.05	0.48 ± 0.03	0.52 ± 0.02	0.61 ± 0.04	0.68 ± 0.02	0.72 ± 0.01	0.69 ± 0.05	0.69 ± 0.03
C. orbiculata	50	0.09 ± 0.01	0.29 ± 0.01	0.34* ± 0.01	0.41* ± 0.07	0.50* ± 0.02	0.53* ± 0.01	0.61* ± 0.04	0.59* ± 0.05	0.58* ± 0.03
	100	0.08 ± 0.05	0.26* ± 0.01	0.31** ± 0.04	0.37** ± 0.01	0.38+ ± 0.02	0.36+ ± 0.03	0.36+ ± 0.02	0.33+ ± 0.01	0.36+ ± 0.04
	200	0.11 ± 0.03	0.22* ± 0.02	0.26+ ± 0.01	0.27+ ± 0.01	0.28+ ± 0.04	0.31+ ± 0.02	0.30 ± 0.02	0.20+ ± 0.01	0.30+ ± 0.01
	400	0.10 ± 0.04	0.19* ± 0.02	0.22+ ± 0.01	0.21+ ± 0.03	0.21+ ± 0.02	0.20+ ± 0.04	0.22+ ± 0.01	0.19+ ± 0.01	0.19+ ± 0.02
Indomethacin	10	0.11 ± 0.02	0.14+ ± 0.02	0.18+ ± 0.04	0.20+ ± 0.06	0.19+ ± 0.03	0.18+ ± 0.01	0.17+ ± 0.02	0.16+ ± 0.03	0.15+ ± 0.04
DMSO	0.25 mL	0.11 ± 0.03	0.36 ± 0.06	0.44 ± 0.04	0.53 ± 0.07	0.64 ± 0.03	0.66 ± 0.04	0.70 ± 0.02	0.69 ± 0.03	0.67 ± 0.01

*$P < 0.05$, **$P < 0.025$, +$P < 0.001$ versus physiological saline control, ANOVA ($n = 8$).
UR: untreated rats.
PS: physiological saline.
DMSO: dimethylsuloxide.

drug [3], significantly attenuated the thermal stimulation or nociception produced by the hot plate. *C. orbiculata* also significantly attenuated the nociception produced by hot plate. It is probable that the plant species may be acting via certain central pain receptors to attenuate the nociception produced by hot plate in this study. According to Koster et al. [9], Williamson et al. [10] and Eddy and Leimback [11], acetic acid writhing and hot plate tests are used to evaluate peripherally and centrally acting analgesic drugs respectively. In this study, *C. orbiculata* attenuated both the acetic acid-induced writhing and the nociception produced by hot plate which may suggest that the plant species may have both peripheral and central antinociceptive effect.

Swingle [17] has shown that prostaglandins, histamine, serotonin, and bradykinin are mediators of different phases of carrageenan-induced oedema. Di Rosa et al. [18], Capasso et al. [19], and Salvemini et al. [20] have also reported the involvement of histamine, 5-hydroxytrptamine, bradykinin, prostaglandin, and nitric oxide in carrageenan-induced paw oedema. Nag-Chaudhuri et al. [21] in their report on their work on the anti-inflammatory and related actions of *Syzygium cuminii* seed extract suggested that prostaglandin E₁,

histamine, serotonin, and bradykinin mediate carrageenan-induced rat paw oedema. Indomethacin has been shown to produce its anti-inflammatory effect by inhibiting the enzyme, cyclooxygenase, thus inhibiting prostaglandin synthesis [22]. It has also been shown that the nonsteroidal anti-inflammatory drugs may antagonize mediators such as serotonin, bradykinin, and capsaicin [23] some of which have been implicated in carrageenan-induced paw oedema. It is not surprising that in this study, indomethacin attenuated carrageenan-induced rat right hind paw oedema. *C. orbiculata* also attenuated the carrageenan-induced rat right hind paw oedema which may suggest that probably, the plant species may be affecting a host of mediators to produce its anti-inflammatory effect.

Amabeoku et al. [8] have shown that the leaves of *C. orbiculata* contain tannins, saponins, triterpene steroid, reducing sugar, and cardiac glycosides. Bruneton [24] reported that saponins have both analgesic and anti-inflammatory properties. It is possible, therefore, that saponins may also be contributing to the antinociceptive and anti-inflammatory activities of *C. orbiculata* in this study. The HPLC fingerprint of the plant species obtained revealed major characteristic peaks at the following retention times (minutes): 6.983, 10.521, 12.088, 12.838, and13.342. The acute toxicity test carried out showed that the LD$_{50}$ value obtained for *C. orbiculata* could be greater than 4000 mg/kg (p.o.).

In conclusion, the data obtained show that *C. orbiculata* has both antinociceptive and anti-inflammatory activities which may be produced by the plant species inhibiting various chemical mediators including prostaglandins and bradykinin. The relatively high LD$_{50}$ value of 4000 mg/kg (p.o.) obtained for the plant species shows that it may be safe in or nontoxic to mice. The result obtained justifies the use of the plant species by traditional medicine practitioners in South Africa for the treatment of painful conditions such as headache, earache, toothache, and inflammation. However, more studies are needed to further elucidate the mechanism of the antinociceptive and anti-inflammatory actions of *C. orbiculata*.

Acknowledgments

The National Research Foundation, South Africa (NRF: 67983) funded the study. The plant materials were donated by Kirstenbosch National Botanical Gardens, Western Cape, South Africa. The authors are grateful to Mr. F. Weitz for authenticating the plant species and Mr. V. Jeaven for his valuable technical assistance.

References

[1] S. K. Raghav, B. Gupta, C. Agrawal, K. Goswami, and H. R. Das, "Anti-inflammatory effect of *Ruta graveolens* L. in murine macrophage cells," *Journal of Ethnopharmacology*, vol. 104, no. 1-2, pp. 234–239, 2006.

[2] H. P. Rang, M. M. Dale, J. M. Ritter, R. J. Flower, and G. Henderson, *Pharmacology*, Elsevier Churchill Livingstone, Edinburgh, UK, 7th edition, 2011.

[3] *South African Medicines Formulary (SAMF)*, Health and Medical Publishing Group of the South African Medical Association, Cape Town, South Africa, 9th edition, 2010.

[4] G. B. Martini-Bettolo, "Present aspects of the use of plants in traditional medicine," *Journal of Ethnopharmacology*, vol. 2, no. 1, pp. 5–7, 1980.

[5] B. E. van Wyk, B. van Oudtshoorn, and N. Gericke, *Medicinal Plants of South Africa*, Briza, Pretoria, South Africa, 1997.

[6] J. M. Watt and M. J. Breyer-Brandwijk, *The Medicinal and Poisonous Plants of Southern and Eastern Africa*, Livingstone, London, UK, 2nd edition, 1962.

[7] R. B. Bhat and T. V. Jacobs, "Traditional herbal medicine in Transkei," *Journal of Ethnopharmacology*, vol. 48, no. 1, pp. 7–12, 1995.

[8] G. J. Amabeoku, I. Green, and J. Kabatende, "Anticonvulsant activity of *Cotyledon orbiculata* L. (Crassulaceae) leaf extract in mice," *Journal of Ethnopharmacology*, vol. 112, no. 1, pp. 101–107, 2007.

[9] R. Koster, M. Anderson, and E. J. De Beer, "Acetic acid for analgesic screening," *Federation Proceedings*, vol. 18, pp. 412–418, 1959.

[10] E. M. Williamson, D. T. Okpako, and F. J. Evans, *Pharmacological Methods in Phytotherapy Research. Vol.1, Selection, Preparation and Pharmacological Evaluation of Plant Material*, John Wiley & Sons, New York, NY, USA, 1996.

[11] N. B. Eddy and D. Leimback, "Synthetic analgesics.II. Dithylenylbutenylamines and dithylenylbutylamines," *Journal of Pharmacology and Experimental Therapeutics*, vol. 3, pp. 131–147, 1953.

[12] C. A. Winter, E. A. Risley, and G. W. Nuss, "Carrageenan-induced oedema in hind paw of rat as an assay for anti-inflammatory drugs," *Proceedings of the Society for Experimental Biology and Medicine*, vol. 111, pp. 544–547, 1962.

[13] D. Lorke, "A new approach to practical acute toxicity testing," *Archives of Toxicology*, vol. 54, no. 4, pp. 275–287, 1983.

[14] J. E. Hilaly, H. Z. Israili, and B. Lyoussi, "Acute and chronic toxicological studies of *Ajugaiva* in experimental animals," *Journal of Ethnopharmacology*, vol. 91, no. 1, pp. 43–50, 2004.

[15] P. S. V. Satyanarayana, N. K. Jain, A. Singh, and S. K. Kulkarni, "Isobolographic analysis of interaction between cyclooxygenase inhibitors and tramadol in acetic acid-induced writhing in mice," *Progress in Neuro-Psychopharmacology and Biological Psychiatry*, vol. 28, no. 4, pp. 641–649, 2004.

[16] R. J. Flower and J. R. Vane, "Inhibition of prostaglandin synthetase in brain explains the anti-pyretic activity of paracetamol (4-acetamidophenol)," *Nature*, vol. 240, no. 5381, pp. 410–411, 1972.

[17] K. F. Swingle, "Evaluation for antiinflammatory activity," in *Antiinflammatory Agents: Chemistry Pharmacology*, R. A. Scherrer and M. W. Whitehouse, Eds., vol. 2, pp. 33–122, Academic Press, New York, NY, USA, 1974.

[18] M. Di Rosa, J. P. Giroud, and D. A. Willoughby, "Studies on the mediators of the acute inflammatory response induced in rats in different sites by carrageenan and turpentine," *Journal of Pathology*, vol. 104, no. 1, pp. 15–29, 1971.

[19] F. Capasso, B. Balestrieri, M. Di Rosa, P. Persico, and L. Sorrentino, "Enhancement of carrageenan foot edema by 1,10-phenanthroline and evidence for bradykinin as endogenous mediator," *Agents Actions*, vol. 5, no. 4, pp. 359–363, 1975.

[20] D. Salvemini, Z. Q. Wang, P. S. Wyatt et al., "Nitric oxide: a key mediator in the early and late phase of carrageenan-induced rat paw inflammation," *British Journal of Pharmacology*, vol. 118, no. 4, pp. 829–838, 1996.

[21] A. K. Nag-Chaudhuri, P. Siddhartha, A. Gomes, and B. Siddhartha, "Anti-inflammatory and related actions of *Syzygiumcuminii* seed extract," *Phytotherapy Research*, vol. 4, no. 1, pp. 5–10, 1990.

[22] H. P. Rang, M. M. Dale, J. M. Ritter, R. J. Flower, and G. Henderson, *Pharmacology*, Elsevier Churchill Livingstone, Edinburgh, UK, 7th edition, 2011.

[23] H. O. Collier, L. C. Dinneen, C. A. Johnson, and C. Schneider, "The abdominal constriction response and its suppression by analgesic drugs in the mouse," *British Journal of Pharmacology*, vol. 32, no. 2, pp. 295–310, 1968.

[24] J. Bruneton, *Pharmacognosy: Phytochemistry, Medicinal Plants*, Intercept, Paris, France, 2nd edition, 1999.

16

The Anti-Inflammatory Role of Vitamin E in Prevention of Osteoporosis

A. S. Nazrun, M. Norazlina, M. Norliza, and S. Ima Nirwana

*Department of Pharmacology, Faculty of Medicine, The National University of Malaysia,
50300 Kuala Lumpur, Malaysia*

Correspondence should be addressed to S. Ima Nirwana, imasoel@medic.ukm.my

Academic Editor: Esra Küpeli Akkol

There is growing evidence that inflammation may be one of the causal factors of osteoporosis. Several cytokines such as IL-1, IL-6, RANKL, OPG, and M-CSF were implicated in the pathogenesis of osteoporosis. These cytokines are important determinants of osteoclast differentiation and its bone resorptive activity. Anticytokine therapy using cytokine antagonists such as IL-receptor antagonist and TNF-binding protein was able to suppress the activity of the respective cytokines and prevent bone loss. Several animal studies have shown that vitamin E in the forms of palm-derived tocotrienol and α-tocopherol may prevent osteoporosis in rat models by suppressing IL-1 and IL-6. Free radicals are known to activate transcription factor NFκB which leads to the production of bone resorbing cytokines. Vitamin E, a potent antioxidant, may be able to neutralise free radicals before they could activate NFκB, therefore suppressing cytokine production and osteoporosis. Vitamin E has also been shown to inhibit COX-2, the enzyme involved in inflammatory reactions. Of the two types of vitamin E studied, tocotrienol seemed to be better than tocopherol in terms of its ability to suppress bone-resorbing cytokines.

1. Introduction

Osteoporosis is a bone disease, characterized by low bone mass and increased risk of fractures [1]. It is well accepted that osteoporosis can be caused by various endocrine, metabolic, and mechanical factors. However, recently, there are opinions that there may be an inflammatory component in the etiology of osteoporosis [2, 3]. There is plenty of evidence linking inflammation to osteoporosis. Epidemiological studies have identified higher incidence of osteoporosis in various inflammatory conditions such as ankylosing spondylitis, rheumatoid arthritis, and systemic lupus erythematosus [4–7]. This association was also observed clinically whereby the degree of osteoporosis was equivalent to the extent of inflammation. If the inflammation was systemic, bone loss will occur at all skeletal sites, whereas if the inflammation was only restricted to a site, bone loss will only occur locally at that site of inflammation [3]. Elderly patients are more prone to osteoporosis, and this was believed to be connected to the elevated production of proinflammatory cytokines with aging [8, 9].

The occurrence of inflammation is indicated by the presence of inflammatory markers such as cytokines and C-reactive protein. Biochemical studies have demonstrated elevation of proinflammatory cytokines TNF-α and IL-6 in arthritic disease such as gouty arthritis, rheumatoid arthritis, and psoriatic arthritis [10, 11]. An obvious relationship between inflammation and osteoporosis was seen in rheumatoid arthritis, whereby proinflammatory cytokines were released causing bone loss around the affected joints [12]. The level of C-reactive protein, a sensitive marker of systemic inflammation, was also found to be associated with bone mineral density [13]. Inflammation may contribute to bone loss by affecting the bone remodeling process, favouring bone resorption activity by osteoclasts rather than bone formation activity by osteoblasts [14, 15]. Bone resorption is determined by the balance between two cytokines, receptor activator of nuclear factor κB ligand (RANKL), and osteoprotegerin (OPG) [16]. RANKL is crucial for the differentiation and activation of osteoclast [17]. Higher RANKL levels were associated with lower bone mineral density in men [18]. Administration of serum

RANKL to mice promoted osteoclast growth and activation, leading to osteoporosis [19]. On the other hand, OPG antagonizes RANKL by binding with RANKL and preventing it from binding to RANK receptors. By doing that, OPG was able to inhibit osteoclastogenesis and bone resorption [20]. Macrophage colony stimulating factor (MCSF) is another important determinant of osteoclastogenesis, but its mechanism to modulate osteoclastogenesis is still not clear [20].

The "upstream" cytokines such as IL-1, IL-6, and TNF-α [21, 22] and "downstream" cytokines such as RANKL, OPG, and M-CSF [23–25] played an important role in bone remodeling. Imbalance in their bioactivity may lead to bone loss and osteoporosis. Cytokines are small- to medium-sized proteins or glycoproteins with molecular weight ranging from 8 to 40,000 dalton. They act as the biological mediator for most cells and function at low concentrations between 10^{-10} and 10^{-5} molar. They have a short half-life of less than 10 minutes, and their serum level can be as low as 10 pg/mL. The cytokine levels increase dramatically during inflammation and infection. The measurement of cytokine levels in close vicinity to bone such as the bone marrow is important for studies on osteoporosis and other bone diseases. In postmenopausal women, cytokine production by the peripheral monocytes correlated well with cytokines secreted by monocytes in the bone marrow. Therefore, cytokine levels in the serum are representative of the local monocytes [26]. Stromal cells and osteoblasts produce interleukin-1, interleukin-6, and tumor necrosis factor-α. These proinflammatory cytokines are also known as the bone-resorbing cytokines or proosteoclast cytokines as they promote osteoclast differentiation and activity [27–30]. The bone resorption activity of these cytokines in ovariectomised rats was reduced with anticytokine therapy such as IL-1 receptor antagonists and TNF-binding protein [31]. Vitamin E, a potent antioxidant vitamin, was also found to inhibit or suppress cytokine production [32, 33]. This vitamin E action may be responsible for its ability to prevent inflammation and osteoporosis, seen in several studies on osteoporosis using animal models [34].

Vitamin E is a group of potent, lipid-soluble, chain-breaking antioxidants. It can be classified into tocopherol and tocotrienol based on the chemical structure. Palm oil, which is extracted from the pulp of the fruit of the oil palm *Elaeis guineensis*, is abundant in tocotrienols. Tocotrienol has an unsaturated farnesyl (isoprenoid) side-chain, while tocopherol has a saturated phytyl side chain [35].

Vitamin E occurs in eight isoforms of α-, β-, γ-, and δ-tocopherols or tocotrienols. It was thought that both the γ and δ isomers of tocopherol have better antioxidant and anti-inflammatory activities than the α isomer [36, 37]. Once vitamin E is absorbed in the intestine, it will enter the circulation via the lymphatic system and be transported to the liver with the chylomicrons [38]. Vitamin E is metabolized by cytochrome P450 and then excreted in the urine [39].

In human subjects and animal models, high doses of vitamin E were found to exhibit anti-inflammatory effects by decreasing C-reactive protein (CRP) and inhibiting the release of proinflammatory cytokines [40]. These were evident in a study on patients with coronary artery disease, whereby the CRP and tumor necrosis factor-α (TNF-α) concentrations were found to be significantly lowered with α-tocopherol supplementation compared to placebo [41]. Since vitamin E was also found to inhibit cyclooxygenase-2 activities, it was thought to be able to exert anti-inflammatory and anticarcinogenic activities, especially in the colon [42]. This was demonstrated by Yang et al. [43], who found that vitamin E was able to significantly lower colon inflammation index and reduced the number of colon adenomas in mice given azoxymethane.

This paper will focus on the effects of vitamin E on bone-resorbing cytokines with special attention on IL-1 and IL-6.

2. Interleukin-1 (IL-1)

IL-1 plays an important role in various reactions towards infection, inflammation, and immune activation. This cytokine is produced by various cells but the main producer is the monocyte. In the physiological condition, monocytes do not secrete IL-1 but, under pathological conditions such as septic shock, IL-1 is rapidly released and acts directly on the blood vessels. Other cytokines such as TNF-α and interferon, bacterial endotoxin, virus, and antigen can also stimulate the release of IL-1. Reactive oxygen species such as superoxide radicals have been shown to induce IL-1 production [32, 44]. IL-1 is involved in the pathogenesis of various diseases associated with bone loss such as osteoporosis [45, 46], cancer-induced osteolysis [47], rheumatoid arthritis [48], and osteolysis of orthopedic implants [49]. IL-1 is also an important factor in both *in vivo* and *in vitro* bone resorption [50, 51]. It stimulates the formation and activity of osteoclasts, leading to excessive bone resorption. Suda et al. [52] demonstrated that the presence of osteoblast and stromal cells was crucial in the formation of osteoclasts by IL-1. Thomson et al. [53] also reported that osteoblasts secrete a factor that stimulates the bone-resorbing activities of rat osteoclasts. However, Xu et al. [54] demonstrated that rat osteoclasts expressed mRNA to IL-1 receptors, while Yu and Ferrier [55] found that osteoclast is one of the target cells for IL-1. These studies proved that IL-1 can act directly on osteoclasts without the presence of osteoblasts or stromal cells. IL-1 may also promote formation of osteoclasts [56]. It acts by activating nuclear factor κB (NFκB) in osteoclast and prevents its apoptosis [57]. It was found that the estrogen-deficient state in postmenopausal women or ovariectomised rats resulted in increased production of IL-1 by monocyte and other bone marrow cells [58, 59]. Estrogen replacement or IL-receptor antagonist was able to prevent the elevation of IL-1 in ovariectomised rats [60, 61]. Vitamin E was also found to have the ability to suppress IL-1 production by activated monocytes [62]. In a different study, combination of superoxide dismutase and vitamin E was effective in inhibiting IL-1 production by human monocytes [32]. The ability of vitamin E to inhibit IL-1 in the bone environment may have prevented bone loss.

3. Interleukin-6 (IL-6)

IL-6 is another cytokine that is associated with various pathophysiological processes in humans. It is produced by the haematopoetic and nonhaematopoetic cells when they were exposed to various types of stimulation. During bone remodeling, IL-6 is produced in nanomolar concentrations by stromal cells and osteoblasts under the influence of parathyroid hormone, vitamin D_3, growth factor, and other cytokines [63]. IL-6 was also reported to be produced by osteoblasts when stimulated by IL-1, TNF-α, and lipopolysaccharide [64]. McSheeny and Chambers [65] reported that osteoblasts were stimulated by local IL-1 to produce IL-6, which was responsible for the activation of osteoclasts. IL-6 promoted the differentiation of osteoclasts from its precursor and played an important role in the pathogenesis of osteoporosis due to estrogen deficiency [66, 67]. The IL-6 elevation in postmenopausal women was reduced by estrogen replacement therapy [68]. The elevation of IL-6 may be related to free radical activities especially reactive oxygen species. Reactive oxygen species was found to elevate the IL-6 levels directly via activation of nuclear factor κB (NFκB) [69]. High cytokine levels would also result in activation of NFκB and promotion of osteoclastogenesis [70].

4. Vitamin E as Anticytokine Agent

The effects of vitamin E on bone resorbing cytokines for prevention and treatment of osteoporosis have been studied using FeNTA and nicotine rat models [34, 71]. These models represent osteoporosis caused by oxidative stress and smoking, respectively. However, similar studies in humans are still lacking. Ferric nitrilotriacetate (FeNTA) is an oxidizing agent which produces free radicals via the Fenton reaction [72, 73]. Oxidative stress can be induced in rats by injecting them with FeNTA, allowing the hazardous effects of free radicals on various organs and tissues including bone to be studied. The bone resorbing cytokines, IL-1 and IL-6, were found to be elevated in this oxidative stress rat model, indicating inflammation. This was accompanied by osteoporotic changes as indicated by the measurement of bone markers and histomorphometric parameters [34]. The elevation of cytokines was probably achieved through the activation of cytokine-encoding genes like STAT3 or nuclear factor-kappaB by the free radicals [74, 75]. Therefore, there exist relationships between free radicals, inflammation, and bone loss which can lead to osteoporosis. When vitamin E in the form of tocotrienols and α-tocopherol were supplemented to these rats, IL-1 and IL-6 elevations were suppressed. Concurrent with this, the osteoporotic changes were also inhibited [34, 71, 76]. Therefore, there is a possibility that vitamin E, a potent antioxidant, has prevented free radicals from causing inflammation and osteoporosis. Tocotrienols seemed to be more superior than α-tocopherol in suppressing proinflammatory cytokines in the FeNTA rat model and in protecting their bone against osteoporosis [34]. Both the tocopherol and tocotrienol may have achieved this by scavenging the free radicals generated by FeNTA before they could activate the monocytes and osteoblasts, cells that produce IL-1 and IL-6.

Cigarette smoking is a modest risk factor for osteoporosis [77]. Nicotine is among the 4,700 chemicals found in the tar phase of cigarette smoke [78]. Nicotine injected into rats can be used as a model for osteoporosis related to smoking. Various animal studies have confirmed the deleterious effects of nicotine on bone remodeling [79–85]. Nicotine inhibited osteoblast activity and growth [86, 87] but stimulated osteoclast activity [83]. Nicotine has also been shown to induce oxidative stress in both *in vitro* and *in vivo* animal studies [88, 89]. Crowley-Weber et al. [90] had reported that other than oxidative stress, nicotine also activated nuclear transcription factor-κB (NF-κB) in the tissues of smokers. The activation of NF-κB-signaling pathway may be the mechanism for bone loss as it is responsible for osteoclast differentiation [76, 91]. Nicotine has been shown to significantly elevate the proinflammatory cytokines IL-1 and IL-6 in rats. Using the same model, tocotrienol was able to prevent nicotine-induced elevation of IL-1 and IL-6, while tocopherol had no significant effects on both cytokines [71]. Tocotrienol was more effective compared to tocopherol in terms of its action on bone resorbing cytokines and therefore was more effective in reducing inflammation and bone loss.

5. Anti-Inflammatory Action of Vitamin E in Prevention of Osteoporosis

Results from studies on cytokines have given us some insight on the mechanisms involved in the protection of vitamin E against osteoporosis. Free radicals are known to activate transcription factor NFκB which leads to the production of bone resorbing cytokines interleukin-1 and interleukin-6. These proinflammatory cytokines were believed to provide the link between inflammation and osteoporosis. Vitamin E may scavenge and neutralize free radicals before they could activate transcription factor NFκB. This was seen in an oxidative stress model (FeNTA model) in which vitamin E had reduced the levels of bone-resorbing cytokines [34]. Alternatively, vitamin E may have prevented the activation of NFκB by enhancing the internal antioxidative enzymes within the bone. This was demonstrated by Maniam et al. [92], whereby vitamin E supplementation reduced the femoral thiobarbituric acid-reactive substance (TBARS) and increased the glutathione peroxidase activity.

Since osteoporosis is associated with inflammation, there is also a possibility that Vitamin E may have some anti-inflammatory action. Yam et al. [93] found that tocotrienol was able to suppress cyclooxygenase-2 (COX-2) expression in RAW 264.7 cells that were exposed to lipopolysaccharide. COX-2 is an inducible enzyme expressed during inflammation. A RAW cell is a macrophage-like cell which transformed into preosteoclasts when RANKL is added. This suggested that vitamin E may act as anti-inflammatory agent in protecting bone against excessive osteoclastic activity. Previous study has shown that aspirin or other nonsteroidal anti-inflammatory drugs (NSAID) inhibited NFκB [94]. Similar to tocotrienol, these anti-inflammatory drugs inhibit COX-2. As the activation of NFκB is linked to proinflammatory cytokines and inflammation, it further provides evidence of the anti-inflammatory role of tocotrienol in preventing osteoporosis.

Based on the results from the studies above, tocotrienol was more superior than tocopherol in terms of its ability to suppress bone resorbing cytokines. The more superior tocotrienol action may be contributed by its more potent antioxidant property. It has better interaction with lipoprotein in membrane lipids and is uniformly distributed in the membrane layer compared to tocopherol [35, 95]. Tocotrienol was also better at maintaining the antioxidant status within the rat bone compared to tocopherol [92]. Thus, the antiosteoporotic effect of tocotrienol may be partly explained by its anti-inflammatory as well as antioxidative effects.

Acknowledgments

The author would like to thank University Kebangsaan Malaysia (UKM) for the grants and Mr. Arizi Aziz and the Pharmacology department staffs for their technical support.

References

[1] P. D. Delmas, "Treatment of postmenopausal osteoporosis," *Lancet*, vol. 359, no. 9322, pp. 2018–2026, 2002.

[2] A. J. Yun and P. Y. Lee, "Maldaptation of the link between inflammation and bone turnover may be a key determinant of osteoporosis," *Medical Hypotheses*, vol. 63, no. 3, pp. 532–537, 2004.

[3] D. Mitra, D. M. Elvins, D. J. Speden, and A. J. Collins, "The prevalence of vertebral fractures in mild ankylosing spondylitis and their relationship to bone mineral density," *Rheumatology*, vol. 39, no. 1, pp. 85–89, 2000.

[4] G. Hougeberg, M. C. Lodder, W. F. Lems et al., "Hand cortical bone mass and its associations with radiographic joint damage and fractures in 50–70 year old female patients with rheumatoid arthritis: cross sectional Oslo-Truro-Amsterdam (OSTRA) collaborative study," *Annals of the Rheumatic Diseases*, vol. 63, no. 10, pp. 1331–1334, 2004.

[5] I. E. M. Bultink, W. F. Lems, P. J. Kostense, B. A. C. Dijkmans, and A. E. Voskuyl, "Prevalence of and risk factors for low bone mineral density and vertebral fractures in patients with systemic lupus erythematosus," *Arthritis and Rheumatism*, vol. 52, no. 7, pp. 2044–2050, 2005.

[6] T. R. Mikuls, K. G. Saag, J. Curtis et al., "Prevalence of osteoporosis and osteopenia among African Americans with early rheumatoid arthritis: the impact of ethnic-specific normative data," *Journal of the National Medical Association*, vol. 97, no. 8, pp. 1155–1160, 2005.

[7] C. Franceschi, M. Bonafè, S. Valensin et al., "Inflamm-aging. An evolutionary perspective on immunosenescence," *Annals of the New York Academy of Sciences*, vol. 908, pp. 244–254, 2000.

[8] J. K. Kiecolt-Glaser, K. J. Preacher, R. C. MacCallum, C. Atkinson, W. B. Malarkey, and R. Glaser, "Chronic stress and age-related increases in the proinflammatory cytokine IL-6," *Proceedings of the National Academy of Sciences of the United States of America*, vol. 100, no. 15, pp. 9090–9095, 2003.

[9] K. Ishihara and T. Hirano, "IL-6 in autoimmune disease and chronic inflammatory proliferative disease," *Cytokine and Growth Factor Reviews*, vol. 13, no. 4-5, pp. 357–368, 2002.

[10] A. R. Moschen, A. Kaser, B. Enrich et al., "The RANKL/OPG system is activated in inflammatory bowel diseases and relates to the state or bone loss," *Gut*, vol. 54, no. 4, pp. 479–487, 2005.

[11] N. Saidenberg-Kermanac'h, M. Cohen-Solal, N. Bessis, M. C. De Vernejoul, and M. C. Boissier, "Role for osteoprotegerin in rheumatoid inflammation," *Joint Bone Spine*, vol. 71, no. 1, pp. 9–13, 2004.

[12] K. Ganesan, S. Teklehaimanot, T. H. Tran, M. Asuncion, and K. Norris, "Relationship of C-reactive protein and bone mineral density in community-dwelling elderly females," *Journal of the National Medical Association*, vol. 97, no. 3, pp. 329–333, 2005.

[13] J. R. Arron and Y. Choi, "Bone versus immune system," *Nature*, vol. 408, no. 6812, pp. 535–536, 2000.

[14] J. Lorenzo, "Interactions between immune and bone cells: new insights with many remaining questions," *Journal of Clinical Investigation*, vol. 106, no. 6, pp. 749–752, 2000.

[15] S. L. Teitelbaum, "Bone resorption by osteoclasts," *Science*, vol. 289, no. 5484, pp. 1504–1508, 2000.

[16] D. L. Lacey, E. Timms, H. L. Tan et al., "Osteoprotegerin ligand is a cytokine that regulates osteoclast differentiation and activation," *Cell*, vol. 93, no. 2, pp. 165–176, 1998.

[17] A. Stern, G. A. Laughlin, J. Bergstrom, and E. Barrett-Connor, "The sex-specific association of serum osteoprotegerin and receptor activator of nuclear factor κB legend with bone mineral density in older adults: the Rancho Bernardo study," *European Journal of Endocrinology*, vol. 156, no. 5, pp. 555–562, 2007.

[18] S. A. J. Lloyd, Y. Y. Yuan, P. J. Kostenuik et al., "Soluble RANKL induces high bone turnover and decreases bone volume, density, and strength in mice," *Calcified Tissue International*, vol. 82, no. 5, pp. 361–372, 2008.

[19] W. J. Boyle, W. S. Simonet, and D. L. Lacey, "Osteoclast differentiation and activation," *Nature*, vol. 423, no. 6937, pp. 337–342, 2003.

[20] R. Pacifici, "Estrogen, cytokines, and pathogenesis of postmenopausal osteoporosis," *Journal of Bone and Mineral Research*, vol. 11, no. 8, pp. 1043–1051, 1996.

[21] S. C. Manolagas and R. L. Jilka, "Mechanisms of disease: bone marrow, cytokines, and bone remodeling - Emerging insights into the pathophysiology of osteoporosis," *New England Journal of Medicine*, vol. 332, no. 5, pp. 305–311, 1995.

[22] K. Fuller, B. Wong, S. Fox, Y. Choi, and T. J. Chambers, "TRANCE is necessary and sufficient for osteoblast-mediated activation of bone resorption in osteoclasts," *Journal of Experimental Medicine*, vol. 188, no. 5, pp. 997–1001, 1998.

[23] R. Pacifici, "Cytokines and osteoclast activity," *Calcified Tissue International*, vol. 56, no. 1, pp. S27–S28, 1995.

[24] R. L. Jilka, "Cytokines, bone remodeling, and estrogen deficiency: a 1998 update," *Bone*, vol. 23, no. 2, supplement 1, pp. 75–81, 1998.

[25] K. Matsuzaki, N. Udagawa, N. Takahashi et al., "Osteoclast differentiation factor (ODF) induces osteoclast-like cell formation in human peripheral blood mononuclear cell cultures," *Biochemical and Biophysical Research Communications*, vol. 246, no. 1, pp. 199–204, 1998.

[26] M. E. Cohen-Solal, F. Boitte, O. Bernard-Poenaru et al., "Increased bone resorbing activity of peripheral monocyte culture supernatants in elderly women," *Journal of Clinical*

Endocrinology and Metabolism, vol. 83, no. 5, pp. 1687–1690, 1998.

[27] J. Pfeilschifter, C. Chenu, A. Bird, G. R. Mundy, and G. D. Roodman, "Interleukin-1 and tumor necrosis factor stimulate the formation of human osteoclastlike cells in vitro," *Journal of Bone and Mineral Research*, vol. 4, no. 1, pp. 113–118, 1989.

[28] M. Kanatani, T. Sugimoto, M. Fukase, and K. Chihara, "Role of interleukin-6 and prostaglandins in the effect of monocyte-conditioned medium on osteoclast formation," *American Journal of Physiology*, vol. 267, no. 6, pp. E868–E876, 1994.

[29] R. Pacifici, "Cytokines and osteoclast activity," *Calcified Tissue International*, vol. 56, no. 1, supplement 1, pp. S27–S28, 1995.

[30] T. Suda, N. Udagawa, I. Nakamura, C. Miyaura, and N. Takahashi, "Modulation of osteoclast differentiation by local factors," *Bone*, vol. 17, no. 2, pp. S87–S91, 1995.

[31] R. Kitazawa, R. B. Kimble, J. L. Vannice, V. T. Kung, and R. Pacifici, "Interleukin-1 receptor antagonist and tumor necrosis factor binding protein decrease osteoclast formation and bone resorption in ovariectomized mice," *Journal of Clinical Investigation*, vol. 94, no. 6, pp. 2397–2406, 1994.

[32] T. Kasama, K. Kobayashi, T. Fukushima et al., "Production of interleukin 1-like factor from human peripheral blood monocytes and polymorphonuclear leukocytes by superoxide anion: the role of interleukin 1 and reactive oxygen species in inflamed sites," *Clinical Immunology and Immunopathology*, vol. 53, no. 3, pp. 439–448, 1989.

[33] S. Devaraj, D. Li, and I. Jialal, "The effects of alpha tocopherol supplementation on monocyte function: decreased lipid oxidation, interleukin 1β secretion, and monocyte adhesion to endothelium," *Journal of Clinical Investigation*, vol. 98, no. 3, pp. 756–763, 1996.

[34] N. S. Ahmad, B. A. K. Khalid, D. A. Luke, and S. I. Nirwana, "Tocotrienol offers better protection than tocopherol from free radical-induced damage of rat bone," *Clinical and Experimental Pharmacology and Physiology*, vol. 32, no. 9, pp. 761–770, 2005.

[35] E. Serbinova, V. Kagan, D. Han, and L. Packer, "Free radical recycling and intramembrane mobility in the antioxidant properties of alpha-tocopherol and alpha-tocotrienol," *Free Radical Biology and Medicine*, vol. 10, no. 5, pp. 263–275, 1991.

[36] Q. Jiang and B. N. Ames, "γ-tocopherol, but not α-tocopherol, decreases proinflammatory eicosanoids and inflammation damage in rats," *FASEB Journal*, vol. 17, no. 8, pp. 816–822, 2003.

[37] A. Patel, F. Liebner, T. Netscher, K. Mereiter, and T. Rosenau, "Vitamin E chemistry. Nitration of non-α-tocopherols: products and mechanistic considerations," *Journal of Organic Chemistry*, vol. 72, no. 17, pp. 6504–6512, 2007.

[38] M. G. Traber and H. Sies, "Vitamin E in humans: demand and delivery," *Annual Review of Nutrition*, vol. 16, pp. 321–347, 1996.

[39] R. Brigelius-Flohé, "Vitamin E and drug metabolism," *Biochemical and Biophysical Research Communications*, vol. 305, no. 3, pp. 737–740, 2003.

[40] U. Singh and S. Devaraj, "Vitamin E: inflammation and atherosclerosis," *Vitamins and Hormones*, vol. 76, pp. 519–549, 2007.

[41] S. Devaraj, R. Tang, B. Adams-Huet et al., "Effect of high-dose α-tocopherol supplementation on biomarkers of oxidative stress and inflammation and carotid atherosclerosis in patients with coronary artery disease," *American Journal of Clinical Nutrition*, vol. 86, no. 5, pp. 1392–1398, 2007.

[42] Q. Jiang, X. Yin, M. A. Lil, M. L. Danielson, H. Freiser, and J. Huang, "Long-chain carboxychromanols, metabolites of vitamin E, are potent inhibitors of cyclooxygenases," *Proceedings of the National Academy of Sciences of the United States of America*, vol. 105, no. 51, pp. 20464–20469, 2008.

[43] C. S. Yang, G. Lu, J. Ju, and G. X. Li, "Inhibition of inflammation and carcinogenesis in the lung and colon by tocopherols," *Annals of the New York Academy of Sciences*, vol. 1203, pp. 29–34, 2010.

[44] S. K. Clinton and P. Libby, "Cytokines and growth factors in atherogenesis," *Archives of Pathology and Laboratory Medicine*, vol. 116, no. 12, pp. 1292–1300, 1992.

[45] R. Pacifici, L. Rifas, and S. Teitelbaum, "Spontaneous release of interleukin 1 from human blood monocytes reflects bone formation in idiopathic osteoporosis," *Proceedings of the National Academy of Sciences of the United States of America*, vol. 84, no. 13, pp. 4616–4620, 1987.

[46] S. H. Ralston, "Analysis of gene expression in human bone biopsies by polymerase chain reaction: evidence for enhanced cytokine expression in postmenopausal osteoporosis," *Journal of Bone and Mineral Research*, vol. 9, no. 6, pp. 883–890, 1994.

[47] M. Kawano, I. Yamamoto, K. Iwato et al., "Interleukin-1 beta rather than lymphotoxin as the major bone resorbing activity in human multiple myeloma," *Blood*, vol. 73, no. 6, pp. 1646–1649, 1989.

[48] S. J. Hopkins, M. Humphreys, and M. I. V. Jayson, "Cytokines in synovial fluid. I. The presence of biologically active and immunoreactive IL-1," *Clinical and Experimental Immunology*, vol. 72, no. 3, pp. 422–427, 1988.

[49] N. Al Saffar and P. A. Revell, "Interleukin-1 production by activated macrophages surrounding loosened orthopaedic implants: a potential role in osteolysis," *British Journal of Rheumatology*, vol. 33, no. 4, pp. 309–316, 1994.

[50] B. F. Boyce, T. B. Aufdemorte, I. R. Garrett, A. J. P. Yates, and G. R. Mundy, "Effects of interleukin-1 on bone turnover in normal mice," *Endocrinology*, vol. 125, no. 3, pp. 1142–1150, 1989.

[51] M. Gowen, D. D. Wood, and E. J. Ihrie, "An interleukin 1 like factor stimulates bone resorption in vitro," *Nature*, vol. 306, no. 5941, pp. 378–380, 1983.

[52] T. Suda, N. Takahashi, and T. J. Martin, "Modulation of osteoclast differentiation," *Endocrine Reviews*, vol. 13, no. 1, pp. 66–80, 1992.

[53] B. M. Thomson, J. Saklatvala, and T. J. Chambers, "Osteoblasts mediate interleukin 1 stimulation of bone resorption by rat osteoclasts," *Journal of Experimental Medicine*, vol. 164, no. 1, pp. 104–112, 1986.

[54] L. X. Xu, T. Kukita, Y. Nakano et al., "Osteoclasts in normal and adjuvant arthritis bone tissues express the mRNA for both type I and II interleukin-1 receptors," *Laboratory Investigation*, vol. 75, no. 5, pp. 677–687, 1996.

[55] H. Yu and J. Ferrier, "Interleukin-1 alpha induces a sustained increase in cytosolic free calcium in cultured rabbit osteoclasts," *Biochemical and Biophysical Research Communications*, vol. 191, no. 2, pp. 343–350, 1993.

[56] E. Jimi, T. Ikebe, N. Takahashi, M. Hirata, T. Suda, and T. Koga, "Interleukin-1α activates an NF-κB-like factor in osteoclast-like cells," *Journal of Biological Chemistry*, vol. 271, no. 9, pp. 4605–4608, 1996.

[57] E. Jimi, I. Nakamura, T. Ikebe, S. Akiyama, N. Takahashi, and T. Suda, "Activation of NF-κB is involved in the survival of osteoclasts promoted by interleukin-1," *Journal of Biological Chemistry*, vol. 273, no. 15, pp. 8799–8805, 1998.

[58] R. Pacifici, C. Brown, E. Puscheck et al., "Effect of surgical menopause and estrogen replacement on cytokine release from human blood mononuclear cells," *Proceedings of the National Academy of Sciences of the United States of America*, vol. 88, no. 12, pp. 5134–5138, 1991.

[59] F. Sato, Y. Ouchi, A. Masuyama et al., "Effects of estrogen replacement on insulin-like growth factor I concentrations in serum and bone tissue and on interleukin 1 secretion from spleen macrophages in oophorectomized rats," *Calcified Tissue International*, vol. 53, no. 2, pp. 111–116, 1993.

[60] R. Pacifici, L. Rifas, R. McCracken et al., "Ovarian steroid treatment blocks a postmenopausal increase in blood monocyte interleukin 1 release," *Proceedings of the National Academy of Sciences of the United States of America*, vol. 86, no. 7, pp. 2398–2402, 1989.

[61] R. B. Kimble, J. L. Vannice, D. C. Bloedow et al., "Interleukin-1 receptor antagonist decreases bone loss and bone resorption in ovariectomized rats," *Journal of Clinical Investigation*, vol. 93, no. 5, pp. 1959–1967, 1994.

[62] S. Devaraj and I. Jialal, "The effects of alpha-tocopherol on critical cells in atherogenesis," *Current Opinion in Lipidology*, vol. 9, no. 1, pp. 11–15, 1998.

[63] S. C. Manolagas, "Role of cytokines in bone resorption," *Bone*, vol. 17, no. 2, pp. 63S–67S, 1995.

[64] G. Girasole, R. L. Jilka, G. Passeri et al., "17β-Estradiol inhibits interleukin-6 production by bone marrow-derived stromal cells and osteoblasts in vitro: a potential mechanism for the antiosteoporotic effect of estrogens," *Journal of Clinical Investigation*, vol. 89, no. 3, pp. 883–891, 1992.

[65] P. M. J. McSheehy and T. J. Chambers, "Osteoblast-like cells in the presence of parathyroid hormone release soluble factor that stimulates osteoclastic bone resorption," *Endocrinology*, vol. 119, no. 4, pp. 1654–1659, 1986.

[66] N. Kurihara, D. Bertolini, T. Suda, Y. Akiyama, and G. D. Roodman, "IL-6 stimulates osteoclast-like multinucleated cell formation in long term human marrow cultures by inducing IL-1 release," *Journal of Immunology*, vol. 144, no. 11, pp. 4226–4230, 1990.

[67] D. A. Papanicolaou and A. N. Vgontzas, "Interleukin-6: the endocrine cytokine," *Journal of Clinical Endocrinology and Metabolism*, vol. 85, no. 3, pp. 1331–1333, 2000.

[68] R. H. Straub, H. W. Hense, T. Andus, J. Schölmerich, G. A. J. Riegger, and H. Schunkert, "Hormone replacement therapy and interrelation between serum interleukin-6 and body mass index in postmenopausal women: a population-based study," *Journal of Clinical Endocrinology and Metabolism*, vol. 85, no. 3, pp. 1340–1344, 2000.

[69] A. S. Baldwin, "Control of oncogenesis and cancer therapy resistance by the transcription factor NF-κB," *Journal of Clinical Investigation*, vol. 107, no. 3, pp. 241–246, 2001.

[70] D. Maggio, M. Barabani, M. Pierandrei et al., "Marked decrease in plasma antioxidants in aged osteoporotic women: results of a cross-sectional study," *Journal of Clinical Endocrinology and Metabolism*, vol. 88, no. 4, pp. 1523–1527, 2003.

[71] M. Norazlina, Y. M. K. Nik-Farideh, A. Arizi, A. Faisal, and S. Ima-Nirwana, "Effects of nicotine on bone resorbing cytokines in male rats," *International Medical Journal*, vol. 3, no. 2, pp. 1–9, 2004.

[72] M. Awai, M. Narasaki, Y. Yamanoi, and S. Seno, "Induction of diabetes in animals by parenteral administration of ferric nitrilotriacetate A model of experimental hemochromatosis," *American Journal of Pathology*, vol. 95, no. 3, pp. 663–673, 1976.

[73] T. Kawabata, M. Awai, and M. Kohno, "Generation of active oxygen species by iron nitrilotriacetate (Fe-NTA)," *Acta Medica Okayama*, vol. 40, no. 3, pp. 163–173, 1986.

[74] M. Carballo, M. Conde, R. El Bekay et al., "Oxidative stress triggers STAT3 tyrosine phosphorylation and nuclear translocation in human lymphocytes," *Journal of Biological Chemistry*, vol. 274, no. 25, pp. 17580–17586, 1999.

[75] F. L. J. Visseren, M. S. A. Verkerk, T. Van Der Bruggen, J. J. M. Marx, B. S. Van Asbeck, and R. J. A. Diepersloot, "Iron chelation and hydroxyl radical scavenging reduce the inflammatory response of endothelial cells after infection with Chlamydia pneumoniae or influenza A," *European Journal of Clinical Investigation*, vol. 32, no. 1, pp. 84–90, 2002.

[76] H. Hermizi, O. Faizah, S. I. Nirwana, S. A. Nazrun, D. A. Luke, and M. Norazlina, "Nicotine impaired bone histomorphometric parameters and bone remodeling biomarkers in Sprague–Dawley male rats," *Annals of Microscopy*, vol. 7, pp. 10–24, 2007.

[77] P. O. Ill and C. Alexandre, "Tobacco as risk factor of osteoporosis, myth or reality?" *Revue du Rhumatisme*, vol. 60, no. 4, pp. 280–286, 1993.

[78] D. Hoffmann, I. Hoffmann, and K. El-Bayoumy, "The less harmful cigarette: a controversial issue. A tribute to Ernst L. Wynder," *Chemical Research in Toxicology*, vol. 14, no. 7, pp. 767–790, 2001.

[79] P. D. Broulik, J. Rosenkrancová, P. Růžička, R. Sedláček, and I. Kurcová, "The effect of chronic nicotine administration on bone mineral content and bone strength in normal and castrated male rats," *Hormone and Metabolic Research*, vol. 39, no. 1, pp. 20–24, 2007.

[80] A. Riesenfeld, "Growth-depressing effects of alcohol and nicotine in two strains of rats," *Acta Anatomica*, vol. 122, no. 1, pp. 18–24, 1985.

[81] P. D. Broulik and J. Jarab, "The effect of chronic nicotine administration on bone mineral content in mice," *Hormone and Metabolic Research*, vol. 25, no. 4, pp. 219–221, 1993.

[82] J. A. Yee, L. Yan, D. M. Cullen, M. P. Akhter, and R. R. Recker, "Nicotine inhibits osteoblast differentiation in cultures of neonatal rat calvarial cells," *Journal of Bone and Mineral Research*, vol. 14, supplement 1, pp. S23–S29, 1999.

[83] C. L. Henemyre, D. K. Scales, S. D. Hokett et al., "Nicotine stimulates osteoclast resorption in a porcine marrow cell model," *Journal of Periodontology*, vol. 74, no. 10, pp. 1440–1446, 2003.

[84] A. R. Kamer, N. El-Ghorab, N. Marzec, J. E. Margarone, and R. Dziak, "Nicotine induced proliferation and cytokine release in osteoblastic cells," *International Journal of Molecular Medicine*, vol. 17, no. 1, pp. 121–127, 2006.

[85] L.W. Zheng, L. K. Ma, and L. K. Cheung, "Effects of nicotine on mandibular distraction osteogenesis: a radiological and immunohistochemical study," *European Cellular Material*, vol. 13, supplement 2, p. 54, 2007.

[86] M. A. Fang, P. J. Frost, A. Iida-Klein, and T. J. Hahn, "Effects of nicotine on cellular function in UMR 106-01 osteoblast-like cells," *Bone*, vol. 12, no. 4, pp. 283–286, 1991.

[87] W. K. Ramp, L. G. Lenz, and R. J. S. Galvin, "Nicotine inhibits collagen synthesis and alkaline phosphatase activity, but stimulates DNA synthesis in osteoblast-like cells," *Proceedings of the Society for Experimental Biology and Medicine*, vol. 197, no. 1, pp. 36–43, 1991.

[88] G. J. Wetscher, M. Bagchi, D. Bagchi et al., "Free radical production in nicotine treated pancreatic tissue," *Free Radical Biology and Medicine*, vol. 18, no. 5, pp. 877–882, 1995.

[89] C. Kalpana and V. P. Menon, "Protective effect of curcumin on circulatory lipid peroxidation and antioxidant status during nicotine-induced toxicity," *Toxicology Mechanisms and Methods*, vol. 14, no. 6, pp. 339–343, 2004.

[90] C. L. Crowley-Weber, K. Dvorakova, C. Crowley et al., "Nicotine increases oxidative stress, activates NF-κB and GRP78, induces apoptosis and sensitizes cells to genotoxic/xenobiotic stresses by a multiple stress inducer, deoxycholate: relevance to colon carcinogenesis," *Chemico-Biological Interactions*, vol. 145, no. 1, pp. 53–66, 2003.

[91] E. Jimi and S. Ghosh, "Role of nuclear factor-κB in the immune system and bone," *Immunological Reviews*, vol. 208, pp. 80–87, 2005.

[92] S. Maniam, N. Mohamed, A. N. Shuid, and I. N. Soelaiman, "Palm tocotrienol exerted better antioxidant activities in bone than α-tocopherol," *Basic and Clinical Pharmacology and Toxicology*, vol. 103, no. 1, pp. 55–60, 2008.

[93] M. L. Yam, S. R. Abdul Hafid, H. M. Cheng, and K. Nesaretnam, "Tocotrienols suppress proinflammatory markers and cyclooxygenase-2 expression in RAW264.7 macrophages," *Lipids*, vol. 44, no. 9, pp. 787–797, 2009.

[94] Y. Yamamoto and R. B. Gaynor, "Therapeutic potential of inhibition of the NF-κB pathway in the treatment of inflammation and cancer," *Journal of Clinical Investigation*, vol. 107, no. 2, pp. 135–142, 2001.

[95] C. Suarna, R. L. Hood, R. T. Dean, and R. Stocker, "Comparative antioxidant activity of tocotrienols and other natural lipid-soluble antioxidants in a homogeneous system, and in rat and human lipoproteins," *Biochimica et Biophysica Acta*, vol. 1166, no. 2-3, pp. 163–170, 1993.

17

Effects of Nicotine on Emotional Reactivity in PTSD and Non-PTSD Smokers: Results of a Pilot fMRI Study

Brett Froeliger,[1] **Jean Crowell Beckham,**[1,2,3] **Michelle Feldman Dennis,**[1,2] **Rachel Victoria Kozink,**[1] **and Francis Joseph McClernon**[1,2]

[1] Department of Psychiatry and Behavioral Sciences, Duke University Medical Center, Durham, NC 27708, USA
[2] Durham Veterans Affairs Medical Center, Durham, NC 27708, USA
[3] VISN 6, Mental Illness Research, Education, and Clinical Center (MIRECC), Durham, NC 27708, USA

Correspondence should be addressed to Francis Joseph McClernon, francis.mcclernon@duke.edu

Academic Editor: Peter J. Winsauer

There is evidence that individuals with posttraumatic stress disorder (PTSD) may smoke in part to regulate negative affect. This pilot fMRI study examined the effects of nicotine on emotional information processing in smokers with and without PTSD. Across groups, nicotine increased brain activation in response to fearful/angry faces (compared to neutral faces) in ventral caudate. Patch x Group interactions were observed in brain regions involved in emotional and facial feature processing. These preliminary findings suggest that nicotine differentially modulates negative information processing in PTSD and non-PTSD smokers.

1. Introduction

Posttraumatic stress disorder (PTSD) is associated with elevated rates of cigarette smoking (40%–63%) compared with population norms (20%–30%) [1–3]. Moreover, smokers with PTSD are significantly more likely to be "heavy" smokers (i.e., smoke >25 cigarettes/day) [4] and take larger puffs [5]. In naturalistic studies, PTSD smokers are more likely to report negative affective (NA) states as an antecedent to smoking [6] and also report significant reductions in NA following smoking [7].

A hallmark phenotype of individuals with PTSD is increased psychophysiological responsivity and NA to idiopathic trauma-related stimuli [8]. Furthermore, individuals with PTSD exhibit aberrant responding to nonspecific, negative emotional stimuli [9]. For instance, individuals with PTSD exhibit biased attention to negative emotional information [10, 11]. Moreover, compared to non-PTSD trauma survivors, PTSD survivors have increased electrocortical responses to sad faces [12]. It has been proposed [13, 14] that dysregulated emotional information processing in PTSD is due to hyperresponsiveness of the amygdala—a region subserving negative emotional information processes [15]—and also hyporesponsiveness of medial prefrontal cortices—a region involved in cognitive control of emotional responses [16]. Support for this hypothesis comes from fMRI studies of PTSD patients showing increased reactivity to fearful faces in amygdala as compared to controls [17, 18] coincident with decreased reactivity in medial prefrontal regions [18].

Laboratory studies show that smoking and nicotine reduces distraction caused by negative stimuli [19] and electrocortical responses [20] to these stimuli among smokers. Moreover, neuroimaging studies show that nicotine acts on limbic (e.g., amygdala) and prefrontal brain areas that subserve emotional information processing [21–23]. Despite evidence regarding smoking/PTSD interactions, no neuroimaging studies to date have evaluated the neurobiological basis of nicotine and/or smoking effects on emotional information processing among individuals with PTSD. Thus, we conducted a preliminary study aimed at evaluating this question. Smokers with and without a PTSD diagnosis underwent fMRI scanning 2 hrs after application of a 21 mg transdermal nicotine or placebo patch. During scanning participants viewed emotional or neutral face stimuli. We

TABLE 1: Participant demographics[ab].

Sub.	Age	Sex	FTND	Cigs/day	Yrs smoked	BDI	PTSD (CAPS)	Psychiatric history	Trauma event	Drug dep. hx
P-1	27	F	5	10	9	1	Yes	MDD, OCD, Adjustment disorder	Witness to assault	Alcohol
P-2	41	F	3	20	25	11	Yes	None	Death of daughter	None
P-3	28	F	8	50	11	24	Yes	Agoraphobia, specific phobia (heights), MDD	Children removed by social services	None
P-4	31	F	6	15	15	9	Yes	MDD	Child sexual abuse	
C-1	68	F	5	60	49	2	No	MDD	Death of husband	Alcohol
C-2	27	M	4	15	8	0	No	None	Hurricane	None
C-3	28	F	3	13	12	1	No	None	None	None
C-4	43	F	10	39	31	10	No	Subthreshold OCD	Death of friend	None

[a]PTSD group subjects are denoted as de-identified subject numbers P-1 through P-4.
[b]Control group subjects are denoted as de-identified subject numbers C-1 through C-4.

hypothesized that nicotine and PTSD, both separately and in combination, would have effects on brain activation, specifically in regions underlying emotional processes.

2. Materials and Methods

2.1. Subjects and Stimuli. Participants ($n = 11$) were adult smokers with and without PTSD recruited from community and clinic sources. Eligibility requirements included being between the ages of 18–75, smoking ≥ 10 cigarettes per day over the past year, abstinence from nicotine delivery other than cigarettes, having 20/20 corrected vision, native English speaking, free of any neurological history, or major medical problems, passing a urine drug screen and pregnancy test if female and not meeting DSM-IV criteria for current drug or alcohol abuse/dependence (except nicotine). Participants read and signed an Institutional Review Board approved informed consent form and were paid $250 upon study completion. Eleven participants completed all aspects of the study. Data from 3 participants were excluded due to computer hardware difficulty ($n = 2$) and data-related problems ($n = 1$).

2.2. Procedure. Participants completed three sessions—one screening/diagnostic and two scanning sessions. PTSD diagnosis was based on the Clinician Administered PTSD Scale [24]. Other psychiatric disorders were diagnosed based on the Structured Clinical Interview for DSM-IV diagnosis [25]. Current alcohol and drug abuse/dependence diagnoses were determined by a 3-month time frame; current diagnoses for major depressive episode and anxiety disorders were determined by a 1-month time frame. Two trained raters (kappa for diagnoses = .97) conducted the interviews under the supervision of a licensed clinical psychologist (JCB). The Beck Depression Inventory (BDI), the Fagerström test for Nicotine Dependence (FTND), and a smoking history form were administered (see Table 1).

On each experimental day, participants were administered either a transdermal nicotine (21 mg NicoDerm) or placebo patch. Placebo patches (resembling nicotine patches)

were manufactured by 1–800-PATCHES. Participants were instructed to smoke as usual up to patch administration. The patch was placed on the lower upper arm to avoid complications during scanning. In the 2 hrs following patch application, participants maintained smoking abstinence and were monitored by study personnel. After 2 hours, participants entered the MRI suite, were placed in the scanner, and then performed an experimental task during fMRI scanning. Patch order was randomly assigned and counterbalanced across participants.

2.3. Experimental Task. The experimental task was a modified version of a face viewing task previously shown to increase activation in brain regions underlying emotion processing [26]; see Figure 1. In brief, neutral and negative (angry and fearful) faces [27] were presented in a dynamic (i.e., morphed) fashion. The morphing caused them to appear to change from neutral to negative in the same actor (emotion morph) or from one neutral identity to another neutral identity (identity morph). Trials were separated by a fixation cross. Participants used a response box to indicate whether each face depicted an emotion or an identity morph. Stimuli were presented in a pseudorandom event-related design. The intertrial interval varied between 12 and 15 s (M = 13.5 s). Each session was divided into eight, 8 min 24 s runs. Run order was counterbalanced across participants.

2.4. Scanning Procedures. MR images were acquired on a 1.5 T General Electric Signa NVi scanner (Milwaukee, WI, USA) equipped with 41 mT/m gradients. The participant's head was immobilized using a cushion and tape. The anterior and posterior commissures were identified in the midsagittal slice of a localizer series. A high-resolution T1-weight anatomical image was then acquired (124 contiguous slices, repetition time, TR = 8.2 s, TE = 3.3 ms, FOV = 24 cm, matrix = 256^2, slice thickness = 1.5 mm). Functional images were collected during the task with an inverse spiral pulse sequence sensitive to blood-oxygenation-level-dependent (BOLD) contrast (30 slices, TR = 1.5 s,

TABLE 2: Brain areas where significant main effects of group were observed.

Side	Brain area	BA	Cluster size (mm³)	MNI coordinates			Tmax
				x	y	z	
PTSD > control							
L	Fusiform gyrus	37	744	−42	−54	−20	6.33
		19		−38	−68	−18	6.25
R	Putamen		200	32	−10	−8	5.48
R	Amygdala			26	−6	−12	4.75
R	Caudate		208	10	−6	22	5.21
				12	−2	14	3.86
L	Caudate		280	−8	4	8	4.85
R	Angular gyrus	19	152	40	−78	44	4.73
L	Thalamus		280	−18	−20	14	4.6
				−12	−26	12	4.45
L	Superior frontal gyrus	8	104	−22	38	48	4.53
R	Inferior frontal gyrus	9	96	60	20	26	4.24
R	Thalamus		104	16	−4	12	4.12
Control > PTSD							
No significant areas of activation							

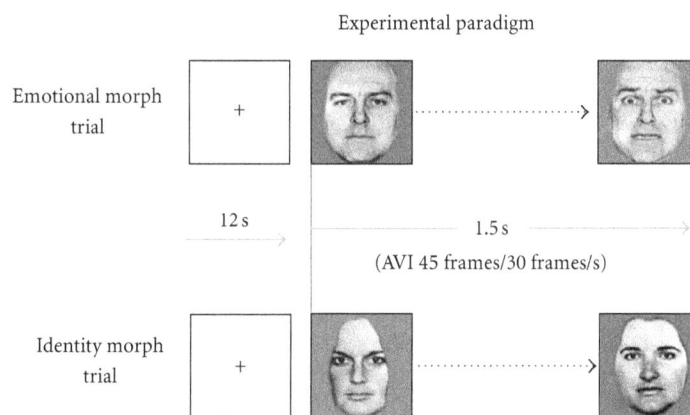

FIGURE 1: fMRI task paradigm.

TE = 10 ms, FOV = 24 cm, matrix = 64^2, flip angle = 81°, slice thickness = 3.8 mm, in-plane resolution = 3.75 mm²).

2.5. Data Analysis. The fMRI data analysis utilized a voxel-based approach implemented in SPM5 (Wellcome Trust Centre for Neuroimaging, London, UK). Preprocessing steps included (1) slice-time correction, (2) realignment using rigid body translation and rotation, (3) normalization into a standard stereotaxic space (Montreal Neurological Institute) with an isotropic 2 mm³ voxel size, and (4) smoothing with an 8 mm Gaussian filter.

For each participant on each session, statistical parametric maps were derived by applying linear contrasts to the parameter estimates for the event of interest (emotional morph > identity morph), resulting in a t-statistic for every voxel. These contrasts were then passed onto the second

level for random-effects analyses. Statistical contrasts were set up to calculate signal differences between patch condition (nicotine versus placebo), group (PTSD versus control), and the 2-way interaction between patch and group. A gray matter mask was applied to statistical parametric maps, and results were thresholded at $P < 0.001$, uncorrected, with a spatial extent of ten contiguous voxels.

3. Results

3.1. Participant Demographics. Participants were adult smokers with ($n = 4$) and without PTSD ($n = 4$). See Table 1 for smoking history and demographic information. Groups were matched on age (sample M = 36.6, SD = 14.2), average number of years smoked (M = 20, SD = 14.3), cigarettes per day (M = 19.2, SD = 6.8), and nicotine dependence (FTND score M = 5.5; SD = 2.4).

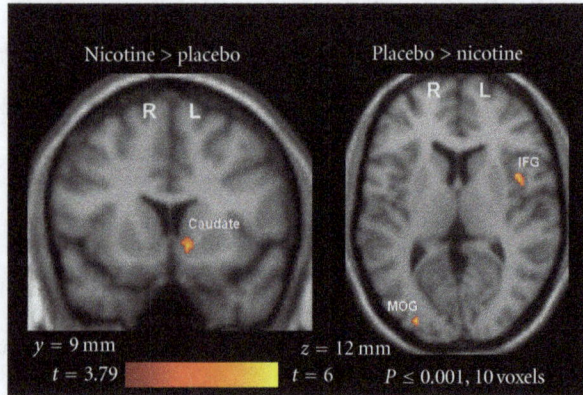

FIGURE 2: fMRI contrast of the main effects of patch type. Across groups, activation (emotion morph > identity morph) was greater for nicotine versus placebo patch in left caudate ($x = -10$, $y = 14$, $z = -6$), whereas greater activation was observed in left inferior frontal gyrus (IFG) ($x = -42$, $y = 8$, $z = 8$) and right middle occipital gyrus (MOG) ($x = 32$, $y = -88$, $z = 4$) for placebo versus nicotine patch.

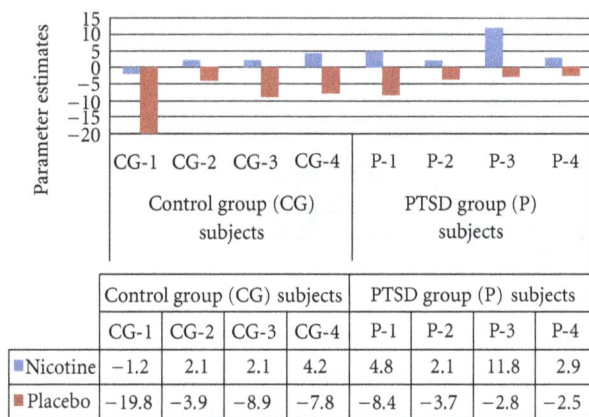

	Control group (CG) subjects				PTSD group (P) subjects			
	CG-1	CG-2	CG-3	CG-4	P-1	P-2	P-3	P-4
■Nicotine	−1.2	2.1	2.1	4.2	4.8	2.1	11.8	2.9
■Placebo	−19.8	−3.9	−8.9	−7.8	−8.4	−3.7	−2.8	−2.5

FIGURE 3: Model parameter estimates of the main effect of patch type on task-related left caudate ($x = -10$, $y = 14$, $z = -6$) BOLD response.

3.2. fMRI Activations. Patch effects Across groups, nicotine patch compared to placebo resulted in increased activation in left ventral caudate (Figures 2 and 3). As represented in Figure 2, significant activations for placebo relative to nicotine patch were observed in right middle occipital gyrus (BA 19) and left inferior frontal gyrus (BA 44).

Group Effects. Across patch conditions, activation was significantly greater in the PTSD as compared to non-PTSD group in striatum, amygdala, and frontal, parietal, and occipital cortices (see Table 2). No activations were greater in the non-PTSD relative to PTSD group.

Patch x Group Interaction. As represented in Figure 4, patch x group interactions were observed in right superior frontal gyrus (SFG) (Figure 5) and left middle temporal gyrus (MTG). In SFG, activation was greatest in the PTSD group

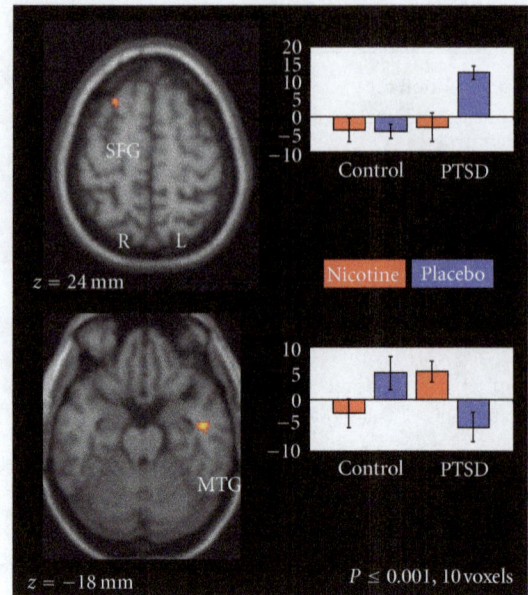

FIGURE 4: fMRI contrast of the patch x group interactions. Significant patch x group interactions were observed in right superior frontal gyrus (SFG) ($x = 24$, $y = 22$, $z = 60$) and left middle temporal gyrus (MTG) ($x = -48$, $y = -10$, $z = -24$).

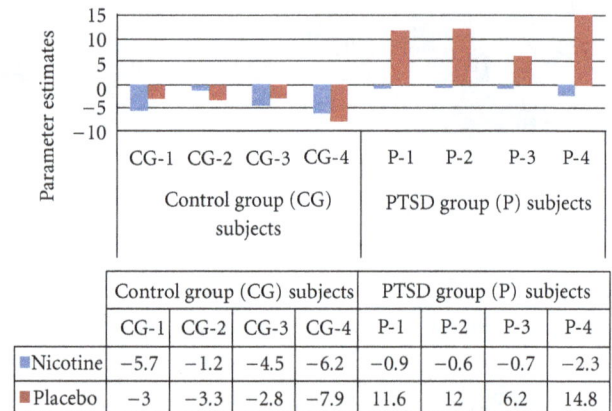

	Control group (CG) subjects				PTSD group (P) subjects			
	CG-1	CG-2	CG-3	CG-4	P-1	P-2	P-3	P-4
■Nicotine	−5.7	−1.2	−4.5	−6.2	−0.9	−0.6	−0.7	−2.3
■Placebo	−3	−3.3	−2.8	−7.9	11.6	12	6.2	14.8

FIGURE 5: Model parameter estimates of the group x patch interaction on task-related right superior frontal gyrus (SFG) ($x = 24$, $y = 22$, $z = 60$) BOLD response.

than that in the placebo condition. In MTG, activation was greater in the PTSD group in the nicotine relative to placebo condition; the opposite pattern was observed in the non-PTSD group.

4. Discussion

This preliminary study is the first to systematically assess the effects of nicotine on neural correlates of emotional information processing in a PTSD sample. As in previous studies [17, 18], PTSD was associated with larger brain responses to emotional face stimuli in amygdala and prefrontal regions.

In evaluating the effects of nicotine, we observed patch x group interactions in several brain areas which suggest nicotine might modulate emotional information processing *via* different neural mechanisms in smokers with and without PTSD. The observed patch x group interaction in SFG suggested greater reactivity to emotional cues in this region when smokers with PTSD were in a nicotine-deprived state. The SFG plays an important role in emotion, memory, and motivational processes. As compared to controls, individuals with PTSD have been shown to exhibit increased activation in SFG upon recall of neutral information that was encoded in an emotional context [28]. A patch x group interaction was also observed in MTG—a region previously shown to be selectively active in response to nonaffective components of face stimuli (e.g., perception and familiarity; [29]). This area was more reactive to emotional face cues in smokers with PTSD when receiving nicotine. Collectively, these findings suggest that nicotine (and nicotine deprivation) may modulate reactivity to the nonaffective and affective components of face stimuli in smokers with PTSD.

In addition to the above interactions, we observed a main effect of nicotine in which activation to emotional face stimuli was greater in left ventral caudate following nicotine patch administration. The ventral caudate is part of the ventral striatum—a brain region that mediates reward processes [30]. Nicotine stimulates the release of dopamine in the ventral striatum in both animals [31] and in human smokers [32]. Likewise, nicotine abstinence results in decreased ventral striatal dopamine functioning [33]. Thus, our novel findings of nicotine-induced increases in reactivity to emotional stimuli in the striatum may be due to increased dopamine transmission in this region brought on by nicotine administration (or decreases in dopamine neurotransmission in the absence of nicotine).

The present study has limitations including a small sample size and a relatively heterogeneous sample with respect to age, psychiatric comorbidity, and smoking history. We manipulated nicotine in the context of brief abstinence so it remains unknown what effect a longer abstinence period would have on emotional information processing. Additional work with larger samples and under other clinically relevant conditions is needed.

5. Conclusion

The present preliminary study provides novel information regarding the effects of nicotine on emotional information processing in smokers with and without PTSD. Smokers with PTSD report greater NA immediately prior to smoking [34] and greater decreases in NA following smoking [35], and these findings are consistent with the observed patterns of brain activation in the current study. Thus, our findings provide a neurobiological basis that helps explain why individuals with PTSD are at greater risk of smoking and also experience greater difficulty quitting. The present study is not without its limitations. Our sample size was small and was predominately represented by female smokers. Moreover, among the female participants, we did not obtain

information regarding menstrual cycle phase in relation to the timing of each of their experimental sessions which may have added some variance to the results. Future work will examine the effects of nicotine and smoking in larger samples of smokers with PTSD, control for sex differences, and among females control for time in menstrual cycle, and relate these findings to smoking-related outcomes (e.g., smoking cessation success/failure).

Acknowledgments

This work was supported K23DA017261 (F. J. McClernon) and by the Office of Research and Development Clinical Science, Department of Veterans Affairs, and by, K24DA016388, 2R01CA081595, R21DA019704, and 2R01MH62482 (J. C. Beckham). The views expressed in this paper are those of the authors and do not necessarily represent the views of the Department of Veterans Affairs or the National Institutes of Health. The authors wish to thank Dr. Kevin Labar who developed and programmed the task that was used in the study.

References

[1] J. C. Beckham, A. A. Roodman, R. H. Shipley et al., "Smoking in Vietnam combat veterans with post-traumatic stress disorder," *Journal of Traumatic Stress*, vol. 8, no. 3, pp. 461–472, 1995.

[2] N. Breslau, G. C. Davis, and L. R. Schultz, "Posttraumatic stress disorder and the incidence of nicotine, alcohol, and other drug disorders in persons who have experienced trauma," *Archives of General Psychiatry*, vol. 60, no. 3, pp. 289–294, 2003.

[3] K. Lasser, J. W. Boyd, S. Woolhandler, D. U. Himmelstein, D. McCormick, and D. H. Bor, "Smoking and mental illness: a population-based prevalence study," *Journal of the American Medical Association*, vol. 284, no. 20, pp. 2606–2610, 2000.

[4] J. C. Beckham, A. C. Kirby, M. E. Feldman et al., "Prevalence and correlates of heavy smoking in Vietnam veterans with chronic posttraumatic stress disorder," *Addictive Behaviors*, vol. 22, no. 5, pp. 637–647, 1997.

[5] F. J. McClernon, J. C. Beckham, S. L. Mozley, M. E. Feldman, S. R. Vrana, and J. E. Rose, "The effects of trauma recall on smoking topography in posttraumatic stress disorder and non-posttraumatic stress disorder trauma survivors," *Addictive Behaviors*, vol. 30, no. 2, pp. 247–257, 2005.

[6] J. C. Beckham, M. E. Feldman, S. R. Vrana et al., "Immediate antecedents of cigarette smoking in smokers with and without posttraumatic stress disorder: a preliminary study," *Experimental and Clinical Psychopharmacology*, vol. 13, no. 3, pp. 219–228, 2005.

[7] J. C. Beckham, M. T. Wiley, S. C. Miller et al., "Ad lib smoking in post-traumatic stress disorder: an electronic diary study," *Nicotine and Tobacco Research*, vol. 10, no. 7, pp. 1149–1157, 2008.

[8] S. P. Orr, L. J. Metzger, and R. K. Pitman, "Psychophysiology of post-traumatic stress disorder," *Psychiatric Clinics of North America*, vol. 25, no. 2, pp. 271–293, 2002.

[9] J. E. Rose, "Nicotine and nonnicotine factors in cigarette addiction," *Psychopharmacology*, vol. 184, no. 3-4, pp. 274–285, 2006.

[10] W. H. Alexander and J. W. Brown, "Competition between learned reward and error outcome predictions in anterior cingulate cortex," *NeuroImage*, vol. 49, no. 4, pp. 3210–3218, 2010.

[11] R. G. Schlösser, G. Wagner, C. Schachtzabel et al., "Fronto-cingulate effective connectivity in obsessive compulsive disorder: a study with fMRI and dynamic causal modeling," *Human Brain Mapping*, vol. 31, no. 12, pp. 1834–1850, 2010.

[12] K. J. Friston, L. Harrison, and W. Penny, "Dynamic causal modelling," *NeuroImage*, vol. 19, no. 4, pp. 1273–1302, 2003.

[13] R. J. McNally, "Cognitive abnormalities in post-traumatic stress disorder," *Trends in Cognitive Sciences*, vol. 10, no. 6, pp. 271–277, 2006.

[14] S. L. Rauch, L. M. Shin, E. Segal et al., "Selectively reduced regional cortical volumes in post-traumatic stress disorder," *NeuroReport*, vol. 14, no. 7, pp. 913–916, 2003.

[15] J. E. LeDoux, "Emotion circuits in the brain," *Annual Review of Neuroscience*, vol. 23, pp. 155–184, 2000.

[16] R. J. Davidson, K. M. Putnam, and C. L. Larson, "Dysfunction in the neural circuitry of emotion regulation—a possible prelude to violence," *Science*, vol. 289, no. 5479, pp. 591–594, 2000.

[17] S. L. Rauch, P. J. Whalen, L. M. Shin et al., "Exaggerated amygdala response to masked facial stimuli in posttraumatic stress disorder: a functional MRI study," *Biological Psychiatry*, vol. 47, no. 9, pp. 769–776, 2000.

[18] L. M. Shin, C. I. Wright, P. A. Cannistraro et al., "A functional magnetic resonance imaging study of amygdala and medial prefrontal cortex responses to overtly presented fearful faces in posttraumatic stress disorder," *Archives of General Psychiatry*, vol. 62, no. 3, pp. 273–281, 2005.

[19] A. Rzetelny, D. Gilbert, J. Hammersley, R. Radtke, N. Rabinovich, and S. Small, "Nicotine decreases attentional bias to negative-affect-related Stroop words among smokers," *Nicotine and Tobacco Research*, vol. 10, no. 6, pp. 1029–1036, 2008.

[20] D. G. Gilbert, C. Sugai, Y. Zuo, N. E. Rabinovich, F. J. McClernon, and B. Froeliger, "Brain indices of nicotine's effects on attentional bias to smoking and emotional pictures and to task-relevant targets," *Nicotine and Tobacco Research*, vol. 9, no. 3, pp. 351–363, 2007.

[21] E. F. Domino, L. Ni, Y. Xu, R. A. Koeppe, S. Guthrie, and J. K. Zubieta, "Regional cerebral blood flow and plasma nicotine after smoking tobacco cigarettes," *Progress in Neuro-Psychopharmacology and Biological Psychiatry*, vol. 28, no. 2, pp. 319–327, 2004.

[22] J. E. Rose, F. M. Behm, E. C. Westman et al., "PET studies of the influences of nicotine on neural systems in cigarette smokers," *American Journal of Psychiatry*, vol. 160, no. 2, pp. 323–333, 2003.

[23] E. A. Stein, J. Pankiewicz, H. H. Harsch et al., "Nicotine-induced limbic cortical activation in the human brain: a functional MRI study," *American Journal of Psychiatry*, vol. 155, no. 8, pp. 1009–1015, 1998.

[24] C. Mueller-Pfeiffer, C. Martin-Soelch, J. R. Blair et al., "Impact of emotion on cognition in trauma survivors: what is the role of posttraumatic stress disorder?" *Journal of Affective Disorders*, vol. 126, no. 1-2, pp. 287–292, 2010.

[25] S. S. Watkins, G. F. Koob, and A. Markou, "Neural mechanisms underlying nicotine addiction: acute positive reinforcement and withdrawal," *Nicotine and Tobacco Research*, vol. 2, no. 1, pp. 19–37, 2000.

[26] J. Fan, P. R. Hof, K. G. Guise, J. A. Fossella, and M. I. Posner, "The functional integration of the anterior cingulate cortex during conflict processing," *Cerebral Cortex*, vol. 18, no. 4, pp. 796–805, 2008.

[27] A. Azizian, L. J. Nestor, D. Payer, J. R. Monterosso, A. L. Brody, and E. D. London, "Smoking reduces conflict-related anterior cingulate activity in abstinent cigarette smokers performing a stroop task," *Neuropsychopharmacology*, vol. 35, no. 3, pp. 775–782, 2010.

[28] CDC, "Annual smoking-attributable mortality, years of potential life lost, and productivity losses—United States, 1995–1999," *Morbidity and Mortality Weekly Report*, vol. 51, pp. 300–313, 2002.

[29] CDC, "Cigarette smoking among adults—United States, 2000," *Morbidity and Mortality Weekly Report*, vol. 51, pp. 642–645, 2000.

[30] R. Elliott, K. J. Friston, and R. J. Dolan, "Dissociable neural responses in human reward systems," *Journal of Neuroscience*, vol. 20, no. 16, pp. 6159–6165, 2000.

[31] H. Garavan, "Insula and drug cravings," *Brain structure & function*, vol. 214, no. 5-6, pp. 593–601, 2010.

[32] M. Guitart-Masip, N. Bunzeck, K. E. Stephan, R. J. Dolan, and E. Düzel, "Contextual novelty changes reward representations in the striatum," *Journal of Neuroscience*, vol. 30, no. 5, pp. 1721–1726, 2010.

[33] E. K. Miller and J. D. Cohen, "An integrative theory of prefrontal cortex function," *Annual Review of Neuroscience*, vol. 24, pp. 167–202, 2001.

[34] H. S. Mayberg, "Limbic-cortical dysregulation: a proposed model of depression," *Journal of Neuropsychiatry and Clinical Neurosciences*, vol. 9, no. 3, pp. 471–481, 1997.

[35] G. A. Croghan, J. A. Sloan, I. T. Croghan et al., "Comparison of nicotine patch alone versus nicotine nasal spray alone versus a combination for treating smokers: a minimal intervention, randomized multicenter trial in a nonspecialized setting," *Nicotine and Tobacco Research*, vol. 5, no. 2, pp. 181–187, 2003.

18

Preclinical Determinants of Drug Choice under Concurrent Schedules of Drug Self-Administration

Matthew L. Banks and S. Stevens Negus

Department of Pharmacology and Toxicology, Virginia Commonwealth University, P.O. Box 980613, Richmond, VA 23298, USA

Correspondence should be addressed to Matthew L. Banks, mbanks7@vcu.edu

Academic Editor: Edward W. Boyer

Drug self-administration procedures have played a critical role in the experimental analysis of psychoactive compounds, such as cocaine, for over 50 years. While there are numerous permutations of this procedure, this paper will specifically focus on choice procedures using concurrent schedules of intravenous drug self-administration. The aims of this paper are to first highlight the evolution of drug choice procedures and then review the subsequent preclinical body of literature utilizing these choice procedures to understand the environmental, pharmacological, and biological determinants of the reinforcing stimulus effects of drugs. A main rationale for this paper is our proposition that choice schedules are underutilized in investigating the reinforcing effects of drugs in assays of drug self-administration. Moreover, we will conclude with potential future directions and unexplored scientific space for the use of drug choice procedures.

1. The Evolution of Drug Choice Procedures

Drug self-administration procedures have played a critical role in the experimental analysis of psychoactive compounds, such as cocaine, for more than 50 years. In general, preclinical drug self-administration procedures are utilized for two main scientific purposes. One purpose is in abuse liability testing of psychoactive compounds for potential scheduling as controlled substances by the Drug Enforcement Agency, and there are already excellent reviews on the use of drug self-administration procedures for this purpose, see [1, 2]. The other main purpose of drug self-administration procedures is in understanding the pharmacological, environmental and biological determinants of drug-taking behavior as a model of drug addiction. This paper will focus on the use of concurrent-choice schedules of drug self-administration to address this latter purpose.

Although there are numerous permutations of drug self-administration procedures, all use the classic 3-term contingency of operant conditioning to investigate the stimulus properties of drugs [3]. This 3-term contingency can be diagrammed as follows:

$$S^D \longrightarrow R \longrightarrow S^C, \tag{1}$$

where S^D designates a *discriminative stimulus*, R designates a *response* on the part of the organism, and S^C designates a *consequent stimulus*. The arrows specify the contingency that, in the presence of the discriminative stimulus S^D, performance of the response R will result in delivery of the consequent stimulus S^C. As a simple and common example from a preclinical laboratory, a rat implanted with a chronic indwelling catheter might be connected to an infusion pump containing a dose of a psychoactive drug and placed into an experimental chamber that contains a stimulus light and a response lever. Contingencies can be programmed such that, if the stimulus light is illuminated (the discriminative stimulus), then depression of the response lever (the response) will result in delivery of a drug injection (the consequent stimulus). Conversely, if the stimulus light is not illuminated, then responding does not result in the delivery of the drug injection. Under these conditions, subjects typically learn to respond when the discriminative stimulus is present. Consequent stimuli that increase responding leading to their delivery are operationally defined as *reinforcers*, whereas stimuli that decrease responding leading to their delivery are defined as *punishers*. The contingencies that relate discriminative stimuli, responses, and consequent stimuli are defined by the schedule of reinforcement [4].

The first published reports of intravenous drug self-administration used exactly this type of single-response procedure described above to examine morphine self-administration in morphine-dependent rats [5, 6]. Furthermore, these seminal studies demonstrated three principles that have been commonly observed in single-response drug self-administration procedures ever since. First, these studies demonstrated that intravenous morphine could maintain schedule-appropriate rates and patterns of responding leading to its delivery, indicating that morphine functioned as a reinforcer. Second, this single-response procedure produced a bitonic, "inverted U shaped" dose-effect function relating the unit dose of morphine in each injection to measures of rate (either rates of responding or injection delivery). Thus, maximal rates of self-administration were maintained by intermediate morphine doses, and lower rates were maintained not only by lower morphine doses, but also by higher doses. Importantly, this pattern of responding indicates a dissociation between rates of self-administration maintained by a given consequent stimulus and the reinforcing efficacy of that stimulus [7, 8], because if the research subject is given a choice between a lower and higher dose of the same drug, the subject will almost always choose the higher drug dose indicating that the higher drug dose is the preferred or more efficacious reinforcer [9, 10]. Why would rates of drug self-administration decrease as dose increases above some apparent optimal level? As is often the case in other pharmacology domains, the presence of a bitonic dose-effect function indicates that multiple and/or opposing drug effects are being integrated into a common dependent variable. For example, measures of self-administration rate can be influenced not only by the reinforcing effects of a drug (which would have the effect of increasing rates), but also by other effects of the self-administered drug that can either increase or decrease rates (e.g., effects that improve or impair motor competence or information processing). These other drug effects will be collectively referred to as "reinforcement-independent rate-altering effects" in this paper to distinguish them from reinforcing effects, and one goal of more recently developed procedures is to dissociate reinforcing drug effects from reinforcement-independent rate-altering effects.

The third and final principle revealed by these early studies was that rates of morphine self-administration could be altered by treatment with other drugs. These effects were interpreted to suggest treatment effects on drug reinforcement (and by extension, to provide evidence regarding mechanisms of drug reinforcement). However, just as self-administration rates can be influenced by multiple effects of the self-administered drug, so these rates can also be influenced by multiple effects of a treatment drug (or of any

other experimental manipulation, such as a lesion or genetic modification) [11, 12]. More specifically, these experimental manipulations can alter rates of self-administration not only by changing the reinforcing effects of the self-administered drug, but also by changing the reinforcer-independent rate-altering effects of the self-administered drug, or by producing its own reinforcement-independent rate-altering effects. Overall, these early studies illustrated the promise of drug self-administration as a model of drug addiction, but they also provided a glimpse of the challenges to interpretation of rate-based measures generated by single-response procedures.

Since the early 1960s, preclinical drug self-administration research has flourished, and techniques for intravenous drug self-administration were rapidly extended to studies with other drug classes and in other species of experimental subjects [13, 14]. However, over the decades, drug reinforcement research has evolved along three divergent paths. One path of self-administration research has retained the use of single-response procedures initially used by Weeks and colleagues [5, 6] and utilized more demanding and complex schedules of reinforcement, such as progressive-ratio and second-order schedules, than the simple fixed-ratio schedules used by Weeks and colleagues. In general, studies using these approaches have demonstrated that numerous drug classes can maintain rates and patterns of responding consistent with the hypothesis that drugs can function as reinforcers [15]. However, these approaches have been less successful in generating dependent measures that clearly dissociate reinforcing drug effects from reinforcement-independent rate-altering drug effects. To highlight the prevalence of single-response procedures in the current drug self-administration literature, we used the keyword "self-administration" in PubMed on April 11, 2012, to retrieve the 50 most recent preclinical studies using intravenous drug self-administration procedures as the primary independent variable. This "snapshot" of the literature revealed that 15 of the 50 most recent studies used a single-response drug self-administration procedure.

A second path of self-administration research has retained the simple fixed-ratio schedules utilized by Weeks and colleagues on one response lever, but incorporated rudimentary aspects of choice by introducing an "inactive" response option in addition to the "active" drug option. For example, an early study by Pickens and Thompson [16] used a two-lever self-administration procedure in which responding on one "active" lever produced intravenous cocaine delivery under an FR1 schedule of reinforcement, whereas responding on a second "inactive" lever had no scheduled consequences. Schedule-appropriate responding was maintained exclusively on the "active" lever, and when the contingencies on the two levers were reversed, rats rapidly reallocated their responding to the newly "active" lever. In our snapshot analysis of the current self-administration literature, the majority of drug self-administration studies (32 out of 50) used an "inactive" manipulandum. Differential rates of responding on "active" and "inactive" manipulanda are useful for investigating the reinforcing effects of consequent stimuli associated with the "active" manipulandum; however, the utility of this simple type of choice procedure is limited for at least two main reasons. First, although "active/inactive-response" procedures technically employ a concurrent schedule capable of generating measures of response allocation and choice, such measures are rarely computed or reported. Rather, investigators more commonly report measures of response or reinforcement rate on the "active" manipulandum as if it were the only response option available, and such rate-based measures of drug reinforcement are vulnerable to all the reinforcement-independent rate-altering drug effects described above. Second, baseline rates of behavior on the "active" and "inactive" manipulanda are normally vastly different, with rates on the "inactive" manipulandum being very low. As a result, data on "inactive" responding are primarily useful for only detecting reinforcement-independent rate-*increasing* effects. However, because "inactive" rates are already low, they are insensitive to reinforcer-independent rate-*decreasing* effects of experimental manipulations. This is a critical issue, because most drug self-administration studies are designed to evaluate the ability of experimental manipulations, such as pharmacological, environmental, or genetic variables, to decrease drug reinforcement as indicated by decreases in drug self-administration rates. Thus, procedures that use "active" and "inactive" manipulanda are not much different than the single-response self-administration procedures described above.

The third and least common path of drug self-administration research has used concurrent schedules in which responding is maintained on two or more manipulanda by two or more motivationally relevant consequent stimuli. For example, responding on one manipulandum might result in delivery of a particular drug dose, and responding on a different, concurrently available manipulandum might result in delivery of a different dose of the same drug, a different drug, or a qualitatively different consequent stimulus such as food (Figure 1). These procedures are often referred to as "choice" procedures, because subjects allocate their behavior, or "choose," between the available consequent stimuli, and the relative reinforcing effects of drug in comparison to an alternative are derived from measures of behavioral allocation (or "drug choice") rather than behavioral rate. As with any other type of self-administration procedure, the self-administered drug or other experimental manipulations might also influence overall self-administration rate by producing reinforcement-independent rate-altering effects; however, the impact of these other effects on choice measures of drug reinforcement can be minimized by appropriate use of manipulanda, discriminative, and alternative reinforcing stimuli, and schedules of reinforcement. A specific example of this dissociation is shown in Figure 1. Cocaine versus food choice increases as the unit cocaine dose increases; however, rates of responding display the prototypic inverted-U shaped dose-effect function. Moreover, choice procedures generate distinct measures of behavioral allocation and behavioral rate that permit dissociation of reinforcing effects from reinforcement-independent rate-altering effects. For example, an experimental manipulation that decreases reinforcing efficacy of a drug might be expected to reduce drug choice but increase choice of the alternative and produce

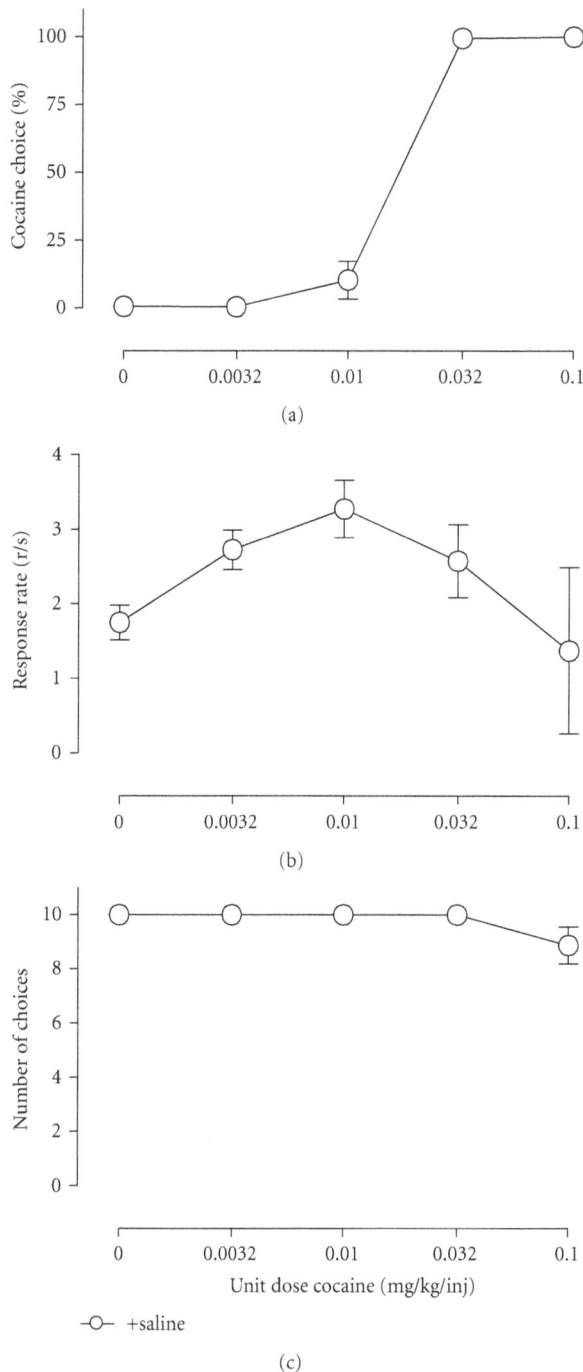

FIGURE 1: Baseline choice between different doses of cocaine (0–0.1 mg/kg/injection) and food pellets in rhesus monkeys ($n = 4$) under a concurrent FR10 : FR100 schedule of cocaine injections and food availability. Abscissae: unit dose of cocaine in milligrams per kilogram per injection. Top ordinate: percent cocaine choice. Middle ordinate: rates of responding in responses per second. Bottom ordinate: number of choices completed. All points represent mean data SEM obtained during the last 3 days of saline treatment. These unpublished data demonstrate two key observations from choice procedures. First, cocaine choice increases in a monotonic function as the unit cocaine dose increases. Second, while rates of responding display the prototypic, inverted-U-shaped dose-effect function, rates of responding are not predictive of cocaine choice, nor are rates of responding predictive of the number of choices completed per component.

no net change in overall reinforcement rates. A specific example of this selective effect from the literature is shown in Figure 2 examining cocaine versus food choice during chronic treatment with the dopamine (DA)-selective releaser *m*-fluoroamphetamine [17]. Conversely, a manipulation that produces reinforcement-independent rate-altering effects (e.g., motor impairment) might be expected to reduce overall reinforcement rates without altering drug choice. An example of this specific effect from the literature is shown in Figure 3 examining cocaine versus food choice during chronic treatment with the mu-opioid agonist methadone [18]. These distinct dependent measures of reinforcing effects (represented in measures of drug choice) and reinforcement-independent rate-altering effects (represented in measures of overall self-administration rates) are analogous to the use of concurrent schedules in the closely related field of drug discrimination research to generate dependent measures that permit dissociation of discriminative stimulus effects (represented in measures of drug-appropriate responding) from discrimination-independent rate-altering effects (represented in measures of overall rates of responding or reinforcement). Despite this apparent advantage, our PubMed search indicated that only 3 of the 50 most recent IV drug self-administration studies used a concurrent schedule of reinforcement. This paucity of research with concurrent schedules in research on the reinforcing stimulus effects of drugs stands in striking contrast to the almost exclusive use of concurrent schedules in drug discrimination research and suggests that concurrent schedules are underutilized in studies of drug self-administration [19].

Although choice procedures have been underutilized, their value has long been appreciated. As noted above, the earliest studies of *intravenous* drug self-administration used single-response procedures, but these studies were predated by choice studies in which drug was delivered by other routes of administration. For example, more than two decades before the studies by Weeks and colleagues, Spragg evaluated choice between intramuscular morphine and fruit in morphine-dependent chimpanzees and demonstrated that choice was largely influenced by the state of morphine withdrawal (such that morphine withdrawal was associated with increased probability of morphine choice) [20]. Similarly, Nichols and colleagues established responding for oral morphine in rats and found that morphine withdrawal increased choice of morphine over water [21]. Intravenous drug delivery subsequently gained prominence in drug self-administration research because it promotes a rapid onset of drug action that facilitates learned contingencies between responding and drug delivery. However, the rise of intravenous drug self-administration was also accompanied by a growing reliance on single-response and "active/inactive"-response procedures, perhaps because the limited lifespan of intravenous catheters selected for procedures that require the least initial training. Nonetheless, the use of choice procedures persisted, especially in studies of oral drug self-administration [13, 22] and in a small but steady series of intravenous drug self-administration studies. The goal here is to review the history and major findings of research on intravenous drug choice.

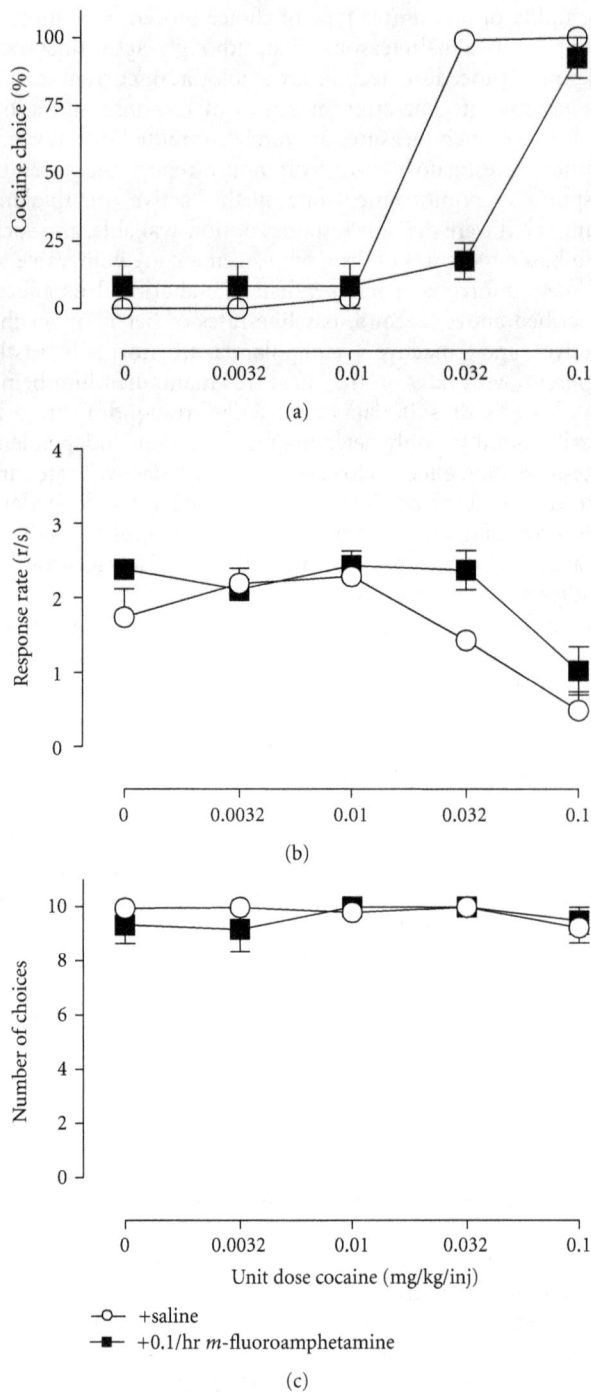

FIGURE 2: Effects of chronic intravenous *m*-fluoroamphetamine (0.1 mg/kg/hr) administration on choice between cocaine and food in rhesus monkeys ($n = 4$). Abscissae: unit dose of cocaine in milligrams per kilogram per injection. Top ordinate: percent cocaine choice. Middle ordinate: rates of responding in responses per second. Bottom ordinate: number of choices completed. All points represent mean data SEM obtained during the last 3 days of *m*-fluoroamphetamine treatment. These published data [17] demonstrate that experimental manipulations can selectively decrease cocaine choice without also decreasing rates of responding and the number of choices completed. This profile would be considered ideal for a candidate medication to treat cocaine dependence.

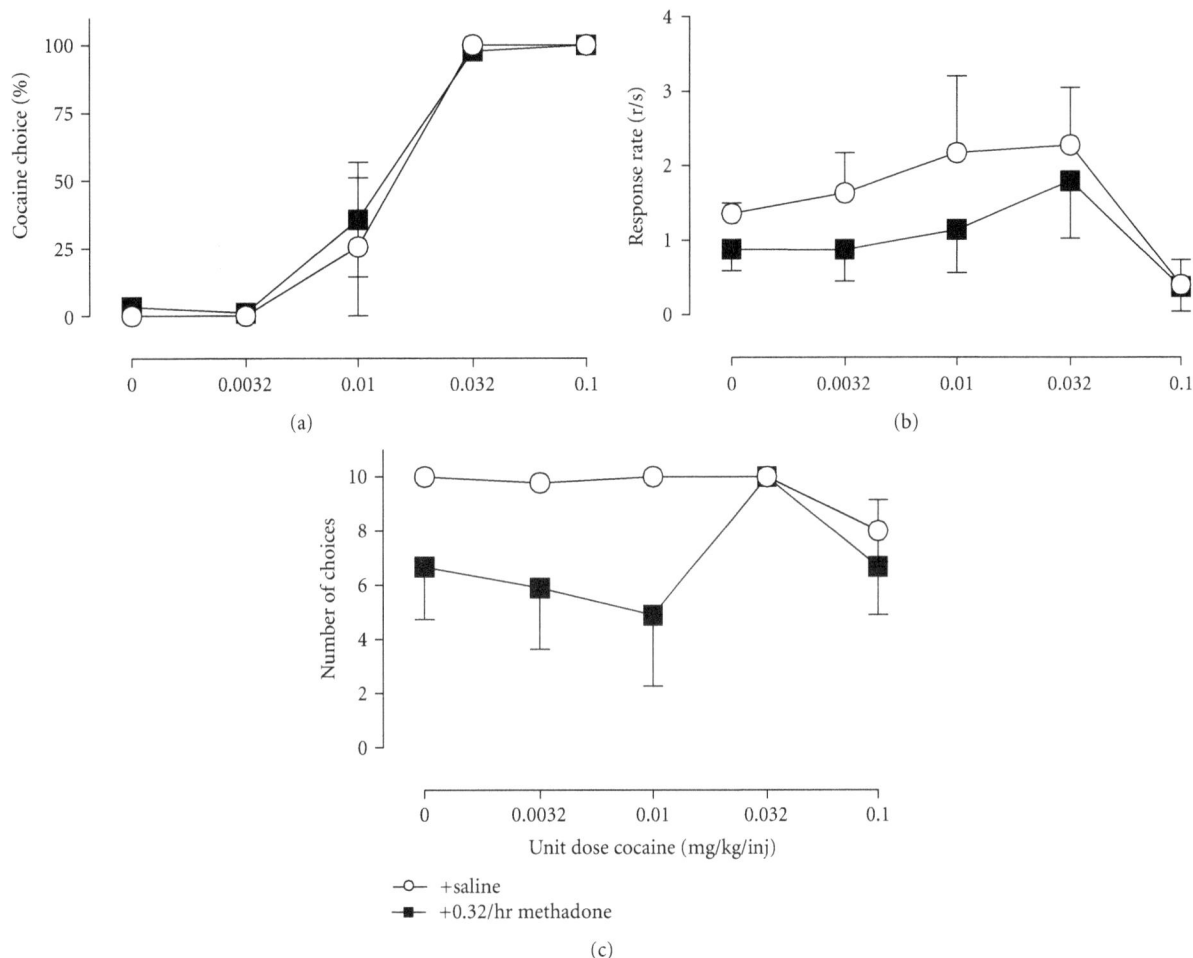

(a)

(b)

(c)

−○− +saline
−■− +0.32/hr methadone

FIGURE 3: Effects of chronic intravenous methadone (0.32 mg/kg/hr) administration on choice between cocaine and food in rhesus monkeys ($n = 3$). Abscissae: unit dose of cocaine in milligrams per kilogram per injection. Top ordinate: percent cocaine choice. Middle ordinate: rates of responding in responses per second. Bottom ordinate: number of choices completed. All points represent mean data SEM obtained during the last 3 days of methadone treatment. These published data [18] demonstrate that experimental manipulations can selectively decrease rates of responding and the number of choices completed without decreasing cocaine choice.

Before proceeding, two other points are worthy of mention. First, although choice procedures are sparingly used in *preclinical* studies of drug reinforcement, they have emerged as the standard approach in *clinical* studies of drug reinforcement [23, 24]. Consequently, increased preclinical use of choice procedures might facilitate translational research on drug reinforcement. Second, scientific interest in drug reinforcement derives in large part from its presumed role in drug addiction, and drug addiction can be defined as a disorder of choice and behavioral allocation [25, 26]. Moreover, 5 of the 7 diagnostic criteria for substance dependence in the revised fourth edition of the Diagnostic and Statistical Manual (DSM) of Mental Disorders are defined by allocation of behavior towards procurement and use of the substance compared to other behavior maintained by nondrug and presumably more adaptive alternative reinforcers [27]. In the fifth edition of the DSM that is still under development, 6 of the 11 diagnostic criteria are defined by behavioral allocations toward the procurement and use of the substance

[28]. Thus, addiction implies excessive drug choice at the expense of more adaptive behaviors. The pharmacological, environmental, and genetic determinants that influence drug choice and contribute to drug addiction can be directly studied using choice procedures.

2. Determinants of Drug Choice

2.1. Overview. While the first drug choice procedure was published in 1940 [20] by Spragg it was not until 1972 that the first intravenous drug choice procedure was published, approximately 10 years after intravenous drug self-administration procedures were introduced [5]. In their seminal study, Findley et al. [29] examined the effects of dependence and withdrawal on secobarbital and chlordiazepoxide preference. Since 1972, there have been 66 publications examining the determinants of drug choice, and these publications are summarized in Table 1. The predominant drugs examined have been cocaine (80%)

TABLE 1: Summary of published manuscripts reporting on IV drug self-administration under concurrent-choice schedules. Columns show the primary drug option(s), the alternative reinforcer(s) (sometimes also a drug), the species in which studies were conducted, the primary effect examined in the study, and the reference. Numbers in parentheses show drug unit doses in mg/kg/injection.

#	Drug (dose in mg/kg/inj)	Alternative reinforcer	Species	Main effect examined	Ref.
1	Cocaine (0.05–0.1)	Cocaine (0.013–0.8)	Rhesus	Effect of drug dose	[9]
2	Cocaine (0.05–0.1)	Cocaine (0.05–0.1)	Rhesus	Effect of schedule type	[30]
3	Cocaine (0.05 or 0.1)	Cocaine (0.013–0.8)	Rhesus	Effect of drug dose	[34]
4	Cocaine (0.025–0.2)	Cocaine (0.025–0.2)	Rhesus	Effects of dose and schedule manipulations	[33]
5	Cocaine (0.03–0.3)	Cocaine (0.03–0.3)	Rhesus	Effect of infusion delay	[32]
6	Cocaine (0.025–0.05)	Cocaine (0.025–0.05) Food pellet	Rhesus	Effect of reinforcement delay	[37]
7	Cocaine (0.05–0.2)	Cocaine (0.05–0.2)	Rhesus	Effect of reinforcement probability	[38]
8	Cocaine (0.025–0.1)	Cocaine (0.025–0.1)	Rhesus	Application of generalized matching law	[40]
9	Cocaine (0.025–0.1)	Cocaine (0.025–0.1)	Rhesus	Effect of schedule type	[39]
10	Cocaine (0.1–0.75)	Cocaine (0.1–0.75)	Rhesus	Effect of punishment (electric shock)	[71]
11	Cocaine (0.3–1)	Cocaine (0.3–1)	Rat	Effect of infusion rate	[35]
12	Nicotine (0.015)	Nicotine (0.015) Cocaine (0.05)	Rat	Effect of infusion rate	[36]
13	Alfentanil (0.001–0.004) Methohexital (0.25–0.5) Cocaine (0.1–0.056)	Alfentanil (0.001–0.004) Methohexital (0.25–0.5) Cocaine (0.1–0.056)	Rhesus	Application of generalized matching law	[41]
14	Remifentanil Methohexital (0.32)	Remifentanil (0.0001–0.00003) Methohexital (0.32) Cocaine (0.1–1.5)	Rhesus	Application of generalized matching law	[42]
15	Cocaine (0.05–1.5)	Methylphenidate (0.075–0.07) Diethylpropion (0.5–1)	Rhesus	Effect of various pharmacological and environmental manipulations	[31]
16	Cocaine (0.05–1.5)	Methylphenidate (0.075–0.7)	Rhesus	Drug versus drug preference	[10]
17	Cocaine (0.05–0.2)	d,l-Cathinone (0.05–0.2)	Rhesus	Drug versus drug preference	[47]

Table 1: Continued.

#	Drug (dose in mg/kg/inj)	Alternative reinforcer	Species	Main effect examined	Ref.
18	Cocaine (0–0.1)	Procaine (0.4–1.6)	Rhesus	Drug versus drug preference	[46]
19	Cocaine (0.01–0.03)	PTT (0.01–0.03)	Rhesus	Drug versus drug preference	[50]
20	Cocaine (0.01–0.03)	Remifentanil (0.0001–0.0003)	Rhesus	Behavioral economic analysis of choice	[51]
21	Cocaine (0.03)	Remifentanil (0.00003)	Rhesus	Effect of chronic morphine administration and withdrawal on drug choice	[78]
22	Cocaine (0.267 or 0.8)	Nicotine (8–75)	Rat	Drug versus drug preference	[49]
23	Cocaine (0.4)	Heroin (0.025)	Rat	Effect of home cage environment	[52]
24	Secobarbital (18–100 mg) Chlordiazepoxide (5–20 mg)	Saline Secobarbital Cocaine (0.01–0.56)	Rhesus	Effect of dependence and withdrawal	[29]
25	Cocaine (0.1)	Remifentanil (0.00003–0.003) Cocaine + Remifentanil	Rhesus	Effect of drug mixtures on drug choice	[69]
26	Cocaine (0.038–3)	Heroin (0.025–0.05) Cocaine + Heroin Cocaine (0.267–2.4)	Rat	Effect of drug mixtures on drug choice	[68]
27	Cocaine (0.8)	SKF82958 (0.003–0.03) (+)-PHNO (0.001–0.01) SKF82958 + (+)-PHNO	Rat	Effect of drug mixtures on drug choice	[48]
28	Cocaine (0.05–0.1)	Cocaine (0.05–0.1) + histamine (0.00037–0.0005)	Rhesus	Effect of punishment (IV histamine) delay on drug choice	[73]
29	Cocaine (0.3)	Food pellet	Rhesus	First study of cocaine versus food choice	[53]
30	Cocaine (0.03–1)	Food pellet	Rhesus	Effect of response requirement	[58]
31	Cocaine (0.03–1)	Food pellet	Rhesus	Effect of food availability conditions	[59]
32	Cocaine (0.05–0.4)	Food pellet	Rhesus	Behavioral economic analysis of choice	[99]
33	Cocaine (0.05–0.2)	Food pellet	Rhesus	Behavioral economic analysis of choice	[100]
34	Cocaine (0.025–0.05)	Food pellet	Rhesus	Application of generalized matching law	[101]
35	Cocaine (0.0032–0.32)	Food pellet	Rhesus	Effect of dose and cocaine pretreatment	[54]
36	Cocaine (0.33)	Food pellet or water	Rat	Effect of alternative reinforcer on drug choice	[63]

TABLE 1: Continued.

#	Drug (dose in mg/kg/inj)	Alternative reinforcer	Species	Main effect examined	Ref.
37	Cocaine (0.25)	Glucose/Saccharin solution	Rat	Effect of alternative reinforcer on drug choice	[62]
38	Cocaine (0.25–1.5)	Saccharin or Sucrose	Rat	Effect of sweet solutions on drug choice	[65]
39	Cocaine (0.1–0.3)	Food pellet	Rhesus	Effect of chronic lithium treatment	[86]
40	Cocaine (0.05–0.3)	Food pellet	Rhesus	Effect of chronic antipsychotic treatment	[85]
41	Cocaine (0.0032–0.1)	Food pellet	Rhesus	Effect of monoamine releasers with varying selectivity for dopamine versus serotonin	[17]
42	Cocaine (0.0032–0.1)	Food pellet	Rhesus	Effect of various pharmacological and environmental manipulations	[55]
43	Cocaine (0.0032–0.1)	Food pellet	Rhesus	Effect of chronic kappa opioid treatment	[84]
44	Cocaine (0.0032–0.1)	Food pellet	Rhesus	Effect of chronic methadone treatment	[18]
45	Cocaine (0.003–0.1)	Food pellet	Squirrel monkey	Effect of acute and chronic aripiprazole treatment	[93]
46	Cocaine (0.003–0.03)	10% Sweet Condensed milk	Cynomolgus	Effect of 8-OH-DPAT treatment	[83]
47	Cocaine (0–1)	Food pellet	Rat	Effect of acute and chronic aripiprazole treatment	[61]
48	Cocaine (0–1)	Ensure liquid food	Rat	Effect of amphetamine treatment and environmental manipulations	[81]
49	Cocaine (0.25)	Ensure liquid food	Rat	Effect of diazepam treatment	[82]
50	Cocaine (0.0032–0.1)	Saccharin	Rhesus	Effect of punishment (IV histamine)	[72]
51	Cocaine (0.0032–0.1)	Food pellet	Rhesus	Effect of exposure to and withdrawal from extended cocaine access	[80]
52	Cocaine (0.003–0.03)	Food pellet	Cynomolgus	Effect of social hierarchy	[91]
53	Cocaine (0.003–0.1)	Food pellet	Cynomolgus	Effect of social hierarchy and environmental stimuli	[56]
54	Cocaine (0.03–0.56) Procaine (1–10) Cocaine (0.003–0.3)	Food pellet	Rhesus	Effect of drug type and food reinforcer magnitude	[57]
	Methylphenidate (0.003–0.1) Amphetamine (0.003–0.1) Atomoxetine (0.01–0.3) Desipramine (0.3–1)	Food pellet	Rhesus	Effects of drug type on drug versus food choice	[102]

TABLE 1: Continued.

#	Drug (dose in mg/kg/inj)	Alternative reinforcer	Species	Main effect examined	Ref.
55	Cocaine (0.0032–0.1) Heroin (0.0032–0.1) Cocaine + Heroin	Food pellet	Rhesus	Effects of drug mixtures on drug choice	[67]
56	Cocaine (0–0.1)	Food pellet	Rhesus	Reinstatement of cocaine choice by dopaminergic compounds	[103]
57	Heroin (0.1)	Food	Baboon	Effect of economic conditions	[60]
58	Heroin (0.055–0.83)	Food pellet ± Heroin (0.055–0.83)	Baboon	Various pharmacological and environmental manipulations	[66]
59	Heroin (0.32–0.96)	Food pellet	Baboon	Effect of methadone, naloxone treatment	[74]
60	Heroin (0.32 or 1)	Food pellet	Baboon	Effect of morphine, naloxone, secobarbital	[75]
61	Heroin (0.0032–0.1) Heroin + SNC80	Food pellet	Rhesus	Effect of drug mixtures on drug choice	[70]
62	Heroin (0.0032–0.1)	Food pellet	Rhesus	Effect of methadone, buprenorphine, naloxone treatment in nondependent and opioid-dependent monkeys	[76]
63	Heroin (0.0032–0.1)	Food pellet	Rhesus	Effect of morphine, amphetamine, clonidine, antalarmin, norbinaltorphimine treatment in opioid-dependent monkeys	[79]
64	MDMA (0.03–0.3)	Food pellet	Rhesus	Effect of ambient temperature	[92]
65	MDMA (0.03–0.3)	Food pellet	Rhesus	Effect of thyroid hormone levels	[94]
66	Methamphetamine (0.06)	Food pellet	Rat	Drug versus food preference	[64]

and heroin (15%). Furthermore, nonhuman primates have been the predominant research subjects (81%) utilized in these studies, with rhesus monkeys (70%) being the most commonly used species. The results and implications of this literature will be reviewed in more detail below.

2.2. Choice between Drug and Itself

2.2.1. Effect of Dose. One of the first fundamental research questions to be answered was whether drug choice was dose-dependent. This question was important in determining whether drug choice varied independently of rates of responding as drug dose increased, such that, choice would increase and response rates decrease as a function of increasing drug doses. Although this specific experimental question has only been explicitly examined using intravenous cocaine as the reinforcer and rhesus monkeys as the research subjects, animals almost always choose the larger drug dose [9, 30–33]. Furthermore, in the manuscripts that did report rates of responding, there was no systematic relationship between cocaine choice and rates of cocaine-maintained responding [30, 34]. Overall, this body of literature supports the conclusion that drug choice is dose-dependent and that drug choice may be less sensitive than single-response procedures to reinforcer-independent rate-altering drug effects.

2.2.2. Effect of Temporal Parameters of Reinforcer Delivery. Another fundamental question to be answered was whether drug choice was sensitive to manipulations in the delivery of the drug. In general, when equal drug doses are available as the consequence for two response options, research subjects will allocate their behavior equally between the two response options. However, if the infusion rate was to be varied between the two response options, subjects will almost exclusively choose the dose associated with the shorter (faster) infusion rate [32, 35, 36]. The delay between response and drug delivery is a related variable that has been manipulated in choice studies [31, 37]. For example, Woolverton and Anderson [37] systematically varied the delay between completing the response requirement and delivery of the intravenous drug injection. When the delay was 0 sec and the choice was between a low (0.025 mg/kg/injection) and high (0.05 mg/kg/injection) unit cocaine dose, the subjects almost exclusively chose the high cocaine dose. However, increasing delays in the delivery of the high cocaine dose produced a monotonic decrease in high cocaine dose choice and a reciprocal increase in choice of the alternative low cocaine dose. Overall, these data support the notion that drug choice is highly sensitive to manipulations that affect the timing or probability of reinforcer delivery and that subjects prefer reinforcers to be delivered quickly and with no delay.

2.2.3. Effect of Schedule of Reinforcement. Finally, a third fundamental question to be addressed was whether the programmed schedules of reinforcement influenced drug choice. For example, when rhesus monkeys were given a choice between identical cocaine doses, but the probability of reinforcement was decreased such that every other FR5 (probability 50%) or every fourth FR5 (probability 25%)

completion resulted in delivery of the cocaine injection on one of the response options, monkeys consistently chose the response option associated with the higher probability of reinforcement [38]. Several laboratories have examined the effects of schedule manipulations under concurrent variable-interval (VI): VI schedules. Under a VI schedule of reinforcement, the first response after a variable amount of time has passed results in presentation of the reinforcer. The variability in time is anchored at some programmed time interval by the investigator such that, on average, the interval of reinforcement is the anchored time, for example 600 sec. Most of the studies have examined cocaine versus cocaine choice [30, 33, 39, 40], but a few have also examined other drugs such as the mu-opioid agonists alfentanil [41] or remifentanil [42] and the barbiturate methohexital [41, 42]. In general, these studies have been used to demonstrate that drug self-administration procedures adhere well to the predictions of the matching law, which posits that the allocation of behavior between two response options will match the frequency of reinforcement associated with those options [30, 33, 39–41]. Moreover, as predicted, subjects will chose reinforcers delivered under shorter versus longer VI schedules. In contrast to concurrent VI: VI schedules, only one published study has examined the effects of manipulating the response requirement under a concurrent fixed-ratio (FR): FR schedule of choice between a drug and itself [31]. In this study, only one of the three monkeys was sensitive to FR manipulations such that increases in the FR requirement decreased choice of the higher unit cocaine dose and produced a reciprocal increase in choice of the lower unit cocaine dose. Thus, choice behavior maintained under concurrent FR: FR schedules appears to be more quantal than choice behavior maintained under current VI: VI schedules. Overall, this body of the literature suggests that subjects prefer schedules of reinforcement that produce the higher probability of reinforcement.

2.3. Choice between Drug and Alternatives

2.3.1. Behavioral Economic Considerations. One method to understand how concurrently available reinforcers interact is to apply conceptual frameworks employed by behavioral economics [43, 44]. Based on economic theories, concurrently available reinforcers can interact in one of three ways [44, 45]. First, concurrently available reinforcers can function as *substitutes*; such that as the price of one reinforcer increases, choice of that reinforcer decreases and is replaced by choice of the substitute. The perfect substitute for a commodity is itself, so that studies summarized above that considered choice between a drug and itself could be conceptualized as choice between substitutes. However, different commodities can also function as economic substitutes for each other. For example, potato chips and pretzels can function as substitutes, such that as the price of potato chips increases, consumption of potato chips decreases and consumption of pretzels increases. Secondly, concurrently available reinforcers can function as *complements*; under this condition, as price of one reinforcer increases, choice of that reinforcer, and choice of a complement also decreases. For example, peanut butter and jelly can function as complements, and as the price of peanut butter increases, choice of both peanut butter and jelly decreases. Finally, concurrently available reinforcers can function as *independents*, such that changes in the price and consumption of one reinforcer would have no effect on choice of an independent reinforcer. For example, peanut butter and shoes typically function as independents, such that as the price of peanut butter increases and choice of peanut butter decreases, and consumption of shoes is unlikely to change. The interaction between two concurrently available reinforcers will be an important consideration in the following sections. In general, alternative reinforcers used in studies of drug choice are expected to function as substitutes, but this is an empirical question.

2.3.2. Drug versus Other Drugs. To ascertain the relative reinforcing efficacy of two different drugs in maintaining behavior, a choice procedure could be programmed. As stated earlier, a significant advantage of choice procedures is that the primary dependent measure (behavioral allocation or choice) is less confounded by reinforcement-independent rate-altering drug effects. Critical factors to consider when assessing the relative reinforcing efficacy between two different drugs are dose, pharmacokinetics, and pharmacodynamics. The entire literature on choice between two drugs has employed cocaine versus "drug X" choice procedures, with "X" being the dopamine (DA) uptake inhibitor methylphenidate [10, 31], the sodium channel blocker procaine [46], the monoamine releaser cathinone [47], DA agonists [48], nicotine [49], the DA uptake inhibitor 2β-propanoyl-3β-(4tolyl)-tropane (PTT) [50], or the mu-opioid agonists remifentanil [51] and heroin [52]. In general, these studies have reported that as dose of the alternative drug reinforcer increased, cocaine choice decreased. Such results are consistent with the conclusion that the alternative drug functioned as a substitute for cocaine. However, there were two notable exceptions. When choice was between cocaine versus procaine [46] or cocaine versus nicotine [49], cocaine choice predominated despite increasing doses of procaine or nicotine or decreasing doses of cocaine. Moreover, only one study has explicitly examined whether two drugs function as substitutes, complements, or independents. In monkeys choosing between cocaine and the mu-opioid agonist remifentanil, remifentanil was found to function as a behavioral economic substitute for cocaine [51]. Overall, drug versus drug choice procedures can be useful for assessing the relative reinforcing efficacy of two different compounds and this procedure may hold utility in abuse liability testing.

2.3.3. Drug versus Nondrug Reinforcers. Analysis of the choice studies in Table 1 revealed that 61% (41/67) used a nondrug alternative reinforcer with 93% (38/41) of these studies using food and 7% (3/41) using saccharin or sucrose as the alternative. In the first drug versus nondrug choice procedure, rhesus monkeys were allowed to choose between cocaine injections and food in a closed economy, such that no other food source was available outside of the choice procedure [53]. Over the 8 experimental days, monkeys almost exclusively choose cocaine over food despite body weight decreases of 6 to 10% over the course of the 8 days. More recent studies have utilized other experimental designs to evaluate the effects of multiple cocaine doses versus food using a within-session choice procedure [17, 54–56]. For example, Figure 1 demonstrates that a complete cocaine versus food dose-effect function can be determined within a single daily experimental session. Cocaine choice increased in a monotonic function demonstrating that the relative reinforcing efficacy of cocaine versus food is dose-dependent. Furthermore, this monotonic increase in cocaine choice was in contrast to rates of responding, which displayed the prototypic inverted U-shaped dose-effect function. Thus, the example shown in Figure 1 clearly demonstrates the dissociation between using dependent measures of behavioral allocation (choice) and behavioral rate discussed above as a main rationale for the use of drug choice procedures.

As was evident in drug versus drug choice procedures described above, the magnitude of the alternative nondrug reinforcer, programmed schedule consequences, and reinforcement delay were also important independent variables that could impact drug choice [37, 55, 57–60]. For example, increasing the magnitude of the alternative food reinforcer was shown to decrease cocaine choice [55, 57]. In another example, heroin versus food choice was decreased by increasing the intertrial interval [60]. These results suggest that under economic conditions where access to reinforcers was restricted, baboons choose food over a low dose of heroin. Moreover, if the reinforcing value of food was decreased by providing supplemental access to food before the cocaine versus food choice procedure, cocaine choice increased [55, 59].

While most of the drug versus nondrug alternative choice procedures discussed so far used nonhuman primates as research subjects, there is a small, but growing body of literature of drug versus food choice procedures in rodents. For example, a recent study by Thomsen et al. [61] established a within-session cocaine dose-effect versus ensure choice procedure similar to the within-session cocaine dose-effect versus food choice procedure shown in Figure 1. Other rodent studies have demonstrated that introduction of an alternative nondrug reinforcer such as a glucose/saccharin solution [62] or food [63, 64] will attenuate cocaine or methamphetamine choice. In contrast to these other rodent studies, rats choosing between cocaine injections and 0.2% saccharin never chose cocaine over the saccharin solution [65]. This later result suggests that 0.2% saccharin is a very strong and highly preferred reinforcer in rats. Overall, this body of literature demonstrates that nondrug reinforcers can decrease drug choice, but that reinforcer selection, reinforcer magnitude, delay of reinforcement, and reinforcer access conditions are all key independent variables to be considered in drug versus nondrug choice procedures.

2.3.4. Drug versus Compound Consequent Stimuli. In general, two categories of studies have investigated drug choice in the context of another compound consequent stimulus. One category has involved assessment of choice involving drug plus another putative reinforcer (e.g., drug + drug or drug + food). For example, when contingencies were programmed such that one response option produced a high heroin dose and a second response option produced a lower heroin dose delivered in combination with food, monkeys reallocated their behavior away from the high dose heroin towards lower heroin doses plus food [66]. Other studies have examined choice between (a) food and either cocaine alone or cocaine + mu-opioid agonist, or (b) choice between food and either mu agonist alone or delta-opioid + mu agonist [67–70] and, in general, reported that the relative reinforcing efficacies of these drug mixtures were additive.

The other category has involved pairing one of the choices with a putative punisher, such as electric shock [71] or intravenous histamine [72, 73]. For example, Johanson [71] examined choice between cocaine alone versus cocaine + electric shock. In all of these studies, the punisher was effective in decreasing choice of the reinforce + punisher and increasing choice of the alternative reinforcer [71–73]. However, effects of punishment on drug choice could be mitigated by increasing the drug dose [71] associated with the punisher, decreasing the intensity of the punisher [72, 73], or increasing the delay between delivery of the reinforcer and delivery of the punisher [73]. Furthermore, pairing the punisher with the alternative reinforcer can also increase drug choice. For example, in a study of cocaine versus food choice, histamine injections paired with cocaine decreased cocaine choice, but if the histamine injections were paired with food, cocaine choice increased [72]. Moreover, these studies highlight the potential for cocaine use to be influenced by environmental contingencies that may govern choice of nondrug alternative reinforcers. Overall, these results highlight the utility of concurrent schedules of reinforcement to understand relatively sophisticated behaviors maintained by complex, compound consequent stimuli. Moreover, the use of choice procedures to understand abuse of multiple drugs, drug mixtures, and drug + other consequent stimuli is a scientific space that remains relatively unexplored.

2.4. Other Factors Affecting Drug Choice

2.4.1. Effect of Drug Dependence and Withdrawal. Most published studies examining effects of dependence and withdrawal on drug choice have focused on opioids [66, 74–78]. In contemporary experimental designs examining choice of mu agonists such heroin or the short-acting opioid remifentanil, the total amount of opioid available during daily choice sessions is sufficiently limited to prevent development of significant opioid dependence. Under these nondependent conditions, opioid choice can be effectively reduced by treatment with opioid antagonists like naloxone [76]. However, if opioid dependence is established by chronic noncontingent opioid treatment or by permitting supplemental daily access to contingent opioid self-administration, then drug effects on opioid choice change dramatically. So long as dependence is maintained by opioid agonist exposure, opioid choice during choice sessions is generally maintained (when the alternative is food, [76, 79]) or reduced in some subjects (when cocaine is the alternative, [78]). However,

either spontaneous withdrawal or antagonist-precipitated withdrawal produce robust increases in opioid choice, and this withdrawal-associated increase in opioid choice can be blocked by opioid agonists such as methadone, which are effective maintenance medications for treatment of opioid addiction [75, 76, 78, 79]. Overall, then, opioid withdrawal in opioid-dependent subjects increases opioid choice, and opioid agonists that are effective maintenance medications for treatment of opioid addiction can block this withdrawal-associated increase in opioid choice.

In contrast to the opioid dependence literature cited above, minimal research has been conducted examining the effects of dependence and withdrawal on drug choice maintained by other drug classes. Consistent with the opioid studies described above, Findley and colleagues [29] reported that withdrawal from the barbiturate secobarbital in secobarbital-dependent subjects increased choice of lower secobarbital doses versus food. However, similar results have not been demonstrated with cocaine. For example, Banks and Negus [80] evaluated cocaine versus food choice when subjects were exposed to and withdrawn from supplemental daily access to cocaine self-administration under conditions identical to those used to establish opioid dependence [76]. During supplemental cocaine access, daily cocaine intake increased more than 10-fold and was sufficient to disrupt performance during choice sessions; however, neither exposure to nor withdrawal from supplemental cocaine significantly altered cocaine versus food choice. The extent to which drug dependence and withdrawal alters drug choice of other drug classes, such as benzodiazepines, monoamine releasers, or N-methyl D-aspartate antagonists, remains to be elucidated.

2.4.2. Effect of Pharmacological Variables. Another important body of literature has examined effects of pharmacological manipulations on drug choice, either to evaluate effects of candidate antiaddiction medications or to evaluate mechanisms of drug reinforcement. Effects of opioid agonists and antagonists on opioid choice in nondependent and opioid-dependent rhesus monkeys was described above, and additional studies have investigated potential mechanisms that may underlie withdrawal-associated increases in opioid choice. For example, opioid withdrawal functions as a stressor to activate endogenous release of the stress-related neurotransmitters dynorphin and corticotrophin releasing factor (CRF). This suggested that the hypothesis that either dynorphin acting at kappa-opioid receptors or CRF acting at CRF1 receptors might contribute to withdrawal-associated increases in opioid reinforcement; however, neither the kappa antagonist 5′-guanidinonaltrindole nor the CRF antagonist antalarmin was as effective as morphine in blocking withdrawal-associated increases in opioid choice [79].

A total of 10 studies have investigated pharmacological modulation of cocaine versus food choice. In studies examining candidate "agonist" medications for cocaine addiction, DA-selective monoamine releasers, such as d-amphetamine and phenmetrazine, significantly decreased cocaine choice, whereas mixed DA-serotonin (5HT) releasers or 5HT-selecitve releasers did not [17, 55, 81]. Importantly, these studies demonstrated a selective decrease in cocaine choice without also decreasing rates of behavior, and a representative example of this selective effect is shown in Figure 2 during treatment with the DA-selective releaser *m*-fluoroamphetamine. The atypical antipsychotic and DA D2 receptor partial agonist aripiprazole also decreased cocaine choice in rats after acute treatment, although this effect was not sustained during repeated treatment, and neither acute nor repeated aripiprazole altered cocaine choice in rhesus monkeys [61, 82]. Treatment with the benzodiazepine agonist diazepam also decreased cocaine choice in rats [83]. In contrast to these studies showing decreases in cocaine choice, cocaine choice was increased by treatment with a 5HT1A agonist, a kappa-opioid, agonist and high doses of dopamine receptor antagonists [55, 84–86]. Finally, other treatments that have failed to alter cocaine choice up to doses that suppress responding include methadone and lithium [18, 87]. Overall, this body of the literature suggests that drug choice is sensitive to both acute and chronic pharmacological manipulations, that pharmacological effects on drug choice can be dissociated from other drug effects, and that there is a clear need for more research in understanding the pharmacological mechanisms of drug choice.

One final point regarding the effects of pharmacological variables on drug choice is worth mentioning. An overarching rationale for preclinical studies investigating the pharmacological determinants of drug self-administration is the development of candidate medications to treat drug addiction. Moreover, a main goal of pharmacotherapy should be not only to *decrease* drug-taking behavior, but also to *reallocate* behavior to activities maintained by more adaptive reinforcers [88]. Thus, in preclinical studies that aspire to evaluate candidate medications for drug addiction, choice procedures can play a critical role in the preclinical drug development process to determine whether a given experimental manipulation produces this critical *reallocation* of behavior [19, 24]. Furthermore, human laboratory studies provide an additional critical step in drug development between animal studies and clinical trials, and human laboratory research to evaluate effects of candidate medications on drug self-administration relies exclusively on drug versus nondrug choice procedures [24]. Consequently, the use of choice procedures in preclinical studies may facilitate translation of results to choice procedures in human laboratory studies at this critical juncture in the drug development process, and existing data suggest excellent concordance between medication effects on drug choice in animals and humans [55, 85, 89–91].

2.4.3. Effect of Other Environmental Variables. An emerging body of research has also addressed the degree to which non-pharmacological environmental variables might alter drug choice. In one example, monkeys were housed in a social context to establish a dominant-subordinate hierarchy to examine the effects of social rank on cocaine versus food choice [92]. One main rationale for this study was that the initial differences between dominant and subordinate monkeys in cocaine-maintained responding under a simple

FR schedule disappeared over time as the cocaine self-administration history progressed. Under the concurrent FR: FR schedule of cocaine and food reinforcement, the differences between dominant and subordinate monkeys were recaptured. Furthermore, cocaine choice in socially housed monkeys was decreased by manipulations of environmental variables that were perceived to be enriching (increased cage size), whereas cocaine choice was decreased by environmental variables that were perceived to be stressful (exposure to rubber snake) [56]. Another study examined the effects of ambient temperature on choice between 3,4-methylenedioxymethamphetamine (MDMA) and food in rhesus monkeys [93]. Compared to room temperature, cool ambient temperatures decreased MDMA choice and warm ambient temperatures increased MDMA choice. Similar studies on these and other environmental variables will play a key role in future research to identify environmental mechanisms that may differentially affect the reinforcing strength of drugs and underlie vulnerability to or protection from drug addiction.

2.4.4. Effect of Subject-Related Biological Variables. Intravenous drug choice procedures have been conducted in various species including, rats [62], squirrel monkeys [82], cynomolgus [92] and rhesus [29] macaques, and baboons [66]. However, there is substantial opportunity for more systematic research on the role of these and other subject-related variables, such as gender, genotype, or physiological state. To the best of our knowledge, there is only one example where a subject-related variable was manipulated in the context of drug choice. In this study, exogenous thyroid hormone was administered to induce a hyperthyroid state during MDMA versus food choice [94]. Although thyroid hormone treatment enhanced the thermogenic effects of MDMA, this treatment did not significantly alter MDMA choice. Moreover, drug choice studies can be expected to contribute important insights that might not be apparent from single-response or active/inactive-response procedures. Specifically, as has been emphasized repeatedly above, drug choice is strongly determined by factors that influence the reinforcing strength of alternative reinforcers. Consequently, it should be anticipated that some subject-related variables would have profound effects on drug choice by modulating the reinforcing strength of alternative reinforcers while producing little or no direct changes in the reinforcing strength of the drug.

3. Implications and Future Directions

Research on the reinforcing effects of drugs has been slow to adopt concurrent schedules of reinforcement; however, this paper has argued that choice procedures can play a useful role in preclinical research on drug reinforcement and determinants of drugs use. There are still critical gaps in our knowledge, and there remains much intellectual space to be explored. One future direction might be the establishment of drug versus nondrug alternative choice procedures involving abused drugs other than the classical compounds cocaine and heroin. The degree to which drug choice can be maintained by other novel drug class such as benzodiazepines, cannabinoids, and nicotine remains to be elucidated. Another future direction might be to examine the impact of nondrug alternative reinforcers other than food. Food is an easy alternative reinforcer to control in preclinical laboratories, but there are certainly other nondrug reinforcers (e.g., access to receptive mate or social interactions) that are available as research tools that have yet to be fully explored. As one example of a choice procedure using a nondrug alternative reinforcer other than food, one intriguing study examined effects of putative anorectic drugs on choice between food and visual access to a room containing other monkeys [95]. This type of social reinforcer has yet to be manipulated in studies of drug choice. Finally, a third potential future direction is the integration of drug reinforcers into decision-making "choice" tasks commonly used to assess cognitive function. For example, impaired delay discounting is a cognitive trait commonly linked to drug abuse [96, 97], and delay discounting is often assessed preclinically in assays that compare choice between a delayed high-magnitude reinforcer and an immediate low-magnitude reinforcer [98]. Strikingly, preclinical research with this type of assay has relied exclusively on food as the consequent stimulus. The introduction of drugs as reinforcers into delay discounting and other cognitive tasks may provide new insights into the relationship between cognitive function and drug use. Overall, the body of literature cited in this paper supports the notion that choice procedures can facilitate data interpretation by providing a rate-independent measure of drug reinforcement, improve concordance between preclinical and clinical studies in translational research, and provide experimental access to critical independent variables that influence drug choice and drug addiction in natural environments.

Acknowledgments

The authors would like to acknowledge funding from the National Institute on Drug Abuse, National Institutes of Health under Grants R01-DA026946 and R01-DA031718.

References

[1] N. A. Ator and R. R. Griffiths, "Principles of drug abuse liability assessment in laboratory animals," *Drug and Alcohol Dependence*, vol. 70, no. 3, pp. S55–S72, 2003.

[2] L. P. Carter and R. R. Griffiths, "Principles of laboratory assessment of drug abuse liability and implications for clinical development.," *Drug and Alcohol Dependence*, vol. 105, supplement 1, pp. S14–S25, 2009.

[3] B. F. Skinner, *The Behavior of Organisms*, Appleton-Century-Crofts, New York, NY, USA, 1938.

[4] C. B. Ferster and B. F. Skinner, *Schedules of Reinforcement*, Appleton-Century-Croft, New York, NY, USA, 1957.

[5] J. R. Weeks, "Experimental morphine addiction: method for automatic intravenous injections in unrestrained rats," *Science*, vol. 138, no. 3537, pp. 143–144, 1962.

[6] J. R. Weeks and R. J. Collins, "Factors affecting voluntary morphine intake in self-maintained addicted rats," *Psychopharmacologia*, vol. 6, no. 4, pp. 267–279, 1964.

[7] A. Young and S. Herling, "Drugs as reinforcers: studies in laboratory animals," in *Behavioral Analysis of Drug Dependence*, S. Goldberg and I. Stolerman, Eds., pp. 9–67, Academic Press, Orlando, Fla, USA, 1986.

[8] J. Katz, "Drugs as reinforcers: pharmacological and behavioral factorsin," in *The Neuropharmacological Basis of Reward*, J. Leibman and S. Cooper, Eds., pp. 164–213, Clarendon Press, Oxford, UK, 1989.

[9] C. Iglauer and J. H. Woods, "Concurrent performances: reinforcement by different doses of intravenous cocaine in rhesus monkeys," *Journal of the Experimental Analysis of Behavior*, vol. 22, no. 1, pp. 179–196, 1974.

[10] C. E. Johanson and C. R. Schuster, "A choice procedure for drug reinforcers: cocaine and methylphenidate in the rhesus monkey," *Journal of Pharmacology and Experimental Therapeutics*, vol. 193, no. 2, pp. 676–688, 1975.

[11] N. K. Mello and S. S. Negus, "Preclinical evaluation of pharmacotherapies for treatment of cocaine and opioid abuse using drug self-administration procedures," *Neuropsychopharmacology*, vol. 14, no. 6, pp. 375–424, 1996.

[12] G. Zernig, G. Wakonigg, E. Madlung et al., "Do vertical shifts in dose-response rate-relationships in operant conditioning procedures indicate 'sensitization' to 'drug wanting'?" *Psychopharmacology*, vol. 171, no. 3, pp. 349–363, 2004.

[13] R. Meisch and G. Lemaire, "Drug self-administration," in *Methods In Behavioral Pharmacology*, F. Van Haaren, Ed., pp. 257–300, Elsevier, Amsterdam, The Netherlands, 1993.

[14] G. Deneau, T. Yanagita, and M. H. Seevers, "Self-administration of psychoactive substances by the monkey-a measure of psychological dependence," *Psychopharmacologia*, vol. 16, no. 1, pp. 30–48, 1969.

[15] R. T. Kelleher and S. R. Goldberg, "General introduction: control of drug taking behavior by schedules of reinforcement," *Pharmacological Reviews*, vol. 27, no. 3, pp. 291–299, 1975.

[16] R. Pickens and T. Thompson, "Cocaine-reinforced behavior in rats: effects of reinforcement magnitude and fixed-ratio size.," *Journal of Pharmacology and Experimental Therapeutics*, vol. 161, no. 1, pp. 122–129, 1968.

[17] M. L. Banks, B. E. Blough, and S. S. Negus, "Effects of monoamine releasers with varying selectivity for releasing dopamine/norepinephrine versus serotonin on choice between cocaine and food in rhesus monkeys," *Behavioural Pharmacology*, vol. 22, no. 8, pp. 824–836, 2011.

[18] S. S. Negus and N. K. Mello, "Effects of chronic methadone treatment on cocaine- and food-maintained responding under second-order, progressive-ratio and concurrent-choice schedules in rhesus monkeys," *Drug and Alcohol Dependence*, vol. 74, no. 3, pp. 297–309, 2004.

[19] S. S. Negus and M. L. Banks, "Making the right choice: lessons from drug discrimination for research on drug reinforcement and drug self-administration," in *Drug DiscrimInation: Applications To MedicInal Chemistry and Drug Studies*, R. A. Glennon and R. Young, Eds., pp. 361–388, John Wiley and Sons, Holboken, NJ, USA, 2011.

[20] S. D. S. Spragg, "Morphine addiction in chimpanzees," in *Comparative Psychology Monographs*, pp. 1–132, The John Hopkins Press, Baltimore, Md, USA, 1940.

[21] J. R. Nichols and W. M. Davis, "Drug addiction. II. Variation of addiction," *Journal of the American Pharmacists Association*, vol. 48, pp. 259–262, 1959.

[22] G. M. Heyman, "Ethanol regulated preference in rats," *Psychopharmacology*, vol. 112, no. 2-3, pp. 259–269, 1993.

[23] S. D. Comer, J. B. Ashworth, R. W. Foltin, C. E. Johanson, J. P. Zacny, and S. L. Walsh, "The role of human drug self-administration procedures in the development of medications," *Drug and Alcohol Dependence*, vol. 96, no. 1-2, pp. 1–15, 2008.

[24] M. Haney and R. Spealman, "Controversies in translational research: drug self-administration," *Psychopharmacology*, vol. 199, no. 3, pp. 403–419, 2008.

[25] G. H. Heyman, *Addiction: A Disorder of Choice*, Harvard University Press, Cambridge, Mass, USA, 2009.

[26] R. Hernstein and D. Prelec, "A theory of addiction," in *Choice Over Time*, G. Loewenstein and J. Elster, Eds., pp. 331–360, Russell Sage Press, New York, NY, USA, 1992.

[27] American Psychiatric Association, *Diagnostic and Statistical Manual of Mental Disorders*, vol. 992, American Psychiatric Association, Washington, DC, USA, Fourth edition, 2000.

[28] America Psychiatric Association, 2012, http://www.dsm5 .org/proposedrevision/Pages/SubstanceUseandAddictiveDisorders.aspx.

[29] J. D. Findley, W. W. Robinson, and L. Peregrino, "Addiction to secobarbital and chlordiazepoxide in the rhesus monkey by means of a self-infusion preference procedure," *Psychopharmacologia*, vol. 26, no. 2, pp. 93–114, 1972.

[30] C. Iglauer, M. E. Llewellyn, and J. H. Woods, "Concurrent schedules of cocaine injection in rhesus monkeys: dose variations under independent and non independent variable interval procedures," *Pharmacological Reviews*, vol. 27, no. 3, pp. 367–383, 1975.

[31] C. E. Johanson, "Pharmacological and environmental variables affecting drug preference in rhesus monkeys," *Pharmacological Reviews*, vol. 27, no. 3, pp. 343–355, 1975.

[32] K. G. Anderson and W. L. Woolverton, "Effects of dose and infusion delay on cocaine self-administration choice in rhesus monkeys," *Psychopharmacology*, vol. 167, no. 4, pp. 424–430, 2003.

[33] K. G. Anderson and W. L. Woolverton, "Dose and schedule determinants of cocaine choice under concurrent variable-interval schedules in rhesus monkeys," *Psychopharmacology*, vol. 176, no. 3-4, pp. 274–280, 2004.

[34] M. E. Llewellyn, C. Iglauer, and J. H. Woods, "Relative reinforcer magnitude under a nonindependent concurrent schedule of cocaine reinforcement in rhesus monkeys," *Journal of the Experimental Analysis of Behavior*, vol. 25, no. 1, pp. 81–91, 1976.

[35] C. W. Schindler, L. V. Panlilio, and E. B. Thorndike, "Effect of rate of delivery of intravenous cocaine on self-administration in rats," *Pharmacology Biochemistry and Behavior*, vol. 93, no. 4, pp. 375–381, 2009.

[36] R. E. Sorge and P. B. S. Clarke, "Rats self-administer intravenous nicotine delivered in a novel smoking-relevant procedure: effects of dopamine antagonists," *Journal of Pharmacology and Experimental Therapeutics*, vol. 330, no. 2, pp. 633–640, 2009.

[37] W. L. Woolverton and K. G. Anderson, "Effects of delay to reinforcement on the choice between cocaine and food in rhesus monkeys," *Psychopharmacology*, vol. 186, no. 1, pp. 99–106, 2006.

[38] W. L. Woolverton and J. K. Rowlett, "Choice maintained by cocaine or food in monkeys: effects of varying probability of reinforcement," *Psychopharmacology*, vol. 138, no. 1, pp. 102–106, 1998.

[39] W. L. Woolverton, "Intravenous self-administration of cocaine under concurrent VI schedules of reinforcement," *Psychopharmacology*, vol. 127, no. 3, pp. 195–203, 1996.

[40] W. L. Woolverton and K. Alling, "Choice under concurrent VI schedules: comparison of behavior maintained by cocaine or food," *Psychopharmacology*, vol. 141, no. 1, pp. 47–56, 1999.

[41] K. G. Anderson and W. L. Woolverton, "Concurrent variable-interval drug self-administration and the generalized matching law: a drug-class comparison," *Behavioural Pharmacology*, vol. 11, no. 5, pp. 413–420, 2000.

[42] M. N. Koffarnus and J. H. Woods, "Quantification of drug choice with the generalized matching law in rhesus monkeys," *Journal of the Experimental Analysis of Behavior*, vol. 89, no. 2, pp. 209–224, 2008.

[43] S. R. Hursh, "Economic concepts for the analysis of behavior," *Journal of the Experimental Analysis of Behavior*, vol. 34, no. 2, pp. 219–238, 1980.

[44] W. K. Bickel, R. J. DeGrandpre, and S. T. Higgins, "The behavioral economics of concurrent drug reinforcers: a review and reanalysis of drug self administration research," *Psychopharmacology*, vol. 118, no. 3, pp. 250–259, 1995.

[45] S. R. Hursh and R. Bauman, "The behavioral analysis of demand," in *Advances In Behavioral Economics*, L. Green and J. Kagel, Eds., pp. 117–165, Ablex Publishing, Norwood, Mass, USA, 1987.

[46] C. E. Johanson and T. Aigner, "Comparison of the reinforcing properties of cocaine and procaine in rhesus monkeys," *Pharmacology Biochemistry and Behavior*, vol. 15, no. 1, pp. 49–53, 1981.

[47] W. L. Woolverton and C. E. Johanson, "Preference in rhesus monkeys given a choice between cocaine and d,l-cathinone.," *Journal of the Experimental Analysis of Behavior*, vol. 41, no. 1, pp. 35–43, 1984.

[48] A. M. Manzardo, J. A. Del Rio, L. Stein, and J. D. Belluzzi, "Rats choose cocaine over dopamine agonists in a two-lever self-administration preference test," *Pharmacology Biochemistry and Behavior*, vol. 70, no. 2-3, pp. 257–265, 2001.

[49] A. M. Manzardo, L. Stein, and J. D. Belluzzi, "Rats prefer cocaine over nicotine in a two-lever self-administration choice test," *Brain Research*, vol. 924, no. 1, pp. 10–19, 2002.

[50] J. A. Lile, D. Morgan, A. M. Birmingham et al., "The reinforcing efficacy of the dopamine reuptake inhibitor 2β-propanoyl-3β-(4-tolyl)-tropane (PTT) as measured by a progressive-ratio schedule and a choice procedure in rhesus monkeys," *Journal of Pharmacology and Experimental Therapeutics*, vol. 303, no. 2, pp. 640–648, 2002.

[51] T. Wade-Galuska, G. Winger, and J. H. Woods, "A behavioral economic analysis of cocaine and remifentanil self-administration in rhesus monkeys," *Psychopharmacology*, vol. 194, no. 4, pp. 563–572, 2007.

[52] D. Caprioli, M. Celentano, A. Dubla, F. Lucantonio, P. Nencini, and A. Badiani, "Ambience and drug choice: cocaine- and heroin-taking as a function of environmental context in humans and rats," *Biological Psychiatry*, vol. 65, no. 10, pp. 893–899, 2009.

[53] T. G. Aigner and R. L. Balster, "Choice behavior in rhesus monkeys: cocaine versus food," *Science*, vol. 201, no. 4355, pp. 534–535, 1978.

[54] C. A. Paronis, M. Gasior, and J. Bergman, "Effects of cocaine under concurrent fixed ratio schedules of food and IV drug availability: a novel choice procedure in monkeys," *Psychopharmacology*, vol. 163, no. 3-4, pp. 283–291, 2002.

[55] S. S. Negus, "Rapid assessment of choice between cocaine and food in rhesus monkeys: effects of environmental manipulations and treatment with d-amphetamine and flupenthixol," *Neuropsychopharmacology*, vol. 28, no. 5, pp. 919–931, 2003.

[56] P. W. Czoty and M. A. Nader, "Individual differences in the effects of environmental stimuli on cocaine choice in socially housed male cynomolgus monkeys," *Psychopharmacology*, vol. 224, no. 1, pp. 69–79, 2012.

[57] M. A. Nader and W. L. Woolverton, "Effects of increasing the magnitude of an alternative reinforcer on drug choice in a discrete-trials choice procedure," *Psychopharmacology*, vol. 105, no. 2, pp. 169–174, 1991.

[58] M. A. Nader and W. L. Woolverton, "Effects of increasing response requirement on choice between cocaine and food in rhesus monkeys," *Psychopharmacology*, vol. 108, no. 3, pp. 295–300, 1992.

[59] M. A. Nader and W. L. Woolverton, "Choice between cocaine and food by rhesus monkeys: effects of conditions of food availability," *Behavioural Pharmacology*, vol. 3, no. 6, pp. 635–638, 1992.

[60] T. F. Elsmore, G. V. Fletcher, D. G. Conrad, and F. J. Sodetz, "Reduction of heroin intake in baboons by an economic constraint," *Pharmacology Biochemistry and Behavior*, vol. 13, no. 5, pp. 729–731, 1980.

[61] M. Thomsen, A. Fink-Jensen, D. P. D. Woldbye et al., "Effects of acute and chronic aripiprazole treatment on choice between cocaine self-administration and food under a concurrent schedule of reinforcement in rats," *Psychopharmacology*, vol. 201, no. 1, pp. 43–53, 2008.

[62] M. E. Carroll, S. T. Lac, and S. L. Nygaard, "A concurrently available nondrug reinforcer prevents the acquisition or decreases the maintenance of cocaine-reinforced behavior," *Psychopharmacology*, vol. 97, no. 1, pp. 23–29, 1989.

[63] S. I. Dworkin, S. Mirkis, and J. E. Smith, "Reinforcer interactions under concurrent schedules of food, water, and intravenous cocaine," *Behavioural Pharmacology*, vol. 1, no. 4, pp. 327–338, 1990.

[64] A. Ping and P. J. Kruzich, "Concurrent access to sucrose pellets decreases methamphetamine-seeking behavior in Lewis rats," *Pharmacology Biochemistry and Behavior*, vol. 90, no. 3, pp. 492–496, 2008.

[65] M. Lenoir, F. Serre, L. Cantin, and S. H. Ahmed, "Intense sweetness surpasses cocaine reward," *PloS one*, vol. 2, no. 1, p. e698, 2007.

[66] R. M. Wurster, R. R. Griffiths, J. D. Findley, and J. V. Brady, "Reduction of heroin self-administration in baboons by manipulation of behavioral and pharmacological conditions," *Pharmacology Biochemistry and Behavior*, vol. 7, no. 6, pp. 519–528, 1977.

[67] S. S. Negus, "Interactions between the reinforcing effects of cocaine and heroin in a drug-vs-food choice procedure in rhesus monkeys: a dose-addition analysis," *Psychopharmacology*, vol. 180, no. 1, pp. 115–124, 2005.

[68] S. J. Ward, D. Morgan, and D. C. S. Roberts, "Comparison of the reinforcing effects of cocaine and cocaine/heroin combinations under progressive ratio and choice schedules in rats," *Neuropsychopharmacology*, vol. 30, no. 2, pp. 286–295, 2005.

[69] K. B. Freeman and W. L. Woolverton, "Self-administration of cocaine and remifentanil by monkeys: choice between single drugs and mixtures," *Psychopharmacology*, vol. 215, no. 2, pp. 281–290, 2011.

[70] G. W. Stevenson, J. E. Folk, K. C. Rice, and S. S. Negus, "Interactions between δ and μ opioid agonists in assays of schedule-controlled responding, thermal nociception, drug self-administration, and drug versus food choice in rhesus monkeys: studies with SNC80 [(+)-4-[(αR)-α-((2S,5R)-4-allyl-2,5-dimethyl-1-piperazinyl) -3-methoxybenzyl]-N,N-diethylbenzamide] and heroin," *Journal of Pharmacology and Experimental Therapeutics*, vol. 314, no. 1, pp. 221–231, 2005.

[71] C. E. Johanson, "The effects of electric shock on responding maintained by cocaine injections in a choice procedure in the rhesus monkey," *Psychopharmacology*, vol. 53, no. 3, pp. 277–282, 1977.

[72] S. S. Negus, "Effects of punishment on choice between cocaine and food in rhesus monkeys," *Psychopharmacology*, vol. 181, no. 2, pp. 244–252, 2005.

[73] W. L. Woolverton, K. B. Freeman, J. Myerson, and L. Green, "Suppression of cocaine self-administration in monkeys: effects of delayed punishment," *Psychopharmacology*, vol. 220, no. 3, pp. 509–517, 2012.

[74] R. R. Griffiths, R. M. Wurster, and J. V. Brady, "Discrete trial choice procedure: effects of naloxone and methadone on choice between food and heroin," *Pharmacological Reviews*, vol. 27, no. 3, pp. 357–365, 1975.

[75] R. R. Griffiths, R. M. Wurster, and J. V. Brady, "Choice between food and heroin: effects of morphine, naloxone, and secobarbital.," *Journal of the Experimental Analysis of Behavior*, vol. 35, no. 3, pp. 335–351, 1981.

[76] S. S. Negus, "Choice between heroin and food in non-dependent and heroin-dependent rhesus monkeys: effects of naloxone, buprenorphine, and methadone," *Journal of Pharmacology and Experimental Therapeutics*, vol. 317, no. 2, pp. 711–723, 2006.

[77] S. S. Negus, "Opioid antagonist effects in animal models related to opioid abuse: drug discrimination and drug self-administration," in *Opiate RecepTors and Antagonists: From Bench To Clinic*, R. Dean, E. J. Bilsky, and S. S. Negus, Eds., pp. 201–226, Humana Press, New York, NY, USA, 2009.

[78] T. Wade-Galuska, C. M. Galuska, and G. Winger, "Effects of daily morphine administration and deprivation on choice and demand for remifentanil and cocaine in rhesus monkeys," *Journal of the Experimental Analysis of Behavior*, vol. 95, no. 1, pp. 75–89, 2011.

[79] S. S. Negus and K. C. Rice, "Mechanisms of withdrawal-associated increases in heroin self-administration: pharmacologic modulation of heroin vs food choice in heroin-dependent rhesus monkeys," *Neuropsychopharmacology*, vol. 34, no. 4, pp. 899–911, 2009.

[80] M. L. Banks and S. S. Negus, "Effects of extended cocaine access and cocaine withdrawal on choice between cocaine and food in rhesus monkeys," *Neuropsychopharmacology*, vol. 35, no. 2, pp. 493–504, 2010.

[81] M. Thomsen, A. Barrett, S. S. Negus, and S. B. Caine, "Cocaine-food choice rats: environmentalmanipulations and effects of amphetamine," *Behavioural Pharmacology*. In press.

[82] E. Augier, C. Vouillac, and S. H. Ahmed, "Diazepam promotes choice of abstinence in cocaine self-administering rats," *Addiction Biology*, vol. 17, no. 2, pp. 378–391, 2012.

[83] P. W. Czoty, C. McCabe, and M. A. Nader, "Effects of the 5-HT1A agonist ($\pm$)-8-hydroxy-2-(di-n- propylamino)tetralin (8-OH-DPAT) on cocaine choice in cynomolgus monkeys," *Behavioural Pharmacology*, vol. 16, no. 3, pp. 187–191, 2005.

[84] S. S. Negus, "Effects of the kappa opioid agonist U50,488 and the kappa opioid antagonist nor-binaltorphimine on choice between cocaine and food in rhesus monkeys," *Psychopharmacology*, vol. 176, no. 2, pp. 204–213, 2004.

[85] W. L. Woolverton and R. L. Balster, "Effects of antipsychotic compounds in rhesus monkeys given a choice between

cocaine and food," *Drug and Alcohol Dependence*, vol. 8, no. 1, pp. 69–78, 1981.

[86] W. L. Woolverton and R. L. Balster, "The effects of lithium on choice between cocaine and food in the rhesus monkey," *Communications in Psychopharmacology*, vol. 3, no. 5, pp. 309–318, 1979.

[87] F. J. Vocci, "Commentary: can replacement therapy work in the treatment of cocaine dependence? and what are we replacing anyway?" *Addiction*, vol. 102, no. 12, pp. 1888–1889, 2007.

[88] M. K. Greenwald, L. H. Lundahl, and C. L. Steinmiller, "Sustained release d-amphetamine reduces cocaine but not speedball-seeking in buprenorphine-maintained volunteers: a test of dual-agonist pharmacotherapy for cocaine/heroin polydrug abusers," *Neuropsychopharmacology*, vol. 35, no. 13, pp. 2624–2637, 2010.

[89] C. R. Rush, W. W. Stoops, R. J. Sevak, and L. R. Hays, "Cocaine choice in humans during D-amphetamine maintenance," *Journal of Clinical Psychopharmacology*, vol. 30, no. 2, pp. 152–159, 2010.

[90] S. L. Walsh, B. Geter-Douglas, E. C. Strain, and G. E. Bigelow, "Enadoline and butorphanol: evaluation of κ-agonists on cocaine pharmacodynamics and cocaine self-administration in humans," *Journal of Pharmacology and Experimental Therapeutics*, vol. 299, no. 1, pp. 147–158, 2001.

[91] P. W. Czoty, C. McCabe, and M. A. Nader, "Assessment of the relative reinforcing strength of cocaine in socially housed monkeys using a choice procedure," *Journal of Pharmacology and Experimental Therapeutics*, vol. 312, no. 1, pp. 96–102, 2005.

[92] M. L. Banks, J. E. Sprague, P. W. Czoty, and M. A. Nader, "Effects of ambient temperature on the relative reinforcing strength of MDMA using a choice procedure in monkeys," *Psychopharmacology*, vol. 196, no. 1, pp. 63–70, 2008.

[93] J. Bergman, "Medications for stimulant abuse: agonist-based strategies and preclinical evaluation of the mixed-action D2 partial agonist aripiprazole (Abilify®)," *Experimental and Clinical Psychopharmacology*, vol. 16, no. 6, pp. 475–483, 2008.

[94] M. L. Banks, P. W. Czoty, J. E. Sprague, and M. A. Nader, "Influence of thyroid hormones on 3,4-methylenedioxymethamphetamine-induced thermogenesis and reinforcing strength in monkeys," *Behavioural Pharmacology*, vol. 19, no. 2, pp. 167–170, 2008.

[95] R. L. Corwin and C. R. Schuster, "Anorectic specificity as measured in a choice paradigm in rhesus monkeys," *Pharmacology Biochemistry and Behavior*, vol. 45, no. 1, pp. 131–141, 1993.

[96] L. A. Marsch and W. K. Bickel, "Toward a behavioral economic understanding of drug dependence: delay discounting processes," *Addiction*, vol. 96, no. 1, pp. 73–86, 2001.

[97] J. Monterosso, P. Piray, and S. Luo, "Neuroeconomics and the study of addiction," *Biological Psychiatry*, vol. 72, no. 2, pp. 107–112, 2012.

[98] C. A. Winstanley, "The utility of rat models of impulsivity in developing pharmacotherapies for impulse control disorders," *British Journal of Pharmacology*, vol. 164, no. 4, pp. 1301–1321, 2011.

[99] W. L. Woolverton, J. A. English, and M. R. Weed, "Choice between cocaine and food in a discrete-trials procedure in monkeys: a unit price analysis," *Psychopharmacology*, vol. 133, no. 3, pp. 269–274, 1997.

[100] W. L. Woolverton and J. A. English, "Further analysis of choice between cocaine and food using the unit price model

of behavioral economics," *Drug and Alcohol Dependence*, vol. 49, no. 1, pp. 71–78, 1997.

[101] K. G. Anderson, A. J. Velkey, and W. L. Woolverton, "The generalized matching law as a predictor of choice between cocaine and food in rhesus monkeys," *Psychopharmacology*, vol. 163, no. 3-4, pp. 319–326, 2002.

[102] M. Gasior, J. Bergman, M. J. Kallman, and C. A. Paronis, "Evaluation of the reinforcing effects of monoamine reuptake inhibitors under a concurrent schedule of food and i.v. drug delivery in rhesus monkeys," *Neuropsychopharmacology*, vol. 30, no. 4, pp. 758–764, 2005.

[103] M. Gasior, C. A. Paronis, and J. Bergman, "Modification by dopaminergic drugs of choice behavior under concurrent schedules of intravenous saline and food delivery in monkeys," *Journal of Pharmacology and Experimental Therapeutics*, vol. 308, no. 1, pp. 249–259, 2004.

19

Biomarkers of Oxidative Stress and Personalized Treatment of Pulmonary Tuberculosis: Emerging Role of Gamma-Glutamyltransferase

Etienne Mokondjimobe,[1] Benjamin Longo-Mbenza,[2] Jean Akiana,[1] Ulrich Oswald Ndalla,[1] Regis Dossou-Yovo,[1] Joseph Mboussa,[1] and Henri-Joseph Parra[1]

[1] *Faculty of Health Sciences, Anti-Tuberculosis Centre, National Laboratory of Public Health, Marien Ngouabi University, Brazzaville, Democratic Republic of Congo*
[2] *Faculty of Health Sciences, Walter Sisulu University, Private Bag X1, Eastern Cape, Mthatha 5117, South Africa*

Correspondence should be addressed to Benjamin Longo-Mbenza, longombenza@gmail.com

Academic Editor: Abdelwahab Omri

Background. The objectives were (i) to evaluate the impact of acute pulmonary tuberculosis (PTB) and anti-TB therapy on the relationship between AST, ALT, and GGT levels in absence of conditions related to hepatotoxicity; (ii) to evaluate the rate and the time of alterations of AST, ALT, and GGT. *Design and Methods.* A prospective followup of 40 adults (21 males; mean age of 34.7 ± 5.8 years) with active PTB on initial phase and continuation phase anti-TB. *Results.* Only 3% ($n = 1$) developed a transient and benign ADR at day 30 without interruption of anti-TB treatment. Within normal ranges, GGT decreased significantly from day 0 to day 60, while AST and ALT increased significantly and respectively. During day 0–day 60, there was a significant, negative, and independent association between GGT and AST. *Conclusion.* The initial two months led to significant improvement of oxidative stress. Values of oxidative markers in normal ranges might predict low rate of ADR.

1. Background

The concept of biomarkers is very important in this paper. The role of biomarkers is now exponentially increasing in guiding decisions in drug development and personalized medicine. A biomarker is not predictive or casual to a disease, but it can predict patients' response to compound by identifying certain patient groups that are more likely to response to the drug therapy or to avoid specific adverse events [1].

In patients with pulmonary tuberculosis (PTB), a significant improvement in oxidative stress and suppression of inflammatory response have been recently reported after the initial two-month therapy [2]. However, the literature showed that even after six months of successful chemotherapy, PTB is still associated with increased levels of circulating lipid peroxides and low plasma concentrations of antioxidants such as vitamin E [2, 3].

Before chemotherapy, Mycobacteria induce reactive oxygen species (ROS) production by activating both mononuclear and polymorphonuclear phagocytes. Tuberculosis is, therefore, characterized by poor antioxidants defence that exposes to oxidative host tissue damage [3, 4]. Yasuda et al. found that more than 50% of 113 PTB cases with normal liver function on admission showed abnormalities of transaminases that were aggravated up to 4th week after administration of drugs, and 80% up to the 8th week [5].

Almost 33% of the world population infected with *Mycobacterium tuberculosis* live in developing countries including Brazzaville, the Republic of Congo [6]. Anti-PTB drug-related adverse reactions [7] include benign or fatal hepatic transaminase elevation without any intervention [8, 9]. World Health Organization (WHO) established a major strategy of directly observed treatment short course (DOTS), which is adopted by the Republic of Congo, our country.

The potentially hepatotoxic anti-TB drugs from the first-line regimen are isoniazide, rifampicin, and pyrazinamide [10].

The following conditions increase the risk of anti-TB drug-induced hepatitis: malnutrition, excessive alcohol intake, aging, chronic hepatic diseases including viral infections (HBV, HCV, and HIV/AIDS), female sex, ethnicity (Asians), concurrent administration of enzyme inducers, and inadequate compliance [7, 9, 11, 12].

1.1. Rationale. There are no data related to the chronological observation of liver enzymes and adverse drug reactions (ADR) in PTB patients. This information is useful to determine whether or not the antituberculosis drugs should be discontinued when hepatic dysfunction occurs. Indeed, Yasuda et al. showed that cases with higher peak values and exacerbation in transaminases had a tendency-delayed normalization [5].

With the current and increasing interest in oxidative stress [3], emphasis is to develop functional biomarkers of oxidative stress with epidemiological and clinical implications such as gamma-glutamyltransferase (GGT) [13–15] and alanine aminotransferase (ALT) [15], except for aspartate aminotransferase (AST) [14]. Therefore, the first objective of this study was to evaluate the impact of acute pulmonary tuberculosis (PTB) and anti-TB therapy on the relationship between AST, ALT and GGT levels in absence of conditions related to hepatotoxicity. The second objective of the study was to evaluate the rate and the time, pattern of alterations in AST, ALT, and GGT associated with ADR in these personalized conditions. The findings from this analysis of clinical courses of PTB patients will help the Anti-TB Centre to establish preventive measures for elevated liver enzymes and the background of oxidative stress activity anti-TB therapy.

2. Materials and Methods

2.1. Study Design. This study was approved by the local Research Ethics committee of the Faculty of Health Sciences of the Marien Ngouabi University of Brazzaville, Republic of Congo. The study was a followup prospectively undertaken according to the Helsinki Declaration after verbal consent was obtained from adult patients referred to the Anti-TB Centre in Brazzaville, Republic of Congo, Central Africa, between September 2003 and September 2004.

Inclusion criteria into the study included typical symptoms and signs of active PTB: chronic cough, chronic fever, sweating, fibrocavitary lung infiltrate on chest radiograph, and at least one sputum specimen staining positive Ziehl-Neelsen for acid fast bacilli. Diagnosis of PTB was based on the WHO criteria including a positive culture for *Mycobacterium tuberculosis* or negative culture associated with clinical and radiological features and response to treatment consistent with TB or histological studies [16].

Exclusion criteria were age <18 years old, age >50 years old, the conditions related to the high risk of anti-TB drug-induced hepatitis [7, 9, 11, 12], cigarette smoking, history of drug usage, blood transfusion previous, treatment for PTB,

coexisting lung pathology, renal failure, diabetes mellitus, suspected multidrug resistant (MDR) and extensively drug resistant (XDR) TB, and additional criteria for women being pregnant or lactating, or females being menstruating at the time of blood collection.

Based on WHO recommended standard [16], patients received a regimen of isoniazid, rifampicin, pyrazinamide, and ethambutol for initial phase, followed by isoniazid and rifampicin at continuation phase. Approximately 10 mL of venous blood was drawn using disposable plastic syringes from PTB patients prior to initiation of anti-TB therapy (time 0 day) and at the ends of first month (time 30 days) and the second month (time 60 days) of the initial phase, and transferred immediately into disposable plain tubes.

2.2. Laboratory Analyses. Venous blood was also drawn at the end of the continuation phase, and at 15 days and 45 days after the end of the continuation phase. The serum was separated after centrifugation of the blood and kept frozen at $-20°C$ before being analyzed at the National Laboratory of Public Health in Brazzaville, Republic of Congo.

Serum AST was evaluated by a kinetic determination. Malate dehydrogenase catalyzes the reaction of oxaloacetic acid with β-NADH$_2$ by forming lactic acid and β-NAD. Serum ALT was evaluated by a kinetic determination. Lactate dehydrogenase catalyzes the reaction of pyruvic acid with β-NADH$_2$ by forming lactic acid and β-NAD. Serum GGT was evaluated by an enzymatic colorimetric method. All laboratory measurements were performed using Biomérieux reagents and automatic analyzer (Visual, Biomérieux, Marcy l'Etoile, France).

The interassay coefficients of variation of these laboratory measurements were as follows: AST: 0.8%; ALT: 0.5%; GGT: 0.6%. The intraassay coefficients of variation were within the 0.87–2.1% interval.

2.3. Monitoring. Also the participants were followed clinically during anti-TB therapy course. Noxious or unintended response to a drug which occurs at doses often used in human beings [16] was reported.

2.4. Statistical Analysis. The data of the study were expressed as mean ± standard deviation for continuous variables and as proportions (%) for categorical variables.

One-way analysis of variance (ANOVA) with Bonferroni post hoc test for multiple comparisons was used to compare AST, ALT, and GGT means across the periods of the initiation phase (day 0, day 30, and day 60) and those of the continuation phase (at the end of treatment, 15 days and 45 days after the end of the continuation phase). Students t-test served to compare the means of liver enzymes before anti-TB treatment and the average of their means after the end of the global treatment. Linear-by-linear association with P for trend served to compare the proportions of ADR across the quintiles of AST, ALT, and GGT.

Simple coefficients "r" were determined between the liver enzymes, while the multiple linear regression was fitted with GGT as dependent variable and Age, AST, and ALT as independent variables for the mean values from the baseline and the end of the initial phase, at the end of 30 days (1 month) and 60 days (2 months) after the ignition of the anti-TB therapy. The assumptions were tested by the residual analysis (difference between the actual and the predicted score): histogram of residuals dependent variable residuals against independent variables, and normal probability. A P value < 0.05 was considered to be statistically significant. SPSS for Windows version 19.0 (SPSS Inc., Chicago, IL, USA) was used for all analyses of data.

3. Results

3.1. Characteristics of the Study Population. The study sample comprised of 40 patients (52.5% $n = 21$ were males, and 47.5% $n = 19$ were females with sex ratio almost 1 man: 1 woman and aged 34.7 ± 5.8 years).

3.2. ADR. At the day 30 after starting the initial phase, 1 patient (3%) experienced pruritus due to self-administration of 2 tablets of cotrimoxazole. His transient mild hepatic dysfunction defined by a peak of serum enzymes (AST, ALT, and GGT greater than two times of the upper limit of their normal range: AST < 26 UI/L, ALT < UI/L, and GGT = 7–34 UI/L), vomiting, diarrhoea, but without jaundice. Because normalisation of the liver enzymes and the relief of pruritus and gastrointestinal symptoms occurred after two-day antihistaminic treatment, the anti-TB drugs were not stopped. However, the day 30 liver enzymes values of this patient were not considered in the all statistical analyses.

3.3. Variations of Liver Enzymes. The mean values of AST (19.5 ± 8.6 UI/L), ALT (7.6 ± 3.2 UI/L), and GGT (20.4 ± 16.8 UI/L) before anti-TB therapy were not different (ANOVA, $P > 0.05$) from those observed at the end of the continuation phase (AST = 19.4 ± 8.5 UI/L; ALT = 7.5 ± 3.5 UI/L; GGT = 20.3 ± 16.8 UI/L), at day 15 after the end of the continuation phase (AST = 19.2 ± 5.8 UI/L; ALT = 9.3 ± 4 UI/L; GGT = 19.7 ± 12.1 UI/L), and at day 45 after the end continuation phase (AST = 19.5 ± 7.3 UI/L; ALT = 11.6 ± 4.7 UI/L; GGT = 21.6 ± 17.7 UI/L).

However, during the two months of the initial phase of anti-TB therapy, values of AST (SD: 3.1 VI/L day 0; 0.1 UI/L day 30; 5.4 UI/L day 60) increased significantly (ANOVA, $P < 0.0001$) across the time, while GGT values (SD: 2.8 UI/L day 0; 5.3 UI/L day 30; 4 UI/L day 60) decreased significantly across the time (ANOVA, $P < 0.0001$), respectively, (Figure 1).

At each time of the initial phase of anti-TB therapy, a significant and positive correlation between liver enzymes was observed (Table 1). The level and the strength of association between GGT and AST was increasing with anti-TB therapy duration. The highest level of association between GGT and ALT, and that between AST and ALT, was observed at day 30 after the starting of the initial phase. During the initial phase of anti-TB therapy and after adjusting for confounding factors (age, sex, either AST or ALT) and identifying the independent determinants of GGT at each assessment time,

TABLE 1: Simple correlation coefficients r between liver enzymes according to the initial phase therapy time.

Initial Phase Time	GGT r coefficient P value	ALT r coefficient P value
Day 0		
AST	0.279 $P = 0.041$	0.735 $P < 0.0001$
ALT	0.353 $P = 0.013$	1
Day 30		
AST	0.397 $P = 0.006$	0.964 $P < 0.0001$
ALT	0.428 $P = 0.003$	1
Day 60		
AST	0.687 $P < 0.0001$	0.791 $P < 0.0001$
ALT	0.382 $P = 0.0007$	1

there was a significant linear relationship between adjusted R square defining the variations of GGT and the different times of assessment (Table 2). At day 0 and day 30 after anti-TB treatment, only increasing ALT was the significant explanatory variable of the variations of GGT. At the day 60 after the anti-Tb therapy, 52% of variations in concentrations of GGT were significantly and independently explained by the increase in AST and the decrease in ALT levels (Figure 2).

Within day 0–day 60, average values of 19.2 ± 7.8 UI/L, 14.8 ± 8.9 UI/L, and 13.3 ± 6.1 UI/L were reported for AST, ALT, and GGT, respectively. There was a negative and significant correlation between day 0–day 60 AST values ($r = -0.494$; $P < 0.0001$) ALT values ($r = -0.472$; $P < 0.0001$), and GGT, respectively. However, a positive and very significant association was noticed between day 0–day 60 AST values ($r = 0.893$; $P < 0.0001$) and day 0–day 60 ALT values. After adjusting for age, ALT, and sex, 23.8% of variations of day 0–day 60 GGT values towards decrease were explained by the increase in day 0–day 60 AST values (standard error = 0.063; $P < 0.0001$) as follows: Y (GGT) = 20.8–0.494 AST. Figure 3 describes the curves for histogram and normal P-P plot with day 0–day 60 GGT values as a dependent variable and a reflection of the impact of the initial phase anti-TB therapy: a multivariate and negative association between GGT and AST.

4. Discussion

In this study, the incidence of ADR was only 3%, accidental, transient, benign and due to self-administration of cotrimoxazole. This rate of elevation of hepatic transaminases was within the traditional interval [7], but lower than the levels of 50–75% ADR reported in Eastern European and

TABLE 2: Multiple linear regression of GGT levels at day 0, day 30, and day 60 after starting initial phase anti-TB therapy.

Initial phase time	Adjusted R^2	Standardized beta	Standard error	P value
Time independent of test variable				
Day 0				
ALT	10.2%	0.353	0.328	0.025
Day 30				
ALT	16.1%	0.428	0.715	0.007
Day 60	51.6%			
AST		1.027	0.134	<0.0001
ALT		−0.430	0.162	0.023

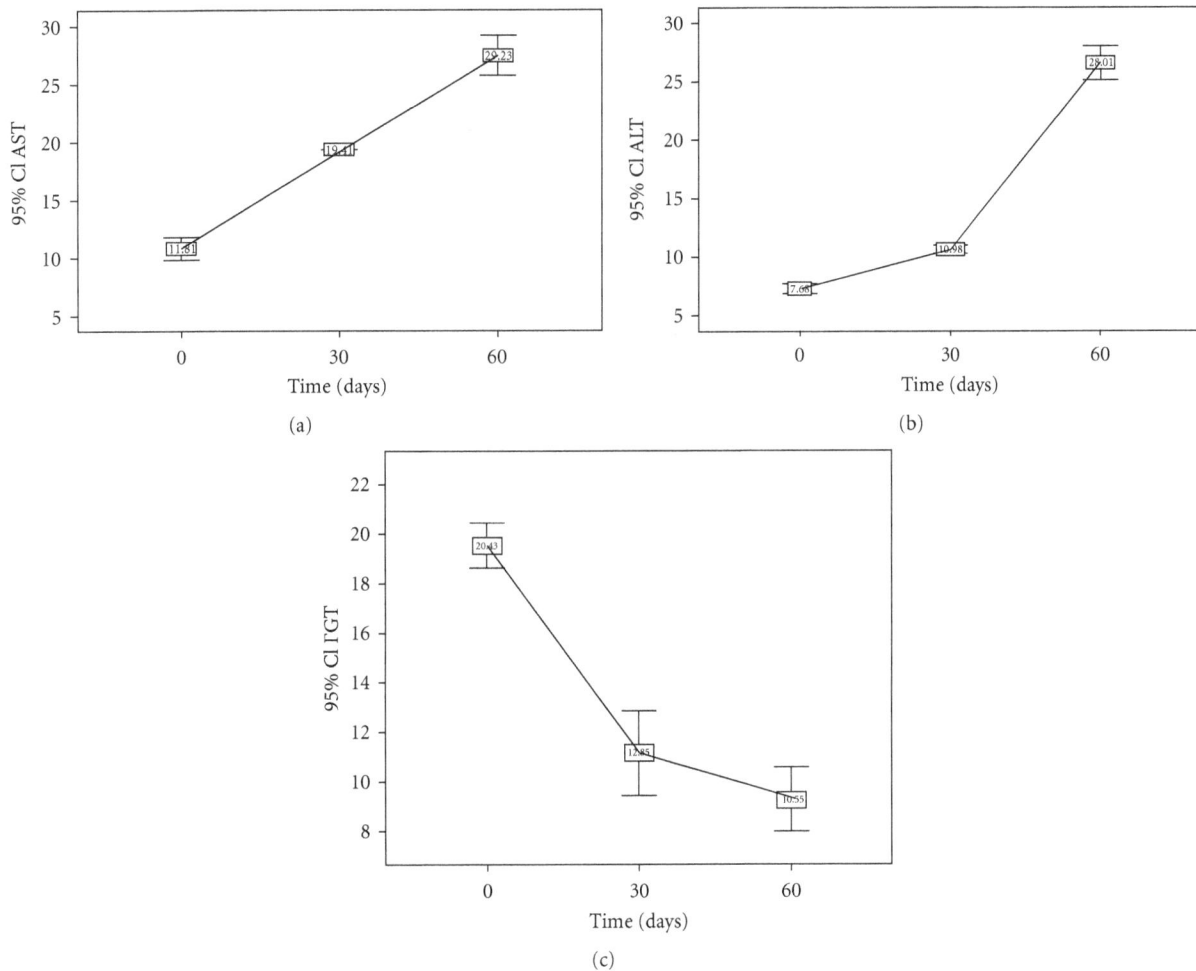

FIGURE 1: Variations of AST, ALT, and GGT during the two months of initial phase with their Bonferroni post hoc tests. *Day 0 versus day 30: $P < 0.0001$; day 0 versus day 60: $P < 0.0001$. *Day 30 versus day 60: $P < 0.0001$.

Asian countries [17]. ADR occurred within the first 30 days of the initiation of anti-TB treatment as usually reported by different studies [17, 18]. Concomitant use of cotrimoxazole or other hepatotoxic drugs is well established as a risk factor for anti-TB-induced liver injury [7, 9, 11, 12].

A significant downward trend in GGT levels was observed from the starting to the end of the initial phase of DOTS. This is because the initial two-month therapy leads to significant improvement in oxidative stress and suppression of inflammation determined by active PTB [2, 3]. Aging, already associated with oxidative stress [19], was one of the exclusion criteria in this study because elderly patients are at a greater risk of oxidative stress and of hepatotoxicity probably because of immunity mechanisms.

In PTB, neutrophils, monocytes, and macrophages are, mobilized to destroy Mycobacteria and generate huge amounts of ROS and lipid peroxidation [20–22]. A series of data obtained from black and white men suggest that serum

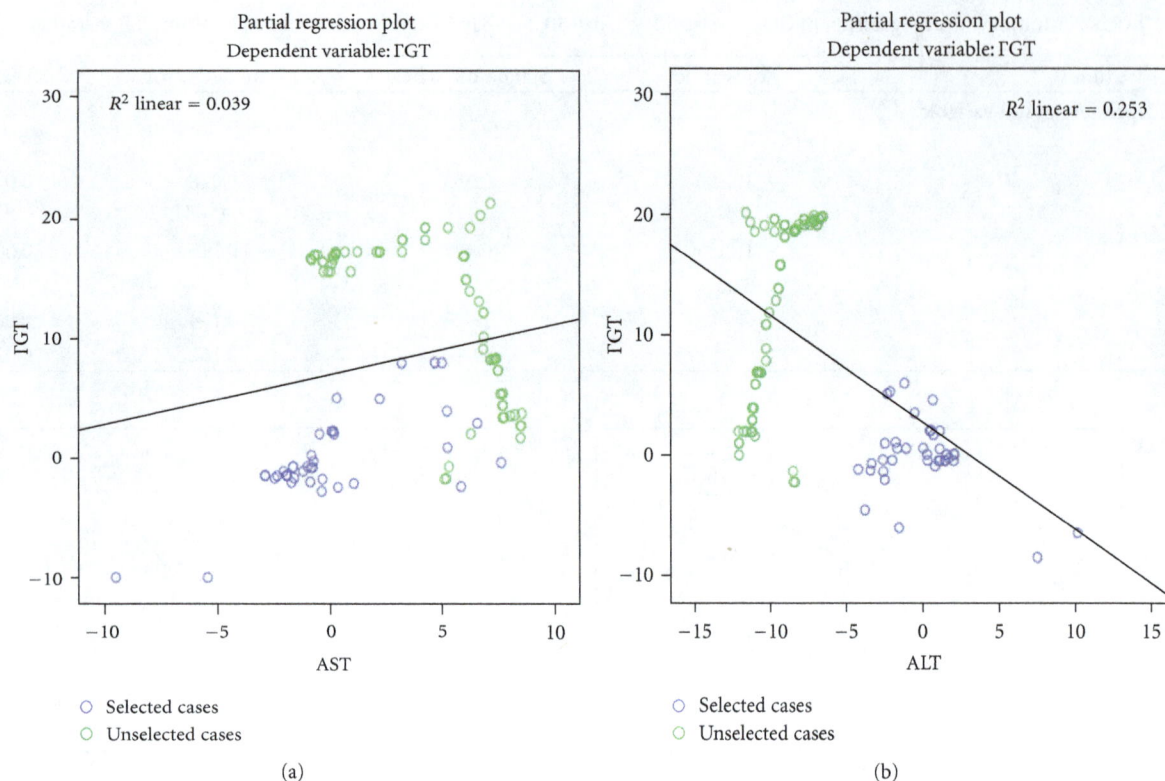

FIGURE 2: Multivariate relation between AST (a), ALT (b), and GGT at day 60 of initial phase of DOTS.

GGT within its normal range might be an early marker of oxidative stress [13]. The variations of serum GGT in this study, except in one patient with benign ADR, were within their normal range before and after DOTS. The deficiency of antioxidants renders PTB patients unable to cope with their increased oxidative stress [21].

With progressive DOTS during the two months of the initial phase, the baseline relationship between GGT and AST, as well between GGT and ALT changed, respectively. The relationship between GGT and ALT become not significant in considering their average values of day 0–day 60. This means that the anti-TB might neutralise the baseline (day 0, day 30, and day 60) synergistic action of GGT and ALT, both markers of oxidative stress [15]. However, in considering the day 0–day 60 average of liver enzymes, only AST was negatively, significantly and independently associated with serum GGT in these black PTB patients.

5. Clinical Implications

The present study will have significant implications in understanding the role of oxidative stress biomarkers and that of liver enzymes in personalizing the DOTS. Systematic steps for prevention of hepatotoxicity are recommended in anti-TB therapy. These recommendations include patient and regimen selection to optimise benefits over risks. Education of patients to avoid self-administration of medications interfering with anti-TB drugs is mandatory.

During the first two months of anti-TB therapy, ALT, AST, and GGT monitoring is recommended. If serum GGT is a marker of oxidative stress targeted by anti-TB during the initial phase, it might have important implications both clinically and epidemiologically because measurement of serum GGT is easy, reliable, and not expensive. It is important to evaluate in tuberculosis patients on DOTS intake of fruits and vegetables, which are rich in antioxidants. Particular attention must be paid in elderly patients at a greater risk of toxicity because of potential poor antioxidant mechanisms [3, 23].

The oxidative stress due to PTB and aggravated by anti-TB therapy hepatotoxicity and the severity of PTB could be reduced by adjuvant therapy with dietary phytochemicals and antioxidants [24, 25].

5.1. Limitations of the Study. The study was limited to some degree, as monitoring of AST, ALT, and GGT was not performed monthly from the end of the initial phase and the end of the continuation phase.

6. Conclusion

This study concludes that oxidative stress markers within normal range before starting anti-TB treatment and considering conditions related to hepatotoxicity in patients admitted for active PTB might predict excellent tolerability of anti-TB drugs and very low rate of ADR.

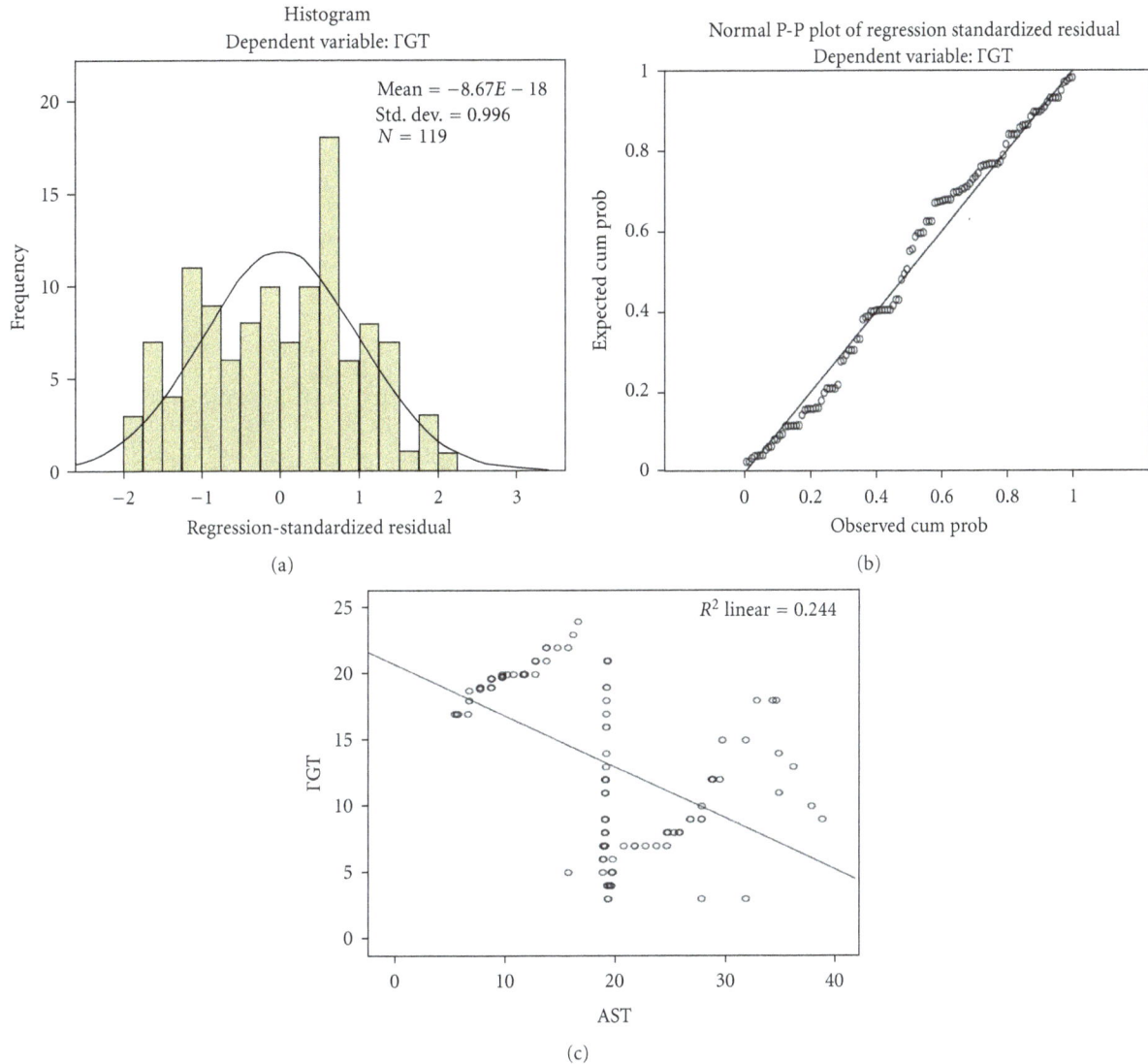

FIGURE 3: Frequency distribution by histogram (a) and normal P-P plot of regression-standardized residual (b) for GGT as dependent variable and AST as the only independent determinant (c) during day 0–day 60 anti-TB therapy of initial phase.

The decrease in serum GGT, contrasting with the increase in serum AST and ALT, should reflect the effect of anti-TB therapy during the intensive and initial two-month phase of DOTS. Cotrimoxazole induces a transient enhancement of oxidative stress due to tuberculosis itself and anti-TB chemotherapy.

Clinicians should educate patients about risk factors of anti-TB treatment-induced hepatotoxicity as well as they should be vigilant for conditions related to oxidative stress and deficiency of antioxidant systems.

Conflict of Interests

The authors declare that they have no conflict of interests.

Acknowledgments

The authors thank all the patients who participated in the study and acknowledge the assistance received from the Anti-TB Centre and the National Laboratory of Public Health in Brazzaville, Congo, during this study.

References

[1] P. Balagopal, S. D. de Ferranti, S. Cook et al., "Nontraditional risk factors and biomarkers for cardiovascular disease: mechanistic, research, and clinical considerations for youth: a scientific statement from the american heart association," *Circulation*, vol. 123, no. 23, pp. 2749–2769, 2011.

[2] D. A. Taha and A.-J. Thanoon, "Antioxidant status, C-reactive protein and iron status in patients with pulmonary

tuberculosis," *Sultan Qaboos University Medical Sciences Journal*, vol. 10, pp. 361–369, 2010.

[3] M. L. Put, A. J. Theron, H. Fickl, C. E. J. van Rensburg, S. Pendel, and R. Anderson, "Influence of antimicrobial chemotherapy and smoking status on the plasma concentrations of vitamin C, vitamin E, β-carotene, acute phase reactants, iron and lipid peroxides in patients with pulmonary tuberculosis," *International Journal of Tuberculosis and Lung Disease*, vol. 2, no. 7, pp. 590–596, 1998.

[4] C. I. A. Jack, M. J. Jackson, and C. R. K. Hind, "Circulating markers of free radical activity in patients with pulmonary tuberculosis," *Tubercle and Lung Disease*, vol. 75, no. 2, pp. 132–137, 1994.

[5] K. Yasuda, A. Sato, K. Chida et al., "Pulmonary tuberculosis with chemotherapy related liver dysfunction," *Kekkaku*, vol. 65, no. 6, pp. 407–413, 1990.

[6] T. F. Brewer and S. J. Heymann, "To control and beyond: moving towards eliminating the global tuberculosis threat," *Journal of Epidemiology and Community Health*, vol. 58, no. 10, pp. 822–825, 2004.

[7] A Tostmann, M. J. Boeree, R. E. Aanoutse, and R. Kedhuijzen, "Anti tuberculosis drug-induced hepatotoxicity: concise up-to-review," *Journal of Gastroenterology and Hepatology*, vol. 23, pp. 192–202, 2008.

[8] E. J. Forget and D. Menzies, "Adverse reactions to first-time antituberculosis drugs," *Expert Opinion on Drug Safety*, vol. 5, no. 2, pp. 231–249, 2006.

[9] Z. Hussain, P. Kar, and S. A. Husain, "Antituberculosis drug-induced hepatitis: risk factors, prevention and management," *Indian Journal of Experimental Biology*, vol. 41, no. 11, pp. 1226–1232, 2003.

[10] T. R. Frieden, T. R. Sterling, S. S. Munsiff, C. J. Watt, and C. Dye, "Tuberculosis," *The Lancet*, vol. 362, no. 9387, pp. 887–899, 2003.

[11] R. A. M. Breen, R. F. Miller, T. Gorsuch et al., "Adverse events and treatment interruption in tuberculosis patients with and without HIV co-infection," *Thorax*, vol. 61, no. 9, pp. 791–794, 2006.

[12] K Krishnaswamy, C. E. Prasad, and K. J. Muthy, "Hepatic dysfunction in under nourished patients receiving isoniazid and rijampia," *Tropical and Geographical Medicine*, vol. 43, pp. 156–160, 1991.

[13] J. S. Lim, J. H. Yang, B. Y. Chun, S. Kam, D. R. Jacobs Jr., and D. H. Lee, "Is serum γ-glutamyltransferase inversely associated with serum antioxidants as a marker of oxidative stress?" *Free Radical Biology and Medicine*, vol. 37, no. 7, pp. 1018–1023, 2004.

[14] S. Bo, R. Gambino, M. Durazzo et al., "Associations between γ-glutamyl transferase, metabolic abnormalities and inflammation in healthy subjects from a population-based cohort: a possible implication for oxidative stress," *World Journal of Gastroenterology*, vol. 11, no. 45, pp. 7109–7117, 2005.

[15] J. Yamada, H. Tomiyama, M. Yambe et al., "Elevated serum levels of alanine aminotransferase and gamma glutamyltransferase are markers of inflammation and oxidative stress independent of the metabolic syndrome," *Atherosclerosis*, vol. 189, no. 1, pp. 198–205, 2006.

[16] World Health Organisation Global Tuberculosis Programme, *Treatment of Tuberculosis: Guidelines for National Programmes*, WHO/CDS/TUBERCULOS, World Health Organization, Geneva, Switzerland, 3rd edition, 2003.

[17] P. V. Kishore, S. Palaian, O. Pradir, and P. R. Shankar, "Pattern of adverse drug reactions experienced by tuberculosis patients in tertiary care teaching hospital in Western Nepal,"

Pakistan Journal of Pharmaceutical Sciences, vol. 21, pp. 51–56, 2008.

[18] V. K. Dhingra, S. Rajpal, N. Aggarwal, J. K. Aggarwal, K. Shadab, and S. K. Jain, "Adverse drug reactions observed during DOTS," *Journal of Communicable Diseases*, vol. 36, no. 4, pp. 251–259, 2004.

[19] M. F. Alexeyev, "Is there more to aging than mitochondrial DNA and reactive oxygen species?" *FEBS Journal*, vol. 276, no. 20, pp. 5768–5787, 2009.

[20] K. Kaur, J. Kishan, G. K. Bedi, and R. S. Ahi, "Oxidants stress and antioxidants in pulmonary tuberculosis," *Chest*, vol. 128, p. 3975, 2005.

[21] Y. N. Reddy, S. V. Murthy, D. R. Krishna, and M. C. Prabhakar, "Role of free radicals and antioxidants in tuberculosis patients," *Indian Journal of Tuberculosis*, vol. 51, pp. 213–218, 2004.

[22] T. Madebo, B. Lindtjørn, P. Aukrust, and R. K. Berge, "Circulating antioxidants and lipid peroxidation products in untreated tuberculosis patients in Ethiopia," *The American Journal of Clinical Nutrition*, vol. 78, no. 1, pp. 117–122, 2003.

[23] A. Walubo, P. J. Smith, and P. I. Folb, "Oxidative stress during antituberculosis therapy in young and elderly patients," *Biomedical and Environmental Sciences*, vol. 8, pp. 106–113, 1995.

[24] A. Agarwal, R. Prasad, and A. Jain, "Effect of green tea extract (catechins) in reducing oxidative stress seen in patients of pulmonary tuberculosis on DOTS Cat I regimen," *Phytomedicine*, vol. 17, no. 1, pp. 23–27, 2010.

[25] E. Sevedrezazadeh, A. Ostradrahini, S. Mahboob, Y. Assadi, J. Ghaemmagami, and M. Poumogaddam, "Effect of vitamin E and selenium supplementation on oxidative stress status in pulmonary tuberculosis patients," *Respirology*, vol. 13, pp. 294–298, 2008.

20

Sedative and Hypnotic Activities of the Methanolic and Aqueous Extracts of *Lavandula officinalis* from Morocco

Rachad Alnamer,[1] **Katim Alaoui,**[2] **El Houcine Bouidida,**[3]
Abdelaziz Benjouad,[1] **and Yahia Cherrah**[2]

[1] *Laboratory of Genetic Immunology and Biochemistry, Department of Biology, Faculty of Science,*
 Mohammed V Agdal University, BP 6203, Rabat Instituts, Agdal, Rabat, Morocco
[2] *Laboratory of Pharmacology and Toxicology, Department of Drugs Sciences, Faculty of Medicine and Pharmacy,*
 Mohammed V Souissi University, ERTP, BP 6203, Rabat Instituts, Agdal, Rabat, Morocco
[3] *National Laboratory of Drugs Controlled, BP 6203, Rabat Instituts, Agdal, Rabat, Morocco*

Correspondence should be addressed to Katim Alaoui, alaouikma@yahoo.fr

Academic Editor: Elaine Cristina Gavioli

We evaluate the sedative and hypnotic activities of the methanolic and aqueous extract of *Lavandula officinalis* L. on central nervous system (CNS). In this study, the effect of the methanolic and aqueous extracts of this plant was investigated in a battery of behavioural models in mice. Stems and flowers of *Lavandula officinalis* L. have several therapeutic applications in folk medicine in curing or managing a wide range of diseases, including insomnia. The methanolic extract produced significant sedative effect at the doses of 200, 400, and 600 mg/kg (by oral route), compared to reference substance diazepam (DZP), and an hypnotic effect at the doses of 800 and 1000 mg/kg while the treatment of mice with the aqueous extract at the doses of 200 and 400 mg/kg via oral pathway significantly reduced in both the reestablishment time and number of head dips during the traction and hole-board tests. In conclusion, these results suggest that the methanolic and aqueous extracts of *Lavandula officinalis* possess potent sedative and hypnotic activities, which supported its therapeutic use for insomnia.

1. Introduction

Morocco is fortunate to have such varied climate that almost any medicinal plant can grow. The varied climate and heterogeneous ecologic condition in Morocco have favoured the proliferation of more than 42,000 species of plants, divided into 150 families and 940 genuses [1–3]. Insomnia defined as persistent difficulty in falling or staying a sleep that affects function can induce significant psychological and physical disorder. Sedatives are drugs that decrease activity and have a calming, relaxing effect. At higher doses, sedatives usually cause sleep. Drugs used mainly to cause sleep are called hypnotics. The difference between sedatives and hypnotics, then, is usually the amount of the dose; lower doses have a calming effect and higher doses cause sleep [4]. Recent studies have shown that herbal drugs exert good sedative and hypnotic effect on the central

nervous system [4–6]. In recent years, *Lavandula officinalis* flowers exhibit such various biological and pharmacological activities as anti-tumour, anti-inflammatory, antihistaminic, antidiabetic, and antimicrobial activity and modulating the central nervous system [2, 7–11]. The aim of this experiment is to evaluate the sedative and hypnotic activities of *Lavandula officinalis* methanolic and aqueous extract, and to, therefore, determine the scientific basis for its use in traditional medicine in the management of central nervous system disorders.

2. Materials and Methods

2.1. Plant Material. Stems and flowers of *Lavandula officinalis* L. were collected based on ethnopharmacological information from the villages around the region Rabat-Sale-Zemour-Zaers, with the agreement from the authorities and respecting the United Nations Convention of Biodiversity and with assistance of traditional medical practitioner. The plant was identified with botanist of scientific institute (Pr. M. Ibn Tatou). A voucher specimen (N°256) was deposited in the Herbarium of Botany Department of the Scientific Institute of Rabat.

2.2. Preparation of Extract.
Stems and flowers of *Lavandula officinalis* were successively extracted with methanol by maceration at room temperature (25°C) over period of 48 hours. 500 g of plant material and one litre of methanol were used in the extraction. Methanol containing the extract was then filtered through Whatman paper and the solvent was vacuum distilled at 65°C in a rotary evaporator. The remaining extract was finally dried in the oven at 30°C for two hours to ensure the removal of any residual solvent (lyophilisation). Final extract was a dark green powder in percentage dry weight 21.8%. For the aqueous extract, 500 g of plant material was extracted by infusion boiled water (500 mL) for three days. The respective aqueous extracts were separated from its residues by gravity filtration. The final crude extract was obtained as yellow greasy powder in percentage from dry weight (15.7% d.w). These extracts were kept in deep freeze at −20°C until use.

2.3. Animals.
Male Swiss mice (20–25 g) (Iffa-credo, France) were used in pharmacological tests and females of the same strain in the LD$_{50}$ calculation. The animals were fed *ad libitum* with standard food and water except when fasting was required in the course of the study. The animals were acquired from the animal experimental centre of Mohammed V Souissi University, Medicine and Pharmacy Faculty, Rabat.

2.4. Acute Toxicity.
Median lethal dose (LD$_{50}$) values were determined as described by Litchfield and Wilcoxon [12]. Seven groups of mice of both sexes ($n = 10$, 5 males and 5 females) received or not single oral doses at different concentrations (500, 1000, 1500, 2000, 3000, and 5000 mg/kg, p.o.). The control group received only the water or saline solution. After a single dose administration, mice were placed in individual clear plastic boxes and continuously observed for 6 h and at 24 h time interval to detect any eventual side effects. The number of animals, which died during this period, was expressed as percentile. The LD$_{50}$ of the extract were estimated by the p.o. route using the procedure reported by Litchfield and Wilcoxon; the method estimated the dose of the extract that would kill 50% of a reduced sample of animals by a given route. In a first phase, the extract was given to ten mice per group at doses of 500 and 1000 mg/kg; when no mortality was observed, the doses were increased to 1500, 2000, 3000, and 5000 mg/kg. Mice were kept under observation for 14 days to register possible mortality, their weights were registered, and at the end of the study they were sacrificed for macroscopic tissue examination [13], and the LD50 was determined by probit test using death percent versus doses log [14–16]. Of note, drugs used as control were given to mice in similar conditions.

2.5. Drugs.
All drugs and extracts were freshly prepared on the day of the experiments. A control group received distilled water (10 mL/kg, p.o.) as vehicle. Diazepam (3 mg/kg, i.p., a conventional sedative) and thiopental (60 mg/kg, i.p., a conventional hypnosis) were used as positive control.

2.6. Pharmacological Evaluations.
The activity of methanolic and aqueous extract from *Lavandula officinalis* on the central nervous system was then studied, using a battery of behavioral tests used in psychopharmacology. We analyzed the effect of different doses of the methanolic extracts (100, 200, 400, and 600 mg/kg, p.o.) and aqueous extracts (100, 200, and 400 mg/kg, p.o.) from Lavandula officinalis for their sedative and hypnotic activities. For testing sedative effect, the effect of extract on mice was qualified in one of the following tests.

2.7. Traction Test.
Mice were individually suspended by anterior limbs to a wire stretched horizontally. Abnormal mice that fail to make a reestablishment at least one of its posterior limbs to reach the wire are considered as subject under a sedative action. When the animals perform normal reestablishment immediately, the reaction is known as positive; other wise, the reaction is called negative; also, the behaviours of animals were recorded during the period of the experiment [17, 18].

2.8. Fireplace Test.
The apparatus used for this test consist of a vertical glass tube 30 cm in length. Mice were individually placed vertically in the glass test tube, a normal mouse typically attempts to escape in thirty seconds, and the mice considered as subject to the sedative effect when performing the rise of cylinder greater than 30 sec [19].

2.9. Hole-Board Test.
Mice were individually placed in the centre of a perforated board, and the number of head dips was registered during a 5 min. The perforated board test was made by using a wood floor board, 40 cm × 40 cm × 25 cm, in which evenly spaced holes were made. The number of explored holes provide a measure of the number of head dips [20, 21].

2.10. Thiopental-Induced Sleep in Mice.
Thiopental (a subhypnotic dose) 60 mg/kg was injected i.p. 30 min after administration of methanolic and aqueous extracts. The mice were treated with different doses of methanolic and aqueous extracts (800, 1000 mg/kg, p.o., $n = 5$), the control group ($n = 5$) was treated with distilled water (10 mL/kg, p.o.), and positive control group ($n = 5$) was administrated with diazepam (3 mg/kg, i.p.), respectively. The effect was recorded for disappearance (latency) and reappearance (duration) of the righting reflex. Hypnotic sleeping time was considered to be the time interval between disappearance and reappearance of the righting reflex [5, 22].

2.11. Statistical Analysis.
The statistical analysis was done using ANOVA. The results with $P < 0.05$ were considered significant. The data are expressed as mean ± SD.

3. Results

3.1. Acute Toxicity of Lavandula officinalis Methanolic and Aqueous Extracts.
Following oral administration of *Lavandula officinalis* extract at the doses of 500, 1000, 1500, 2000, 3000, and 5000 mg/kg, p.o., no toxicity and no significant changes in the body weight between the control and treated group were demonstrated at these doses. This result indicates that, the LD_{50} was higher than 5000 mg/kg.

3.2. Sedative Activity of the Methanolic and Aqueous Extract on the Central Nervous System (CNS).
The results of psychotropic effects of methanolic and aqueous extracts were expressed by comparison with control groups. Pharmacological tests were then performed at nontoxic doses (i.e., 100, 200, 400, and 600 mg/kg, p.o.), for the methanolic extract and (100, 200, and 400 mg/kg, p.o.), for the aqueous extract.

3.3. Traction Test.
The methanolic extract of *Lavandula officinalis* given by oral route at 100 mg/kg did not significantly alter the reestablishment time; all animals performed normal reestablishment immediately ($P > 0.05$). However, the extract at the dose of 200 mg/kg produced significant sedative effect on the central nervous system (CNS) as indicated by the relatively high time for the reestablishment of the mice (Table 1). By increasing the doses to 400 and 600 mg/kg, the average reestablishment time was increased. The reestablishment time was notably higher than control group ($P < 0.001$) (Table 1). For the aqueous extract, after oral administration at the dose of 100 mg/kg, all animals performed normal reestablishment time (notably decreased the reestablishment time). This indicates that this extract produced no significant sedative effect on mice behavior at this dose ($P > 0.05$) (Table 2). By increasing the doses to 200 and 400 mg/kg, the reestablishment time was increased; the mice fail to make a reestablishment immediately ($P < 0.001$). So, the aqueous extract of *Lavandula officinalis* produced significant sedative effect at the doses of 200 and 400 mg/kg p.o. (Table 2). In addition, the dose of 100 mg/kg of both extracts did not decreased the reestablishment time.

3.4. Fireplace Test.
Animal treated with the methanolic extract of *Lavandula officinalis* at the dose of 100 mg/kg via oral route do not show loss of initiative and curiosity. By increasing the doses to 200, 400, and 600 mg/kg, all mice lose initiative and curiosity; that is, animal did not attempt to mount the tube for escape ($P < 0.01$) (Table 1). While, the aqueous extract, at the doses of 100 mg/kg, produced no sedative effect, at the doses of 200 and 400 mg/kg p.o., all animals treated showed loss of initiative and curiosity ($P < 0.001$) (Table 2).

3.5. Hole-Board Test.
In the hole-board test, a significant reduction in the number of head dips at the doses of 200, 400, and 600 mg/kg by oral route administration; with the exception at the dose of 100 mg/kg, the methanolic extract did not reduce the number of head dips. However, animal treated with the aqueous extract at the doses of 100 mg/kg did not reduce the number of head dips ($P > 0.05$). By increasing the doses to 200 and 400 mg/kg, this extract reduced the cumulative number of holes explored and the number of spaces between two holes explored (en relation with motor activity) ($P < 0.001$) (Table 1). The data lead to conclude that the methanolic and aqueous extract of *Lavandula officinalis* possess potential sedative effects on the central nervous system at the doses of 200, 400, and 600 mg/kg via oral route administration (Tables 1 and 2).

3.6. Thiopental-Induced Sleep in Mice.
We observed that the lavender methanolic extract (ME) had induced hypnotic effect significant ($P < 0.001$). Hypnosis induced by methanolic extract (800 and 1000 mg/kg, p.o.) was evaluated by observation of the duration of thiopental-induced sleeping time. The extract showed a reduction in the time of onset of sleep induced by thiopental. The effects of the extract on onset of sleep at 800 and 1000 mg/kg were comparable to that of diazepam at 3 mg/kg. The highest prolongation of sleep produced by the methanolic extract was comparable to that of diazepam (3 mg/kg). Only the highest dose tested for ME significantly increased from 45 ± 2 to 112 ± 3 min; the duration of hypnos is induced by thiopental (Table 3). However, the aqueous extract of *Lavandula officinalis* at the doses of 800 and 1000 mg/kg, p.o., produced no hypnotic activity significant on the central nervous system confirming, thus, the hypnotic action of lavender methanolic extract at high doses by oral pathway (Table 3).

4. Discussion

In aromatherapy, the methanolic and aqueous extracts of *Lavandula officinalis* are believed to possess anticonvulsive, sedative, hypnosis, and antidepressive effects and to be useful for treating nervous breakdown, nervous tension, depression, and insomnia [23–25]. In this paper, we observed the sedative and hypnotic properties of methanolic and aqueous extract from *Lavandula officinalis* L. in mice. Therefore, in order to study the comprehensive effect of our drugs, the following targets were observed: reestablishment time, number of head dips, and loss of initiative and curiosity in mice.

Diazepam is central nervous system depressant used in the management of sleep disorders such as insomnia; these compounds have a binding site on GABA receptor type-A ionophore complex ($GABA_A$) [4, 5]. It decreases activity, moderates excitement, and calms the recipient. Substances like diazepam (which has been chosen as the standard reference drug in this study) reduce onset of and increase duration of barbiturate-induced sleep and reduce exploratory activity possessing potentials as sedative [21, 26]. Lavender extract increased the time of reestablishment by mice in the traction test (Table 1), after oral administration of 200, 400, and 600 mg/kg dosages, producing sedative effect similar to that observed with 3 mg/kg diazepam. Diazepam is a very well-known anxiolytic benzodiazepine (BDS) which produces not only anxiolytic-like effect but also important sedative action. In this respect, lavender extract produced

TABLE 1: Sedative action of *Lavandula officinalis* methanolic extract. p.o. means oral route; i.p. means intraperitoneal route; *n* means number of mice per group; sec means seconds; ME: mean methanolic extract; DZP means diazepam. Data are expressed as mean ± SD; $P < 0.001$ versus the control group.

Test		Control	Diazepam i.p. DZP (3 mg/kg)	Methanolic extract of *Lavandula officinalis* in mg/kg p.o.			
				ME (100 mg/kg)	ME (200 mg/kg)	ME (400 mg/kg)	ME (600 mg/kg)
Traction test	Re-establishment time	0.09 sec ± 0.0	10 sec ± 0.3	0.08 sec ± 0.5	5 sec ± 0.5*	18 sec ± 0.5*	27 sec ± 1*
		n = 5	*n* = 5	*n* = 5	*n* = 5	*n* = 5	*n* = 5
Fireplace test	Time to go back the tube in seconds	7 sec ± 0.5	>2 min	sec ± 0.5	30 sec ± 1*	0.58 sec ± 1*	>2 min*
		n = 5	*n* = 5	*n* = 5	*n* = 5	*n* = 5	*n* = 5
Hole-board test	Explored holes during 5 minutes	10 ± 1	0.0 ± 0.0	8 ± 0.1	2 ± 0.0*	1 ± 0.0*	0.0 ± 0.0*
		n = 5	*n* = 5	*n* = 5	*n* = 5	*n* = 5	*n* = 5

TABLE 2: Sedative effect of aqueous extract of *Lavandula officinalis*. p.o. means oral route; i.p. means intraperitoneal route; *n* means number of mice per group; sec means seconds; AE means aqueous extract; DZP means diazepam. Data are expressed as mean ± SD; $P < 0.001$ versus the control group.

Test		Control	Diazepam i.p. DZP (3 mg/kg)	Aqueous extract of *Lavandula officinalis* p.o.		
				AE (100 mg/kg)	AE (200 mg/kg)	AE (400 mg/kg)
Traction test	Re-establishment time	0.09 sec ± 0.0	10 sec ± 0.3	2 sec ± 0.3	12 sec ± 0.5*	30 sec ± 1*
		n = 5	*n* = 5	*n* = 5	*n* = 4	*n* = 5
Fireplace test	Time to go back the tube in seconds	7 sec ± 0.5	>2 min	12 sec ± 0.1	45 sec ± 1*	>2 min*
		n = 5	*n* = 5	*n* = 5	*n* = 5	*n* = 4
Hole-board test	Explored holes during 5 minutes	10 ± 1	0.0 ± 0.0	6 ± 0.2	1 ± 0.0*	0.0 ± 0.0*
		n = 5	*n* = 5	*n* = 5	*n* = 4	*n* = 4

TABLE 3: Effect of the methanolic extract of *Lavandula officinalis* on the onset and duration of sleep in thiopental-treated mice. Mice received thiopental (60 mg/kg, i.p.) 30 min after the pretreatment of methanolic extract (800 and 1000 mg/kg, p.o.) and diazepam (3 mg/kg, i.p.). i.p. means intraperitoneal route; p.o. means oral route; (*n* = 5) means number of mice per group; ME means methanolic extract; D ZP means diazepam. Data are expressed as mean ± SD; $P < 0.001$ versus the control group.

Group	Dose (mg/kg)	Sleep latency (min)	Sleeping time (min)
Normal	60	8 ± 1	36 ± 3
DZP	3	6 ± 1*	75 ± 3*
ME	800	12 ± 0.5*	45 ± 2*
ME	1000	6 ± 1*	112 ± 3*

a dose-dependent reduction in the number of head dips in the hole-board test similar and/or greater than diazepam (Tables 1 and 2). It is generally believed that locomotor activity results from brain activation, which is manifested as an excitation of central neurons involving different neurochemical mechanism and an increase in cerebral metabolism. It is possible that the sedative activity of methanolic and aqueous extract of Lavandula officinalis is mediated by GABAergic pathway, since GABAergic transmission can produce profound sedation in mice [27]. The inhibitory action of GABA consists in the opening of chloride channels to allow hyperpolarizing the membrane, leading to CNS depression and resulting in sedative and hypnosis activity. Glutamate and GABA are quantitatively the most important excitatory and inhibitory neurotransmitters, respectively, in the mammalian brain [28]. Thus, receptors for these two neurotransmitters are regarded as important targets for psychotropic drugs. In the test of thiopental-induced sleep in mice, the potentiated effect of lavender extract in mice was represented. It not only prolonged the sleeping time but also decreased the latency of falling asleep and increases the rat of sleep onset. The lavender extract has produced hypnosis at high doses' that is, 800 and 1000 mg/kg. Since the effect of thiopental on the CNS involves the activation of the inhibition GABAergic system [29, 30], this finding suggests that some constituents in lavender extract produce facilitation of this inhibitory system (Table 3). Phytochemical studies have identified active components in this plant such as coumarin, chalcones, flavanones, flavones, flavonols, quercetin, and kaempferol derivatives, suggesting that they are the main responsible for sedative and hypnotic activities [4, 6, 31]. Further chemical and pharmacological analysis of the extract will be conducted to isolate and characterize the active principles responsible for the sedative and hypnotic effect. In conclusion, p.o. administration of methanolic and aqueous extract of Lavandula officinalis induces similar sedative effects, supporting its use in folk medicine. Given that the LD$_{50}$ value for these extracts was beyond 5000 mg/kg for oral administration, as determined by Litchfield and Wilcoxon [12]; our results suggest a remote risk of acute toxicity and good tolerance of these extracts in traditional medicine. To sum up, this work represents that the methanolic and aqueous extracts of *Lavandula officinalis* have obvious sedative and hypnotic activity; these data provide pharmacological basis for its therapeutic efficacy on insomnia.

Acknowledgments

The authors wish to thank all the individuals and institutions who made this survey possible.

References

[1] J. Bellakhdar, *La pharmacopée Marocaine traditionnelle*, Ibis Press, 1997.

[2] A. Tahraoui, J. El-Hilaly, Z. H. Israili, and B. Lyoussi, "Ethnopharmacological survey of plants used in the traditional treatment of hypertension and diabetes in south-eastern Morocco (Errachidia province)," *Journal of Ethnopharmacology*, vol. 110, no. 1, pp. 105–117, 2007.

[3] J. El-Hilaly, M. Hmammouchi, and B. Lyoussi, "Ethnobotanical studies and economic evaluation of medicinal plants in Taounate province (Northern Morocco)," *Journal of Ethnopharmacology*, vol. 86, no. 2-3, pp. 149–158, 2003.

[4] F. Huang, Y. Xiong, L. Xu, S. Ma, and C. Dou, "Sedative and hypnotic activities of the ethanol fraction from Fructus Schisandrae in mice and rats," *Journal of Ethnopharmacology*, vol. 110, no. 3, pp. 471–475, 2007.

[5] M. Herrera-Ruiz, C. Gutiérrez, J. Enrique Jiménez-Ferrer, J. Tortoriello, G. Mirón, and I. León, "Central nervous system depressant activity of an ethyl acetate extract from Ipomoea stans roots," *Journal of Ethnopharmacology*, vol. 112, no. 2, pp. 243–247, 2007.

[6] G. Pérez-Ortega, P. Guevara-Fefer, M. Chávez et al., "Sedative and anxiolytic efficacy of Tilia americana var. mexicana inflorescences used traditionally by communities of State of Michoacan, Mexico," *Journal of Ethnopharmacology*, vol. 116, no. 3, pp. 461–468, 2008.

[7] J. Bellakhdar, R. Claisse, J. Fleurentin, and C. Younos, "Repertory of standard herbal drugs in the Moroccan pharmacopoea," *Journal of Ethnopharmacology*, vol. 35, no. 2, pp. 123–143, 1991.

[8] M. Haloui, L. Louedec, J.-B. Michel, and B. Lyoussi, "Experimental diuretic effects of Rosmarinus officinalis and Centaurium erythraea," *Journal of Ethnopharmacology*, vol. 71, no. 3, pp. 465–472, 2000.

[9] K. Tawaha, F. Q. Alali, M. Gharaibeh, M. Mohammad, and T. El-Elimat, "Antioxidant activity and total phenolic content of selected Jordanian plant species," *Food Chemistry*, vol. 104, no. 4, pp. 1372–1378, 2007.

[10] K. Munchid, F. Sadiq, A. Tissent et al., "P214 Cytotoxicité De L'huile Essentielle De Rosmarinus Officinalis," *Transfusion Clinique et Biologique*, vol. 12, no. S1, pp. S135–S136, 2005.

[11] V. Hajhashemi, A. Ghannadi, and B. Sharif, "Anti-inflammatory and analgesic properties of the leaf extracts and essential oil of Lavandula angustifolia Mill," *Journal of Ethnopharmacology*, vol. 89, no. 1, pp. 67–71, 2003.

[12] J. T. Litchfield and F. Wilcoxon, "A simplified method of evaluating dose-effect experiments," *Journal of Pharmacology and Experimental Therapeutics*, vol. 96, pp. 99–113, 1949.

[13] D. Lorke, "A new approach to practical acute toxicity testing," *Archives of Toxicology*, vol. 54, no. 4, pp. 275–287, 1983.

[14] K. Alaoui, M. Belabbes, Y. Cherrah et al., "Acute and chronic toxicity of saponins of Argania spinosa," *Annales Pharmaceutiques Francaises*, vol. 56, no. 5, pp. 213–219, 1998.

[15] W. R. Thompson and C. S. Weil, "On the construction of tables for moving-average interpolation," *Biometrics*, vol. 8, no. 1, pp. 51–54, 1952.

[16] F. F. Perazzo, J. C. T. Carvalho, J. E. Carvalho, and V. L. G. Rehder, "Central properties of the essential oil and the crude ethanol extract from aerial parts of Artemisia annua L," *Pharmacological Research*, vol. 48, no. 5, pp. 497–502, 2003.

[17] S. Courvoisier, R. Ducrot, and L. Julou, *Psychotropic Drugs*, S. Garattini and V. Ghetti, Eds., Elsevier, Amsterdam, The Netherlands, 1957.

[18] M. J. Laroche and F. Rousselet, *Les animaux de laboratoire: éthique et bonnes pratiques*, Masson, Paris, France, 1990.

[19] G. Hoffman, *Les animaux de laboratoire (précis)*, Vigot Frères, Paris, France, 1963.

[20] G. Clark, A. G. Koester, and D. W. Pearson, "Exploratory behavior in chronic disulfoton poisoning in mice," *Psychopharmacologia*, vol. 20, no. 2, pp. 169–171, 1971.

[21] S. E. File and A. G. Wardill, "Validity of head dipping as a measure of exploration in a modified hole board," *Psychopharmacologia*, vol. 44, no. 1, pp. 53–59, 1975.

[22] E. Williamson, D. Okpako, and F. J. Evans, *Selection, Preparation, and Pharmacological Evaluation of Plant Material*, John Wiley & Sons, Chichester, UK, 1996.

[23] R. Tisserand, *The Art of Aromatherapy*, C. W. Daniel, Essex, UK, 1993.

[24] J. Lehrner, G. Marwinski, S. Lehr, P. Johren, and L. Deecke, "Ambient odors of orange and lavender reduce anxiety and improve mood in a dental office," *Physiology and Behavior*, vol. 86, no. 1-2, pp. 92–95, 2005.

[25] T. Umezu, K. Nagano, H. Ito, K. Kosakai, M. Sakaniwa, and M. Morita, "Anticonflict effects of lavender oil and identification of its active constituents," *Pharmacology Biochemistry and Behavior*, vol. 85, no. 4, pp. 713–721, 2006.

[26] P. P. Roy-Byrne, "The GABA-benzodiazepine receptor complex: structure, function, and role in anxiety," *Journal of Clinical Psychiatry*, vol. 66, no. 2, pp. 14–20, 2005.

[27] C. Gottesmann, "GABA mechanisms and sleep," *Neuroscience*, vol. 111, no. 2, pp. 231–239, 2002.

[28] H. P. Rang, M. M. Dale, J. M. Ritter, and P. K. Moore, *Pharmacology*, Churchill Livingstone, Edinburgh, UK, 2007.

[29] J. H. Steinbach and G. Akk, "Modulation of GABAA receptor channel gating by pentobarbital," *Journal of Physiology*, vol. 537, no. 3, pp. 715–733, 2001.

[30] S. P. Sivam, T. Nabeshima, and I. K. Ho, "Acute and chronic effects of pentobarbital in relation to postsynaptic GABA receptors: a study with muscimol," *Journal of Neuroscience Research*, vol. 7, no. 1, pp. 37–47, 1982.

[31] G. Zapata-Sudo, T. C. F. Mendes, M. A. Kartnaller et al., "Sedative and anticonvulsant activities of methanol extract of Dorstenia arifolia in mice," *Journal of Ethnopharmacology*, vol. 130, no. 1, pp. 9–12, 2010.

21

Allosteric Modulation of Beta1 Integrin Function Induces Lung Tissue Repair

Rehab AlJamal-Naylor,[1] Linda Wilson,[2] Susan McIntyre,[3] Fiona Rossi,[4] Beth Harrison,[3] Mark Marsden,[4] and David J. Harrison[3]

[1] *Avipero Ltd., 5th Floor, 125 Princes Street, Edinburgh EH2 4AD, UK*
[2] *School of Biomedical Sciences, The University of Edinburgh, Hugh Robson Building, George Square, Edinburgh EH8 9XD, UK*
[3] *Division of Pathology, Institute of Genetics and Molecular Medicine, The University of Edinburgh, Western General Hospital, Edinburgh EH4 2XU, UK*
[4] *MRC Centre for Inflammation Research, The Queen's Medical Research Institute, The University of Edinburgh, 47 Little France Crescent, Edinburgh EH16 4TJ, UK*

Correspondence should be addressed to Rehab AlJamal-Naylor, r.aljamal.naylor@avipero.com

Academic Editor: Chi Hin Cho

The cellular cytoskeleton, adhesion receptors, extracellular matrix composition, and their spatial distribution are together fundamental in a cell's balanced mechanical sensing of its environment. We show that, in lung injury, extracellular matrix-integrin interactions are altered and this leads to signalling alteration and mechanical missensing. The missensing, secondary to matrix alteration and cell surface receptor alterations, leads to increased cellular stiffness, injury, and death. We have identified a monoclonal antibody against β1 integrin which caused matrix remodelling and enhancement of cell survival. The antibody acts as an allosteric dual agonist/antagonist modulator of β1 integrin. Intriguingly, this antibody reversed both functional and structural tissue injury in an animal model of degenerative disease in lung.

1. Introduction

Tissue regeneration comprises dedifferentiation of adult cells into a stem cell state and the development of these cells into new remodelled tissue, identical to the lost one. Tissue repair is defined as replacement of normal tissue by fibrous tissue and integrins are crucial in these processes.

Integrins are membrane spanning proteins facilitating the two-way communication between the inside and outside of a cell. Integrins have the capacity to bind a multitude of molecules both inside and outside of the cell. The binding of these molecules results in the transmission of information into and out of the cell, which can influence a host of different cellular functions, including the cells metabolic activity.

Of the many types of integrin receptors, the β1 integrin is by far the most ubiquitous allowing cells to detect a vast array of stimuli ranging between toxins, protein hormones, neurotransmitters, and macromolecules. There have been numerous publications documenting a potential role of β1 integrin in tissue development and repair in several tissue types (reviewed in [1]). It is clear that β1 integrin plays a crucial role during postnatal skin development and wound healing, with the loss of epithelial β1 integrin causing extensive skin blistering and wound healing defects. More recently, there has been active interest in the cosmeceutical development of β1 integrin targeting formulations. One such example is following the discovery of fucoidans from *Fucus vesiculosus* and its effect on skin scarring and ageing [2, 3] which was later found to be mainly attributed to alpha2 and β1 integrin [4].

Integrins in general, including β1 integrin, exhibit global structural rearrangement and exposure of ligand binding sites upon activation [5]. The overall strength of cellular adhesiveness, or avidity, is governed by affinity and valency (which is in turn governed by the density of the receptor and its ligand on the cell surface, as well as the spatial and geometric arrangement and movement) [5]. Recent evidence has demonstrated that both affinity and avidity of integrins are strongly related to the size of the focal adhesion clusters [6, 7]. Overall, integrins have three main possible conformations of the extracellular domain; a low affinity, bent conformation; extended conformation with closed headpiece representing an intermediate affinity state; the ligand-binding-induced high-affinity extended form, with an open headpiece [8–10].

Altered conformation of integrins rather than expression levels have been reported both during physiological and pathological remodelling processes which include neurite outgrowth, fibrosis, asthma, cancer, and wound healing amongst many [11–14]. To successfully develop disease modifying therapy, it should be beneficial to rescue or replenish dying or dead cells by activating inherent repair processes other than simply stem cell regeneration. In other words, altering the interaction of the cells with other cells and their abnormal surroundings to promote their survival and continued function may alleviate chronic, ongoing cell loss, a hallmark of many progressive degenerative diseases. We hypothesised that tissue repair might be achieved by rescueing cells from death by mechanically dampening the signals cells receive from their abnormal environment. One key cell surface receptor for adhesion is β1 integrin. We considered that conformational modulation of β1 integrin may cause alteration in cytoskeletal organization and cell stiffness leading to increase susceptibility to oxidative stress and death and thus that prevention of these changes may have therapeutic benefit. Here, we show how we have identified a specific β1 integrin targeting modality using a monoclonal antibody, which we have demonstrated, both protects from tissue injury and facilitates repair. The antibody acts as an allosteric dual agonist/antagonist modulator of β1 integrin and resulted in increased matrix remodelling and enhancement of cell survival.

2. Results

2.1. The Effects of β1 Integrin Modulation on Elastase-Induced Signalling. As a model of tissue remodelling in disease, we investigated the activity of β1 integrin using an *in vitro* model of elastase-induced injury. A coculture of primary, adult human lung fibroblasts was overlayered with NCI-H441 lung cells, under cyclic mechanical stimulation, and subjected to elastase treatment.

To investigate the involvement of β1 integrin activation in elastase-induced signalling, we used three different monoclonal antibodies against β1 integrin. The first was the adhesion blocking clone, JB1a, which is said to target primarily the amino acids 82–87 comprising part of the hybrid domain [15]. We also used the adhesion blocking clone, AIIB2, which binds amino acid residues 207–218 within the A-domain [16], and K20, widely reported to have no functional effects which binds the hybrid/EGF repeat region [17].

Addition of elastase to cell culture induced an increased phosphorylation of signalling proteins known to act downstream of β1 integrin (Figure 1(a)). During the course of injury, pAKT levels increased, followed by transient increases in phospho-cJUN and phospho-JNK (Figure 1(a)). No significant changes were detected for 12 other phosphoproteins at the sampled time points.

When β1 integrin was bound by antibody clone JB1a in the absence of injury, there was no significant effect on downstream signalling. However, when JB1a was added during elastase-induced injury, it abrogated all elastase-induced changes in phosphorylation of signalling proteins. This effect was not seen with either AIIB2 or K20 (Figure 2(a)).

2.2. The Effects of Elastase-Induced Injury on β1 Integrin Activity and Localisation. We next examined the effects of elastase on ligand-binding activity of β1 integrin using the ligand competent specific anti-β1 integrin antibody 9EG7. Ligand competent state can be any of the intermediate physiological conformations or the fully activated extended conformation [19]. Elastase caused an increase in ligand competent/active β1 integrin expression as evident from the staining pattern in Figure 1(b). Modulation of β1 integrin, using JB1a, abrogated the elastase-induced increase in ligand-competent β1 integrin (Figure 1(b)). However, the anti-β1 integrin clone K20 potentiated the elastase-induced increase in the ligand-competent conformation (Figure 2(b)).

The effects of elastase and JB1a on the level of ligand-competent receptor were not simply a result of change in cell surface expression (Figure 1(c)). However, preliminary measurements showed that elastase increased the cytosolic fraction-associated β1 integrin which might be attributed to recycling or degradation. To address that we conducted a time course analyses of β1 integrin in membrane fractions. Elastase induced a change in β1 integrin recycling, an effect inhibited by JB1a but not K20 (Figure 3). Further evidence of elastase-induced β1 integrin activation was the increase of caveolin-1 phosphorylation after two hours of exposure to elastase; changes once again inhibited by JB1a (Figure 4).

2.3. The Conformational Effects of JB1a on β1 Integrin. To further determine the pharmacological mode of action of JB1a action, we questioned whether the effect seen with JB1a is due to its effect on β1 integrin chain allostery. We first estimated the location of the epitope of JB1a on the basis of the theoretical 3-dimensional structure of β1 integrin (Figure 5(a)). We then conducted FRET studies using nonadherent Jurkat cells. FITC-labelled LDV cyclic peptide was used to label the head of alpha4β1 integrin, and the lipophilic dye R18 was used to label the cell membrane. LDV-FITC acts as a donor and R18 as an acceptor [20]. FACS was used for the FRET acquisition and measurement. JB1a caused a conformational activation when added at baseline and inhibited the full conformational activation induced by the divalent cation, Mn^{2+}. The JB1a-induced change resulting in FRET efficiency was indicative of an intermediate partially extended conformation when compared to Mn^{2+} and other known inhibitory or activating antibodies (Figures 5(b)–5(e)).

Taking together these findings indicated that the pharmacological mode of action of JB1a-mediated effect on β1 integrin is as an allosteric dual agonist/antagonist.

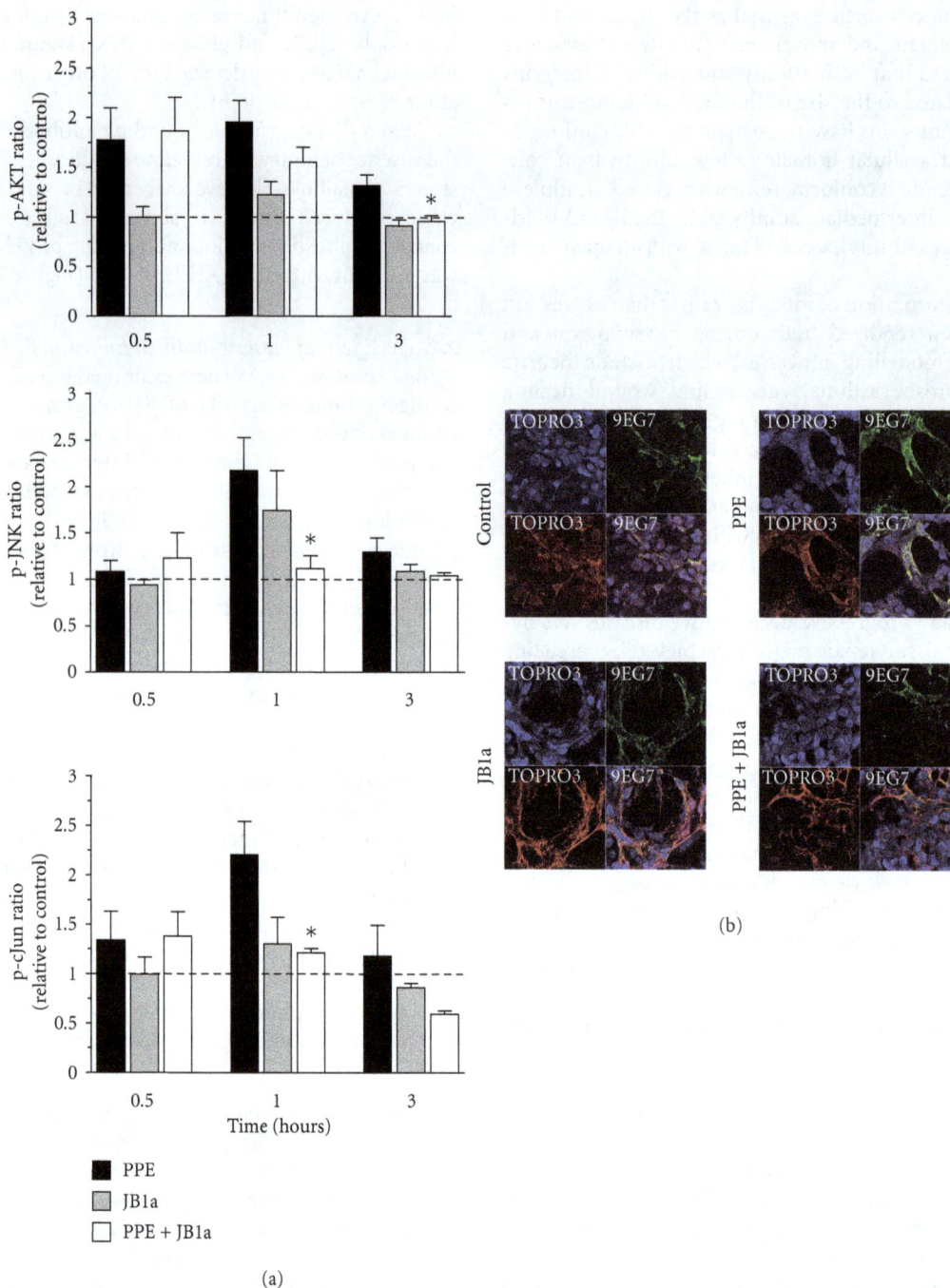

FIGURE 1: The effects of PPE-induced injury and JB1a treatment on (a) activation of signalling downstream of beta1 integrin during mechanical stretch (asterisks denote statistical significance with $P < 0.05$ in comparison to PPE) and (b) beta1 integrin conformational activation indicated by increase in staining using the anti-β1 integrin antibody 9EG7 recognising the ligand competent receptor in comparison to staining using nonconformation dependent antibody (K20).

2.4. Conformational Modulation of β1 Integrin Inhibits Elastase-Induced Changes in Cell Membrane Composition. Using mixed epithelial-mesenchymal in vitro cultures, we found that elastase increased neutral sphingomyelinase activity transiently; an effect inhibited by β1 integrin binding by antibody JB1a (Figure 6(a)). No effect on acid sphingomyelinase was detected under the same conditions.

2.5. Conformational Modulation of β1 Integrin Inhibits Elastase-Induced Changes in Actin Polymerisation and Cellular Impedance. Using our in vitro culture system, we tracked incorporation of labelled monomeric actin, and demonstrated an increase in de novo F-actin formation during the course of elastase-induced injury (Figures 6(b), 12, and S1–S3 in Supplementary Material available online at

(a)

(b)

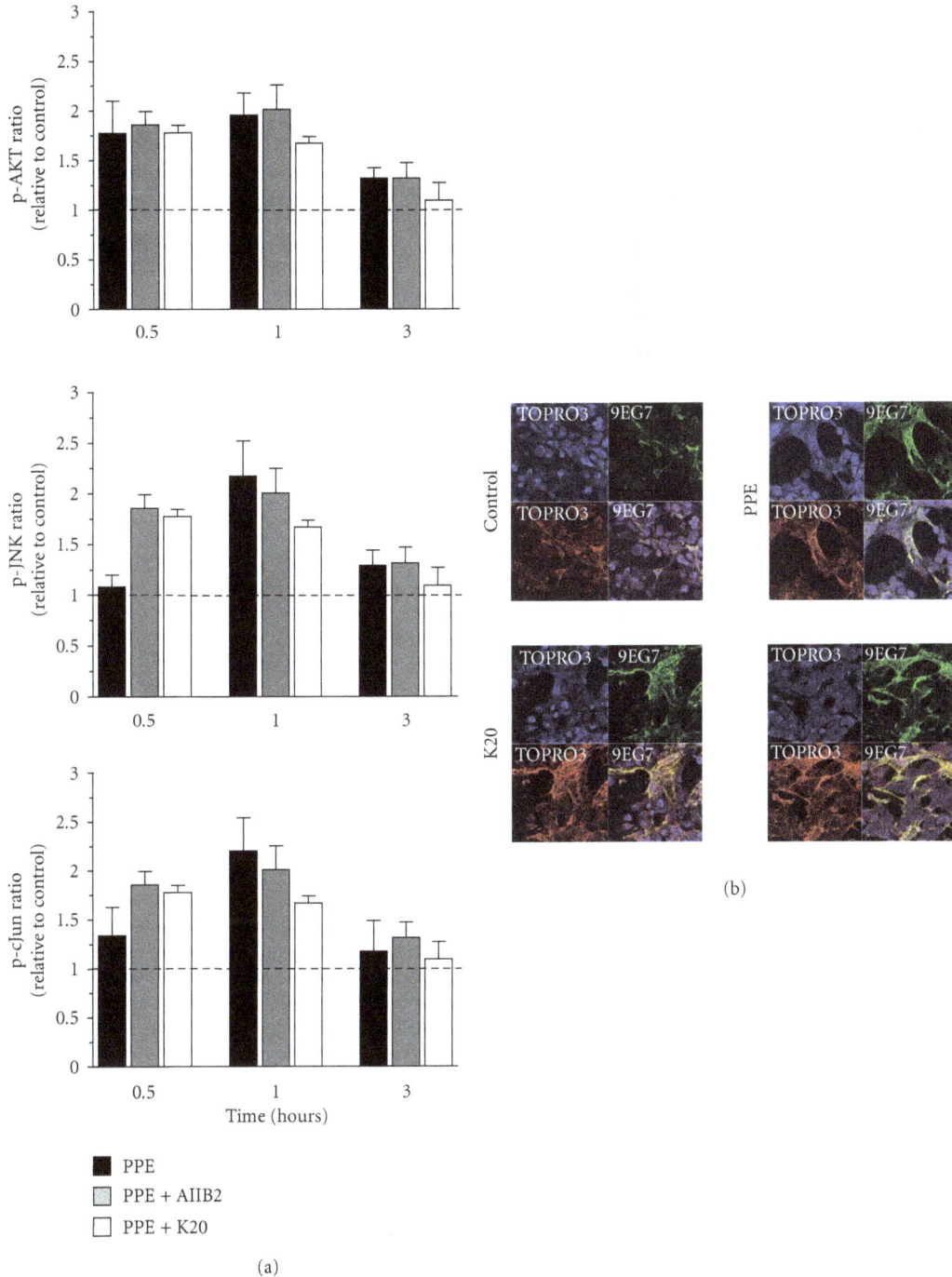

FIGURE 2: The effects of PPE-induced injury and targeting beta1 integrin using AIIB2 and K20 clones on (a) activation of signalling downstream of beta1 integrin during mechanical stretch (asterisks denotes statistical significance with $P < 0.05$ in comparison to PPE) and (b) beta1 integrin conformational activation indicated by increase in staining using the anti-β1 integrin antibody 9EG7 recognising the ligand competent receptor in comparison to staining using nonconformation dependent antibody (K20).

doi:10.1155/2012/768720). Formation of F-actin from monomeric G-actin is energy dependent, and, under ATP depletion conditions, there is a net conversion of monomeric G-actin to polymeric F-actin. In cocultures, elastase reduced the levels of ATP, but this response was inhibited by JB1a (Figure 6(c)).

To corroborate the finding on cellular mechanical properties, we investigated the effect of elastase on cellular impedance. There was an initial drop and recovery in impedance after change of media consistent with responses to sudden stretch, as reported previously [21]. JB1a inhibited the elastase-induced decrease in cellular impedance (Figure 6(d)).

(a)

(b)

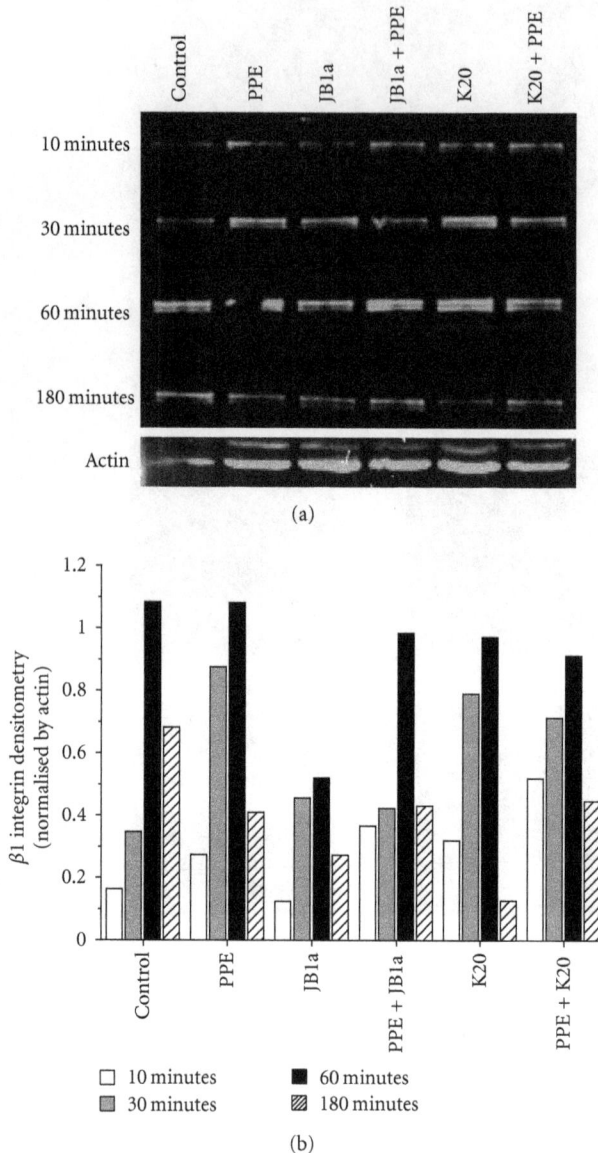

FIGURE 3: The effects of PPE-induced injury (0.6 U/mL) and targeting beta1 integrin using JB1a (1 ug/mL) in comparison to K20 (1 ug/mL) clone on the kinetics of beta1 integrin levels on cell membrane *in vitro* using human lung coculture. (a) Western blot of the cell membrane expression of $\beta 1$ integrin over time. Protein extracts were loaded at equal protein concentration (25 μg). (b) Densitometric analyses of the blot corrected using actin as an internal control.

2.6. Conformational Modulation of $\beta 1$ Integrin Inhibits Elastase-Induced Caspase Activation.

We then investigated the effect of elastase on caspase activation and the role of $\beta 1$ integrin in elastase-induced cell death. Elastase induced caspase activation after 3-hour exposure and led to detachment induced apoptosis of epithelial cells (anoikis) (Figures 7(a) and S1–S3). Modulation of $\beta 1$ integrin using JB1a prevented caspase activation. However, the potently inhibitory anti-$\beta 1$ integrin antibody 6S6, which is also known to induce homotypic aggregation, induced caspase activation (Figure 7(b)).

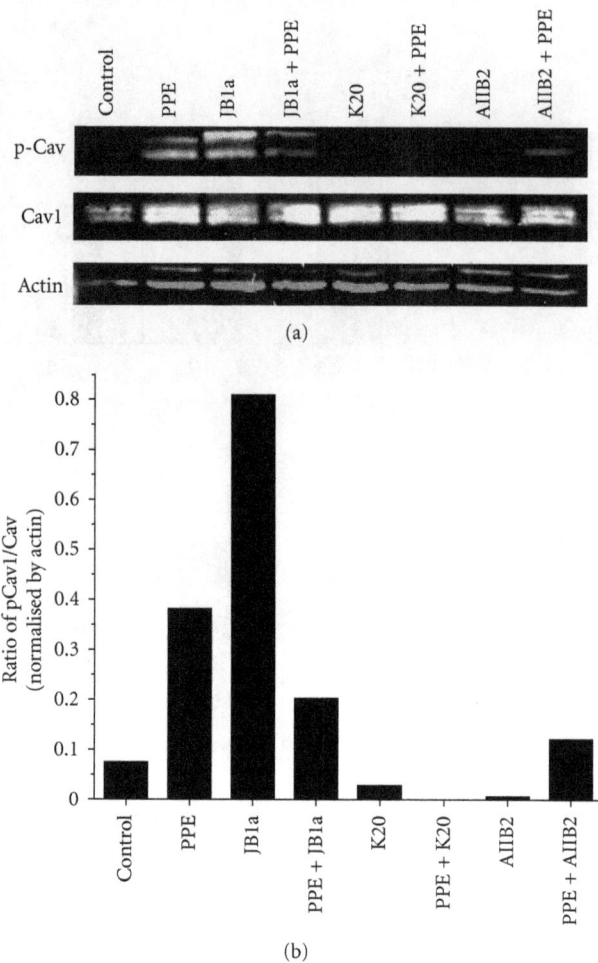

(a)

(b)

FIGURE 4: The effects of PPE-induced injury (0.6 U/mL) and targeting beta1 integrin using AIIB2 (1 ug/mL) and K20 (1 ug/mL) clones on phosphorylated caveolin-1 levels in membrane fractions. (a) Representative blots from $n = 4$. Loading controlled by total amount of protein (50 μg). (b) Densitometric analyses of the blot corrected using actin as an internal control.

2.7. Conformational Modulation of $\beta 1$ Integrin Reversed Elastase-Induced Emphysema in Mice.

To investigate the significance of $\beta 1$ integrin in injury in a disease setting in which remodelling is a key component, we established a murine model of emphysema caused by intratracheal installation of elastase. Mice were instilled with elastase on day 1 and lung injury ensued. At later timepoints, they were treated with the anti-$\beta 1$ integrin monoclonal antibody, JB1a which binds $\beta 1$ integrin in mouse tissues [22], or vehicle, either once on day 14 (21 day group, 21 d) or on days 21 and 28 (35 day group, 35 d). In a subsequent investigation, severe emphysema was induced and JB1a and B44 clones were instilled on days 21 and 28 before lung function assessment on day 35. Both clones demonstrated cross-reactivity with murine $\beta 1$ integrin (Figure 8).

By 21 days after elastase injury, there was a marked progressive leftward shift in the respiratory pressure-volume curve (PV) of close-chested mice, particularly in the 35 day

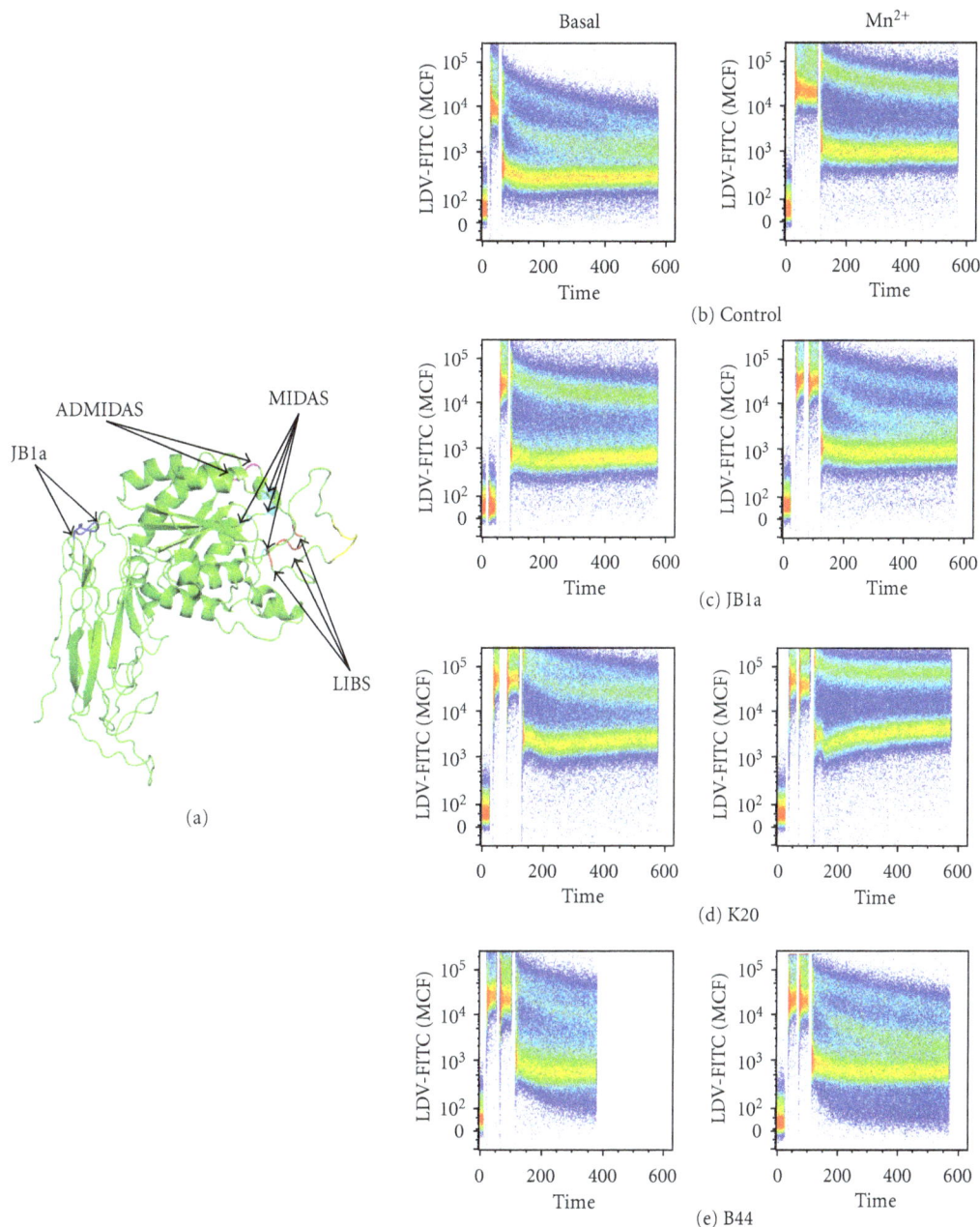

FIGURE 5: (a) The location of JB1a epitope as mapped by Ni and Wilkins [15] produced using polyview 3D as described in [18] http://polyview.cchmc.org/polyview3d.html FRET analyses demonstrating. (b) the baseline conformation of beta1 integrin and following Mn^{2+}-induced integrin activation. The effect of JB1a (c), K20 (d), and B44 (e) on integrin at baseline and on Mn^{2+}-induced integrin activation detected by FRET using the LDV-FITC small molecule and R18 in Jurkat cells. LDV binding is plotted as mean channel fluorescence (MCF) versus time.

group (Figure 9(a)). JB1a, given as a single intratracheal dose at this time point, reversed the loss of respiratory elastic recoil induced by elastase treatment (Figure 9(b)).

In addition to the reversal of functional characteristics, treatment with JB1a was associated by structural repair, assessed by histology and morphometry (Figure 9(c)). In elastase-treated lungs, apoptosis was demonstrated by the TUNEL assay at 21 and 35 days, even in the absence of inflammation. This was prevented by JB1a treatment (Figure 9(d)). There was no change in cellular proliferation as assessed by immunostaining for Ki67. The efficacy of $\beta 1$ integrin modulation using the clone JB1a was evident even in more severe injury when a higher dose of elastase was used. (Figure 10).

When we tested the effect of $\beta 1$ integrin modulation using JB1a in comparison to the clone B44 following the same

(a)

Control   PPE

PPE + JB1a

(b)

(c)

(d)

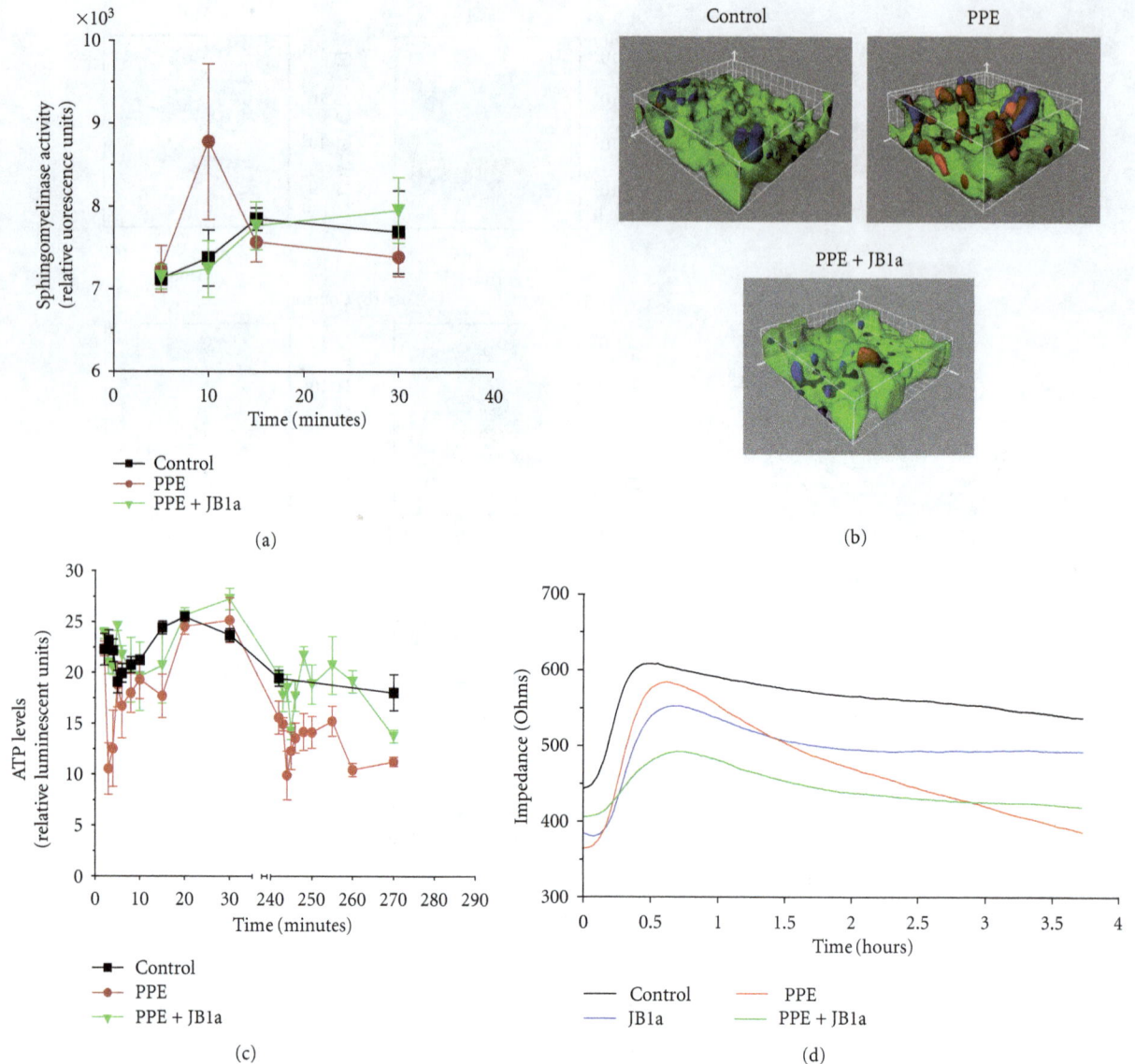

FIGURE 6: The effects of PPE-induced injury (0.6 U/mL) and JB1a treatment (1 ug/mL) *in vitro* using human lung coculture cultured on collagen-coated surfaces. The effects measured were on (a) neutral sphingomyelinase activity one on cultures subjected to mechanical stretch of 2–10% amplitude at 1 Hz ($n = 3$), (b) F-actin using 3D reconstruction of images of human lung coculture after injury using elastase demonstrating the formation of F-actin (blue) and caspase 3/7 activation (red). Ganglioside GM1 for the cell membrane-green and its inhibition by JB1a done on cells cultured on glass ($n = 3$), (c) ATP levels ($n = 3$ and each included separate measurements of cells cultured in 8 wells in 96-well plates). (d) Cellular electrical impedance ($n = 3$).

protocol of the 35 day group, B44 had no significant effect at a comparable dose (Figures 11(a) and 11(b)). The clone B44 bears the closest resemblance in its conformational effect to the JB1a from our FRET results. In parallel studies, we tested the potent inhibitory antibody, 6S6 known to induce homotypic aggregation. Whilst 6S6 had no effect in control animals, its effect on elastase-treated animals was detrimental and worsened injury corroborating it proapoptotic effect *in vitro*.

3. Discussion

In this paper we have investigated the role of $\beta 1$ integrin in lung injury and repair in emphysema. We demonstrated that

$\beta 1$ integrin becomes allosterically activated in epithelial-mesenchymal cells, with the corollary that allosteric modulation inhibited elastase-induced injury. We further demonstrate a potential cellular mechanism for this $\beta 1$ integrin-mediated effect. In order to do so, we established an *in vitro* model system which replicated features of elastase-induced emphysema *in vivo*. We identified that allosteric modulation of $\beta 1$ integrin inhibited caspase activation, F-actin aggregate formation, and abnormal fluctuations in cellular ATP levels, under conditions in which the total $\beta 1$ expression was changed and activation inhibited. The key finding of our investigation was that, by direct allosteric modulation of $\beta 1$ integrin with a specific monoclonal antibody, both functional and structural reversal of elastase-induced tissue injury was induced *in vivo*.

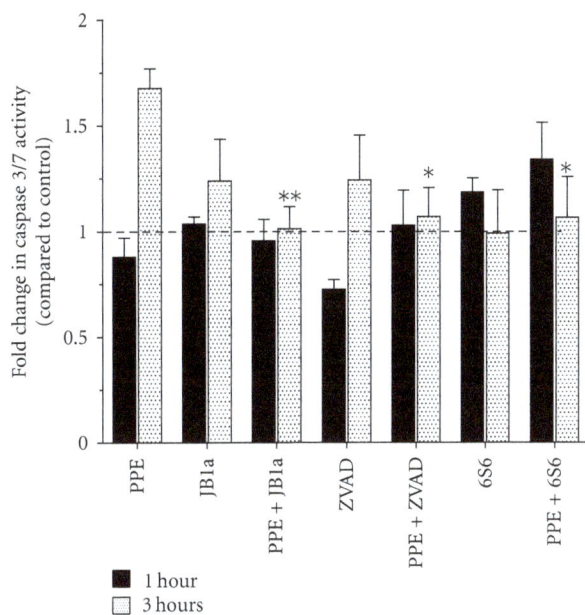

FIGURE 7: The effects of PPE-induced injury (0.6 U/mL) and targeting beta1 integrin using JB1a (1 ug/mL) in comparison to 6S6 clone (1 ug/mL) and the broad spectrum caspase inhibitor, ZVAD-fmk, on caspase 3/7 activation *in vitro* using human lung coculture during mechanical stretch ($n = 3$). Asterisks denotes statistical significance with $*P < 0.05$ and $**P < 0.005$ in comparison to PPE.

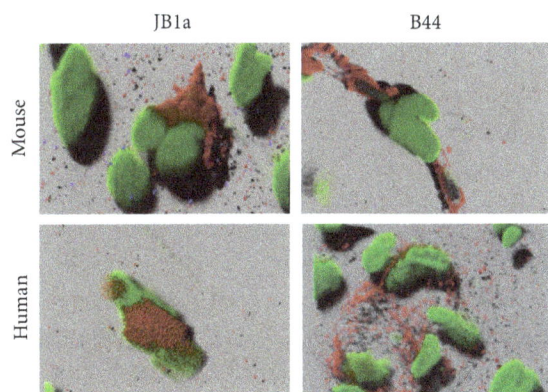

FIGURE 8: JB1a and B44 immunoreactivity with beta1 integrin verification on human tissues and their cross-reactivity with beta1 integrin in mouse tissue. Images were collected using ×40 oil lens and Zeiss LSM510 CLSM microscope with nyquist settings. The resulting images were deconvolved, and three-dimensional images were reconstructed using Huygens software (Scientific Volume Imaging (SVI), The Netherlands).

Our findings support the notion that cytomechanics are important determinants of cell fate and effect repair.

Upon activation, integrin-linked kinase (ILK) binds to the cytoplasmic domain of the $\beta1$ integrin subunit [23]. In turn, ILK activates multiples signalling pathways such as protein kinase B (PKB/AKT) and inhibits glycogen synthase kinase-3β (GSK-3β) activity affecting transcription factor binding to their DNA sequences [23–25]. We demonstrated

that elastase-induced injury activated signalling downstream of $\beta1$ integrin and this effect was modulated by targeting $\beta1$ integrin using the clone JB1a. Although JB1a is known as an inhibitory antibody, the effect on elastase-induced signalling was specific to JB1a since targeting $\beta1$ integrin using the inhibitory clone AIIB2 did not have the same effect nor did the clone K20. The elastase-induced activation of $\beta1$ integrin was corroborated by demonstrating that there was an increased detection of ligand-competent $\beta1$ integrin which was not caused by increased protein level but rather increased recycling. By contrast, the anti-$\beta1$ integrin clone K20 induced an increase in the ligand-competent conformation; an effect previously noted [26].

The separation of the alpha and β subunit legs is a critical step in integrin activation to transform the bent structure to an extended conformation, thus allowing headpiece-ligand engagement [8]. Therefore, we questioned whether the effect seen with JB1a is due to its effect on $\beta1$ integrin chain allostery. Indeed, targeting amino acid sequences within the same epitope of JB1a in the hybrid domain region using other antibodies has been reported to stabilise the physiological intermediate state of the receptor in a similar fashion as an allosteric antagonist [8]. We adopted an assay method used to detect conformational changes in integrin [20, 27] and found that, under baseline conditions, JB1a had an activating effect whilst it acted as a conformational antagonist when $\beta1$ integrin was activated with manganese. We have examined 8 other clones and determined that the clones closest to JB1a in its conformational effect were the B44 and HUTS 21 clones; both of which bind to the second hybrid domain of $\beta1$ integrin (reviewed in [1]). Therefore, adding to the reported effects of JB1a, we have shown that it functions both as an agonist and antagonist.

We then sought to elucidate the significance of integrin activation in response injury. Receptor clustering is, in part, aided by interactions with cellular proteins such as caveolins cell membrane fluidity. The composition of cell plasma membrane directly affects $\beta1$ integrin function and membrane fluidity in response to other types of injury [28, 29], reviewed in [1]. In using *in vitro* mixed epithelial-mesenchymal cultures, we found that elastase increased neutral sphingomyelinase activity transiently; an effect inhibited by $\beta1$ integrin binding by antibody JB1a. The association of neutral sphingomyelinase has been shown recently in cigarette smoke models of lung injury [30].

Gene disruption of caveolin-1, which is known to be involved in integrin clustering and activation, results in pulmonary fibrosis and impairment in liver regeneration after partial hepatectomy which was reversible by treatment with glucose [31], indicating the probable importance of energy preservation. Interestingly, previous reports have shown that $\beta1$ integrin-mediated adhesion regulates cholesterol-rich membrane microdomain internalisation mediated by phosphocaveolin-1 [32] and caveolar endocytosis can be blocked by small interfering RNA knockdown of $\beta1$ integrin [33]. Our finding that allosteric modulation inhibits elastase-induced caveolin phosphorylation reinforces the idea that, in injury, abnormal integrin activation and clustering contribute to cellular damage in elastase-induced injury.

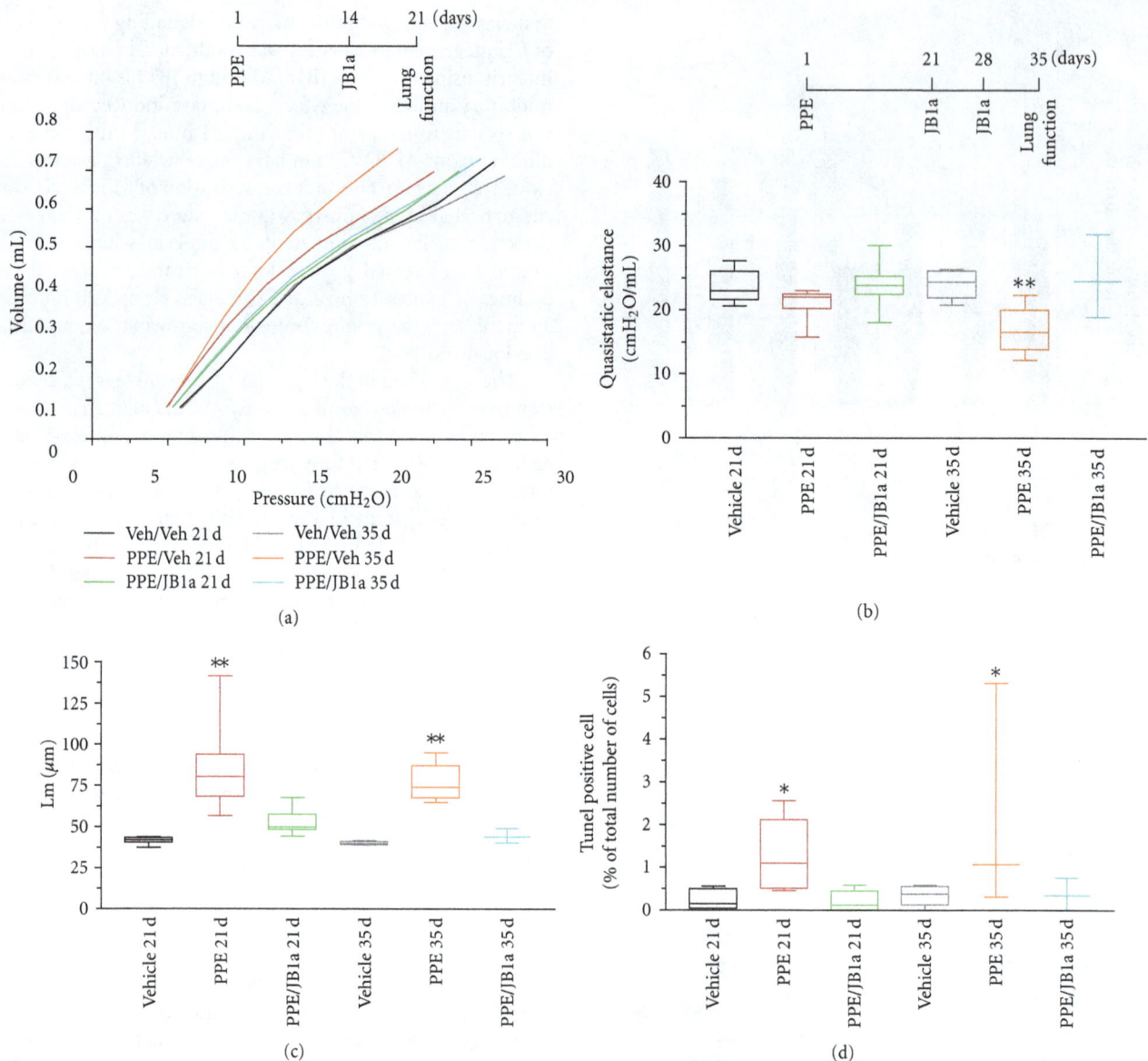

FIGURE 9: The effect of porcine pancreatic elastase (PPE, 0.2 U/g) on respiratory function in mice and its reversal using the anti-beta1 integrin antibody JB1a (3 mg/kg). (a) The effect of PPE on mean respiratory pressure-volume curves in mice from the 21days (21 d) and 35 days (35 d) after instillation and its reversal by JB1a (vehicle = Veh). (b) Reversal of PPE-induced increase in the quasistatic elastance between 5 and 9 cm H_2O by JB1a treatment at different time points after injury. (c) Mean linear intercept (Lm) measurements from the 21 d and 35 d groups. n = 5-6 in 35 d groups and n = 10 in 21 d groups. (d) TUNEL staining demonstrating the effect of JB1a treatment after PPE-induced lung injury. (c) quantification of TUNEL positive cells in lung tissue sections from 21 d and 35 d group following PPE-induced injury and JB1a treatment (n = 5-6 per group). Asterisks denote statistical significance with *$P < 0.05$, **$P < 0.005$ and ***$P < 0.0005$ in comparison to vehicle.

Integrin activation can occur via outside-inside and/or inside-outside signalling. We postulate from our results that outside-inside β1 integrin signalling and activation are induced during injury, possibly as a result of extracellular matrix degradation (reviewed in [1]). Matrix integrity has been shown to play a key role in various injuries including emphysema [34] and amyloid β neurotoxicity [35]. Indeed, unpublished data from our laboratory have shown that β1 integrin allosteric modulation using JB1a, but not 6S6 or TS2/16, caused an increase in perlecan [36]; a change

partially sensitive to pretreatment with cycloheximide and the nonspecific metalloproteinase (MMPs) activator aminophenylmercuric acetate (APMA). The changes in perlecan in response to JB1a were accompanied by an increase in tissue inhibitors of metalloproteinase-1 (TIMP1) initially and pro-MMP-9 subsequently.

Integrin activation can also occur due to cellular changes [37, 38]. Various reports highlighted the effect of plasma membrane lipid composition on β1 integrin function [29, 39, 40]. Ceramide increase during elastase-induced injury

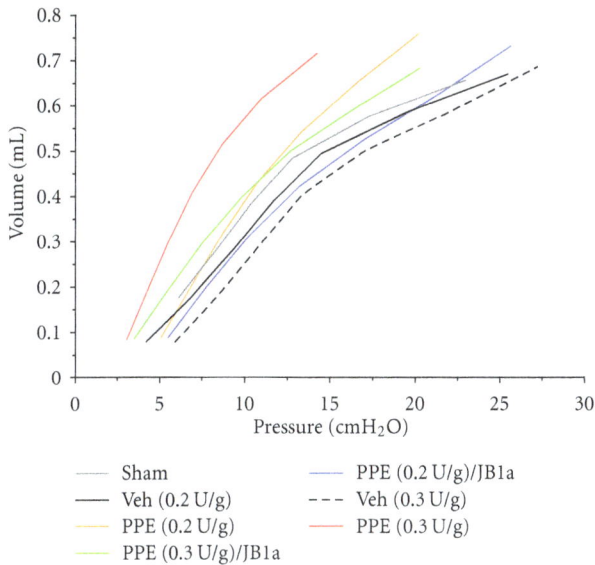

FIGURE 10: Dose-response of the effects of porcine pancreatic elastase (PPE, 0.2 U/g and 0.3 U/g) on respiratory function in mice and its reversal using the anti-beta1 integrin antibody JB1a. The effect of PPE on mean respiratory pressure-volume curves in mice from 35 days (35 d) after instillation and its reversal by JB1a (vehicle = Veh).

has been shown to cause apoptosis [30, 41]. We have shown that, upon the onset of elastase-induced injury, neutral sphingomyelinase increased which may have contributed to $\beta1$ integrin activation; an effect inhibited by modulation of $\beta1$ integrin using JB1a.

Integrin activation is associated with increased engagement with the actin cytoskeleton [42, 43]. More recently, actin polymerisation has been shown to be affected in cigarette smoke models [44]. We have investigated actin polymerisation in our *in vitro* system during the course of elastase-induced injury and the effect of $\beta1$ integrin modulation on the process. We used live cell imaging of labelled monomeric actin incorporation to ascertain de novo increase in the formation of actin aggregates since the phalloidin staining fails to demonstrate the newly formed aggregate. We were able to show an increase in actin aggregates during the course of elastase-induced injury. This effect was inhibited by modulation of $\beta1$ integrin.

We then investigated how elastase-induced injury impacted on ATP. Under ATP depletion conditions, there is a net conversion of monomeric G-actin to polymeric F-actin resulting from an alteration in the ratio of ATP-G-actin and ADP-G-actin with the resultant F-actin forming dispersed aggregates [45]. We chose to characterise ATP dynamic changes *in vitro* following elastase-induced injury. We found not only the levels were reduced after prolonged exposure but preceding this reduction, abnormal fluctuations were detected at the onset of exposure to elastase. These responses were inhibited by allosteric modulation of $\beta1$ integrin.

With changes in cell membrane composition and actin cytoskeleton, we sought to confirm if those changes have impacted on cellular mechanical properties. We have shown

that cellular impedance is altered during the course of elastase-induced injury and this effect was inhibited by modulation of $\beta1$ integrin. Although this measurement does not distinguish between effects caused by changes in cellular composition and cell-cell interaction, when taken together with evidence of alteration in actin polymerisation and cell membrane composition, it further supports our notion. There is strong evidence for the role of the state of the actin cytoskeleton on cell survival and differentiation which mainly came from studies focused on thymosin $\beta4$. Thymosin $\beta4$ functions mainly as a sequestering protein of actin monomers and promotes wound healing and cardiac repair by affecting cell survival [46].

Furthermore, we were able to show caspase activation in both end-point assays and real time. Elastase-induced caspase activation was inhibited by the modulation of $\beta1$ integrin. However, complete inhibition of $\beta1$ integrin using 6S6 clone (potent inhibitor and inducer of homotypic aggregation) has activated caspase.

Our findings support the hypothesis that cellular mechanics play a key part in cell fate and therefore affect repair. To investigate this in a disease setting in which remodelling is a key component, we established a murine model of emphysema caused by intratracheal instillation of elastase. Emphysema is an irreversible component of chronic obstructive pulmonary disease, a major cause of morbidity and mortality worldwide.

We hypothesised that, in irreversible moderately severe emphysema, $\beta1$ integrin becomes allosterically activated, with the corollary that only then might allosteric modulation become therapeutically beneficial. The expression of activation epitopes of $\beta1$ integrin, hence a fully extended active conformation, in human disease is poorly understood due to the technical limitations. However, recently, the presence of ligand competent $\beta1$ integrin in eosinophils from induced sputum samples of asthmatic patients was investigated and found to correlate with airway hyperresponsiveness [47]. Modulation of $\beta1$ integrin using JB1a reversed elastase-induced emphysema when administered at the two different time points after the onset and stabilisation of emphysema. It had no effect on vehicle instilled animals. This was confirmed by both unconscious lung function testing and structural analyses using the mean linear intercept. We have also previously determined that modulating $\beta1$ integrin function allows septation to proceed in damaged lungs by altering the pool of GATA-6 and TTF-1 expressing cells [48].

Although, the clone B44, which had the closest effect to JB1a-induced conformational effect, showed some effect on elastase-induced lung function abnormalities, it has decreased lung compliance in normal animals. We have not yet determined whether the clone B44 has induced fibrosis or alteration in airway responsiveness to account for the observed functional effects.

Thus targeting $\beta1$ integrin with JB1a induced previously unseen disease-modifying effects. The key event, evident from our research, is the synergistic alteration of cell surface receptor distribution leading to alteration in receptor activity state and changes in the cell membrane composition. This effect makes cells more adaptable to their altered mechanical

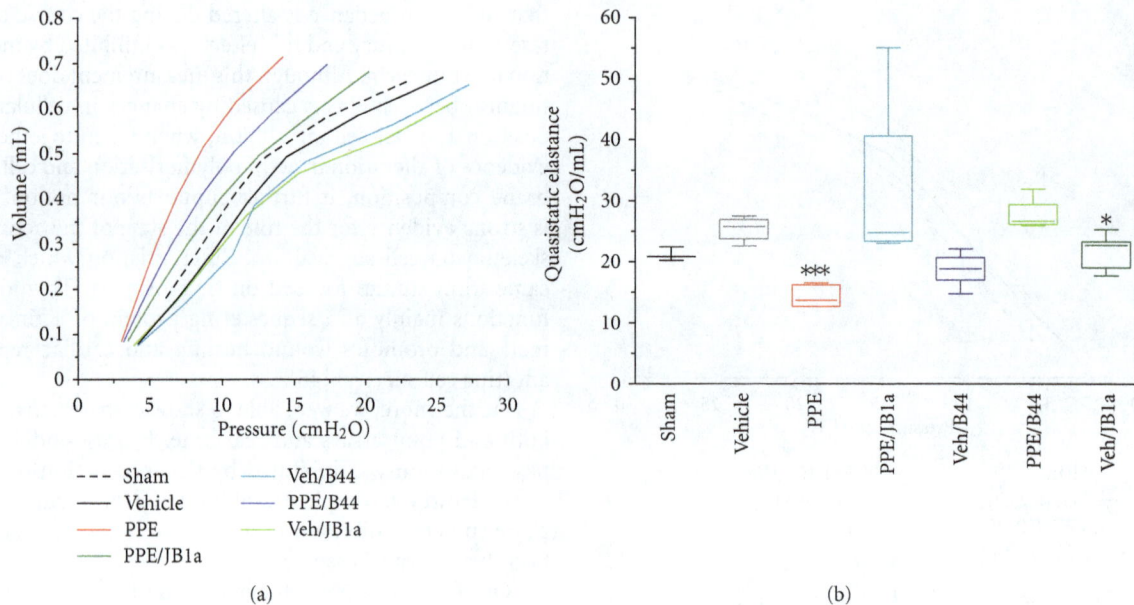

(a)

(b)

FIGURE 11: The effects of porcine pancreatic elastase (PPE, 0.3 U/g) on respiratory function in mice and its reversal using the anti-beta1 integrin antibody JB1a (3 mg/kg) in comparison to the anti-beta1 integrin clone B44 (3 mg/kg). (a) The effect of PPE on mean respiratory pressure-volume curves in mice from 35 days (35 d) after instillation and its reversal by JB1a and not B44. (b) Reversal of PPE-induced increase in the quasi-static elastance between 5 and 9 cm H_2O by JB1a treatment ($n = 6$–10). Asterisks denote statistical significance with *$P < 0.05$, **$P < 0.005$, and ***$P < 0.0005$ in comparison to vehicle.

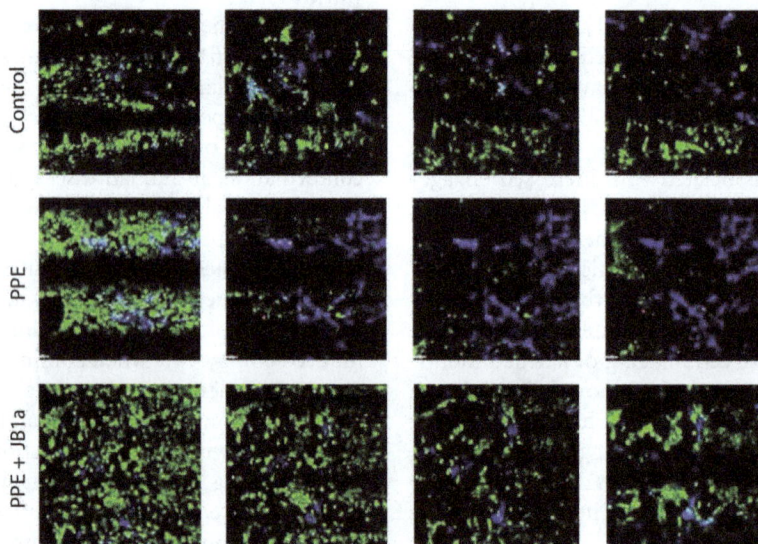

FIGURE 12: Selected frames from time lapse videos of epithelial-mesenchymal cultures during stretch (compressed videos) demonstrating the formation of F-actin (blue) and caspase 3/7 activation (red) in reponse to elastase (PPE, 0.6 U/mL) and its inhibition by JB1a done on cells cultured on glass. Sytox green was used for cell tracking. (a) control, (b) PPE (0.6 U/mL), and (c) PPE + JB1a (1 ug/mL).

environment, thereby reducing the tendency of injury to cause increased cell stiffness, loss of energy, and ultimately death.

4. Material and Methods

4.1. Signalling. Adult human lung fibroblasts (ATCC, CCD-8Lu) were seeded onto collagen-I-coated BioFlex 6-well plates at 0.5×10^6/well. The following day, NCI-H441 cells were seeded on top of the fibroblasts at the same density. Cells were starved with media containing 0.1% FCS. The plates were subjected to stretching at 2–10% sinusoidal stretch at 1 Hz for 2, 4, or 6 hours. PPE was added at 0.3 U/mL alone or in combination with JB1a (1 μg/mL, gift from John Wilkins, Manitoba), AIIB2 (1 μg/mL, Developmental Studies Hybridoma Bank of University of Iowa), or

K20 (1 μg/mL, Santa Cruz). At the end of the stretch, the media was aspirated and protein extracted from the cell layer using Bio-Plex cell lysis kit (Bio-Rad). The protein concentration in the lysates was measured using BCA method. Lysates were analysed for phosphoproteins (50 μg/sample) using Bio-Plex Phospho 15-Plex assay kit (Bio-Rad) for Akt, c-Jun, CREB, ERK1/2, GSK3, histone H3, HSP27, IκB, IRS-1, JNK, MEK1, P38 MAPK, Src, and STAT3 and 6. Measurements were according to manufacturer instructions.

4.2. β1 Integrin Imaging.

Adult human lung fibroblasts (CCD-8Lu, ATCC, Rockville, MD) were seeded onto collagen-I-coated glass coverslips. The following day, NCI-H441 (ATCC, Rockville, MD) was seeded on top of the fibroblasts at the same density. Cells were starved with media containing 0.1% FCS. The plates were subjected PPE at 0.3 U/mL alone or in combination with JB1a (1 μg/mL) or K20 (1 μg/mL) for 1 and 3 hours. The cells were then fixed using ice-cold 4% paraformaldehyde. The cells were blocked using SuperBlock (Pierce) and double immunostained using antibodies against ligand competent β1 integrin (9EG7, BD Biosciences) and JB1a followed by Alexa 488 anti-rat and Alexa 555-anti-mouse, respectively, and nuclear staining with TO-PRO3. Images were acquired using Zeiss LSM 510 using $\times$40 oil lens and raw images presented using LSM image browser.

4.3. Fluorescence Resonance Energy Transfer (FRET).

The human leukemia Jurkat (clone E6-1) cell line was purchased from ATCC (Rockville, MD). Octadecyl rhodamine B chloride (R18) was from molecular probes. The FITC-conjugated analog of α4 specific peptide 4-((n'-2-methylphenyl)ureido)-phenylacetyl-L-leucyl-L-aspartyl-L-valyl-L-prolyl-L-alanyl-L-alanyl-L-lysine (LDV-FITC) was synthesized at Commonwealth Biotechnologies (Richmond, VA).

Cell- and bead-based fluorescence measurements were performed using BD LSRFortessa. The detailed analysis of LDV-FITC binding was described previously [20]. Cells were treated with a range of concentrations of the fluorescent ligand (typically 0–12 nM) in the presence of divalent cations (1 mM Mn^{2+}), eventually choosing 4 nM for experiments. Similar studies were done for R18 and 10 um concentration achieved saturable binding. All experiments were performed in HEPES buffer (110 mM NaCl, 10 mM KCl, 10 mM glucose, 1 mM $MgCl_2$, and 30 mM HEPES, pH 7.4) containing 0.1% FCA. Jurkat cells were used at a density of 1 $\times$ 10^6 cells/mL. Kinetic analysis was done as described previously [20]. Briefly, cells were preincubated in HEPES buffer with or without divalent cations for 10 min at 37°C. Samples were analyzed for 30 s to establish a baseline, then the fluorescent ligand LDV-FITC was added and FACS ad. Additional measurements were carried out in the presence of anti-β1 integrin antibodies at 1–10 μg/mL. studies were done where the antibody was added 1 minute before the commencement of the measurements or 30 seconds after the addition of LDV-FITC without any difference observed. Data were acquired up 600 seconds to a total of 200,000 events. The data were converted to mean channel fluorescence over time using FlowJo software (Tree Star, Inc., Oregon, USA).

4.4. Cell Fractionation

4.4.1. β1 Integrin.

Adult human lung fibroblasts (CCD-8Lu) were seeded onto collagen-I-coated culture dishes. The following day, NCI-H441 cells were seeded on top of the fibroblasts at the same density. Cells were starved with media containing 0.1% FCS. The plates were subjected PPE at 0.3 U/mL alone or in combination with JB1a (1 μg/mL) or K20 (1 μg/mL) for 1 and 3 hours. At the end of the experiment, media was aspirated and cell layer extracted using MEM-PER protein extraction kit (Pierce), protein assayed in the membrane fraction using the BCA methods, and 50 μg separated onto 10% SDS-PAGE, transferred onto Hybond-ECL (GE Healthcare). All membranes were stained with Ponceau S (Sigma) to assess the quality of the transfer and loading and probed for β1 integrin (JB1a) followed by HRP-labelled secondary antibody and developed using ECL-Plus (GE Healthcare) and exposed to Hyperfilm ECL (GE Healthcare). Densitometric analyses was carried out using Image J (NIH).

4.4.2. Caveolin.

In an additional set of experiments, cells were cultured as described onto collagen-I-coated Bioflex plates and subjected to stretch at 2–10% for 10, 30 minutes, 1 or 3 hours. PPE was added at 0.3 U/mL alone or in combination with PPE was added at 0.3 U/mL alone or in combination with JB1a (1 μg/mL), AIIB2 (1 μg/mL), or K20 (1 μg/mL). At the end of the stretch, the media was aspirated, and protein extracted from the cell layer was fractionated using the compartmental protein extraction kit (CNMCS, Biochain). Protein content was measured using the BCA methods. Lysates were separated onto 10% SDS-PAGE using Biorad's Mini Protean 3 Dodeca electrophoresis cell which allows running 12 gels simultaneously to ensure validity for densitometric analyses. The gels were transferred onto ECL-hybond ECL. All membranes were stained with Ponceau S (Sigma) to assess the quality of the transfer and loading. ECL membranes were probed for β1 integrin using JB1a (generous gift from John Wilkins, Manitoba) and mouse actin antibody (NH3, Abcam), or caveolin (rabbit anti-human, BD Biosciences) and phosphocaveolin 1 (BD Biosciences). Secondary detection was done using 680 nm and 800 nm fluorescent antibodies (LiCor), and images of the blots were acquired using LiCor system. Densitometric analyses was carried out using ImageJ (NIH).

4.4.3. Sphingomyelinase Activity.

Adult human lung fibroblasts (CCD-8Lu) were seeded onto collagen-I-coated BioFlex 6 well plates at 0.5 $\times$ 10^6/well. The following day, NCI-H441 cells were seeded on top of the fibroblasts at the same density. Cells were starved with media containing 0.1% FCS. The plates were subjected to stretching at 2–10% sinusoidal stretch at 1 Hz for 2, 4, or 6 hours. PPE was added at 0.3 U/mL alone or in combination with JB1a (1 μg/mL). At the end of the stretch, the media was aspirated, snap frozen in liquid nitrogen, and lyophilised and enzyme activities assayed using Amplex red sphingomyelinase assay kit (Invitrogen) according to the manufacturers' instructions.

4.4.4. Time-Lapse Studies. Cells were cultured as described in methods at 50,000 cell/membrane onto collagen I Bioflex membranes using silicone gaskets of 10 mm diameter. Cells were starved with media containing 0.1% FCS and Syto 16 (Molecular Probes). The media was removed, and Alexa-Fluor 647 labelled G-actin (100 μg/membrane) from rabbit was loaded using Influx (Molecular Probes). The cells were loaded with PhiPhiLux-G_2D_2 for visualisation of caspase activation (OncoImmune). The membrane was then mounted onto the StageFlexer (FlexCell), placed on the stage of an upright Leica-TCS-NT confocal microscope system (Leica Microsystems GmbH, Heidelberg, Germany), and subjected to 2–10% cyclic stretch at 1 Hz for up to 6 hours. Images were collected simultaneously from 3 channels at 1-minute intervals, using the $\times 10$ lens. The resulting time-lapse movies were collated and analysed with Imaris software (Bitplane AG, Switzerland). At various time points during the study, the membrane was held static while serial optical sections were acquired the three fluorescent channels supplemented by the collection of the brightfield channel image.

4.4.5. Three-Dimensional Confocal Microscopy. NCI-H441 cells and human lung fibroblasts were cultured as described above onto collagen-I-coated glass coverslips at 20,000 cells within an area of 5 mm in diameter. The media was removed and Alexa-Fluor 647 labelled G-actin (30 μg/coverslip) from rabbit was loaded using Influx (Molecular Probes). The cells were loaded with PhiPhiLux-G_2D_2 for visualisation of caspase activation (OncoImmune) and FL-ganglioside 1 (GM1, Molecular probes) to visualise the plasma membrane. Images were collected through 4 separate channels (GM1: $\lambda = 488$, caspase $\lambda = 568$, actin: $\lambda = 647$ and brightfield) using x63 water lens and Zeiss LSM510 CLSM microscope. The resulting images were analysed with Imaris software (Bitplane AG, Switzerland). Three-dimensional images were reconstructed.

4.4.6. ATP Measurments. In a separate set of experiments lung fibroblasts and epithelial cells were seeded onto 96 multi-well plates as described above. The cells were starved in media containing 0.1% FCS then in DMEM-glucose-free with 0.1% FCS for 45 minutes before treating with (i) PPE at 0.3 U/mL alone or (ii) PPE preceded by JB1a (1 μg/mL). At the end of the experiment, ATP levels were measured using a bioluminescent ATP kit (Perkin Elmer).

4.4.7. Electrical Impedance. ECIS monitors the impedance of small 250-micrometer diameter electrodes used as substrates for cell growth. When cells grow on the electrode, they impede current flow. Cells were layered as described before onto slides (8W10E, Applied Biophysics) which contain 8 wells each containing ten circular 250 μm diameter active electrodes connected in parallel on a common gold pad. PPE was added at 0.3 U/mL alone or in combination with JB1a (1 μg/mL). Impedance was monitored using ECIS controller model 1600 (Applied Biophysics).

4.5. Caspase Activation Measurements in Human Mesenchymal and Epithelial Cell Coculture. Adult human lung fibroblasts (CCD-8Lu) were seeded onto collagen-I-coated BioFlex 6-well plates at 0.5×10^6/well. The following day, NCI-H441 cells were seeded on top of the fibroblasts at the same density. Cells were starved with media containing 0.1% FCS. The plates were subjected to stretching at 0–5%, 0–10%, or 2–10% sinusoidal stretch at 1 Hz for 6 hours. Control plates on plastic or bioflex plates without stretch were also included. PPE was added at 0.3 U/mL alone or in combination with JB1a (1 μg/mL), 6S6 (1 mg/mL), or ZVAD-fmk at 10 μM. At the end of exposure period which was 1, 3, and 6 hours, the media was aspirated and caspase 3 activity assayed using Caspase-Glo 3/7 (Promega) according to the manufacturers' instructions.

4.6. Cross-Reactivity of β1 Integrin Antibodies. Human and murine neuronal cells were fixed in formaldehyde. The cells were blocked using SuperBlock (Pierce) and immunostained using antibodies against β1 integrin (JB1a and B44, gift from John Wilkins, Manitoba) followed by Alexa 647 anti-mouse (Molecular Probes) and nuclear staining with 7-AAD (Molecular Probes). Image z stacks were acquired using Zeiss LSM 510 with Nyquist calculator settings (http://www.svi.nl/NyquistCalculator) using Plan-Neofluar 40x/1.30 Oil DIC lens and raw images deconuolved and presented in 3d using Huygens software (Scientific Volume Imaging SVI, The Netherlands).

4.7. PPE-Induced Air Space Enlargement Model in Mice. Female C57/BL6 mice (6–8 weeks old) were instilled intratracheally with porcine pancreatic elastase (Roche) as detailed before [49] at 0.2 U/g. All procedures were approved by the Ethical Review Committee of the University of Edinburgh. The procedures were carried out under a project licence number PPL60/3984 issued by the Home Office under the UK Animals (Scientific Procedures) Act 1996. At day 14 (21 d group) or 21 and 28 days (35 d group), mice were treated intratracheally with the anti-integrin antibody JB1a at 3 mg/kg in sterile PBS. The dose chosen is equivalent to the dose of clinically used antibodies against $\alpha 4 \beta 1$ integrin [50]. Control group was instilled initially with PBS with either JB1a or B44 at day 14 (21 d) or at days 21, and 28 (35 d). Additional vehicle control groups were instilled with PBS at days 1 and 14 (21 d) or days 1, 21 and 28 (35 d). We have carried out studies where control groups were instilled with an isotype control (MOPC21, Sigma-Aldrich) and no effect was seen. For the group treated at day 14, the animals were terminated at day 21 (21 d), and, for the group treated on days 21 and 28, the animals were terminated on day 35 (35 d) as follows. The animals were anaesthetised using sodium pentobarbitone (45 mg/kg), paralysed using pancuronium bromide (0.8 mg/kg), and tracheostomised and ventilated using a small animal ventilator (Flexivent, SCIREQ, Montreal) at 8 mL/kg and a rate of 150 breaths/minute and positive end expiratory pressures (PEEP) of 3 cmH$_2$O.

The pressure-volume curve was obtained during inflation and deflation in a stepwise manner by applying volume perturbation incrementally during 16 seconds. The pressure signal was recorded and the pressure-volume (P-V) curve calculated from the plateau of each step. The constant K was obtained using the Salazar-Knowles equation and reflects the curvature of the upper portion of the deflation P-V curve. Quasistatic elastance reflects the static elastic recoil pressure of the lungs at a given lung volume. It was obtained by calculating the slope of the linear part of P-V curve.

In an additional study, female C57/BL6 mice (6–8 weeks old) were instilled intratracheally with 0.3 U/g porcine pancreatic elastase (Elastin products) as detailed above. At days 21 and 28, mice were treated intratracheally with either the anti-integrin antibody JB1a or B44 at 3 mg/kg in sterile PBS. Control group was instilled initially with PBS with either JB1a or B44 at days 21 and 28. An additional vehicle control group was instilled with PBS at days 1, 21, and 28. Lung function was assessed as described above.

4.8. Histochemistry. After the measurements, the animals were sacrificed and lungs were removed and formalin-fixed at a pressure of 25 cm H_2O, paraffin-embedded, and sectioned at 4 μm thickness. Sagittal sections were used from each animal for histological and immunohistochemical assessment of damage and morphometric analysis (mean linear intercept, Lm). Images from 10 fields per section were digitised using Image-Pro plus (version 5.1) and micropublisher 3.3 RTV camera connected to a Zeiss Axioskope with 10x objective. The field size was 0.83 μm $\times$ 0.63 μm. Mean linear intercept was calculated from each field (horizontal and vertical) by dividing the length of the line by the number of alveolar intercepts.

4.9. Apoptosis Measurement. Terminal deoxyribonucleotidyl transferase- (TdT-) mediated dUTP Nick End Labelling (TUNEL) was assessed in sections using the Red ApopTagTM Kit (Chemicon). Data for the quantification of positively stained apoptotic nuclei was acquired using the $\times$40 oil objective of a Zeiss 510 Axiovert confocal microscope system (Carl Zeiss Ltd, Welwyn Gardens City, Herts, UK). The stage-tiling utility was employed for the collection of 4 $\times$ 4 tiled images, equivalent to a total area of 0.921 mm $\times$ 0.921 mm, imaged from a lung section of ~8 mm $\times$ 8 mm (two tiles each from right and left lobes). Images of mainly alveolar tissue were constructed. The images were then converted to 8-bits grey scale, and Image J was used to count total number of cells. TUNEL positive cells were counted manually.

4.10. Statistical Analyses. All data were analysed using SPSS for windows. Data were analysed using the general linear model and multivariate ANOVA with post hoc *t*-test.

Disclosure

R. AlJamal-Naylor and D. Harrison are the inventors for the intellectual property detailing the therapeutic effects of the modulation of β1 integrin function owned by R.

AlJamal-Naylor and Robert J. Naylor (WO2005037313 (17th October 2003) and WO2008104808 (27th February 2007)). The inventors are cofounders and shareholders of AVIPERO Ltd which is developing anti-β1 integrin humanised leads for Parkinson's disease, emphysema, and arthritis (http://www.avipero.com/). The funders had no role in study design, data collection and analysis, decision to publish, or preparation of the paper.

Authors' Contributions

R. AlJamal-Naylor and D. Harrison contributed to the intellectual property, scientific input, planning and carrying out the experiments, and paper preparation. L. Wilson participated in the confocal imaging and time lapse experiments in the investigation of mechanisms of injury and repair. B. Harrison carried out the preliminary β1 integrin clustering (immunofluorescence) and fractionation experiments. S. McIntyre performed the ATP experiments. F. Rossi contributed to flow cytometry in the FRET studies. M. Marsden provided technical assistance in the pilot *in vivo* studies.

Acknowledgments

The authors also wish to thank Robert J. Naylor for the scientific and editorial guidance and James G. Martin for his valuable scientific advice. This work was supported in part by the Chief Scientist Office, Scottish Government. All work was funded by the Chief Scientific Office (Scotland) under Grants CZB4/129 and CZB4/602 in addition to endowment funding from the Division of Pathology of Edinburgh University.

References

[1] R. Al-Jamal and D. J. Harrison, "Beta1 integrin in tissue remodelling and repair: from phenomena to concepts," *Pharmacology and Therapeutics*, vol. 120, no. 2, pp. 81–101, 2008.

[2] T. Fujimura, Y. Shibuya, S. Moriwaki et al., "Fucoidan is the active component of Fucus vesiculosus that promotes contraction of fibroblast-populated collagen gels," *Biological and Pharmaceutical Bulletin*, vol. 23, no. 10, pp. 1180–1184, 2000.

[3] T. Fujimura, K. Tsukahara, S. Moriwaki, T. Kitahara, and Y. Takema, "Effects of natural product extracts on contraction and mechanical properties of fibroblast populated collagen gel," *Biological and Pharmaceutical Bulletin*, vol. 23, no. 3, pp. 291–297, 2000.

[4] T. Fujimura, S. Moriwaki, G. Imokawa, and Y. Takema, "Crucial role of fibroblast integrins α2 and β1 in maintaining the structural and mechanical properties of the skin," *Journal of Dermatological Science*, vol. 45, no. 1, pp. 45–53, 2007.

[5] M. Shimaoka and T. A. Springer, "Therapeutic antagonists and conformational regulation of integrin function," *Nature Reviews Drug Discovery*, vol. 2, no. 9, pp. 703–716, 2003.

[6] J. C. Friedland, M. H. Lee, and D. Boettiger, "Mechanically activated integrin switch controls α5β1 function," *Science*, vol. 323, no. 5914, pp. 642–644, 2009.

[7] M. Kato and M. Mrksich, "Using model substrates to study the dependence of focal adhesion formation on the affinity of integrin-ligand complexes," *Biochemistry*, vol. 43, no. 10, pp. 2699–2707, 2004.

[8] B. H. Luo, K. Strokovich, T. Walz, T. A. Springer, and J. Takagi, "Allosteric β1 integrin antibodies that stabilize the low affinity state by preventing the swing-out of the hybrid domain," *Journal of Biological Chemistry*, vol. 279, no. 26, pp. 27466–27471, 2004.

[9] M. Shimaoka, J. Takagi, and T. A. Springer, "Conformational regulation of integrin structure and function," *Annual Review of Biophysics and Biomolecular Structure*, vol. 31, pp. 485–516, 2002.

[10] J. Takagi, B. M. Petre, T. Walz, and T. A. Springer, "Global conformational earrangements in integrin extracellular domains in outside-in and inside-out signaling," *Cell*, vol. 110, no. 5, pp. 599–611, 2002.

[11] H. Xia, D. Diebold, R. Nho et al., "Pathological integrin signaling enhances proliferation of primary lung fibroblasts from patients with idiopathic pulmonary fibrosis," *Journal of Experimental Medicine*, vol. 205, no. 7, pp. 1659–1672, 2008.

[12] N. Koyama, J. Seki, S. Vergel et al., "Regulation and function of an activation-dependent epitope of the β1 integrins in vascular cells after balloon injury in baboon arteries and in vitro," *American Journal of Pathology*, vol. 148, no. 3, pp. 749–761, 1996.

[13] M. W. Johansson, S. R. Barthel, C. A. Swenson et al., "Eosinophil β1 integrin activation state correlates with asthma activity in a blind study of inhaled corticosteroid withdrawal," *Journal of Allergy and Clinical Immunology*, vol. 117, no. 6, pp. 1502–1504, 2006.

[14] S. Wright, N. L. Malinin, K. A. Powell, T. Yednock, R. E. Rydel, and I. Griswold-Prenner, "α2β1 and αVβ1 integrin signaling pathways mediate amyloid-β-induced neurotoxicity," *Neurobiology of Aging*, vol. 28, no. 2, pp. 226–237, 2007.

[15] H. Ni and J. A. Wilkins, "Localisation of a novel adhesion blocking epitope on the human β1 integrin chain," *Cell Adhesion and Communication*, vol. 5, no. 4, pp. 257–271, 1998.

[16] D. L. Brown, D. R. Phillips, C. H. Damsky, and I. F. Charo, "Synthesis and expression of the fibroblast fibronectin receptor in human monocytes," *Journal of Clinical Investigation*, vol. 84, no. 1, pp. 366–370, 1989.

[17] M. Ticchioni, C. Aussel, J. P. Breittmayer, S. Manie, C. Pelassy, and A. Bernard, "Suppressive effect of T cell proliferation via the CD29 molecule: the CD29 mAb 1 "K20" decreases diacylglycerol and phosphatidic acid levels in activated T cells," *Journal of Immunology*, vol. 151, no. 1, pp. 119–127, 1993.

[18] A. A. Porollo, R. Adamczak, and J. Meller, "POLYVIEW: a flexible visualization tool for structural and functional annotations of proteins," *Bioinformatics*, vol. 20, no. 15, pp. 2460–2462, 2004.

[19] A. Chigaev, A. Waller, O. Amit, L. Halip, C. G. Bologa, and L. A. Sklar, "Real-time analysis of conformation-sensitive antibody binding provides new insights into integrin conformational regulation," *Journal of Biological Chemistry*, vol. 284, no. 21, pp. 14337–14346, 2009.

[20] A. Chigaev, T. Buranda, D. C. Dwyer, E. R. Prossnitz, and L. A. Sklar, "FRET detection of cellular α4-integrin conformational activation," *Biophysical Journal*, vol. 85, no. 6, pp. 3951–3962, 2003.

[21] X. Trepat, L. Deng, S. S. An et al., "Universal physical responses to stretch in the living cell," *Nature*, vol. 447, no. 7144, pp. 592–595, 2007.

[22] U. Cavallaro, J. Niedermeyer, M. Fuxa, and G. Christofori, "N-CAM modulates tumour-cell adhesion to matrix by inducing FGF-receptor signalling," *Nature Cell Biology*, vol. 3, no. 7, pp. 650–657, 2001.

[23] G. E. Hannigan, C. Leung-Hagesteijn, L. Fitz-Gibbon et al., "Regulation of cell adhesion and anchorage-dependent growth by a new β1-integrin-linked protein kinase," *Nature*, vol. 379, no. 6560, pp. 91–96, 1996.

[24] M. D'Amico, J. Hulit, D. F. Amanatullah et al., "The integrated-linked kinase regulates the cyclin D1 gene through glycogen synthase kinase 3β and cAMP-responsive element-binding protein-dependent pathways," *Journal of Biological Chemistry*, vol. 275, no. 42, pp. 32649–32657, 2000.

[25] M. Delcommenne, C. Tan, V. Gray, L. Rue, J. Woodgett, and S. Dedhar, "Phosphoinositide-3-OH kinase-dependent regulation of glycogen synthase kinase 3 and protein kinase B/AKT by the integrin-linked kinase," *Proceedings of the National Academy of Sciences of the United States of America*, vol. 95, no. 19, pp. 11211–11216, 1998.

[26] Y. Shikata, K. Shikata, M. Matsuda et al., "Integrins mediate the inhibitory effect of focal adhesion on angiotensin II-induced p44/42 mitogen-activated protein (MAP) kinase activity in human mesangial cells," *Biochemical and Biophysical Research Communications*, vol. 261, no. 3, pp. 820–823, 1999.

[27] A. Chigaev, A. M. Blenc, J. V. Braaten et al., "Real time analysis of the affinity regulation of α 4-integrin: the physiologically activated receptor is intermediate in affinity between resting and Mn2+ or antibody activation," *Journal of Biological Chemistry*, vol. 276, no. 52, pp. 48670–48678, 2001.

[28] R. Barsacchi, C. Perrotta, P. Sestili, O. Cantoni, S. Moncada, and E. Clementi, "Cyclic GMP-dependent inhibition of acid sphingomyelinase by nitric oxide: an early step in protection against apoptosis," *Cell Death and Differentiation*, vol. 9, no. 11, pp. 1248–1255, 2002.

[29] D. K. Sharma, J. C. Brown, Z. Cheng, E. L. Holicky, D. L. Marks, and R. E. Pagano, "The glycosphingolipid, lactosylceramide, regulates β1- integrin clustering and endocytosis," *Cancer Research*, vol. 65, no. 18, pp. 8233–8241, 2005.

[30] S. Filosto, S. Castillo, A. Danielson et al., "Neutral sphingomyelinase 2: a novel target in cigarette smoke-induced apoptosis and lung injury," *American Journal of Respiratory Cell and Molecular Biology*, vol. 44, no. 3, pp. 350–360, 2011.

[31] M. A. Fernàndez, C. Albor, M. Ingelmo-Torres et al., "Caveolin-1 is essential for liver regeneration," *Science*, vol. 313, no. 5793, pp. 1628–1632, 2006.

[32] M. A. del Pozo, N. Balasubramanian, N. B. Alderson et al., "Phospho-caveolin-1 mediates integrin-regulated membrane domain internalization," *Nature Cell Biology*, vol. 7, no. 9, pp. 901–908, 2005.

[33] R. D. Singh, E. L. Holicky, Z. J. Cheng et al., "Inhibition of caveolar uptake, SV40 infection, and β1-integrin signaling by a nonnatural glycosphingolipid stereoisomer," *Journal of Cell Biology*, vol. 176, no. 7, pp. 895–901, 2007.

[34] A. M. Houghton, P. A. Quintero, D. L. Perkins et al., "Elastin fragments drive disease progression in a murine model of emphysema," *Journal of Clinical Investigation*, vol. 116, no. 3, pp. 753–759, 2006.

[35] S. Wright, C. Parham, B. Lee et al., "Perlecan domain V inhibits α2 integrin-mediated amyloid-β neurotoxicity," *Neurobiology of Aging*. In press.

[36] R. Al-Jamal and D. G. Harrison, "Tissue repair," WO2005037313, 2003, http://v3.espacenet.com/publicationDetails/biblio?DB=EPODOC&adjacent=true&locale=en_GB&FT=D&date=20050428&CC=WO&NR=2005037313A2&KC=A2.

[37] R. O. Hynes, "Integrins: bidirectional, allosteric signaling machines," *Cell*, vol. 110, no. 6, pp. 673–687, 2002.

[38] S. J. Shattil, C. Kim, and M. H. Ginsberg, "The final steps of integrin activation: the end game," *Nature Reviews Molecular Cell Biology*, vol. 11, no. 4, pp. 288–300, 2010.

[39] R. Pankov, T. Markovska, R. Hazarosova, P. Antonov, L. Ivanova, and A. Momchilova, "Cholesterol distribution in plasma membranes of $\beta1$ integrin-expressing and $\beta1$ integrin-deficient fibroblasts," *Archives of Biochemistry and Biophysics*, vol. 442, no. 2, pp. 160–168, 2005.

[40] G. Pande, "The role of membrane lipids in regulation of integrin functions," *Current Opinion in Cell Biology*, vol. 12, no. 5, pp. 569–574, 2000.

[41] I. Petrache, V. Natarajan, L. Zhen et al., "Ceramide upregulation causes pulmonary cell apoptosis and emphysema-like disease in mice," *Nature Medicine*, vol. 11, no. 5, pp. 491–498, 2005.

[42] B. Butler, C. Gao, A. T. Mersich, and S. D. Blystone, "Purified integrin adhesion complexes exhibit actin-polymerization activity," *Current Biology*, vol. 16, no. 3, pp. 242–251, 2006.

[43] J. D. Whittard and S. K. Akiyama, "Activation of $\beta1$ integrins induces cell-cell adhesion," *Experimental Cell Research*, vol. 263, no. 1, pp. 65–76, 2001.

[44] N. Minematsu, A. Blumental-Perry, and S. D. Shapiro, "Cigarette smoke inhibits engulfment of apoptotic cells by macrophages through inhibition of actin rearrangement," *American Journal of Respiratory Cell and Molecular Biology*, vol. 44, no. 4, pp. 474–482, 2011.

[45] J. L. Daniel, I. R. Molish, L. Robkin, and H. Holmsen, "Nucleotide exchange between cytosolic ATP and F-actin-bound ADP may be a major energy-utilizing process in unstimulated platelets," *European Journal of Biochemistry*, vol. 156, no. 3, pp. 677–684, 1986.

[46] I. Bock-Marquette, A. Saxena, M. D. White, J. M. DiMaio, and D. Srivastava, "Thymosin $\beta4$ activates integrin-linked kinase and promotes cardiac cell migration, survival and cardiac repair," *Nature*, vol. 432, no. 7016, pp. 466–472, 2004.

[47] M. W. Johansson, S. R. Barthel, C. A. Swenson et al., "Eosinophil $\beta1$ integrin activation state correlates with asthma activity in a blind study of inhaled corticosteroid withdrawal," *Journal of Allergy and Clinical Immunology*, vol. 117, no. 6, pp. 1502–1504, 2006.

[48] R. Al-Jamal and D. J. Harrison, "Compounds and methods for the modulation of integrin function to mediate tissue repair," WO2008104808, 2007, http://v3.espacenet.com/publication Details/biblio?DB=EPODOC&adjacent=true&locale=en_GB &FT=D&date=20080904&CC=WO&NR=2008104808A2&KC =A2.

[49] E. C. Lucey, R. H. Goldstein, R. Breuer, B. N. Rexer, D. E. Ong, and G. L. Snider, "Retinoic acid does not affect alveolar septation in adult FVB mice with elastase-induced emphysema," *Respiration*, vol. 70, no. 2, pp. 200–205, 2003.

[50] D. H. Miller, O. A. Khan, W. A. Sheremata et al., "A controlled trial of natalizumab for relapsing multiple sclerosis," *New England Journal of Medicine*, vol. 348, no. 1, pp. 15–23, 2003.

22

Effect of a CNS-Sensitive Anticholinesterase Methane Sulfonyl Fluoride on Hippocampal Acetylcholine Release in Freely Moving Rats

Tamotsu Imanishi,[1,2] Muhammad Mubarak Hossain,[1,3] Tadahiko Suzuki,[1] Ping Xu,[1,4] Itaru Sato,[1] and Haruo Kobayashi[1,5]

[1] *Department of Veterinary Medicine, Faculty of Agriculture, Iwate University, Ueda, Morioka 020-8550, Japan*
[2] *Department of Food Safety, Pharmaceutical and Medical Safety Bureau, Ministry of Health, Labour and Welfare, Kasumigaseki, Chiyoda, Tokyo 100-8916, Japan*
[3] *Department of Environmental and Occupational Medicine, Robert Wood Johnson Medical School, University of Medicine and Dentistry of New Jersey, 170 Frelinghuysen Road, Piscataway, NJ 08854, USA*
[4] *Sciences of Cryobiosystems, United Graduate School of Agricultural Sciences of Iwate University, Ueda, Morioka 020-8550, Japan*
[5] *7-272 Aza-Mukaishinden, Ukai, Takizawa-mura, Iwate-gun, Iwate Prefecture 020-0172, Japan*

Correspondence should be addressed to Haruo Kobayashi, yhkoba@ictnet.ne.jp

Academic Editor: Karim A. Alkadhi

Anticholinesterases (antiChEs) are used to treat Alzheimer's disease. The comparative effects of two antiChEs, methanesulfonyl fluoride (MSF) and donepezil, on the extracellular levels of ACh in the hippocampus were investigated by *in vivo* microdialysis in freely moving rats. MSF at 1 and 2 mg/kg produced a dose-dependent increase in ACh efflux from 10 min to at least 3 hrs after injection. At 2 mg/kg, the increase was still present at 24 hr. Donepezil at 1 mg/kg showed a similar but smaller effect, and, paradoxically, 2 mg/kg showed no consistent effect. MSF at 1 and 2 mg/kg decreased acetylcholinesterase activity in the hippocampus to 54.8 and 20.1% of control, respectively. These results suggest that MSF is a suitable candidate for the treatment of Alzheimer's disease.

1. Introduction

Alzheimer's disease (AD) is a slowly progressive neurodegenerative illness characterized by the presence of senile plaques containing β-amyloid protein (Aβ) in brain tissue, tau-neurofibrillary tangles in neurons and, the loss of different transmitter-containing axons, especially cholinergic nerves [1, 2]. Unfortunately, therapeutic strategies targeting amyloid plaques with plaque-removing vaccines or gamma-secretase modulators have been disappointing [3, 4].

It is generally accepted that progressive neurodegeneration of the cholinergic system underlies, at least in part, the cognitive deterioration of Alzheimer's disease (AD) [5–7]. This hypothesis is supported by findings of encouraging symptomatic improvements in clinical trials by the use of AChE inhibitors [8, 9], theoretically by enhancing central cholinergic function by permitting acetylcholine (ACh) to remain in the synaptic cleft longer. Interestingly, some AChE inhibitors have also been reported to be effective also in diminishing amyloid plaques [10, 11].

Methanesulfonyl fluoride (MSF), a long-acting and highly specific inhibitor of brain AChE [12, 13], has been proposed as a safe and effective palliative treatment for senile dementia of the Alzheimer type [14] as well as a method to attenuate stroke-induced deficits in a simple learning and memory task [13]. Therefore, the main aim of this study was to compare MSF-induced increases in extracellular ACh in the hippocampus, one of the target regions for the treatment of AD, with the effects of donepezil, a reference drug widely used for symptomatic treatment of AD. For this purpose, the present study was carried out by measuring extracellular ACh in the hippocampus by *in vivo* microdialysis in freely moving rats following administration of MSF and donepezil.

2. Materials and Methods

Male Sprague-Dawley rats (Japan SLC, Hamamatsu, Japan) weighting 200–250 g were housed one per cage under the standard laboratory conditions (23 ± 1°C, 55 ± 5% humidity) with free access to standard pellet diet (MEQ, Oriental Yeast Co., Tokyo) and drinking water ad libitum with lights on at 08:00 and off at 20:00. Animal handling and procedures were conducted in accordance with the Animal Welfare Act and with the Guide for the Care and Use of Laboratory Animals approved by the Animal Experiment Committee in Iwate University, Japan. Five rats were used in each group.

All reagents used were analytical grade. MSF was purchased from Sigma-Aldrich (Milwaukee, USA) and (R,S-1-benzyl-4-[(5,6-dimethoxy-1-indanon-2-yl)] methylpiperidine hydrochloride (donepezil) was a gift from Eisai Co., Ltd., (Tokyo, Japan).

Microdialysis experiments were conducted according to Hossain et al. [15]. Briefly, the rats were anesthetized with sodium pentobarbital (50 mg/kg, i.p.) and then placed in a stereotaxic apparatus (Kopf instrument). The microdialysis guide cannula (AG-8, Eicom, Kyoto, Japan) was implanted into the left hippocampus with the following coordination (from the bregma): A − 5.8 mm, L + 4.8 mm and, V − 4.5 mm. Following surgery, the animals were returned to their home cage and allowed to recover for at least 3 days before the beginning microdialysis.

ACh and choline content in the dialysate from the different animals were quantified by high-performance liquid chromatograph (HPLC) with electrochemical detection (ECD). The day of the experiment, the microdialysis probe (A-1-8-02, Eicom, Kyoto) was carefully inserted into the hippocampus through the guide cannula. The inlet of the microdialysis probe was connected to a 2.5 mL gastight syringe and perfused with Ringer's solution (NaCl 147 mM, KCl 4.0 mM and, CaCl$_2$ 2.3 mM) containing 1 μM eserine salicylate at a constant flow 2 μL/min using a microperfusion pump, allowing the rats to move freely in a cubic Plexiglas box (30 cm × 30 cm × 40 cm).

The dialysate collected during the first 30 min was discarded to ensure a stable baseline of ACh release. Thereafter, 20 μL samples of perfusate were collected at 10 min intervals. Upon collection, 20 μL of 1 μM ethylhomocholine containing 10 mM EDTA 2Na was added to each sample as an internal standard. Levels of ACh and choline in the dialysate (20 μL/injection) were determined by electrochemical detection with HPLC (Eicom, Kyoto, Japan) equipped with an enzyme column (AC-ENZ, Eicom, Kyoto, Japan). A 20 μL sample of the perfusate/ethylhomocholine solution was then injected into a HPLC equipped with ECD (HPLC-ECD, Eicom, Kyoto) and enzyme column (AC-ENZ, Eicom, Kyoto).

ACh and choline were separated on a cation exchange column (EICOMPAK AC-GEL, Eicom, Kyoto) with sodium lauryl sulfate (0.5 mg/mL). The mobile phase consisted of 0.05 M phosphate buffer (Na$_2$HPO$_4$ 12 H$_2$O) pH 8.2 containing 0.13 mM EDTA 2Na, 0.6 mM tetramethylammonium chloride and, 1.2 mM SDS pumped at 1 mL/min. The retention times for choline and ACh were 7.3 and 13.2 min, respectively.

The basal efflux was defined as the average output of three samples prior to drug administration, and the results were calculated as the percentage of the baseline choline and ACh.

After establishing the basal efflux, the animals received one of the following IP injections: MSF (1 or 2 mg/kg) or donepezil (1 or 2 mg/kg) dissolved in vehicle (80 μL ethanol + 88 μL Tween 20) and prepared to a 1 mL total volume with isotonic sodium chloride. All control animals were injected with the same isotonic sodium chloride/vehicle solution by the same route and volume (1 mL/kg) as the drug.

At the end of the microdialysis experiment, the rats were euthanized with chloroform, the brains were removed, and the position of the probe in the hippocampus was verified by visual examination of 20 μm frozen sections.

For acetylcholinesterase assays, rats in a parallel group received the same injections of MSF, donepezil, or vehicle on the same schedule as the animals used in microdialysis experiment. Three brain regions, hippocampus, striatum, and cerebral cortex (cortex) were quickly dissected on ice at 180 min and 24 hr after injection of MSF or donepezil and then homogenized in 0.1 M phosphate buffer solution (0.1 M Na$_2$PO$_4$+0.1 M KH$_2$PO$_4$, pH 8.0), followed by dilution with the same buffer to 200, 400, and 200 times of tissue weight, respectively, for the analysis of AChE activity by the method of Ellman et al. [16] with 0.48 mM acetylthiocholine iodide as substrate for 2 min at 25°C using UV-240 spectrophotometer (Shimadzu Corporation, Kyoto, Japan) at 412 nm.

The extracellular levels of ACh and choline from individual rats were calculated relative to the mean basal release (the average of three 10 min sequential samples before drug administration was taken as 100% basal release). Analysis of variance, followed by Dunnett's post hoc test for repeated measurements (treatment versus time), was used to analyze changes from ACh and choline baselines as well as for tests of significant differences over time. A level of $P < 0.05$ was taken to indicate a statistically significant effect.

3. Results

The injections of MSF and donepezil (1 and 2 mg/kg i.p.) did not produce any observable clinical signs or symptoms in the rats. The basal rates of efflux from the hippocampus of vehicle-only injected control rats were 5.2 ± 0.2 pmol ACh/10 μL/10 min and 180.8 ± 2.6 pmol choline/10 μL/10 min (n = 15). The response of ACh in the hippocampus to vehicle treatment was not significantly different throughout the experiment.

As shown in Figure 1, MSF increased the release of ACh in a dose-dependent manner. MSF, at 1 mg/kg, caused a significant ($P < 0.05$, $P < 0.01$) and prolonged increase of

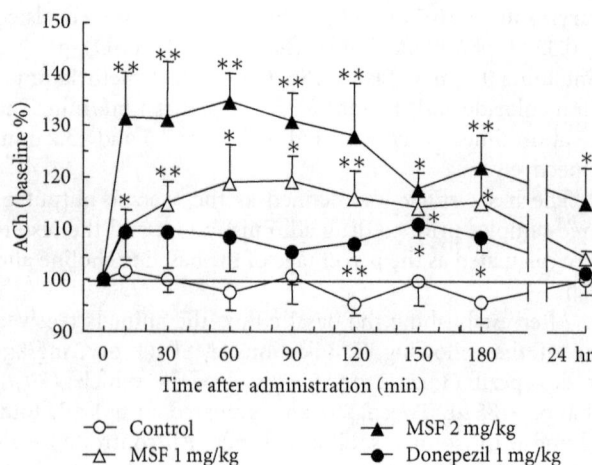

FIGURE 1: Effect of MSF and donepezil on the level of extracellular ACh in the freely moving rats. Data are expressed as percentage changes from baseline. Each value represents the mean ± S.E.M. of five experiments. Asterisks indicate effects significantly different from time course vehicle control ($^*P < 0.05$, $^{**}P < 0.01$).

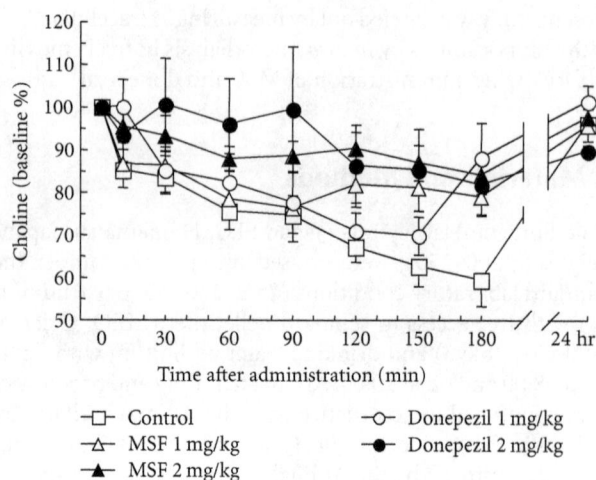

FIGURE 2: Effect of MSF and donepezil on the level of extracellular choline in the freely moving rats. Data are expressed as percentage changes from baseline. Each value represents the mean ± S.E.M. of five experiments.

ACh efflux in the hippocampus from 10 to 180 min which returned to control levels at 24 hr after the administration of MSF. At the higher dose of 2 mg/kg, MSF produced a consistent and proportionately larger increase in ACh release between 10 to 90 min ($P < 0.01$), decreasing progressively from 120 to 180 min ($P < 0.05$, $P < 0.01$) after the treatment. At 2 mg/kg MSF, the elevation of ACh efflux remained elevated at 24 hr after injection ($P < 0.05$).

The effects of donepezil on ACh efflux are also shown in Figure 1. A dose of 1 mg/kg donepezil produced a small but consistent increase in ACh efflux over the first 180 minutes. However, the dose of 2 mg/kg did not produce a dose-dependent effect, and ACh efflux over the 180 min experiment was not different from animals received the dose of 1 mg/kg (data not shown).

As shown in Figure 2, the choline efflux decreased progressively from basal levels throughout the course of the first 180 min after injection for every group, MSF, donepezil, and controls but returned to basal levels by 24 hr. The decreases were less significant in the groups that received MSF or donepezil than in the control group.

The effect of MSF and donepezil on AChE activity in the hippocampus, striatum, and cortex at 180 min (Figure 3(a)) and 24 hr (Figure 3(b)) after drug administration is shown in Figure 3. MSF at 1 mg/kg decreased AChE activity in hippocampus, striatum, and cortex by about 50%, to 55, 51, and 49% of the respective control activities. At 2 mg/kg, MSF produced 80–90% inhibition, bringing AChE activity to about 20, 12, and 11% of the respective control activities. Donepezil at 1 mg/kg did not produce any significant effect on AChE activity in the three brain regions at 180 min after injection. The dose of 2 mg/kg, however, produced a significant decrease in AChE activity in the cortex but not in the hippocampus or striatum 180 min after administration (Figure 3(a)). Figure 3(b) also shows the brain regional AChE activity 24 hr after 1 mg/kg of MSF or donepezil. The

activity of AChE in the hippocampus, striatum, and cortex of rats administered MSF was about 44, 36 and 41% ($P < 0.05$ to 0.001) of control values, respectively. At 24 hr, no other significant differences were not observed in the activity of AChE in any of the three brain regions between the rats treated with donepezil or vehicle.

4. Discussion

We have previously reported that a single dose of MSF at 1.5 mg/kg s.c. significantly increased the concentrations of extraterminal ACh and cytoplasmic ACh in the cortex of mice [17]. In these experiments, an increase in the fractional ACh content of brain tissues taken *ex vivo* and homogenized for analysis was found to be elevated at 180 min, and the increase persisted to 24 hr. The extraterminal ACh determined in that earlier *ex vivo* experiment may approximately correspond to extracellular ACh in the current *in vivo* experiment at those same time points. The present experiment confirmed the earlier results and showed that doses of either 1 mg/kg or 2 mg/kg MSF strongly increase extracellular ACh during the first 180 min after administration and the effect persists for 24 hr after the higher dose of 2 mg/kg.

Corresponding to the increases in ACh efflux found after MSF, the present study also found that the same doses reduced AChE activity in the hippocampus to about 55% and 20% of control 180 min after 1 mg/kg and 2 mg/kg of MSF, respectively, and to about 44% of control 24 hr after 1 mg/kg of MSF (the only dose studied at 24 hr). These results support several studies on the effects of drugs for Alzheimer's disease that show that increasing levels of extracellular ACh in various brain regions are found with decreasing AChE activity [8, 9, 18–22].

Donepezil (1.66 mg/kg), rivastigmine (0.4 mg/kg), and huperzine A (more than 0.6 and 3 mg/kg) have been found to increase extracellular ACh in the hippocampus, and the

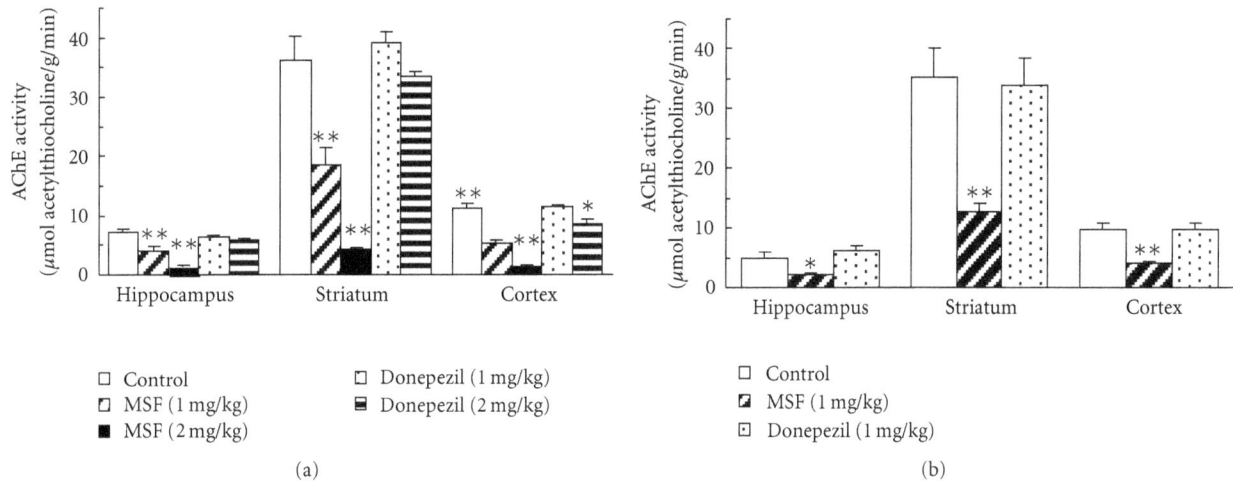

Figure 3: Effect of MSF and donepezil on the activity of AChE in brain regions 180 min (a) and 24 hr (b) after administration. Each value represents the mean ± S.E.M. of five experiments. Asterisks indicate effects significantly different from time course vehicle control ($*P < 0.05$, $**P < 0.01$).

results are generally not so different between the oral or intraperitoneal administration [8, 18]. All three of these drugs produced the maximal increase in extracellular ACh within 3 hrs, mostly around 30 to 60 min, after administration. On the other hand, the present study shows that MSF increased the level of extracellular ACh for at least 3 hrs without showing significant peaks. After 2 mg/kg MSF, a significant increase was still present at 24 hr.

Although donepezil is generally accepted to be effective in increasing the release of ACh from hippocampus in freely moving animals [8, 9], the present study, however, found that donepezil succeeded in increasing extracellular ACh only at a dose of 1 mg/kg. Surprisingly, it failed to demonstrate a dose-dependent effect at a dose of 2 mg/kg. Although the doses of donepezil, 1 mg/kg and 2 mg/kg, were selected for comparison to the MSF results, a possible explanation for our failure to find a dose-dependent effect of donepezil on extracellular ACh may be that the dose of 2 mg/kg was not sufficiently greater than the 1 mg/kg dose to produce a clear difference. The dose-dependent effects of donepezil on increasing the level of extracellular ACh in the striatum achieved by previous reports [18] were obtained by using doses at 1, 3, and 5 mg/kg.

In the present study, donepezil at doses of 1 and 2 mg/kg did not show any significant inhibitory effect on the activity of AChE in the hippocampus at 180 min after administration (Figure 3(a)). Donepezil is a reversible AChE inhibitor [9, 23] and the AChE inhibition it produces may disappear when the tissues are homogenized as the donepezil will be diluted.

5. Conclusions

The present study showed that MSF at doses 1 and 2 mg/kg produced a consistent increase in the efflux of ACh in freely moving rats as measured by microdialysis throughout the first 3 hrs at both doses and a persistent increase was still present at 24 hr. Since ChE inhibitors

are the major therapeutic agents used in AD patients, the agent-like MSF, which increases extracellular ACh in the hippocampus with a long-lasting efficacy but without excess stimulation, may serve as an effective therapy to alleviate or prevent the central cholinergic deficits which are reported to cause cognitive impairments.

Acknowledgment

The authors would like to thank Dr. Moss, D.E., Department of Psychology, University of Texas at El Paso, USA. for reviewing the paper and valuable suggestions.

References

[1] H. Braak and E. Braak, "Neuropathological stageing of Alzheimer-related changes," *Acta Neuropathologica*, vol. 82, no. 4, pp. 239–259, 1991.

[2] D. R. Thal, U. Rüb, M. Orantes, and H. Braak, "Phases of Aβ-deposition in the human brain and its relevance for the development of AD," *Neurology*, vol. 58, no. 12, pp. 1791–1800, 2002.

[3] P. E. Potter, "Investigational medications for treatment of patients with Alzheimer disease," *Journal of the American Osteopathic Association*, vol. 110, supplement 8, pp. S27–S36, 2010.

[4] D. W. Ethell, "An amyloid-notch hypothesis for Alzheimer's disease," *Neuroscientist*, vol. 16, no. 6, pp. 614–617, 2010.

[5] P. Davies and A. J. F. Maloney, "Selective loss of central cholinergic neurons in Alzheimer's disease," *The Lancet*, vol. 2, no. 8000, p. 1403, 1976.

[6] E. J. Mufson, A. D. Kehr, B. H. Wainer, and M. M. Mesulam, "Cortical effects of neurotoxic damage to the nucleus basalis in rats: persistent loss of extrinsic cholinergic input and lack of transsynaptic effect upon the number of somatostatin-containing, cholinesterase-positive, and cholinergic cortical neurons," *Brain Research*, vol. 417, no. 2, pp. 385–388, 1987.

[7] P. J. Whitehouse, D. L. Price, A. W. Clark, J. T. Coyle, and M. R. DeLong, "Alzheimer disease: evidence for selective

loss of cholinergic neurons in the nucleus basalis," *Annals of Neurology*, vol. 10, no. 2, pp. 122–126, 1981.

[8] Y. Q. Liang and X. C. Tang, "Comparative studies of huperzine A, donepezil, and rivastigmine on brain acetylcholine, dopamine, norepinephrine, and 5-hydroxytryptamine levels in freely-moving rats," *Acta Pharmacologica Sinica*, vol. 27, no. 9, pp. 1127–1136, 2006.

[9] H. Sugimoto, H. Ogura, Y. Arai, Y. Iimura, and Y. Yamanishi, "Research and development of donepezil hydrochloride, a new type of acetylcholinesterase inhibitor," *Japanese Journal of Pharmacology*, vol. 89, no. 1, pp. 7–20, 2002.

[10] M. Rosini, E. Simoni, M. Bartolini et al., "Inhibition of acetylcholinesterase, β-amyloid aggregation, and NMDA receptors in Alzheimer's disease: a promising direction for the multi-target-directed ligands gold rush," *Journal of Medicinal Chemistry*, vol. 51, no. 15, pp. 4381–4384, 2008.

[11] H. Sugimoto, "The new approach in development of anti-Alzheimer's disease drugs via the cholinergic hypothesis," *Chemico-Biological Interactions*, vol. 175, no. 1–3, pp. 204–208, 2008.

[12] D. E. Moss, H. Kobayashi, G. Pacheco, R. Paracios, and R. G. Perez, "Methanesulfonyl fluoride: a CNS selective inhibitor," in *Current Research in Alzheimer Theory: Cholinesterase Inhibitors*, E. Giacobini and R. Becher, Eds., pp. 305–314, Taylor and Francis, New York, NY, USA, 1988.

[13] G. Pacheco, R. Palacios-Esquivel, and D. E. Moss, "Cholinesterase inhibitors proposed for treating dementia in Alzheimer's disease: selectivity toward human brain acetylcholinesterase compared with butyrylcholinesterase," *Journal of Pharmacology and Experimental Therapeutics*, vol. 274, no. 2, pp. 767–770, 1995.

[14] D. E. Moss, P. Berlanga, M. M. Hagan, H. Sandoval, and C. Ishida, "Methanesulfonyl fluoride (MSF): a double-blind, placebo-controlled study of safety and efficacy in the treatment of senile dementia of the Alzheimer type," *Alzheimer Disease and Associated Disorders*, vol. 13, no. 1, pp. 20–25, 1999.

[15] M. M. Hossain, T. Suzuki, I. Sato, T. Takewaki, K. Suzuki, and H. Kobayashi, "The modulatory effect of pyrethroids on acetylcholine release in the hippocampus of freely moving rats," *NeuroToxicology*, vol. 25, no. 5, pp. 825–833, 2004.

[16] G. L. Ellman, K. D. Courtney, V. Andres, and R. M. Featherstone, "A new and rapid colorimetric determination of acetylcholinesterase activity," *Biochemical Pharmacology*, vol. 7, no. 2, pp. 88–95, 1961.

[17] H. Kobayashi, T. Nakano, D. E. Moss, and T. Suzuki, "Effects of a central anticholinesterase, methanesulfonyl fluoride on the cerebral cholinergic system and behavior in mice: comparison with an organophosphate DDVP," *Journal of Health Science*, vol. 45, no. 4, pp. 191–202, 1999.

[18] K. Isomae, M. Ishikawa, M. Ohta et al., "Effects of T-82, a new quinoline derivative, on cholinesterase activity and extracellular acetylcholine concentration in rat brain," *Japanese Journal of Pharmacology*, vol. 88, no. 2, pp. 206–212, 2002.

[19] T. Kosasa, Y. Kuriya, and Y. Yamanishi, "Effect of donepezil hydrochloride (E2020) on extracellular acetylcholine concentration in the cerebral cortex of rats," *Japanese Journal of Pharmacology*, vol. 81, no. 2, pp. 216–222, 1999.

[20] E. Shearman, S. Rossi, B. Szasz et al., "Changes in cerebral neurotransmitters and metabolites induced by acute donepezil and memantine administrations: a microdialysis study," *Brain Research Bulletin*, vol. 69, no. 2, pp. 204–213, 2006.

[21] K. Takashina, T. Bessho, R. Mori, J. Eguchi, and K. I. Saito, "MKC-231, a choline uptake enhancer: (2) Effect on synthesis and release of acetylcholine in AF64A-treated rats," *Journal of Neural Transmission*, vol. 115, no. 7, pp. 1027–1035, 2008.

[22] K. Yano, K. Koda, Y. Ago et al., "Galantamine improves apomorphine-induced deficits in prepulse inhibition via muscarinic ACh receptors in mice," *British Journal of Pharmacology*, vol. 156, no. 1, pp. 173–180, 2009.

[23] M. Živin and P. Pregelj, "Prolonged treatment with donepezil increases acetylcholinesterase expression in the central nervous system," *Psychiatria Danubina*, vol. 20, no. 2, pp. 168–173, 2008.

23

Protective Effects of Methylsulfonylmethane on Hemodynamics and Oxidative Stress in Monocrotaline-Induced Pulmonary Hypertensive Rats

Sadollah Mohammadi,[1,2,3] Moslem Najafi,[1] Hossein Hamzeiy,[1,4] Nasrin Maleki-Dizaji,[1,5] Masoud Pezeshkian,[6] Homayon Sadeghi-Bazargani,[7] Masoud Darabi,[8] Sara Mostafalou,[9] Shahab Bohlooli,[3] and Alireza Garjani[1,4,5]

[1] Department of Pharmacology and Toxicology, School of Pharmacy, Tabriz University of Medical Sciences, Tabriz 5165665931, Iran
[2] Division of Molecular Toxicology, Institute of Environmental Medicine, Karolinska Institutet (KI), Box 210, 17177 Stockholm, Sweden
[3] Department of Pharmacology and Physiology, School of Medicine, Ardabil University of Medical Sciences, Ardabil 56135665, Iran
[4] Research Center for Pharmaceutical Nanotechnology (RCPN), Tabriz University of Medical Sciences, Tabriz 5165691749, Iran
[5] Drug Applied Research Center (DARC), Tabriz University of Medical Sciences, Tabriz 5165665811, Iran
[6] Department of Cardiac Surgery and Cardiovascular Research Center, School of Medicine, Tabriz University of Medical Sciences, Tabriz 5166615573, Iran
[7] Department of Statistics and Epidemiology, School of Health and Nutrition, Tabriz University of Medical Sciences, Tabriz 5166614711, Iran
[8] Department of Biochemistry and Clinical Laboratories, School of Medicine, Tabriz University of Medical Sciences, Tabriz 5166615731, Iran
[9] Department of Toxicology, Pharmaceutical Sciences Research Center (PSRC) and School of Pharmacy, Tehran University of Medical Sciences, Tehran 141556451, Iran

Correspondence should be addressed to Alireza Garjani, garjania@tbzmed.ac.ir

Academic Editor: Mustafa F. Lokhandwala

Methylsulfonylmethane (MSM) is naturally occurring organic sulfur that is known as a potent antioxidant/anti-inflammatory compound. The aim of this study was to investigate the effect of MSM on hemodynamics functions and oxidative stress in rats with monocrotaline- (MCT-) induced pulmonary arterial hypertension (PAH). Wistar rats were randomly assigned to 38-days treatment. MSM was administered to rats at 100, 200, and 400 mg/kg/day doses 10 days before a single dose of 60 mg/kg, IP, MCT. Hemodynamics of ventricles were determined by Powerlab AD instrument. Blood samples were obtained to evaluate changes in the antioxidative system including activities of catalase (CAT), superoxide dismutase (SOD), glutathione peroxidase (GPx), and the level of reduced glutathione (GSH) and malondialdehyde (MDA). Improvements in cardiopulmonary hemodynamics were observed in the MSM-treated pulmonary arterial hypertensive rats, with a significant reduction in right ventricular systolic pressure (RSVP) and an increase in the mean arterial pressure (MAP). The values of CAT, SOD, GSH-px activities, and GSH were significantly lower in MCT-induced PAH ($P < 0.01$), but they were recovered to control levels of MSM-treated groups. Our present results suggest that long-term administration of the MSM attenuates MCT-induced PAH in rats through modulation of oxidative stress and antioxidant defense.

1. Introduction

Pulmonary arterial hypertension (PAH) is a pathophysiological state characterized by a progressive increase in pulmonary vascular resistance. In addition to inducing myocardial hypertrophy, it also induces marked interstitial fibrosis to compensate for the increased ventricular workload. These adaptive changes often clinically lead to heart failure and sudden cardiac death [1]. Despite all current progress in the diagnosis and therapeutics, PAH continues to be a devastating disease with a high morbidity and mortality [2].

Recent reports have implicated increased oxidative stress as a mediator in the pathogenesis and the development of PAH [3]. Accordingly, antioxidant therapy has been effective in the treatment of right ventricle (RV) dysfunction in PAH [4].

Methylsulfonylmethane (MSM) is naturally occurring organic sulfur that is known as a potent antioxidant/anti-inflammatory compound [5, 6]. MSM is widely used as an arthritis remedy with potential anti-inflammatory effects [7, 8]. MSM may also be beneficial in PAH due to its anti-inflammatory and antiproliferative effects [9]. Despite an increasing clinical use, the mechanisms by which MSM exerts its effects remain largely unknown.

Monocrotaline (MCT) is a toxic pyrrolizidine alkaloid and has a selective toxic effect on pulmonary vessels without an effect on systemic vessels. Recently, we have observed that the expression of oxidative stress-related substances such as angiotensin II and endotheline 1 is increased in rats after exposure to MCT and that treatment with MSM suppresses these responses (unpublished findings). MSM was shown to act directly as free radical scavenger, which would further add to the efficiency of MSM as an antioxidant [7]. Thus, it is possible that MSM exerts its effect on PAH by interfering with oxidative events that may be associated with the heart failure. To investigate whether MSM may provide preventive effects on PAH, an experimental study was conducted examining the activity of antioxidative enzymes, including superoxide dismutase (SOD), catalase (CAT), and glutathione peroxidase (GSH-Px) in the serum samples from rats with MCT-induced PAH subjected to pretreatment. Moreover, we analyzed the nonenzymatic antioxidants reduced glutathione (GSH)/oxidized glutathione (GSSG) and the levels of malondialdehyde (MDA) as a lipid peroxidation biomarker.

2. Methods and Materials

2.1. Animals. Two-month-old male Wistar rats (200 ± 20 g) were, fed with standard laboratory chow ad libitum, used in the experiment, as previously described by us [10]. Animals were obtained from the Pasteur Institute of Iran (Tehran, Iran). Tabriz University of Medical Sciences Animal Ethics Committee approved the study protocol. Injections were all administered intraperitoneally (i.p.) to rats. Invasive experimental procedures were carried out on pentobarbital anaesthetized rats (60 mg/kg body weight, i.p.). At the end of the experiment, blood samples were obtained from the inferior vena cava under general anesthesia [11] for determination of serum SOD, GPx, GSH, and CAT. Then animals were sacrificed by pentobarbital overdose [12], and heart and lung tissues were excised to calculate tissue wet-to-body and wet-to-dry weight ratios.

2.2. Experimental Protocol. PAH was induced by means of a single dose of MCT (Sigma-Aldrich; 60 mg/kg) [13]. The effective doses of MSM (Fluka/Sigma-Aldrich) were determined according to a significant improvement in hemodynamic status of MCT-induced PAH rats [14]. Rats were subjected to treatment with MSM (0–400 mg/kg/day) 10 days before MCT injection ($n = 48$) and continued until 4 weeks after the MCT injection. Saline was used as vehicle in control experiments. MSM was well tolerated by the rats and no abnormal behavior was observed.

2.3. Hemodynamic Measurements. All hemodynamic measurements were carried out in rats, as described previously [10]. Right ventricular systolic pressure (RVSP), mean arterial pressure (MAP), and heart rate (HR) were measured under pentobarbital (60 mg/kg; i.p.) anesthesia and artificial respiration via a trachea cannula. The peak rate of right ventricular pressure (RV dP/dt_{max}) and relaxation time constant (τ), as indices of myocardial contractility, were also calculated from RVSP. All parameters were continuously recorded using Powerlab system (AD Instruments, Australia).

2.4. Tissue Weights. Following the hemodynamic measurements, animals were sacrificed by an overdose of pentobarbital. The hearts and lungs were removed and weighed. Then, the tissues were cut into small pieces for drying at $55°$C until a constant weight was reached. Wet-to-body weight ratios and wet-to-dry weight ratios of the tissues were calculated to assess the degree of the congestion [10]. The ratio of the wet weight of the RV to that of the LV + S [RV/(LV + S)] was calculated as an indicator of RV hypertrophy.

3. Measurements of Blood Oxidants and Antioxidative Enzymes

The enzyme activities of CAT (Cayman, Chemical Company, MI), SOD, and GSH-Px (RANDOX Laboratories Ltd., UK) were determined by using spectrophotometric assay kits. Serum glutathione (GSH) and glutathione disulfide (GSSG) contents were measured using colorimetric enzymatic kits from Assay Designs/Stressgen Bioreagents. The MDA levels were measured spectrophotometrically based on the coupling of MDA with thiobarbituric acid [15].

3.1. Statistics. Data were presented as mean $\pm$ SE. Comparisons between groups were made with Student's paired t-test or one-way ANOVA as appropriate. If ANOVA analysis indicated significant differences, a Tukey's multiple-comparison posttest was performed to compare mean values between treatment groups and control. In addition to the ANOVA, a standard regression analysis for linear response in the dose groups was performed. A P value of <0.05 was considered statistically significant.

4. Results

4.1. Morphometric and Hemodynamic Evaluation. Table 1 shows a comparison of the morphometric and hemodynamic parameters of rats in the control group and the MCT groups. There were no significant differences in either LV + S or lung dry/wet ratio among groups. Compared to the control group, MCT administration caused a significant increase in lung

TABLE 1: Morphometric parameters and hemodynamic data of control and monocrotaline-injected male rats.

| | Control | MCT-induced pulmonary hypertension groups. MSM (mg/kg/day) | | | | r^2 | P |
		0	100	200	400		
Morphometric parameters							
Body wt (g)	265 ± 8	204 ± 12*	230 ± 10	244 ± 21	262 ± 11	0.39	<0.01
Heart (g)	0.71 ± 0.13	0.81 ± 0.19	0.78 ± 0.18	0.75 ± 0.20	0.74 ± 0.17	0.09	0.21
Heart/body wt (mg/g)	2.67 ± 0.11	3.4 ± 0.14**	3.44 ± 0.27	3.23 ± 0.53	2.84 ± 0.054	0.36	<0.01
RV wt (g)	0.16 ± 0.01	0.31 ± 0.04**	0.25 ± 0.02	0.22 ± 0.03	0.18 ± 0.01	0.38	<0.01
RV/body wt (mg/g)	0.59 ± 0.04	1.54 ± 0.15**	1.09 ± 0.15*	0.92 ± 0.27	0.70 ± 0.38	0.46	<0.01
LV + S wt (g)	0.55 ± 0.02	0.50 ± 0.01	0.53 ± 0.02	0.53 ± 0.01	0.56 ± 0.02	0.23	0.04
LV + S /body wt (mg/mg)	2.08 ± 0.08	2.46 ± 0.08	2.33 ± 0.15	2.24 ± 0.26	2.15 ± 0.07	0.15	0.11
RV /LV + S	0.28 ± 0.02	0.62 ± 0.07**	0.47 ± 0.04*	0.42 ± 0.06	0.33 ± 0.03	0.50	<0.01
Lung wet (g)	1.11 ± 0.06	3.09 ± 0.14**	2.23 ± 0.36*	1.99 ± 0.26	1.28 ± 0.09	0.60	<0.01
Lung dry (g)	0.25 ± 0.01	0.52 ± 0.02**	0.46 ± 0.06*	0.41 ± 0.06	0.27 ± 0.02	0.50	<0.01
Lung dry/wet	0.22 ± 0.03	0.17 ± 0.02**	0.20 ± 0.09	0.21 ± 0.03	0.21 ± 0.03	0.36	0.01
Lung wet/body wt (mg/g)	4.19 ± 0.18	15.17 ± 1.15**	9.35 ± 2.06*	8.17 ± 2.38	4.83 ± 0.20	0.60	<0.01
Hemodynamic data							
HR (beats/min)	397 ± 31	274 ± 19*	312 ± 16	326 ± 24	406 ± 31	0.47	<0.01
MAP (mmHg)	83.28 ± 7.42	54.07 ± 7.13**	53.100 ± 2.76**	58.68 ± 3.149*	77.83 ± 1.31	0.62	<0.01
RVSP (mmHg)	22.56 ± 1.65	35.87 ± 1.76**	29.21 ± 2.79	27.65 ± 2.60	22.62 ± 2.11	0.53	<0.01
RV dP/dt_{max} (mmHg/s)	1958 ± 40	2376 ± 116*	2196 ± 25	2130 ± 50	2027 ± 39	0.39	<0.01
τ (ms)	14.43 ± 0.92	22.62 ± 0.83**	19.05 ± 1.43*	17.44 ± 0.91	15.65 ± 0.97	0.53	<0.01

Data are mean ± SE. Significant Tukey's post hoc differences compared with controls are indicated by asterisks (**$P < 0.01$ and *$P < 0.05$) and r^2 is the regression coefficient of the dose-response effect. MCT: monocrotaline; MSM: methylsulfonylmethane; RV: right ventricle; LV: left ventricle; S: septum; wt: weight; HR: heart rate; MAP: mean arterial pressure; RVSP: right ventricular systolic pressure; RV dP/dt_{max}: peak rate of right ventricular pressure; τ: relaxation time constant.

TABLE 2: Effects of different doses of methylsulfonylmethane (MSM) on the activities of antioxidant enzymes in rats with monocrotaline- (MCT-) induced pulmonary hypertension.

| | Control | MCT-induced pulmonary hypertension groups, MSM (mg/kg/day) | | | | r^2 | P |
		0	100	200	400		
CAT (U/mL)	6.10 ± 0.83	2.02 ± 0.33*	4.16 ± 0.57	5.02 ± 0.75	7.98 ± 1.68	0.48	<0.001
SOD (U/mL)	203.33 ± 3.80	168.33 ± 6.67**	206.67 ± 5.11	210.00 ± 7.30	220.83 ± 3.96	0.50	<0.001
GSH-px (U/mL)	10.01 ± 0.12	7.05 ± 0.62**	8.14 ± 1.09	9.80 ± 0.25	10.20 ± 0.20	0.40	0.001

Significant Tukey's post hoc differences compared with controls are indicated by asterisks (**$P < 0.01$ and *$P < 0.05$) and r^2 is the regression coefficient of the dose-response effect. MCT: monocrotaline; MSM: methylsulfonylmethane; SOD: superoxide dismutase; GSH-Px: glutathione peroxidase; CAT: catalase; GSH: reduced glutathione; GSSG: oxidized glutathione; MDA: malondialdehyde.

wet and lung/body weight. The MCT-induced increase in lung/body weight was significantly attenuated by MSM in a dose-dependent manner ($P < 0.01$). The RV/LV + S ratio was calculated as an index of right ventricular hypertrophy. The value of RV/LV + S ratio was significantly higher in rats exposed to MCT, which was significantly reversed by MSM treatment ($r^2 = 0.50$; $P < 0.01$).

Levels of right ventricular systolic pressure (RSVP), peak rate of right ventricular pressure (RV dP/dt_{max}), and relaxation time constant (τ) were significantly increased at week 4 of MCT treatment. All the hemodynamics parameters were significantly improved in all MSM-treated rats when compared with those in the saline-treated pulmonary hypertensive rats (Table 1).

4.2. Activities of Antioxidant Enzymes. Levels of CAT, SOD, and GSH-Px in the serum of hypertensive rats were significantly decreased at week 4 of MCT treatment (Table 2). The effects of MSM (0–400 mg/kg/day) given from the 10th day prior to MCT-induced hypertension on the activities of serum antioxidant enzymes are shown in Table 2. The activities of all CAT, SOD, and GSH-Px were significantly increased ($P < 0.01$) in MSM-treated rats. Both ANOVA and linear regression demonstrated a dose-proportional rise in activities of antioxidant enzymes in MCT-induced hypertensive rats that were treated with MSM.

4.3. Levels of GSH and GSSG. The effect of MSM treatment on the serum content of GSH and GSSG is shown in

TABLE 3: Effects of different doses of methylsulfonylmethane (MSM) on the levels of reduced glutathione (GSH) and disulfide-oxidized glutathione (GSSG) and MDA in rats with monocrotaline- (MCT-) induced pulmonary hypertension.

| | Control | MCT-induced pulmonary hypertension groups, MSM (mg/kg/day) | | | | | |
		0	100	200	400	r^2	P
GSH (nmol/mL)	543.54 ± 16.22	347.33 ± 41.54*	551.65 ± 93.28	695.95 ± 106.36	774.62 ± 45.62	0.41	<0.01
GSSG (nmol/mL)	50.71 ± 2.17	76.19 ± 6.51*	62.98 ± 9.36	59.05 ± 4.80	51.31 ± 2.41	0.26	0.01

Significant Tukey's post hoc differences compared with controls are indicated by asterisks (**P < 0.01 and *P < 0.05) and r^2 is the regression coefficient of the dose-response effect. MCT: monocrotaline; MSM: methylsulfonylmethane; SOD: superoxide dismutase; GSH-Px: glutathione peroxidase; CAT: catalase; GSH: reduced glutathione; GSSG: oxidized glutathione; MDA: malondialdehyde.

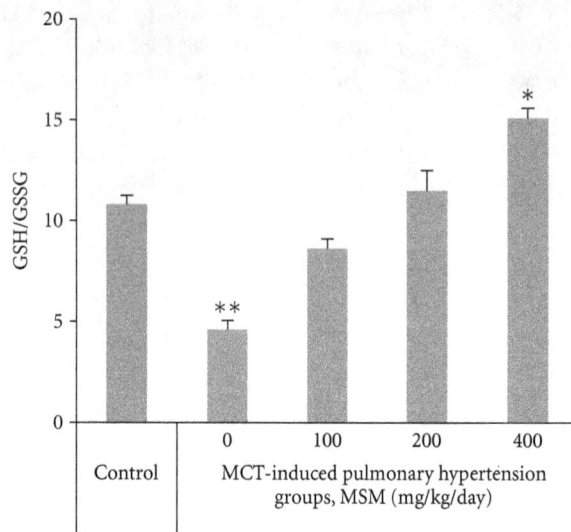

FIGURE 1: Effects of different doses (0–400 mg/kg/day) of methyl-sulfonylmethane (MSM) on the reduced to oxidized glutathione (GSH/GSSG) in rats with monocrotaline- (MCT-) induced pulmonary hypertension (regression coefficient r^2 = 0.84, P < 0.01). Data are means ± SE, n = 6. Significant Tukey's post hoc differences compared with controls are indicated by asterisks (**P < 0.01 and *P < 0.05).

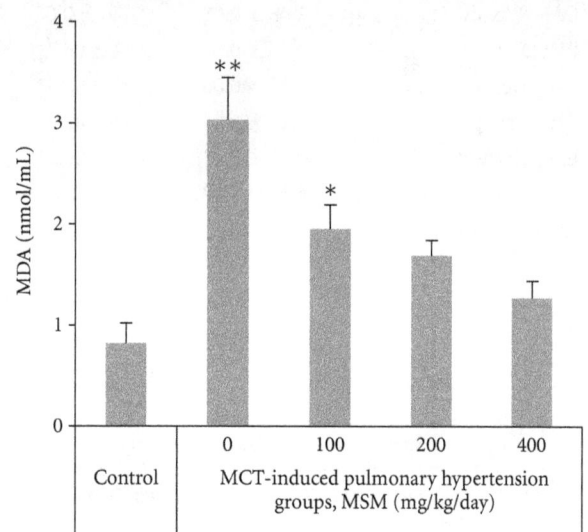

FIGURE 2: Effects of different doses (0–400 mg/kg/day) of methyl-sulfonylmethane (MSM) on lipid peroxidation expressed as the contents of malondialdehyde (MDA) in rats with monocrotaline- (MCT-) induced pulmonary hypertension (regression coefficient r^2 = 0.44, P < 0.01). Data are means ± SE, n = 6. Significant Tukey's post hoc differences compared with controls are indicated by asterisks (**P < 0.01 and *P < 0.05).

Table 3. MSM administration at 100 mg/kg/day significantly restored the levels of GSH and GSSG by +58% and −17%, respectively. The ratio of GSH/GSSG was calculated as an index of the redox state. The value of GSH/GSSG ratio was significantly lower in MCT-induced PAH (P = 0.002), but it was recovered to control levels after the treatment with 200 mg/kg/day MSM (Figure 1) and further enhanced by treatment with 400 mg/kg/day MSM (r^2 = 0.84; P < 0.01).

4.4. Level of Lipid Peroxidation. The serum levels of MDA were assayed as index of lipid peroxidation. Levels of MDA in the serum of hypertensive rats were significantly increased versus control (Figure 2). In MCT-induced hypertensive rats, MSM treatment led to a significant decrease in serum MDA level. MSM caused a dose-dependent decrease in MDA, with a maximal suppression of 60% in response to 400 mg/kg/day MSM.

5. Discussion

In this study, significant changes in the hemodynamics, serum antioxidative enzymes, glutathione, and MDA were observed in MCT-induced pulmonary hypertensive rats, and these changes were modulated with MSM in the experimental treatments.

Our findings are in agreement with previous reports showing adverse effects on the hemodynamics and lower final body weight gain in rats treated with MCT [16]. In the animals that received MSM, the hemodynamics were maintained at control levels, indicating prevention from the effects of MCT.

Consistent with the current study, several studies have reported that cardiovascular system of MCT-induced pulmonary hypertensive rats showed inflammatory alterations similar to those observed in human PAH [17, 18]. The effects of PAH on myocardium include hypertrophy and interstitial inflammatory cell infiltration. The RV tissue in the rat model of PAH was generally characterized by oxidative stress generation and showed elevation in stress markers MDA and nitrotyrosine [18]. Oxidative events observed in patients with chronic heart failure included markedly increased serum levels of the MDA and decreased GSH-px [19].

Furthermore, the finding of increased RAAS and ET-1 in rats with MCT-induced pulmonary hypertension supports the presence of enhanced oxidative stress in the RV of PAH rats. The PAH-induced increase in RAAS and ET-1 was reverted by treatment of MSM, indicating an improvement in the oxidative status of the cells.

In this study, enzymatic activity assay showed reduced CAT, SOD, and GSH-Px in serum of PAH rats compared with control. Biphasic changes in antioxidant enzymes have been described in association with the time point of sampling during MCT-induced PAH. These changes include an increase in antioxidant enzymes during hypertrophy stage and a decrease during heart failure stage [20]. Overall concordance between changes in hemodynamics and codirectional changes in oxidative markers in the current study implicates a role of oxidative stress in the pathogenesis of PAH.

In this study, CAT and SOD activities were higher in 400 mg/kg/day MSM-treated pulmonary hypertensive rats than in either the normotensive controls or the MCT-induced pulmonary hypertensive rats. A similar observation was previously made by Jin et al. [21] who showed that CAT, SOD, and GSH-Px activities in the plasma increased obviously in the MCT-induced hypertensive rats with the use of a sulfur dioxide (SO2) donor. These results imply that the SO2 can, at least partly, increase the antioxidative capacity of rats. These results are consistent with previous reports showing antioxidative effects of MSM through inhibition of oxidant production [22].

Recent reports have implicated increased lipid peroxidation as a mediator in the pathogenesis and the development of PAH [23]. Accordingly, antilipid peroxidation treatment therapy has been effective in the treatment of pulmonary arterial pressure and pulmonary resistance in PAH [24]. The finding of decreased lipid peroxidation marker MDA in rats with MCT-induced pulmonary hypertension supports the presence of enhanced oxidative stress in the RV of PAH rats. The PAH-induced increase in MDA was reverted by treatment of MSM, indicating an improvement in the oxidative status of the cells. Kim et al. [22] have recently shown that MSM inhibits LPS-induced release of oxidative stress biomarkers such as nitric oxide and prostaglandin E2 in macrophages through downregulation of NF-κB signaling. Moreover, MSM may act directly as free radical scavenger, which would further add to the efficiency of MSM as an antioxidant [7].

In pretreatment assessments, a decrease in circulating elevation of oxidative markers and an improved overall antioxidant potential with MSM treatment were evident. To the authors' knowledge, there are no specific data regarding the effect of MSM on oxidative parameters in pulmonary hypertensive rats. Although no mechanistic interpretation can be made at this point, the results obtained in the present study provide evidence for the first time that the MSM could limit oxidative response following pulmonary hypertension.

Future studies regarding the effects of MSM treatment on antioxidative defense function in PAH are clearly warranted.

6. Conclusion

MSM could exert protective antioxidative effects through the induction of CAT, SOD, and GSH-px activities along with associated reducing agents, such as GSH. In addition, these results suggest that MCT-induced PAH could induce harmful effects on the RV function, probably due to a decrease in antioxidant enzyme activity and subsequent oxidative damage.

Acknowledgment

This study was partially supported by a Grant from the Tabriz University of Medical Sciences (1388/4/20-5/4/3255).

References

[1] G. Simonneau, I. M. Robbins, M. Beghetti et al., "Updated clinical classification of pulmonary hypertension," *Journal of the American College of Cardiology*, vol. 54, no. 1, pp. S43–S54, 2009.

[2] R. L. Benza, D. P. Miller, M. Gomberg-Maitland et al., "Predicting survival in pulmonary arterial hypertension: insights from the registry to evaluate early and long-term pulmonary arterial hypertension disease management (REVEAL)," *Circulation*, vol. 122, no. 2, pp. 164–172, 2010.

[3] C. E. Huggins, A. A. Domenighetti, T. Pedrazzini, S. Pepe, and L. M. D. Delbridge, "Elevated intracardiac angiotensin II leads to cardiac hypertrophy and mechanical dysfunction in normotensive mice," *Journal of the Renin-Angiotensin-Aldosterone System*, vol. 4, no. 3, pp. 186–190, 2003.

[4] E. M. Redout, A. Van Der Toorn, M. J. Zuidwijk et al., "Antioxidant treatment attenuates pulmonary arterial hypertension-induced heart failure," *American Journal of Physiology*, vol. 298, no. 3, pp. H1038–H1047, 2010.

[5] K. Amirshahrokhi, S. Bohlooli, and M. M. Chinifroush, "The effect of methylsulfonylmethane on the experimental colitis in the rat," *Toxicology and Applied Pharmacology*, vol. 253, no. 3, pp. 197–202, 2011.

[6] K. Ebisuzaki, "Aspirin and methylsulfonylmethane (MSM): a search for common mechanisms, with implications for cancer prevention," *Anticancer Research*, vol. 23, no. 1, pp. 453–458, 2003.

[7] S. Parcell, "Sulfur in human nutrition and applications in medicine," *Alternative Medicine Review*, vol. 7, no. 1, pp. 22–44, 2002.

[8] E. M. Debbi, G. Agar, G. Fichman et al., "Efficacy of methylsulfonylmethane supplementation on osteoarthritis of the knee: a randomized controlled study," *BMC Complementary and Alternative Medicine*, vol. 11, article 50, 2011.

[9] E. J. Lim, D. Y. Hong, J. H. Park et al., "Methylsulfonylmethane suppresses breast cancer growth by down-regulating STAT3 and STAT5b pathways," *PLoS ONE*, vol. 7, no. 4, Article ID e33361, 2012.

[10] A. Garjani, A. Afrooziyan, H. Nazemiyeh, M. Najafi, A. Kharazmkia, and N. Maleki-Dizaji, "Protective effects of hydroalcoholic extract from rhizomes of Cynodon dactylon (L.) Pers. on compensated right heart failure in rats," *BMC Complementary and Alternative Medicine*, vol. 9, article 28, 2009.

[11] Y. L. Chang, H. S. Sohn, K. C. Chan, C. D. Berdanier, and J. L. Hargrove, "Low dietary protein impairs blood coagulation in BHE/cdb rats," *Journal of Nutrition*, vol. 127, no. 7, pp. 1279–1283, 1997.

[12] F. Squadrito, D. Altavilla, G. Squadrito et al., "Genistein supplementation and estrogen replacement therapy improve endothelial dysfunction induced by ovariectomy in rats," *Cardiovascular Research*, vol. 45, no. 2, pp. 454–462, 2000.

[13] U. R. Kodavanti, D. L. Costa, and P. A. Bromberg, "Rodent models of cardiopulmonary disease: their potential applicability in studies of air pollutant susceptibility," *Environmental Health Perspectives*, vol. 106, supplement 1, pp. 111–130, 1998.

[14] "Methylsulfonylmethane (MSM). Monograph," *Alternative Medicine Review*, vol. 8, pp. 438–441, 2003.

[15] M. Uchiyama and M. Mihara, "Determination of malonaldehyde precursor in tissues by thiobarbituric acid test," *Analytical Biochemistry*, vol. 86, no. 1, pp. 271–278, 1978.

[16] C. Carlino, J. D. Tobias, R. I. Schneider et al., "Pulmonary hemodynamic response to acute combination and monotherapy with sildenafil and brain natriuretic peptide in rats with monocrotaline-induced pulmonary hypertension," *American Journal of the Medical Sciences*, vol. 339, no. 1, pp. 55–59, 2010.

[17] F. Akhavein, E. Jean St-Michel, E. Seifert, and C. V. Rohlicek, "Decreased left ventricular function, myocarditis, and coronary arteriolar medial thickening following monocrotaline administration in adult rats," *Journal of Applied Physiology*, vol. 103, no. 1, pp. 287–295, 2007.

[18] P. Dorfmüller, M.-C. Chaumais, M. Giannakouli et al., "Increased oxidative stress and severe arterial remodeling induced by permanent high-flow challenge in experimental pulmonary hypertension," *Respiratory Research*, vol. 12, article 119, 2011.

[19] P. Joppa, D. Petrasova, B. Stancak, Z. Dorkova, and R. Tkacova, "Oxidative stress in patients with COPD and pulmonary hypertension," *Wien Klin Wochenschr*, vol. 119, pp. 428–434, 2007.

[20] F. Farahmand, M. F. Hill, and P. K. Singal, "Antioxidant and oxidative stress changes in experimental cor pulmonale," *Molecular and Cellular Biochemistry*, vol. 260, no. 1, pp. 21–29, 2004.

[21] H. F. Jin, S. X. Du, X. Zhao et al., "Effects of endogenous sulfur dioxide on monocrotaline-induced pulmonary hypertension in rats," *Acta Pharmacologica Sinica*, vol. 29, no. 10, pp. 1157–1166, 2008.

[22] Y. H. Kim, D. H. Kim, H. Lim, D. Y. Baek, H. K. Shin, and J. K. Kim, "The anti-inflammatory effects of methylsulfonylmethane on lipopolysaccharide-induced inflammatory respons-es in murine macrophages," *Biological and Pharmaceutical Bulletin*, vol. 32, no. 4, pp. 651–656, 2009.

[23] J. L. Cracowski, C. Cracowski, G. Bessard et al., "Increased lipid peroxidation in patients with pulmonary hypertension," *American Journal of Respiratory and Critical Care Medicine*, vol. 164, no. 6, pp. 1038–1042, 2001.

[24] Z. C. Li, F. Q. Zhang, J. C. Song, Q. B. Mei, and D. H. Zhao, "Therapeutic effects of DCDDP, a calcium channel blocker, on chronic pulmonary hypertension in rat," *Journal of Applied Physiology*, vol. 92, no. 3, pp. 997–1003, 2002.

24

Effect of Aqueous Extract of *Crocus sativus* L. on Morphine-Induced Memory Impairment

Sayede Maryam Naghibi,¹ Mahmoud Hosseini,¹ Fatemeh Khani,¹ Motahare Rahimi,¹ Farzaneh Vafaee,¹ Hassan Rakhshandeh,² and Azita Aghaie²

¹ *Neuroscience Research Center and Department of Physiology, School of Medicine, Mashhad University of Medical Sciences, Mashhad, Iran*
² *Pharmacological Research Center of Medicinal Plants and Department of Pharmacology, School of Medicine, Mashhad University of Medical Sciences, Mashhad 9177948564, Iran*

Correspondence should be addressed to Mahmoud Hosseini, hosseinim@mums.ac.ir

Academic Editor: Karim A. Alkadhi

In the present study, the effect of aqueous extracts of saffron on morphine-induced memory impairment was investigated. On the training trial, the mice received an electric shock when the animals were entered into the dark compartment. Twenty-four and forty-eight hours later, the time latency for entering the dark compartment was recorded and defined as the retention trial. The mice were divided into (1) control, (2) morphine which received morphine before the training in the passive avoidance test, (3–5) three groups treated by 50, 150 and 450 mg/kg of saffron extract before the training trial, and (6 and 7) the two other groups received 150 and 450 mg/kg of saffron extract before the retention trial. The time latency in morphine-treated group was lower than control ($P < 0.01$). Treatment of the animals by 150 and 450 mg/kg of saffron extract before the training trial increased the time latency at 24 and 48 hours after the training trial ($P < 0.05$ and $P < 0.01$). Administration of both 150 and 450 mg/kg doses of the extract before retention trials also increased the time latency ($P < 0.01$). The results revealed that the saffron extract attenuated morphine-induced memory impairment.

1. Introduction

Crocus sativus L. is a plant with green and hairy leaves and funnel-shaped reddish-purple flowers, which is cultivated in some countries including China, Spain, Italy, Greece, and especially Iran. It is commonly known as saffron or "Zaaferan" in Iran and is added to food for its color and taste [1, 2]. The part used for medication is the central part of the flower or the female sexual organ which is also called stigma or style. The main active constituents of this plant are picrocrocin and its derivatives include safranal, flavonoid derivatives, and crocin [3]. Safranal is the main aromatic component of saffron which comprises about 60% of the volatile ingredients in saffron [4]. *Crocus sativus* is used in folk medicine as an antispasmodic, eupeptic, anticatarrhal, carminative, diaphoretic, expectorant, stimulant, stomachic, aphrodisiac, emmenagogue gingival, and sedative [3].

It has been reported that extracts of *Crocus sativus* prevent from scopolamine and ethanol-induced memory impairment in Morris water maze and passive avoidance tests. It also protects against ethanol-induced inhibition of hippocampal long-term potentiation (LTP) [5, 6]. In addition, it has been reported that crocin counteracts the ethanol inhibition of NMDA receptor-mediated responses in rat hippocampal neurons [7]. It has been also shown that saffron attenuates cerebral ischemia [8] and reduces the extracellular hippocampal levels of glutamate and aspartate [9]. Saffron extracts or its active constituents have other activities on the central nervous system including antidepressant [10, 11], anticonvulsant [12, 13], and anxiolytic and hypnotic [14]. Some actions of saffron on central nervous system have been attributed to its effects on opioid system [12]. It has been also demonstrated that aqueous and ethanolic extracts of

Crocus sativus stigma and its constituent crocin can suppress morphine withdrawal syndrome [1].

Learning and memory in laboratory animals are known to be affected by opioids and their antagonists [15]. For example, pretraining administration of morphine impairs memory retrieval in passive avoidance tests which will be restored by pretest administration of the same dose of morphine [16]. Hippocampus is one of the areas involved in learning and memory in which both opioid peptides and opioid receptors are expressed [17]. Endogenous opioid peptides consider important neuromodulators in the brain, which are rich in the hippocampus and cerebral cortex [18]. Using different animal models, it was shown that repeated administering morphine can impair memory and learning processes [17, 19, 20].

With regard to the effects of saffron on learning and memory and its interactions with opioid system, the aim of the present study was to evaluate the effect of aqueous extract of *Crocus sativus* L. on morphine-induced memory impairment in mice using the passive avoidance test.

2. Materials and Methods

2.1. Preparing the Plant Extract. In this study, saffron was kindly provided by Novin Zaafran Company, Mashhad, Iran. The powder (100 g) of saffron was extracted with distilled water in a Soxhlet apparatus for 72 h. The resulting extract was concentrated under reduced pressure and kept at −20°C until being used (yielded 33.2%). The extract was dissolved in saline and was then applied [21–23].

2.2. Animals and the Experimental Protocol. Seventy-two male mice (30 ± 5 g, 10 weeks old) were kept at 22 ± 2°C and 12 h light/dark cycle (light on at 7:00 AM). All behavioral experiments were carried out between 10 AM and 2 PM The experiments were conducted in accordance with the Guide for the Care and Use of Laboratory Animals and the study was approved by Mashhad University of Medical Sciences. In the present study, the effects of the extract were examined in 2 experiments. In Experiment 1, the extract was injected before training phase (pretraining effect), while in Experiment 2 the extract was administered 24 and 48 hours after training phase (before the test phase, pretest effect).

Experiment 1. In this experiment the pretraining effect of the extract was examined. The animal groups were as follows. (1) Control group (*n* = 8): the animals in this group received saline instead of both the saffron extract and morphine. (2) Morphine group (*n* = 8): the animals were treated by saline instead of saffron extract, but morphine was injected to them (5 mg/kg, s.c.) 30 min before the training phase. (3–5) Pretraining treated groups (*n* = 8 in each group) (pretrain 50, pretrain 150, and pretrain 450): the animals in these groups were daily treated by 50, 150, and 450 mg/kg of saffron extract (i.p.), respectively, for 3 days before the training phase.

Experiment 2. In this experiment the pretest effect of the extract was examined. The animal groups were as follows. (1) Control group (*n* = 8): the animals in this group received saline instead of both saffron extract and morphine. (2) Morphine group (*n* = 8): the animals were treated by saline instead of saffron extract before the retention phase, but morphine was injected to them (5 mg/kg, s.c.) 30 min before the training phase. (3–4) Pretest groups (*n* = 8 in each group) (pretest 150 and pretest 450): the animals in these groups received 150 and 450 mg/kg of saffron extract (i.p.), respectively, before the test phase (24 and 48 hours after training phase).

2.3. Behavioral Procedures. The animals were handled for 1 week before starting the experiments. A passive avoidance learning test based on negative reinforcement was used to examine the memory. The apparatus consisted of a light and a dark compartment with a grid floor adjoining each other through a small gate. The animals were accustomed to the behavioral apparatus during two consecutive days (5 min in each day) before the training session. On the third day, the animals were placed in the light compartment, and the time latency for entering the dark compartment was recorded. In the training phase, the mice were placed in the light compartment facing away from the dark compartment. When the animals were entered completely into the dark compartment, they received an electric shock (1 MA, 2 s duration). The mice were then returned to their home cage. Twenty-four and forty-eight hours later (the retention phase or test phase), the animals were placed in the light compartment, and the time latency for entering the dark compartment as well as the time spent by the animals in the dark and light compartments was recorded and defined as the retention trial [24, 25].

2.4. Statistical Analysis. The data were expressed as mean ± SEM. The statistical analysis was done by one-way ANOVA followed by a tukey post hoc comparison test. The criterion for statistical significance was considered ($P < 0.05$).

3. Results

Experiment 1. In the morphine group, the time latency for entering the dark compartment was lower than that of the control group (Figure 1, $P < 0.01$). The treatment of the animals by 150 and 450 mg/kg of saffron extract significantly increased the time latency for entering the dark compartment Twenty-four and forty-eight h after receiving a shock (Figure 1, $P < 0.05$ and $P < 0.01$). Administration of 50 mg/kg of saffron extract was not effective for changing the time latency for entering the dark compartment. The results also showed that the total time spent in the dark compartment by the animals of the morphine group was higher than that of the saline group (Figure 2, $P < 0.01$). Twenty-four and forty-eight h after receiving the shock, the total time spent in the dark compartment by the animals of the pretrain 150 group was lower than that of the morphine group (Figure 2, both $P < 0.01$). The results also indicated

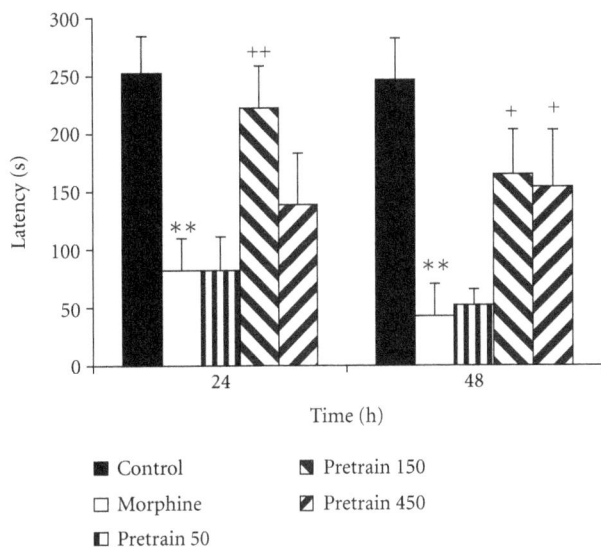

FIGURE 1: The effects of pretraining injection of saffron extract on time latency for entering the dark compartment 24 and 48 h after receiving the shock in the experimental groups. The animals of control group received saline instead of both saffron extract and morphine. The animals of morphine group were treated by saline instead of SE but received morphine (5 mg/kg, s.c.) 30 min before the training phase. Pretrain 50, pretrain 150, and pretrain 450 groups were treated by 50, 150, and 450 mg/kg of SE (i.p.), respectively, for 3 days before the training phase. The data were presented as mean ± SEM of the time latency (8 animals in each group). **$P < 0.01$ compared with the control group; +$P < 0.05$ and ++$P < 0.01$ compared with the morphine group.

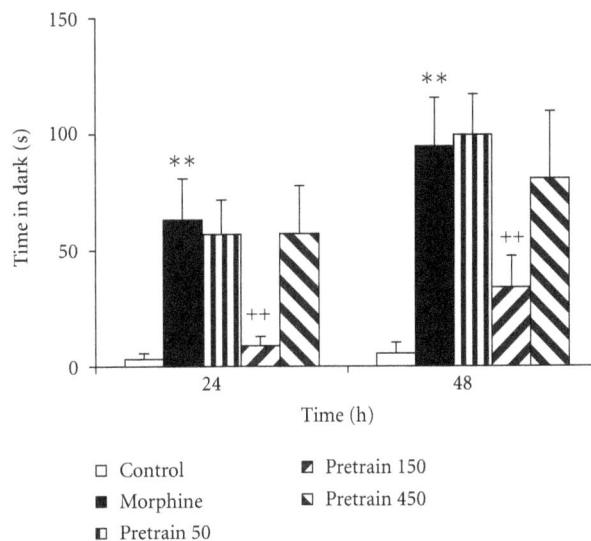

FIGURE 2: The effects of pretraining injection of saffron extract on the time spent in the dark compartment 24 and 48 h after receiving the shock. The animals of control group received saline instead of both saffron extract and morphine. The animals of morphine group were treated by saline instead of SE but received morphine (5 mg/kg, s.c.) 30 min before the training phase. Pretrain 50, Pretrain 150, and pretrain 450 groups were treated by 50, 150, and 450 mg/kg of saffron extract (i.p.), respectively, for 3 days before the training phase. The data were presented as mean ± SEM of the total time spent in the dark compartment (8 animals in each group). **$P < 0.01$ compared with the control group; ++$P < 0.01$ compared with the morphine group.

that the total time spent in the light compartment by the animals of the morphine group was lower than that of the saline group at 24 and 48 h after receiving the shock (Figure 3, $P < 0.05$ and $P < 0.01$). In the pretrain 150 group, the total time spent in the light compartment was higher than that of the morphine group at 48 h after receiving the shock (Figure 3, $P < 0.05$).

Experiment 2. Treatment of the animals by 150 and 450 mg/kg of saffron before retention phases (24 and 48 h after the shock) increased the time latency for entering the dark compartment (Figure 4, $P < 0.01$). The total time spent in the dark compartment by the animals treated by 450 mg/kg of saffron extract was lower than that of the morphine group (Figure 5, $P < 0.05$ and $P < 0.01$). However, there was no significant difference in the total time spent in the light compartment between these groups (Figure 6).

4. Discussion

The results of the present study showed that saffron extract attenuated memory impairment induced by morphine. The results were in agreement with the results of previous studies showing the beneficial effects of saffron on memory [5, 26, 27]. Haghighizad et al. also suggested the protective effect of the saffron extract against morphine-induced inhibition

of spatial learning and memory in rats. The used doses were lower than that in the present study [28]. It has been recently found that the alcoholic extract of the pistils of *Crocus sativus* L. affects learning and memory in mice [27]. In another study, oral administration of 125–500 mg/kg of *Crocus sativus* extract alone had no effect on the learning behavior of mice in passive avoidance test but significantly improved ethanol-induced impairment of memory acquisition [27]. It has been also shown that treatment of animals by 50–200 mg/kg crocin alone had no effect but significantly improved ethanol-induced impairment of memory acquisition in mice [5]. Intracerebroventricular administration of crocin significantly prevented from ethanol-induced inhibition of hippocampal LTP in anaesthetized rats *in vivo* [26, 29]. The results of the present study also showed that *Crocus sativus* extract inhibited of the deleterious effect morphine on memory.

There is accumulating evidence that opiates modulate synaptic transmission and plasticity in the brain. Opiates have been shown to alter glutamatergic transmission [30], neurogenesis [31], dendritic stability [32], and long-term potentiation [33–35]. The passive avoidance paradigm used in the present study depends upon both the amygdala and hippocampal systems [36–38]. It has been also shown that both the amygdala and hippocampus are involved in the effects of opioids on memory [39–41]. The exact mechanism(s) of morphine induced impairment of memory

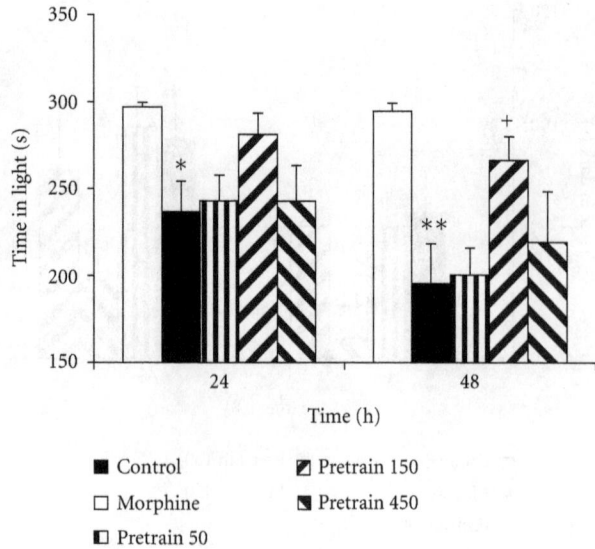

FIGURE 3: The effects of pretraining injection of saffron extract on the total time spent in the light compartment 24 and 48 h after receiving the shock between the groups. The animals of control group received saline instead of both saffron extract and morphine. The animals of morphine group were treated by saline instead of SE but received morphine (5 mg/kg, s.c.) 30 min before the training phase. Pretrain 50, pretrain 150, and pretrain 450 groups were treated by 50, 150, and 450 mg/kg of SE (i.p.), respectively, for 3 days before the training phase. The data were presented as mean $\pm$ SEM of the total time spent in the light compartment (8 animals in each group). $*P < 0.05$ and $**P < 0.01$ compared to control; $+P < 0.05$ compared to morphine group.

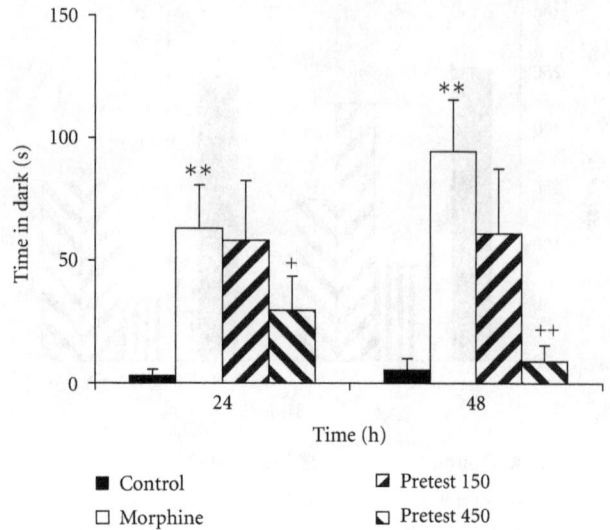

FIGURE 5: Comparison of the total time spent in the dark compartment in the experimental groups. The animals of the control group received saline instead of both saffron extract and morphine. The animals of morphine group were treated by saline instead of SE but received morphine (5 mg/kg, s.c.) 30 min before the training phase. Pretest 150 and pretest 450 groups were treated by 150 and 450 mg/kg of SE (i.p.), respectively, before the recall phase. The data were presented as mean $\pm$ SEM of the total time spent in the dark compartment (8 animals in each group). $**P < 0.01$ compared with the control; $+P < 0.05$ and $++P < 0.01$ compared with the morphine group.

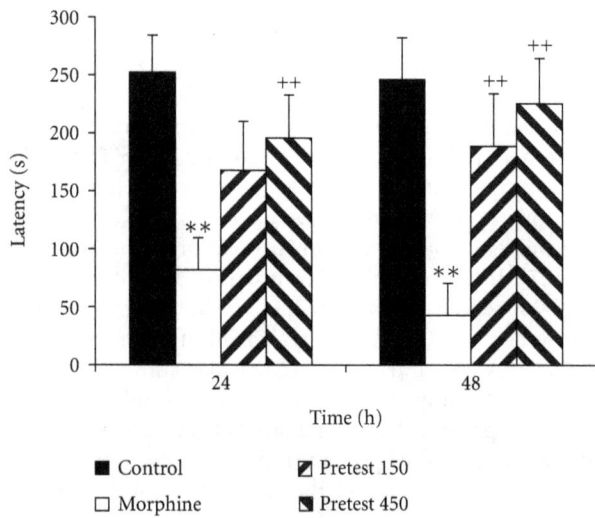

FIGURE 4: The effects of pretest injection of saffron extract on time latency for entering the dark compartment. The animals of the control group received saline instead of both saffron extract and morphine. The animals of morphine group were treated by saline instead of SE but received morphine (5 mg/kg, s.c.) 30 min before the training phase. Pretest 150 and pretest 450 groups were treated by 150 and 450 mg/kg of SE (i.p.), respectively, before the recall phase. The data were presented as mean $\pm$ SEM of the time latency (8 animals in each group). $**P < 0.01$ compared with the control group and $++P < 0.01$ compared with the morphine group.

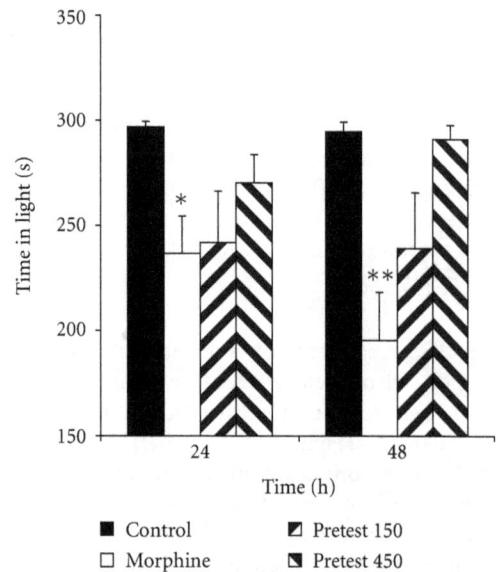

FIGURE 6: Comparison of the total time spent in the light compartment 24 and 48 h after receiving the shock between the groups. The animals of the control group received saline instead of both saffron extract and morphine. The animals of morphine group were treated by saline instead of SE but received morphine (5 mg/kg, s.c.) 30 min before the training phase. Pretest 150 and pretest 450 groups were treated by 150 and 450 mg/kg of SE (i.p.), respectively, before the recall phase. The data were presented as mean $\pm$ SEM of the total time spent in the light compartment (8 animals in each group).

formation have not been completely elucidated [42]. The role of NMDA receptors in morphine state-dependent learning has been suggested [43, 44]. These receptors are also involved in post-training memory processing by the amygdala and hippocampus [45]. Furthermore, NMDA receptors may have a role in the effect of saffron or its constituents on memory [46, 47]. Moreover, the analgesic effect of saffron is attenuated by NMDA receptor antagonists [48]. It has been suggested that opioid-induced impairment of memory formation may be accompanied by a decreased activity level in nitric oxide/cyclic guanosine monophosphate (NO/cGMP) signaling pathway [16]. The interaction of saffron with nitric oxide has been also reported [49]. It has been shown that morphine-induced memory recall might be influenced by the central cholinergic activity [50]. Beneficial effects of saffron on memory in inhibited cholinergic system animal models [2, 51] may be another explanation for the effect of the extract on memory in the present study. The sedative-effects of as well as the protective effects in pentylenetetrazole (PTZ-) induced seizure in mice and rats may imply that saffron affects the GABAergic system [12, 27, 52] in which the latter has a role in memory impairment by the opioids [53, 54]. It is believed that saffron extract, crocetin or crocin, could be useful in the treatment of brain neurodegenerative disorders because of its powerful antioxidant activities [55]. Considering the possible role of oxidative damage in the deleterious effect of morphine [56], the antioxidant activity of the extract can be considered as another explanation for the beneficial effects of saffron on morphine-induced memory impairments [56, 57]. A functional interaction between dopamine and opioid system in memory storage processes has been suggested [58]. This mechanism may also have a role in the effect of saffron on memory impairment by opioids [59]. There are also other pieces of evidence which confirm the interaction of the opioid system with saffron or its constituents. It has been indicated that crocin produces a dose-dependent antinociceptive effect and also increases morphine-induced antinociception [60]. The analgesic effects of saffron ethanolic extract have been attributed to its effect on the opioid system [48]. Hosseinzadeh and Jahanian. also showed that the aqueous extracts in doses 80–320 mg/kg and ethanolic ones in doses 400–800 mg/kg attenuated morphine withdrawal signs induced by naloxone in mice [1]. It was also shown that injection of 100 mg/kg of Crocus sativus extract inhibited the acquisition and expression of morphine-induced conditioned place preference [61, 62]. In the present study, 50–450 mg/kg of the saffron extract inhibited morphine-induced memory impairment; however, it seems that the medium dose was more effective. The results of the present study added evidence for the effects of saffron on the brain opioid system.

In the present study, the chemical compound(s) for the beneficial effects of saffron was not indentified. The presence of crocin as a water-soluble carotenoid, as well as the monoterpene aldehyde and its glucosides including safranal and picrocrocin, and flavonoids including quercetin and kaempferol in saffron, has been well documented [63]. The beneficial effects of saffron on memory have been repeatedly attributed to crocin [7, 51, 55, 63]. Therefore, the

results of present study may at least in part be due to this component. However, the memory enhancing effect as well as the protective effects of safranal on PTZ-induced seizure model may also be a good evidence for the interaction of safranal with GABAergic system [6, 12, 13]. It was also shown that safranal affects the extracellular levels of glutamate and aspartate in hippocampal tissues of kainic acid-treated rats [9]. On the other hand, the interaction of safranal with opioid system has been suggested [1, 62]. For example it has been shown that safranal affects morphine-induced conditioned place preference [62]. The injection of safranal to morphine-dependent animals also acted as an opioid antagonist and induced-morphine withdrawal like behaviors including jumping, seizure, diarrhea, ptosis, irritability, and wet-dog shake [1]. Therefore, it seems that this constituent may also have a role in the results of present study. The precise compound(s) and mechanism(s) responsible for the efficacy of saffron extract on memory impairments elicited by morphine still remain as an important issue and need to be clarified by further studies.

5. Conclusion

The results of the present study showed that the aqueous extract of Crocus sativus prevented from morphine induced memory deficits in mice. Further studies are needed to confirm this protective effect of Crocus sativus.

Acknowledgment

The authors would like to thank the Vice Presidency of Research, Mashhad University of Medical Sciences, for its financial supports.

References

[1] H. Hosseinzadeh and Z. Jahanian, "Effect of Crocus sativus L. (saffron) stigma and its constituents, crocin and safranal, on morphine withdrawal syndrome in mice," Phytotherapy Research, vol. 24, no. 5, pp. 726–730, 2010.

[2] N. Pitsikas and N. Sakellaridis, "Crocus sativus L. extracts antagonize memory impairments in different behavioural tasks in the rat," Behavioural Brain Research, vol. 173, no. 1, pp. 112–115, 2006.

[3] M. H. Boskabady, M. Ghasemzadeh Rahbardar, H. Nemati, and M. Esmaeilzadeh, "Inhibitory effect of Crocus sativus (saffron) on histamine (H1) receptors of guinea pig tracheal chains," Pharmazie, vol. 65, no. 4, pp. 300–305, 2010.

[4] F. I. Abdullaev and J. J. Espinosa-Aguirre, "Biomedical properties of saffron and its potential use in cancer therapy and chemoprevention trials," Cancer Detection and Prevention, vol. 28, no. 6, pp. 426–432, 2004.

[5] M. Sugiura, Y. Shoyama, H. Saito et al., "Crocin improves the ethanol-induced impairment of learning behaviors of mice in passive avoidance tasks," Proceedings of the Japan Academy B, vol. 71, no. 10, pp. 319–324, 1995.

[6] H. Hosseinzadeh and T. Ziaei, "Effects of Crocus sativus stigma extract and its constituents, crocin and safranal, on intact memory and scopolamine-induced learning deficits in rats

performing the Morris water maze task," *Journal of Medicinal Plants*, vol. 5, no. 19, pp. 40–60, 2006.

[7] K. Abe, M. Sugiura, Y. Shoyama, and H. Saito, "Crocin antagonizes ethanol inhibition of NMDA receptor-mediated responses in rat hippocampal neurons," *Brain Research*, vol. 787, no. 1, pp. 132–138, 1998.

[8] H. Hosseinzadeh and H. R. Sadeghnia, "Safranal, a constituent of *Crocus sativus* (saffron), attenuated cerebral ischemia induced oxidative damage in rat hippocampus," *Journal of Pharmacy and Pharmaceutical Sciences*, vol. 8, no. 3, pp. 394–399, 2005.

[9] H. Hosseinzadeh, H. R. Sadeghnia, and A. Rahimi, "Effect of safranal on extracellular hippocampal levels of glutamate and aspartate during kainic acid treatment in anesthetized rats," *Planta Medica*, vol. 74, no. 12, pp. 1441–1445, 2008.

[10] S. Akhondzadeh, N. Tahmacebi-Pour, A. A. Noorbala et al., "*Crocus sativus* L. in the treatment of mild to moderate depression: a double-blind, randomized and placebo-controlled trial," *Phytotherapy Research*, vol. 19, no. 2, pp. 148–151, 2005.

[11] H. Hosseinzadeh, V. Motamedshariaty, and F. Hadizadeh, "Antidepressant effect of kaempferol, a constituent of saffron (*Crocus sativus*) petal, in mice and rats," *Pharmacologyonline*, vol. 2, pp. 367–370, 2007.

[12] H. Hosseinzadeh and H. R. Sadeghnia, "Protective effect of safranal on pentylenetetrazol-induced seizures in the rat: involvement of GABAergic and opioids systems," *Phytomedicine*, vol. 14, no. 4, pp. 256–262, 2007.

[13] H. Hosseinzadeh and F. Talebzadeh, "Anticonvulsant evaluation of safranal and crocin from *Crocus sativus* in mice," *Fitoterapia*, vol. 76, no. 7-8, pp. 722–724, 2005.

[14] H. Hosseinzadeh and N. B. Noraei, "Anxiolytic and hypnotic effect of *Crocus sativus* aqueous extract and its constituents, crocin and safranal, in mice," *Phytotherapy Research*, vol. 23, no. 6, pp. 768–774, 2009.

[15] I. Izquierdo, M. A. M. R. De Almeida, and V. R. Emiliano, "Unlike β-endorphin, dynorphin1-13 does not cause retrograde amnesia for shuttle avoidance or inhibitory avoidance learning in rats," *Psychopharmacology*, vol. 87, no. 2, pp. 216–218, 1985.

[16] S. Khavandgar, H. Homayoun, and M. R. Zarrindast, "The effect of L-NAME and L-arginine on impairment of memory formation and state-dependent learning induced by morphine in mice," *Psychopharmacology*, vol. 167, no. 3, pp. 291–296, 2003.

[17] F. Motamedi, M. Ghasemi, F. Davoodi, and N. Naghdi, "Comparison of learning and memory in morphine dependent rats using different behavioral models," *Iranian Journal of Pharmaceutical Research*, vol. 2, no. 4, pp. 225–230.

[18] A. L. Vaccarino, G. A. Olson, R. D. Olson, and A. J. Kastin, "Endogenous opiates: 1998," *Peptides*, vol. 20, no. 12, pp. 1527–1574, 1999.

[19] K. Saadipour, A. Sarkaki, H. Alaei, M. Badavi, and F. Rahim, "Forced exercise improves passive avoidance memory in morphine-exposed rats," *Pakistan Journal of Biological Sciences*, vol. 12, no. 17, pp. 1206–1211, 2009.

[20] H. Alaei, L. Borjeian, M. Azizi, S. Orian, A. Pourshanazari, and O. Hanninen, "Treadmill running reverses retention deficit induced by morphine," *European Journal of Pharmacology*, vol. 536, no. 1-2, pp. 138–141, 2006.

[21] A. R. Ebrahimzadeh Bideskan, M. Hosseini, T. Mohammadpour et al., "Effects of soy extract on pentylenetetrazol-induced seizures in ovariectomized rats," *Journal of Chinese Integrative Medicine*, vol. 9, no. 6, pp. 611–618, 2011.

[22] H. Rakhshandah and M. Hosseini, "Potentiation of pentobarbital hypnosis by Rosa damascena in mice," *Indian Journal of Experimental Biology*, vol. 44, no. 11, pp. 910–912, 2006.

[23] M. Hosseini, M. G. Rahbardar, H. R. Sadeghnia, and H. Rakhshandeh, "Effects of different extracts of rosa damascena on pentylenetetrazol-induced seizures in mice," *Journal of Chinese Integrative Medicine*, vol. 9, no. 10, pp. 1118–1124, 2011.

[24] M. Nassiri-Asl, F. Zamansoltani, A. Javadi, and M. Ganjvar, "The effects of rutin on a passive avoidance test in rats," *Progress in Neuro-Psychopharmacology and Biological Psychiatry*, vol. 34, no. 1, pp. 204–207, 2010.

[25] J. W. Wright, J. A. Clemens, J. A. Panetta et al., "Effects of LY231617 and angiotensin IV on ischemia-induced deficits in circular water maze and passive avoidance performance in rats," *Brain Research*, vol. 717, no. 1-2, pp. 1–11, 1996.

[26] M. Sugiura, Y. Shoyama, H. Saito, and K. Abe, "Crocin (crocetin di-gentiobiose ester) prevents the inhibitory effect of ethanol on long-term potentiation in the dentate gyrus in vivo," *Journal of Pharmacology and Experimental Therapeutics*, vol. 271, no. 2, pp. 703–707, 1994.

[27] Y. Zhang, Y. Shoyama, M. Sugiura, and H. Saito, "Effects of *Crocus sativus* L. on the ethanol-induced impairment of passive avoidance performances in mice," *Biological and Pharmaceutical Bulletin*, vol. 17, no. 2, pp. 217–221, 1994.

[28] H. Haghighizad, A. Pourmotabbed, and H. Sahraei, "Protective effect of Saffron extract on morphine-induced inhibition of spatial learning and memory in rat," *Physiology and Pharmacology*, vol. 12, no. 3, pp. 170–179, 2008.

[29] M. Sugiura, Y. Shoyama, H. Saito, and K. Abe, "Crocin (crocetin di-gentiobiose ester) prevents the inhibitory effect of ethanol on long-term potentiation in the dentate gyrus in vivo," *Journal of Pharmacology and Experimental Therapeutics*, vol. 271, no. 2, pp. 703–707, 1994.

[30] N. J. Xu, L. Bao, H. P. Fan et al., "Morphine withdrawal increases glutamate uptake and surface expression of glutamate transporter GLT1 at hippocampal synapses," *Journal of Neuroscience*, vol. 23, no. 11, pp. 4775–4784, 2003.

[31] A. J. Eisch, M. Barrot, C. A. Schad, D. W. Self, and E. J. Nestler, "Opiates inhibit neurogenesis in the adult rat hippocampus," *Proceedings of the National Academy of Sciences of the United States of America*, vol. 97, no. 13, pp. 7579–7584, 2000.

[32] D. Liao, H. Lin, Y. L. Ping, and H. H. Loh, "Mu-opioid receptors modulate the stability of dendritic spines," *Proceedings of the National Academy of Sciences of the United States of America*, vol. 102, no. 5, pp. 1725–1730, 2005.

[33] F. A. Mansouri, F. Motamedi, Y. Fathollahi, N. Atapour, and S. Semnanian, "Augmentation of LTP induced by primed-bursts tetanic stimulation in hippocampal CA1 area of morphine dependent rats," *Brain Research*, vol. 769, no. 1, pp. 119–124, 1997.

[34] F. A. Mansouri, F. Motamedi, and Y. Fathollahi, "Chronic in vivo morphine administration facilitates primed-bursts-induced long-term potentiation of Schaffer collateral-CA1 synapses in hippocampal slices in vitro," *Brain Research*, vol. 815, no. 2, pp. 419–423, 1999.

[35] L. Pu, G. B. Bao, N. J. Xu, L. Ma, and G. Pei, "Hippocampal long-term potentiation is reduced by chronic opiate treatment and can be restored by re-exposure to opiates," *Journal of Neuroscience*, vol. 22, no. 5, pp. 1914–1921, 2002.

[36] L. Stubley-Weatherly, J. W. Harding, and J. W. Wright, "Effects of discrete kainic acid-induced hippocampal lesions on spatial and contextual learning and memory in rats," *Brain Research*, vol. 716, no. 1-2, pp. 29–38, 1996.

[37] M. Sakurai, M. Sekiguchi, K. Zushida et al., "Reduction in memory in passive avoidance learning, exploratory behaviour and synaptic plasticity in mice with a spontaneous deletion in the ubiquitin C-terminal hydrolase L1 gene," *European Journal of Neuroscience*, vol. 27, no. 3, pp. 691–701, 2008.

[38] R. J. McDonald and N. M. White, "A triple dissociation of memory systems: hippocampus, amygdala, and dorsal striatum," *Behavioral Neuroscience*, vol. 107, no. 1, pp. 3–22, 1993.

[39] H. Miladi-Gorji, A. Rashidy-Pour, Y. Fathollahi, M. M. Akhavan, S. Semnanian, and M. Safari, "Voluntary exercise ameliorates cognitive deficits in morphine dependent rats: the role of hippocampal brain-derived neurotrophic factor," *Neurobiology of Learning and Memory*, vol. 96, no. 3, pp. 479–491, 2011.

[40] M. Gallagher and B. S. Kapp, "Manipulation of opiate activity in the amygdala alters memory processes," *Life Sciences*, vol. 23, no. 19, pp. 1973–1977, 1978.

[41] M. R. Zarrindast, F. Asadi, and A. Rezayof, "Repeated pretreatment of morphine prevents morphine-induced amnesia: a possible involvement for dorsal hippocampal NMDA receptors," *Archives of Iranian Medicine*, vol. 14, no. 1, pp. 32–38, 2011.

[42] L. A. Bruins Slot and F. C. Colpaert, "Opiate states of memory: receptor mechanisms," *Journal of Neuroscience*, vol. 19, no. 23, pp. 10520–10529, 1999.

[43] M. R. Zarrindast, M. Jafari-Sabet, M. Rezayat, B. Djahanguiri, and A. Rezayof, "Involvement of NMDA receptors in morphine state-dependent learning in mice," *International Journal of Neuroscience*, vol. 116, no. 6, pp. 731–743, 2006.

[44] V. Cestari and C. Castellano, "MK-801 potentiates morphine-induced impairment of memory consolidation in mice: involvement of dopaminergic mechanisms," *Psychopharmacology*, vol. 133, no. 1, pp. 1–6, 1997.

[45] I. Izquierdo, C. Da Cunha, R. Rosat, D. Jerusalinsky, M. B. C. Ferreira, and J. H. Medina, "Neurotransmitter receptors involved in post-training memory processing by the amygdala, medial septum, and hippocampus of the rat," *Behavioral and Neural Biology*, vol. 58, no. 1, pp. 16–26, 1992.

[46] M. Lechtenberg, D. Schepmann, M. Niehues, N. Hellenbrand, B. Wünsch, and A. Hensel, "Quality and functionality of saffron: quality control, species assortment and affinity of extract and isolated saffron compounds to NMDA and σ_1 (Sigma-1) receptors," *Planta Medica*, vol. 74, no. 7, pp. 764–772, 2008.

[47] K. Abe, M. Sugiura, S. Yamaguchi, Y. Shoyama, and H. Saito, "Saffron extract prevents acetaldehyde-induced inhibition of long-term potentiation in the rat dentate gyrus in vivo," *Brain Research*, vol. 851, no. 1-2, pp. 287–289, 1999.

[48] S. Nasri, H. Sahraei, and H. Zardooz, "Inhibition of pain and inflamation induced by formalin in male mice by ethanolic extract of saffron (*Crocus sativus*) and its constituents crocin and safranal," *Kowsar Medical Journal*, vol. 15, no. 4, pp. 189–195, 2011.

[49] F. Nabavizadeh, E. Salimi, Z. Sadroleslami, S. M. Karimian, and J. Vahedian, "Saffron (*Crocus sativus*) increases gastric acid and pepsin secretions in rats: role of nitric oxide (NO)," *African Journal of Pharmacy and Pharmacology*, vol. 3, no. 5, pp. 181–184, 2009.

[50] M. R. Jafari, M. R. Zarrindast, and B. Djahanguiri, "Influence of cholinergic system modulators on morphine state-dependent memory of passive avoidance in mice," *Physiology and Behavior*, vol. 5, supplement, article S163, 2006.

[51] M. R. Ghadami and A. Pourmotabbed, "The effect of crocin on scopolamine induced spatial learning and memory deficits in rats," *Physiology and Pharmacology*, vol. 12, no. 4, pp. 287–295, 2009.

[52] N. Pitsikas, A. Boultadakis, G. Georgiadou, P. A. Tarantilis, and N. Sakellaridis, "Effects of the active constituents of *Crocus sativus* L., crocins, in an animal model of anxiety," *Phytomedicine*, vol. 15, no. 12, pp. 1135–1139, 2008.

[53] J. D. Brioni, A. H. Nagahara, and J. L. McGaugh, "Involvement of the amygdala GABAergic system in the modulation of memory storage," *Brain Research*, vol. 487, no. 1, pp. 105–112, 1989.

[54] M. R. Zarrindast, M. Noorbakhshnia, F. Motamedi, A. Haeri-Rohani, and A. Rezayof, "Effect of the GABAergic system on memory formation and state-dependent learning induced by morphine in rats," *Pharmacology*, vol. 76, no. 2, pp. 93–100, 2006.

[55] K. Abe and H. Saito, "Effects of saffron extract and its constituent crocin on learning behaviour and long-term potentiation," *Phytotherapy Research*, vol. 14, no. 3, pp. 149–152, 2000.

[56] D. C. Guzmán, I. E. Vázquez, N. O. Brizuela et al., "Assessment of oxidative damage induced by acute doses of morphine sulfate in postnatal and adult rat brain," *Neurochemical Research*, vol. 31, no. 4, pp. 549–554, 2006.

[57] M. A. Papandreou, M. Tsachaki, S. Efthimiopoulos, P. Cordopatis, F. N. Lamari, and M. Margarity, "Memory enhancing effects of saffron in aged mice are correlated with antioxidant protection," *Behavioural Brain Research*, vol. 219, no. 2, pp. 197–204, 2011.

[58] C. Castellano, V. Cestari, S. Cabib, and S. Puglisi-Allegra, "The effects of morphine on memory consolidation in mice involve both D1 and D2 dopamine receptors," *Behavioral and Neural Biology*, vol. 61, no. 2, pp. 156–161, 1994.

[59] P. S. Widdowson and R. B. Holman, "Ethanol-induced increase in endogenous dopamine release may involve endogenous opiates," *Journal of Neurochemistry*, vol. 59, no. 1, pp. 157–163, 1992.

[60] E. Tamaddonfard and N. Hamzeh-Gooshchi, "Effect of crocin on the morphine-induced antinociception in the formalin test in rats," *Phytotherapy Research*, vol. 24, no. 3, pp. 410–413, 2010.

[61] N. Mojabi, A. Eidi, M. Kamalinejad et al., "Study of the effects of intra-nucleus accumbens shell injections of alcohlic extract of *Crocus sativus* on the acquisition and expression of morphine-induced conditioned place preference in rats," *Physiology and Pharmacology*, vol. 12, no. 2, pp. 121–128, 2008.

[62] H. Sahraei, M. Mohammadi, M. Kamalinejad, J. Shams, H. Ghoshooni, and A. Noroozadeh, "Effects of the *Crocus sativus* L. extract on the acquisition and expression of morphine-induced conditioned place preference in female mice," *Journal of Medicinal Plants*, vol. 7, no. 25, pp. 29–38, 2008.

[63] H. Hosseinzadeh, H. R. Sadeghnia, F. A. Ghaeni, V. S. Motamedshariaty, and S. A. Mohajeri, "Effects of saffron (*Crocus sativus* L.) and its active constituent, crocin, on recognition and spatial memory after chronic cerebral hypoperfusion in rats," *Phytotherapy Research*, vol. 26, no. 3, pp. 381–386, 2012.

25

Anti-Inflammatory Activity of *Delonix regia* (Boj. Ex. Hook)

Vaishali D. Shewale,[1,2] **Tushar A. Deshmukh,**[1,2] **Liladhar S. Patil,**[1,3] **and Vijay R. Patil**[1,2]

[1] Tapi Valley Education Society, Hon'ble, Loksevak Madhukarrao Chaudhari College of Pharmacy,
 Faizpur 425 503, India
[2] Department of Pharmacognosy, Hon'ble, Loksevak Madhukarrao Chaudhari College of Pharmacy,
 Faizpur 425 503, Maharashtra, India
[3] Department of Biotechnology, Hon'ble, Loksevak Madhukarrao Chaudhari College of Pharmacy,
 Faizpur 425 503, Maharashtra, India

Correspondence should be addressed to Tushar A. Deshmukh, deshmukhta@rediffmail.com

Academic Editor: Lutfun Nahar

The present work was to evaluate the anti-inflammatory activity of *Delonix regia* leaves (Family: Caesalpiniaceae). The powder of *Delonix regia* leaves was subjected to extraction with ethanol in soxhlet extractor. The ethanol extract after preliminary phytochemical investigation showed the presence of sterols, triterpenoids, phenolic compounds and flavonoids. The anti-inflammatory activity was studied using carrageenan-induced rat paw edema and cotton pellet granuloma at a three different doses (100, 200, and 400 mg/kg b.w. p.o.) of ethanol extract. The ethanol extract of *Delonix regia* leaves was exhibited significant anti-inflammatory activity at the dose of 400 mg/kg in both models when compared with control group. Indomethacin (10 mg/kg b.w. p.o) was also shown significant anti-inflammatory activity in both models.

1. Introduction

Inflammation is a series of pathological changes associated with local vascular reaction and cellular response, the living tissue, an injury insufficient to kill the tissue. This is distinguished from the wider problem of generalized reactions of the body. However, it is related to infection caused by microorganisms, and various pathological changes are associated with it [1]. Traditional medicines play an important role in health services around the globe. About three-quarters of the world population relies on plants and plant extracts for healthcare. The rational design of novel drugs from traditional medicine offers new prospects in modern healthcare. *Delonix regia* (Boj. Ex. Hook) (Family: Caesalpiniaceae) is a medium-sized tree found in greater parts of India. The decoction of the leaves is traditionally used in treating gastric problems, body pain, and rheumatic pains of joints [2, 3]. Ethanolic extracts of flower and bark were investigated to anti-inflammatory activity in rats [4]. The leaves are reported to antibacterial [5] and antimalarial [6]. *Delonix regia* contains proteins, flavonoids, tannins,

phenolic compounds, glycosides, sterols, and triterpenoids. However, no data were found regarding the pharmacological and phytochemical evaluation of the leaves of the plant. The aim of the present study was to investigate the anti-inflammatory activity of the ethanol extract of the leaves of *Delonix regia* (Boj. Ex. Hook).

2. Materials and Methods

2.1. Plant Material. *Delonix regia* leaves were procured from the local market in Jalgaon, Maharashtra, India, identified, and authenticated. A voucher specimen (voucher specimen number-Vaishu 9200) was deposited in the herbarium of the Department of Botany, Rashtrasant Tukdoji Maharaj, Nagpur University, Nagpur.

2.2. Extraction of Plant Material. The leaves were dried under a shade and pulverized. The coarse powder (1000 g) was extracted with ethanol using a soxhlet apparatus. The extract was dried using a rotary vacuum evaporator and stored in a desiccator until further use. The percentage yield of ethanol extract of *Delonix regia* (EEDR) was 25.0% w/w.

2.3. Phytochemical Screening. A preliminary phytochemical screening of *Delonix regia* was carried out [7]. The presence of alkaloid (Dragendorff reagent and Mayer's reagent), flavonoids (Shinoda test), steroids (Liberman Burchard test), and terpenes (Vanillin sulfuric acid reagent) were analyzed.

2.4. Drugs and Chemicals. Indomethacin was purchased from Themis Pharmaceutical Ltd. India. Carrageenan was purchased from Sigma Aldrich, USA. Tween 80 and other reagents of analytical grade were purchased from S. D. Fine Chem. Ltd, India.

2.5. Animals. Wistar albino rats (150–200 g) and mice (20–25 g) of either sex were purchased from Calcutta Fish Aquarium, Indore, India and were housed under standard conditions of temperature and light. Animals had free access to food (Amrut Feeds, Pune, India) and water. The Institutional Animal Ethics Committee approved the protocol of the study.

2.6. Acute Toxicity Studies. Healthy adult Swiss albino mice of either sex weighing between 20 and 25 g were subjected to acute toxicity studies as per guidelines (AOT no. 425) suggested by the Organization for Economic Cooperation and Development [8]. Groups of six mice each were administered orally graded doses ranging from 0.1 to 5 g/kg. The mice were observed continuously for 2 h for behavioral, neurological, and autonomic profiles for any lethality or death for the next 48 h.

2.7. Anti-Inflammatory Activity

2.7.1. Carrageenan-Induced Paw Edema. The anti-inflammatory activity of the extract was carried out using Wistar albino rats (150–200 g) of either sex [9, 10]. The rats were divided into five groups of six rats each. The control group received 1% (v/v) Tween 80 in water, p.o. at a dose of 10 mL/kg. The positive control group was treated orally with the standard drug, indomethacin (10 mg/kg). Ethanol extract was administered orally to the other groups in doses of 100, 200, and 400 mg/kg as shown in Table 1. All the suspensions were administered 30 min before the induction of oedema by administering 0.1 mL of 1% w/v carrageenan in saline [11, 12]. The degree of paw oedema of all the groups was measured using a plethysmometer at 0, 1, 3, 5, and 7 h after the administration of carrageenan to each group.

2.8. Cotton Pellet Granuloma. Two autoclaved cotton pellets weighing 10 ± 1 mg were implanted subcutaneously into both sides of the groin region of each rat. The rats were divided into five groups of six rats each. The control group received 1% (v/v) Tween 80 in water, p.o. at a dose of 10 mL/kg. The positive control group was treated orally with the standard drug, indomethacin (10 mg/kg). Ethanol extract

was administered to the other groups in doses of 100, 200, and 400 mg/kg orally for 7 days. After 7 days, the animals were sacrificed, and the pellets together with the granuloma tissues were carefully removed, dried in an oven at 60°C, weighed, and compared with control [13].

2.9. Statistical Analysis. All values are expressed as Mean ± SEM. Statistical analysis was performed by one-way analysis of Variance (ANOVA), and individual comparisons of the group mean values were done using Dunnet's t-test, with the help of Graph Pad prism 4.0 software. The value of P lower than 0.05 was considered as significant (P is probability) [14, 15].

3. Results

3.1. Phytochemical Studies. The preliminary phytochemical studies of ethanol extract of *Delonix regia* was indicated the presence of sterols, triterpenoids, phenolic compounds, and flavonoids.

3.2. Acute Toxicity Studies. In acute oral toxicity study, mice given graded doses ranging from 0.1 to 5 g/kg appeared normal. *Delonix regia* was safe up to a dose level of 5000 mg/kg of body weight. No lethality or any toxic reactions were found up to the end of the study period.

3.3. Anti-inflammatory Activity

3.3.1. Carrageenan-Induced Paw Edema. The ethanol extract (400 mg/kg) significantly inhibited carrageenan-induced paw oedema. The ethanol extract produced a dose-dependent inhibition of carrageenan oedema which was comparable with known anti-inflammatory drugs. The ethanol extract of *Delonix regia* produced significant ($P < 0.01$) anti-inflammatory activity. Significant reduction of paw oedema was observed at 3 h after carrageenan injection. The reduction in carrageenan-induced paw oedema by 400 mg/kg of ethanol extract after 3 h was 48.1%, while oedema reduction by the standard drug, indomethacin (10 mg/kg), was 65.8% (Table 1).

3.3.2. Cotton Pellet Granuloma. The ethanol extract significantly inhibited cotton pellet granuloma. The percent inhibition of ethanol extract was 42.4% at dose of 400 mg/kg, and this inhibition was less than that produced by indomethacin (61.6%) (Table 2).

4. Discussion

Carrageenan-induced oedema of rat foot is used widely as a working model of inflammation in the search for new anti-inflammatory agents [16] and appeared to be the basis for the discovery of indomethacin, the anti-inflammatory drug [17]. The oedema which develops in rat paw after carrageenan injection is a biphasic event. The initial phase is attributed to the release of histamine and serotonin, the oedema maintained between the first and second phase to kinin, and

TABLE 1: Effect of ethanol extract of *Delonix regia* (100, 200, and 400 mg/kg) on paw volume in carrageenan-induced paw edema rats.

Treatment	Dose mg kg^{-1}	Carrageenan-induced rat paw edema Mean ± SEM*			
		+1 h	+3 h	+5 h	+7 h
Control	—	0.36 ± 0.06	0.79 ± 0.05	0.64 ± 0.04	0.68 ± 0.01
Indomethacin	10	0.18 ± 0.03^a	0.27 ± 0.04 (65.82)^b	0.29 ± 0.03 (54.68)^b	0.33 ± 0.06 (51.47)^b
EEDR	100	0.28 ± 0.02 (22.22)^{NS}	0.46 ± 0.03 (41.77)^b	0.39 ± 0.03 (39.06)^b	0.41 ± 0.03 (35.93)^b
EEDR	200	0.25 ± 0.01 (30.55)^{NS}	0.43 ± 0.01 (45.56)^b	0.38 ± 0.03 (40.62)^b	0.39 ± 0.03 (42.64)^b
EEDR	400	0.21 ± 0.02 (41.66)^{NS}	0.41 ± 0.02 (48.10)^b	0.37 ± 0.01 (42.18)^b	0.4 ± 0.01 (41.17)^b

*The number of animal was 6 in each group. Figure in parenthesis indicates percent inhibition in paw volume. The probability values were calculated using one way ANOVA followed by Dunnet's t-test: a < 0.05, b < 0.01, NS: not significant.

TABLE 2: Effect of ethanol extract of *Delonix regia* (100, 200 and 400 mg/kg) on cotton pellet granuloma in rats.

Treatment	Dose mg kg^{-1}	Cotton pellet granuloma Weight of pellets Mean ± SEM
Control	0.3 mL	51.73 ± 2.35
Indomethacin	10	19.82 ± 2.52 (61.68)^b
EEDR	100	37.24 ± 2.00 (27.99)^{NS}
EEDR	200	30.85 ± 3.72 (40.36)^b
EEDR	400	29.77 ± 3.76 (42.44)^a

*The number of animal was 6 in each group. Figure in parenthesis indicate percent inhibition in cotton pellet granuloma. The probability values were calculated using one way ANOVA followed by Dunnet's t-test: a < 0.05, b < 0.01, NS: not significant.

the second phase to prostaglandin [18]. All the mediators appear to be dependent upon an intact complement system for their activation and release [19]. It has been shown that, in the early phase of the oedema, the dominant cells are polymorphonuclears whereas in advanced stages mononuclears predominate. In this study, indomethacin (nonsteroidal) anti-inflammatory drug was tested on carrageenan oedema [20]. Phytochemical studies on *Delonix regia* revealed that it contains β-sitosterol, tannin, lupeol, and flavonoids [21]. Hentriacontane, hentriacontanol and it's D-glucoside, and campesterol were identified as constituents of *Delonix regia* [22].

Most of the anti-inflammatory triterpenes isolated have lupane, oleanane, ursane, and taraxastane. Lupeol and ursolic acid showed significant anti-inflammatory activity in various models [23, 24]. Lupeol has been reported to possess dose-dependent suppression of PGE$_2$ without any effect of LTC$_4$ release. Thus, ursolic acid and lupeol [25] were able to prevent the production of some inflammatory mediators which likely contributed to anti-inflammatory effect of *Delonix regia*. Jiang and Dusting have reported that phenolic compounds have potential role in inflammatory conditions [26]. Satya Prasad et al. have further shown that phenolics inhibit polymorphonuclear lipoxygenase, an enzyme involved in inflammatory conditions [27]. The cotton pellet granuloma method has been widely employed to assess the transductive, exudative, and proliferative components of chronic inflammation and is a typical feature of established chronic inflammatory reaction. The fluid absorbed by the pellet greatly influences the wet weight of the granuloma, and dry weight correlates well with the granuloma of the granulomatous tissue formed [28, 29]. Administration of ethanol extract at the doses of 400 mg/kg significantly reduced the granulomatous tissue formation when compared to control.

5. Conclusion

Preliminary phytochemical analysis indicated that the ethanol extract of *Delonix regia* contains sterols, triterpenoids, flavonoids, and phenolic compounds. The anti-inflammatory activity of ethanol extract of *Delonix regia* may probably be due to the presence of several bioactive anti-inflammatory principals. However, it needs isolation, structural elucidation, and screening of any of the above-mentioned active principle/s to pin point activity of drug. It is thus apparent that ethanol extract of *Delonix regia* possesses anti-inflammatory activity.

References

[1] N. C. Dey and T. K. Dey, *A Text Book of Pathology*, Messrs Allied Agency, Calcutta, India, 3rd edition, 1970.

[2] J. A. Parrota, *Healing of Plants of Peninsular India*, CABI Publication, New York, NY, USA, 2000.

[3] Anonymous, *The Wealth of India, A Dictionary of Indian Raw Material and Industrial Product*, vol. 3, CSIR, New Delhi, India, 2002.

[4] K. Srinivasan, K. N. Muruganandan, and S. Chandra, "Anti-inflammatory and analgesic activity of some medicinal plants," *Journal of Medicinal and Aromatic Plant Sciences*, pp. 56–58, 2001.

[5] J. Parekh, D. Jadeja, and S. Chanda, "Efficacy of aqueous and methanol extracts of some medicinal plants for potential antibacterial activity," *Turkish Journal of Biology*, vol. 29, pp. 203–210, 2005.

[6] N.-A. Ankrah, A. K. Nyarko, P. G.A. Addo et al., "Evaluation of efficacy and safety of a herbal medicine used for the treatment of malaria," *Phytotherapy Research*, vol. 17, no. 6, pp. 697–701, 2003.

[7] H. Wagner, S. Bladt, and E. M. Zgainski, *Plant Drug Analysis*, Springer, Berlin, Germany, 1984.

[8] Organization for Economic Co-operation and Development, "OECD Guidelines for the Testing of Chemicals. OECD Guideline 425," Acute Oral Toxicity. Up-and-Down Procedure, 1998.

[9] W. Borgi, K. Ghedira, and N. Chouchane, "Antiinflammatory and analgesic activities of Zizyphus lotus root barks," *Fitoterapia*, vol. 78, no. 1, pp. 16–19, 2007.

[10] H. G. Vogel and B. A. Scholliens, *Drug Discovery and Evaluation*, Springer, Berelin, Germany, 2nd edition, 2002.

[11] A. J. Akindele and O. O. Adeyemi, "Antiinflammatory activity of the aqueous leaf extract of *Byrsocarpus coccineus*," *Fitoterapia*, vol. 78, no. 1, pp. 25–28, 2007.

[12] T. Dimo, A. Fotio, T. Nguelefack, E. Asongalem, and P. Kamtchouing, "Antiinflammatory activity of leaf extracts of *Kalanchoe crenata* Andr," *Indian Journal of Pharmacology*, vol. 38, no. 2, pp. 115–119, 2006.

[13] P. F. D'Arcy, E. M. Haward, and P. W. Muggleton, "The anti-inflammatory action of griseofulvin in experimental animals," *Journal of Pharmacy and Pharmacology*, vol. 12, pp. 659–665, 1960.

[14] A. Osel, A. R. Gennaro, and A. N. Martin, *Remington's Pharmaceutical Science*, Mark Publishing Company, 15th edition, 1975.

[15] C. W. Dunnet, "New tables for multiple comparisons with a control," *Biometrics*, vol. 20, pp. 482–491, 1964.

[16] E. Valencia, M. Feria, J. G. Diaz, A. Gonzalez, and J. Bermejo, "Antinociceptive, anti-inflammatory and antipyretic effects of lapidin, a bicyclic sesquiterpene," *Planta Medica*, vol. 60, no. 5, pp. 395–399, 1994.

[17] C. A. Winter, E. A. Risley, and G. W. Nuss, "Antiinflammatory, Antipyretic activities of indomethacin, 1-(p- chlorobenzyl) - 5-methoxy -2-Methylindole 3-acetic acid," *Journal of Pharmacology and Experimental Therapeutics*, vol. 141, no. 3, pp. 369–376, 1963.

[18] M. DiRosa and D. A. Willoughby, "Anti-inflammatory drugs," *Journal of Pharmacy and Pharmacology*, vol. 23, pp. 297–298, 1971.

[19] J. P. Giroud and D. A. Willoughby, "The interrelations of complement and a prostaglandin-like substance in acute inflammation," *Journal of Pathology*, vol. 101, no. 3, pp. 241–249, 1970.

[20] R. J. Perper, M. Sanda, G. Chinea, and A. L. Oronsky, "Leukocyte chemotaxis in vivo. I. Description of a model of cell accumulation using adoptively transferred 51Cr labeled cells," *Journal of Laboratory and Clinical Medicine*, vol. 84, no. 3, pp. 378–393, 1974.

[21] V. Lakshmi, "Constituents of wood of *Delonix regia*," *National Academy Science Letters*, vol. 10, no. 6, p. 197, 1987.

[22] R. P. Rastogi and B. N. Mehrotra, *Compendium of Indian Medicinal Plants*, vol. 4, PID, New Delhi, INdia, 1995.

[23] D. Baricevic, S. Sosa, R. Della Loggia et al., "Topical anti-inflammatory activity of Salvia officinalis L. leaves: the relevance of ursolic acid," *Journal of Ethnopharmacology*, vol. 75, no. 2-3, pp. 125–132, 2001.

[24] T. Geetha and P. Varalakshmi, "Anti-inflammatory activity of lupeol and lupeol linoleate in adjuvant-induced arthritis," *Fitoterapia*, vol. 69, no. 1, pp. 13–19, 1998.

[25] A Fernandez, A Alvarez, and MD. Garcia, "Anti-inflammatory effect of Pimenta racemosa var. ozua and isolation of triterpene lupeole," *Il Farmaco*, vol. 56, pp. 335–338, 2001.

[26] F. Jiang and G. J. Dusting, "Natural phenolic compounds as cardiovascular therapeutics: potential role of their antiinflammatory effects," *Current vascular pharmacology*, vol. 1, no. 2, pp. 135–156, 2003.

[27] N. Satya Prasad, R. Raghavendra, B. R. Lokesh, and K. Akhilender Naidu, "Spice phenolics inhibit human PMNL 5-lipoxygenase," *Prostaglandins Leukotrienes and Essential Fatty Acids*, vol. 70, no. 6, pp. 521–528, 2004.

[28] O. A. Olajide, J. M. Makinde, and S. O. Awe, "Effects of the aqueous extract of Bridelia ferruginea stem bark on carrageenan-induced oedema and granuloma tissue formation in rats and mice," *Journal of Ethnopharmacology*, vol. 66, no. 1, pp. 113–117, 1999.

[29] O. A. Olajide, S. O. Awe, and J. M. Makinde, "Studies on the anti-inflammatory, antipyretic and analgesic properties of the Aistonia boonei stems bark," *Journal of Ethnopharmacology*, vol. 1, pp. 179–186, 2007.

26

Perisynaptic GABA Receptors: The Overzealous Protector

Andrew N. Clarkson

Departments of Anatomy and Psychology, University of Otago, P.O. Box 913, Dunedin 9013, New Zealand

Correspondence should be addressed to Andrew N. Clarkson, andrew.clarkson@otago.ac.nz

Academic Editor: John Atack

An attempt to find pharmacological therapies to treat stroke patients and minimize the extent of cell death has seen the failure of dozens of clinical trials. As a result, stroke/cerebral ischemia is the leading cause of lasting adult disability. Stroke-induced cell death occurs due to an excess release of glutamate. As a consequence to this, a compensatory increased release of GABA occurs that results in the subsequent internalization of synaptic GABA$_A$ receptors and spillover onto perisynaptic GABA$_A$ receptors, resulting in increased tonic inhibition. Recent studies show that the brain can engage in a limited process of neural repair after stroke. Changes in cortical sensory and motor maps and alterations in axonal structure are dependent on patterned neuronal activity. It has been assumed that changes in neuronal excitability underlie processes of neural repair and remapping of cortical sensory and motor representations. Indeed, recent evidence suggests that local inhibitory and excitatory currents are altered after stroke and modulation of these networks to enhance excitability during the repair phase can facilitate functional recovery after stroke. More specifically, dampening tonic GABA inhibition can afford an early and robust improvement in functional recovery after stroke.

1. γ-Aminobutyric Acid (GABA)

GABA is the major inhibitory neurotransmitter within the mammalian brain. Twenty to 50% of all synapses within the CNS use GABA as a neurotransmitter, mediating both fast and slow inhibitory synaptic transmission [1]. GABA is an endogenous ligand for the GABA$_A$, GABA$_B$, and GABA$_C$ receptors [2], and these receptor subtypes have been classified according to differences in both structure and pharmacology. GABA$_A$Rs are ligand-gated chloride channels [2, 3] formed from 5 subunits arranged around a central ion pore. At least nineteen mammalian genes encoding for the various GABA$_A$R subunits exist: α_{1-6}, β_{1-3}, γ_{1-3}, δ, ε, φ, π, and ρ_{1-3}, with slice variants also contributing to variations in receptor functions [4–9]. The most common subunit combinations are believed to be composed of 2α, 2β, and γ, with the γ-subunit being able to be substituted for either an ε- or a δ-subunit [7–9].

Depolarization of inhibitory interneurons produces a phasic release of GABA and inhibition of postsynaptic neurons. Extrasynaptic GABA$_A$R's respond to ambient levels of GABA present in the extracellular space to regulate baseline pyramidal neuron excitability and show reduced desensitization remaining active for long periods of time [10]. Tonic GABA$_A$R's in the hippocampus and cortex contain either $\alpha5$ or δ-subunits [6, 10]. Reduced activity of $\alpha5$ or δ-subunits enhances pyramidal neuron firing to afferent inputs [10–12], enhances neuronal network excitability [13], and facilitates LTP and cognitive performance [14–17]. GABA transporters modulate the level of tonic GABA$_A$R activity [18] with the uptake of GABA into neurons and astrocytes for recycling. Low GABA concentrations activate extrasynaptic GABA$_A$R's, leading to persistent or tonic inhibition [19, 20]. Synaptic and extrasynaptic GABA$_A$R's exhibit distinct pharmacological and biophysical properties that differentially influence brain physiology and behavior [19].

Synaptic GABA$_A$R's are composed of α_{1-3}, β_{1-3}, and γ_{1-3}, subunits, and the site of action for a variety of clinically important drugs, such as benzodiazepines, neurosteroids, and anesthetics. Where as extrasynaptic GABA$_A$R's are composed of subunit combinations containing α_{4-6},

β_{1-3}, and γ_2- or δ-subunits. Of these receptors, the δ-containing GABA$_A$R's coassembled as $\alpha_4\beta\delta$—located in the cortex, hippocampus and thalamus—or $\alpha_6\beta\delta$—located in the cerebellum—that are emerging as unique and fundamental players in GABAergic neurotransmission [19]. In addition to δ-containing GABA$_A$R's having a functional role in the cortex, the α5-containing GABA$_A$R's coassembled primarily as $\alpha_5\beta\gamma_2$ have also been implicated in poststroke repair [21]. Even though the expression of the α5-subunit is low in the cortex compared to the δ-subunit, greater functional improvements in motor recovery are seen following modulation of the α5-subunit [21]. The pharmacology of these extrasynaptic receptors is inconsistent between research groups [22] and has been hampered by the lack of selective agents to probe function in recombinant, native, and whole animal systems [23]. Conflicting data is also present with respect for the ability of these receptors to desensitize [19, 24]. Determining the composition and pharmacology of this receptor will enable the development of much needed therapies for use in stroke.

1.1. Disability in Stroke. Stroke is the leading cause of death and long-term disability in adults worldwide. Stroke-induced sensory and motor loss of limb function, in particular, prevents patients from returning to work and accounts for the statistic that almost one-third of stroke survivors become institutionalized after having a stroke [25–28]. Recent studies have shown that the brain has a limited capacity to repair after stroke. In both humans and animals, neural repair after stroke has been shown to involve remapping of cognitive functions and sprouting of new connections in tissue adjacent to the stroke site, the peri-infarct cortex [29, 30]. However, mechanisms associated with poststroke neural repair and recovery have not been well characterized, and it has been assumed that changes in cortical representational maps underlying the recovery involve changes in neuronal excitability. Consistent with this, animal studies suggest that therapies associated with rehabilitation can promote plasticity changes in tissue that survives the stroke [31].

Functional recovery within the peri-infarct cortex involves changes in neuronal excitability. Clinical studies using direct current stimulation of the peri-infarct cortex, with protocols that boost local neuronal excitability, have been shown to improve use of the affected limb in stroke patients [32, 33]. Furthermore, forced use or task-specific repetition of the affected limb have also been shown to activate the peri-infarct cortex and improve functional recovery [34]. Studies suggest that decreases in γ-aminobutyric acid GABA activity within the motor cortex could facilitate structural changes [35] and promote recovery of motor function [36]. Alterations in neuronal excitability underlie fundamental changes in information transfer in neuronal circuits [37] such as long-term potentiation and depression (LTP and LTD) as well as the unmasking of quiescent synaptic connections and remodeling of cortical maps [38]. Furthermore, changes in LTP and cortical map formation

occur within the peri-infarct cortex adjacent to the stroke [29]. These data suggest a critical role for modulating cortical excitability as a means for promoting functional recovery after stroke.

1.2. Brain Excitability in Learning, Memory, and Repair. The processes of neurorehabilitation involve physical, occupational, and cognitive therapies [27, 28]. Further changes in poststroke cortical plasticity play a critical role in mediating repair mechanisms. While these modalities clearly promote functional recovery, no drug treatments exist that promote poststroke brain repair and recovery. Recent evidence suggests that suppression of either cortical tonic GABA inhibition or stimulation of α-amino-3-hydroxy-5-methyl-4-isoxazolepropionic acid (AMPA) receptor currents can promote poststroke function gain [21, 39]. This ability to regain function relies heavily on the ability to learn or relearn after stroke and likely follows classical activity-dependent processes associated with motor learning and memory [40, 41]. In addition to these behavioral links, stroke recovery and classical learning and memory pathways share similar molecular and cellular links. For instance, genes that are important for learning and memory are also elevated during periods of poststroke repair and include membrane-associated phosphoproteins GAP43 and MARCKS, the transcription factor c-jun, and the cell adhesion molecule L1 [42].

Modulation of learning and memory pathways have previously been shown to promote functional recovery and poststroke axonal sprouting following administration of pharmacological agents such as amphetamines and phosphodiesterase type-4 inhibitors that boost cAMP/CREB signaling and learning and memory function [43, 44]. These data indicate that manipulating learning and memory pathways can offer a novel means for promoting recovery. As with stroke recovery, the processes of learning and memory can be enhanced by manipulations that increase neuronal excitability, which has also been shown to promote function recovery [21]. Significant data is accumulating indicating an imbalance in inhibitory and excitatory pathways after stroke, and modulation of these pathways by either enhancing glutamate-mediated transmission or dampening the tonic form of GABA can facilitate functional recovery [21, 39, 45–48]. α5GABA$_A$R negative allosteric modulators are part of a broad class of drugs that boost learning and memory function by influencing key elements in neuronal memory storage, such as LTP [14, 16]. α5GABA$_A$R negative allosteric modulators, and indeed any mechanism that dampens tonic GABA signaling, could significantly improve poststroke recovery [21]. This suggests that the similarities between neuronal mechanisms of learning and memory and those of functional recovery after stroke extend to common treatment strategies for both.

Most strategies that promote functional recovery after stroke, such as axonal sprouting, neurogenesis, or angiogenesis, focus or rely on inducing structural changes in the brain as a means to promote functional recovery after stroke [49–53]. In order to promote structural change in the brain, however, these treatments take time to develop a functional effect. Blocking tonic GABA inhibition induces a rapid improvement in behavioral recovery in the absence of any change in axonal sprouting within the peri-infarct cortex [21]. This data suggests that treatments that focus on inducing molecular memory systems after stroke may have the advantage of promoting synaptic plasticity in peri-infarct cortex rapidly and without altering the tissue reorganization that normally occurs after stroke. These therapies are highly translatable into the clinic due to their timing of drug administration, 3–7 days after stroke in rodents, and with the early effects seen with functional recovery, will aid in the huge social and economical burdens seen after stroke.

1.3. Attenuating GABAA Receptor Function in Neural Repair after Stroke. As with stroke recovery, the processes of learning and memory can be enhanced by manipulations that increase neuronal excitability. However, unlike the stroke recovery field, basic science studies in learning and memory have defined specific cellular pathways that lead to enhanced neuronal excitability and improved function.

Recent work has shown that enhanced neuronal excitability occurs following the dampening of the baseline level of inhibition in neurons. This baseline inhibition is in part set by a tonic, always present, degree of inhibitory signaling from the major inhibitory neurotransmitter, GABA. Unlike the phasic nature of synaptically released GABA, the action of GABA via extrasynaptic receptors is to tonically suppress neuronal excitability and to help regulate neuronal action potential firing. These extrasynaptic GABA receptors consist of $\alpha5$ and δ-subunit containing GABA$_A$R's. Recent evidence using $\alpha5$GABA$_A$R "knock-out", and point-mutated mice have clearly shown that the $\alpha5$-subunit plays a key role in cognitive processing [15, 17]. In addition, *in vitro* and *in vivo* work has shown that $\alpha5$GABA$_A$R negative allosteric modulators can enhance cognition within the Morris water maze, enhance hippocampal LTP and do not have any proconvulsant effects [14, 16]. Using pharmacological and genetic manipulations of extrasynaptic GABA$_A$R's, we have shown marked improvements in functional recovery when starting treatments from 3 days after the stroke [21]. These data are consistent for offering a potential role for extrasynaptic GABA$_A$R's in processes involving synaptic plasticity and learning and memory and more recently poststroke recovery.

Neuronal inhibition and network function is disturbed in peri-infarct tissue during periods of cortical plasticity, re-mapping, and recovery. The increase in tonic inhibition in cortical pyramidal neurons reported by Clarkson and colleagues [21] occurs at precisely the same time as cortical map plasticity and recovery [54]. Behavioral recovery in stroke is closely correlated with functional plasticity in peri-infarct and connected cortical regions. In human stroke patients, an expansion in motor representation maps is seen in tissue adjacent to or connected to stroke [29, 55]. In animal models, when stroke damages primary motor or somatosensory areas, motor and sensory representations

remap in peri-infarct cortex [54, 56]. These processes of recovery identify plasticity in the cortical circuits in peri-infarct cortex as key elements in functional recovery.

2. GABA and Cerebral Ischemia

A large body of work has been devoted to developing and exploring neuroprotectants that act to block glutamate-mediated neurotransmission in animal models of cerebral ischemia [57, 58]. Increased inhibitory neurotransmission associated with GABA has been shown to normalize the balance of glutamate-mediated excitation. Therefore, pharmacological enhancement of GABA$_A$R neurotransmission provides an alternative means for neuroprotection. Indeed, over recent years, changes in GABA function following cerebral ischemia and possible protective benefits of GABAergic drugs have been extensively assessed [59–65]. Even though it has been proposed that enhancing GABA transmission may elicit protection against cerebral ischemia [60–62, 65], the exact mechanisms that are associated with these neuroprotectants have, as yet, not been fully elucidated and increasing GABA function may be protective during cerebral ischemia for different reasons [59–65]. However, even though GABA agonists have shown great promise in animal model, these compounds have failed to translate into the clinic [66, 67]. The failure of these compounds highlights the need to firstly establish better preclinical rodent models of stroke that better mimic what occurs in humans. Secondly, the use of subunit specific GABA compounds is more likely to show an effect, due to them having less side effects, such as drug-induced hypothermia and sedation. However, even with recent developments in this area, studies are lacking. The need to assess subunit-specific GABA compounds to help understand what is happening after stroke in terms of GABA function is highlighted with clinical reports showing that zolpidem, an $\alpha1$ subunit GABA$_A$R modulator, can result in transiently improves in aphasia in chronic stroke survivors [68].

During situations of cerebral ischemia, it has been shown that the extracellular concentrations of GABA increase (approx. 50 fold compared to basal levels) to the micromolar range [59, 69] and remain elevated for at least 30 minutes during periods of reperfusion. Prolonged exposure of the GABA$_A$Rs to high concentrations of GABA agonists *in vitro* has routinely been shown to become desensitized and/or downregulated [70–72]. Similarly, the GABA$_A$R is also downregulated in the gerbil hippocampus following transient cerebral ischemia [63]. In this model, receptor downregulation was shown to be via internalization, as there was a rapid decrease in binding of the hydrophilic ligand [3H]-SR-95531, but not the hydrophobic ligand [3H]-flunitrazepam [63]. This increase in extracellular GABA is likely to result in the spill over onto peri-synaptic GABA$_A$R's resulting in an increase in tonic inhibition. Indeed, recent evidence showing an increase in tonic inhibition after stroke supports this notion [21]. This increase in tonic inhibition is most likely a safety mechanism imposed by the brain as a means to minimize neuronal damage. However, as this increase in tonic inhibition persists for at least 2 weeks after the stroke, this safety mechanism which is likely to have either wrong or no feedback mechanism has been formed to compensate for such a change in tonic GABA.

3. Poststroke Tonic Inhibition

Changes in neuronal excitability, loss of GABAergic inhibition, enhanced glutamatergic transmission, and synaptic plasticity all contribute to neuronal reorganization after stroke. Studies that promote an increase in local brain excitability result in improved function [21, 34, 39, 45] and suggest that decreasing GABA activity within the brain could facilitate structural changes that promote functional recovery [21, 34, 45]. In particular, this enhancement of neuronal excitability involves dampening baseline levels of inhibition.

Tonic or continuous signaling from GABA sets baseline inhibition. GABA acts via extrasynaptic $GABA_A R$'s to tonically suppress neuronal excitability and regulate neuronal action potential firing. Therefore, in order to facilitate functional recovery, an increase in brain excitability is required to overcome this hypofunctionalism [34]. Recently Clarkson and colleagues have demonstrated marked improvements in poststroke functional recovery using pharmacological manipulations of extrasynaptic $GABA_A R$'s, implicating $\alpha5$ or δ-containing $GABA_A R$'s as novel targets for developing agents to help stroke sufferers.

GABA has been shown to mediate both fast and slow inhibitory synaptic transmission [1]. During development, however, the $GABA_A R$s have been shown to mediate excitation as well as play an important role in neural migration and synaptogenesis [73, 74]. During situations of cerebral ischemia, extracellular concentrations of GABA are significantly elevated [59, 69], resulting in $GABA_A$ receptor desensitization and/or downregulation [63, 71]. This is supported by immunohistochemical and autoradiographic data showing decreased expression of $\alpha1$, $\alpha2$, $\alpha3$, $\alpha5$, and $\gamma2$ subunits following photothrombotic stroke and freeze-lesion-induced cortical injury [75–77].

Recent work has shown that epileptogenesis results in the suppression of functionally active $\alpha5 GABA_A R$s and results in an increase/substitution of other $GABA_A R$'s with a subsequent increase in rather than suppression of tonic inhibitory currents [78]. A similar compensatory increase in $\alpha4\delta$-mediated tonic currents has been seen in the $\alpha5$ knockout mice within region CA1 of the hippocampus [11]. Extracellular GABA concentrations and thus tonic inhibition have been shown to increase as the excitatory drive increases resulting in the modulation of neuronal excitability and prevention of neuronal saturation [79]. Consistent with these findings, Clarkson and colleagues reported an increase in GABA tonic inhibitory currents from 3–14 days poststroke in layer II cortical pyramidal neurons [21]. This poststroke increase in tonic inhibition may act as a compensatory mechanism to prevent further neuronal injury. However, this prolonged increase in tonic inhibition during the repair phase is acting as a hindrance by preventing cortical expansion and improvements in functional recovery. This

is supported by findings by Clarkson and colleagues who show that both pharmacological and genetic modulation of tonic inhibition, dampening either $\alpha5$ or δ-mediated increase in tonic GABA currents, results in early and marked improvements in functional recovery [21].

Understanding the profile for which cortical plasticity occurs, altered after a stroke, is critical for fully determining when to start treatments and with what therapeutic compound to use. Based on our findings, we have clearly shown that dampening of tonic GABA currently from 3 days results in robust functional improvements of motor recovery [21]. These improvements, however, may not be the same if treatments are started weeks after stroke onset as previously shown in humans using zolpidem, which was shown to transiently improve aphasia in chronic stroke survivors [68]. The $\alpha1$ and $\beta2$ $GABA_A R$ subunits are densely localized within the cortex and coassembly with the $\gamma2$-subunit accounts for about 40% of all $GABA_A R$s within the cortex [80]. Assembly of $GABA_A R$s containing $\alpha1\beta2\gamma2$ has been shown to be enriched at synaptic sites throughout the cortex [81] and involved in changes in synaptic plasticity. However, studies have also shown that the δ subunit can coassemble with $\alpha1$ subunits to form functional recombinant receptors[82, 83]. Furthermore, immunoprecipitation studies have shown that δ subunits can associate with $\alpha1$ subunits [84], and $GABA_A R\alpha1$ subunits have also been found extrasynaptically [85, 86] consistent with the typical localization of δ-containing $GABA_A R$s[81]81. These data could suggest an alternative method for why zolpidem was having an effect in chronic stroke patients to alleviate the burden of aphasia. However, further studies are needed, as one previous study would suggest that the $\gamma2$-subunit is required in order for zolpidem to have an effect [87].

4. Dampening Cortical Inhibition Alters Cortical Responsiveness

Disinhibition of cortical connections within the peri-infarct or regions associated with the peri-infarct cortex have been argued as either occurring as a direct consequence of the stroke or as a potential compensatory mechanism related to the recovery [88]. This argument has come about based on a number of observations such as local blockage of GABAergic inhibition unmasking preexisting horizontal connections within the rat motor cortex [38]; LTP of adult rat motor cortex horizontal connections is dependent on GABA disinhibition during theta burst stimulation, unlike other regions such as the hippocampus or somatosensory cortex [35]; and finally modulation of GABA has been shown to be involved in learning in healthy humans as shown using imaging studies showing a correlation between a decrease in GABA concentration in motor cortex and motor skill learning [89]. Consistent with the notion that cortical disinhibition is occurring as a compensatory mechanism, Clarkson and colleagues have shown a robust and persistent increase in tonic inhibition in the peri-infarct cortex after stroke and blockade of this tonic inhibition at the time of stroke with the extrasynaptic GABA$_A$R negative allosteric modulator, L655-708, exacerbated the lesion [21]. Further to this, Clarkson and colleagues showed for the first time that delayed treatment L655-708, which has previously been shown to induce LTP [14], provides an early and robust reversal in behavioral deficits [21]. Given the early behavioral effects seen and the lack of effect on sprouting of new connections, cortical disinhibition following L655-708-treatment seems a logical argument. To support the notion that dampening GABA activity is having a beneficial effect, no improvement in motor function was observed after stroke following administration of the GABA agonist, muscimol [21]. This is backed by clinical studies illustrating the reemergence of stroke symptoms following administration of the GABA agonist midazolam in chronic stroke patients that have shown significant improvements in function [90]. The peri-infarct cortex exhibits neuronal metabolic dysfunction over a one-month period [91], which would indicate a therapeutic time window for blockade of tonic GABA signaling of at least one month after stroke. Consistent with this is the fact, when L655-708 treatment is discontinued after a two-week period of administration after stroke, a slight rebound effect/reversal in functional recovery is observed compared to animals that received treatment for the six-week period [21].

5. Conclusions

Therapies that promote functional recovery after stroke are limited to physical rehabilitation measures. While specific measures, such as constraint-induced therapies, promote recovery of motor function, no pharmacological therapies are available that aid in recovery. Functional recovery after stroke follows psychological learning rules [41] that indicate learning and memory principles may underlie behavioral recovery. At the cellular level, learning and memory are mediated by specific excitatory neuronal responses, such as LTP, and are potentiated by drugs that facilitate aspects of excitatory neuronal signaling [13], such as tonic GABA$_A$R antagonists [10]. Recent data shows that stroke alters the balance of excitatory and inhibitory inputs to neurons in the peri-infarct cortex, by increasing inhibitory tone. This altered excitatory balance occurs through a decrease in the normal cellular uptake of GABA. Dampening GABA-mediated tonic inhibition restores the excitatory/inhibitory balance in peri-infarct motor cortex *ex vivo* and promotes recovery of motor function *in vivo*. These effects occur through blockade of α5 or δ-containing GABA$_A$R's. This data indicates a novel role for tonic GABA$_A$R function in promoting poststroke recovery most likely via cortical disinhibition [38, 92, 93] and suggests a new avenue for pharmacological treatment of neurorehabilitation in stroke. This early effect on stroke recovery opens the possibility for treatments that block tonic GABA signaling and may be used in conjunction with later-acting stroke repair therapies in a combinatorial manner. More generally, tonic GABA signaling has a biphasic role in stroke. Early tonic GABA signaling limits stroke size, later tonic GABA signaling limits stroke recovery. These data identify a promising molecular system for future stroke recovery therapies and implicate molecular memory systems as likely key players in recovery from stroke.

Acknowledgments

This paper was completed during tenure of a Repatriation Fellowship from the New Zealand Neurological Foundation and the Sir Charles Hercus Fellowship from the Health Research Council of New Zealand.

References

[1] W. Sieghart, "Structure and pharmacology of γ-aminobutyric acid(A) receptor subtypes," *Pharmacological Reviews*, vol. 47, no. 2, pp. 181–234, 1995.

[2] M. Chebib and G. A. R. Johnston, "The "ABC" of GABA receptors: a brief review," *Clinical and Experimental Pharmacology and Physiology*, vol. 26, no. 11, pp. 937–940, 1999.

[3] C. D'Hulst, J. R. Atack, and R. F. Kooy, "The complexity of the GABA$_A$ receptor shapes unique pharmacological profiles," *Drug Discovery Today*, vol. 14, no. 17-18, pp. 866–875, 2009.

[4] R. L. Macdonald and R. W. Olsen, "GABAA receptor channels," *Annual Review of Neuroscience*, vol. 17, pp. 569–602, 1994.

[5] R. W. Olsen and W. Sieghart, "International Union of Pharmacology. LXX. Subtypes of γ-aminobutyric acidA receptors: classification on the basis of subunit composition, pharmacology, and function. Update," *Pharmacological Reviews*, vol. 60, no. 3, pp. 243–260, 2008.

[6] R. W. Olsen and W. Sieghart, "GABA$_A$ receptors: subtypes provide diversity of function and pharmacology," *Neuropharmacology*, vol. 56, no. 1, pp. 141–148, 2009.

[7] N. P. Barrera, J. Betts, H. You et al., "Atomic force microscopy reveals the stoichiometry and subunit arrangement of the $\alpha_4\beta_3\delta$ GABA$_A$ receptor," *Molecular Pharmacology*, vol. 73, no. 3, pp. 960–967, 2008.

[8] P. J. Whiting, "The GABAA receptor gene family: new opportunities for drug development," *Current Opinion in Drug Discovery and Development*, vol. 6, no. 5, pp. 648–657, 2003.

[9] P. J. Whiting, "GABA-A receptor subtypes in the brain: a paradigm for CNS drug discovery?" *Drug Discovery Today*, vol. 8, no. 10, pp. 445–450, 2003.

[10] J. Glykys and I. Mody, "Activation of GABA$_A$ receptors: views from outside the synaptic cleft," *Neuron*, vol. 56, no. 5, pp. 763–770, 2007.

[11] J. Glykys and I. Mody, "Hippocampal network hyperactivity after selective reduction of tonic inhibition in GABA$_A$ receptor α5 subunit-deficient mice," *Journal of Neurophysiology*, vol. 95, no. 5, pp. 2796–2807, 2006.

[12] K. R. Drasbek and K. Jensen, "THIP, a hypnotic and antinociceptive drug, enhances an extrasynaptic GABA$_A$ receptor-mediated conductance in mouse neocortex," *Cerebral Cortex*, vol. 16, no. 8, pp. 1134–1141, 2006.

[13] M. C. Walker and A. Semyanov, "Regulation of excitability by extrasynaptic GABAA receptors," *Results and Problems in Cell Differentiation*, vol. 44, pp. 29–48, 2008.

[14] J. R. Atack, P. J. Bayley, G. R. Seabrook, K. A. Wafford, R. M. McKernan, and G. R. Dawson, "L-655,708 enhances cognition

in rats but is not proconvulsant at a dose selective for $\alpha 5$-containing GABAA receptors," *Neuropharmacology*, vol. 51, no. 6, pp. 1023–1029, 2006.

[15] N. Collinson, F. M. Kuenzi, W. Jarolimek et al., "Enhanced learning and memory and altered GABAergic synaptic transmission in mice lacking the $\alpha 5$ subunit of the GABAA receptor," *Journal of Neuroscience*, vol. 22, no. 13, pp. 5572–5580, 2002.

[16] G. R. Dawson, K. A. Maubach, N. Collinson et al., "An inverse agonist selective for $\alpha 5$ subunit-containing GABA A receptors enhances cognition," *Journal of Pharmacology and Experimental Therapeutics*, vol. 316, no. 3, pp. 1335–1345, 2006.

[17] F. Crestani, R. Keist, J. M. Fritschy et al., "Trace fear conditioning involves hippocampal $\alpha 5$ GABAA receptors," *Proceedings of the National Academy of Sciences of the United States of America*, vol. 99, no. 13, pp. 8980–8985, 2002.

[18] S. Keros and J. J. Hablitz, "Subtype-specific GABA transporter antagonists synergistically modulate phasic and tonic GABAA conductances in rat neocortex," *Journal of Neurophysiology*, vol. 94, no. 3, pp. 2073–2085, 2005.

[19] D. Belelli, N. L. Harrison, J. Maguire, R. L. Macdonald, M. C. Walker, and D. W. Cope, "Extrasynaptic GABAa receptors: form, pharmacology, and function," *Journal of Neuroscience*, vol. 29, no. 41, pp. 12757–12763, 2009.

[20] I. Mody, "Distinguishing between GABAA receptors responsible for tonic and phasic conductances," *Neurochemical Research*, vol. 26, no. 8-9, pp. 907–913, 2001.

[21] A. N. Clarkson, B. S. Huang, S. E. MacIsaac, I. Mody, and S. T. Carmichael, "Reducing excessive GABA-mediated tonic inhibition promotes functional recovery after stroke," *Nature*, vol. 468, no. 7321, pp. 305–309, 2010.

[22] C. M. Borghese and R. A. Harris, "Studies of ethanol actions on recombinant δ-containing γ-aminobutyric acid type A receptors yield contradictory results," *Alcohol*, vol. 41, no. 3, pp. 155–162, 2007.

[23] K. A. Wafford, M. B. van Niel, Q. P. Ma et al., "Novel compounds selectively enhance δ subunit containing GABAA receptors and increase tonic currents in thalamus," *Neuropharmacology*, vol. 56, no. 1, pp. 182–189, 2009.

[24] D. P. Bright, M. Renzi, J. Bartram et al., "Profound desensitization by ambient GABA limits activation of δ-containing GABA$_A$ receptors during spillover," *Journal of Neuroscience*, vol. 31, no. 2, pp. 753–763, 2011.

[25] Y. S. Ng, J. Stein, M. Ning, and R. M. Black-Schaffer, "Comparison of clinical characteristics and functional outcomes of ischemic stroke in different vascular territories," *Stroke*, vol. 38, no. 8, pp. 2309–2314, 2007.

[26] S. M. Lai, S. Studenski, P. W. Duncan, and S. Perera, "Persisting consequences of stroke measured by the stroke impact scale," *Stroke*, vol. 33, no. 7, pp. 1840–1844, 2002.

[27] B. H. Dobkin, "Training and exercise to drive poststroke recovery," *Nature Clinical Practice Neurology*, vol. 4, no. 2, pp. 76–85, 2008.

[28] B. H. Dobkin, "Strategies for stroke rehabilitation," *Lancet Neurology*, vol. 3, no. 9, pp. 528–536, 2004.

[29] S. T. Carmichael, "Cellular and molecular mechanisms of neural repair after stroke: making waves," *Annals of Neurology*, vol. 59, no. 5, pp. 735–742, 2006.

[30] R. J. Nudo, "Mechanisms for recovery of motor function following cortical damage," *Current Opinion in Neurobiology*, vol. 16, no. 6, pp. 638–644, 2006.

[31] M. A. Maldonado, R. P. Allred, E. L. Felthauser, and T. A. Jones, "Motor skill training, but not voluntary exercise,

[32] improves skilled reaching after unilateral ischemic lesions of the sensorimotor cortex in rats," *Neurorehabilitation and Neural Repair*, vol. 22, no. 3, pp. 250–261, 2008.

[32] M. Alonso-Alonso, F. Fregni, and A. Pascual-Leone, "Brain stimulation in poststroke rehabilitation," *Cerebrovascular Diseases*, vol. 24, no. 1, supplement 1, pp. 157–166, 2007.

[33] F. C. Hummel and L. G. Cohen, "Non-invasive brain stimulation: a new strategy to improve neurorehabilitation after stroke?" *Lancet Neurology*, vol. 5, no. 8, pp. 708–712, 2006.

[34] G. F. Wittenberg and J. D. Schaechter, "The neural basis of constraint-induced movement therapy," *Current Opinion in Neurology*, vol. 22, no. 6, pp. 582–588, 2009.

[35] G. Hess, C. D. Aizenman, and J. P. Donoghue, "Conditions for the induction of long-term potentiation in layer II/III horizontal connections of the rat motor cortex," *Journal of Neurophysiology*, vol. 75, no. 5, pp. 1765–1778, 1996.

[36] P. Cicinelli, P. Pasqualetti, M. Zaccagnini, R. Traversa, M. Olivefi, and P. M. Rossini, "Interhemispheric asymmetries of motor cortex excitability in the postacute stroke stage: a paired-pulse transcranial magnetic stimulation study," *Stroke*, vol. 34, no. 11, pp. 2653–2658, 2003.

[37] A. Citri and R. C. Malenka, "Synaptic plasticity: multiple forms, functions, and mechanisms," *Neuropsychopharmacology*, vol. 33, no. 1, pp. 18–41, 2008.

[38] K. M. Jacobs and J. P. Donoghue, "Reshaping the cortical motor map by unmasking latent intracortical connections," *Science*, vol. 251, no. 4996, pp. 944–947, 1991.

[39] A. N. Clarkson, J. J. Overman, S. Zhong, R. Mueller, G. Lynch, and S. T. Carmichael, "AMPA receptor-induced local brain-derived neurotrophic factor signaling mediates motor recovery after stroke," *Journal of Neuroscience*, vol. 31, no. 10, pp. 3766–3775, 2011.

[40] J. M. Conner, A. A. Chiba, and M. H. Tuszynski, "The basal forebrain cholinergic system is essential for cortical plasticity and functional recovery following brain injury," *Neuron*, vol. 46, no. 2, pp. 173–179, 2005.

[41] J. W. Krakauer, "Motor learning: its relevance to stroke recovery and neurorehabilitation," *Current Opinion in Neurology*, vol. 19, no. 1, pp. 84–90, 2006.

[42] S. T. Carmichael, I. Archibeque, L. Luke, T. Nolan, J. Momiy, and S. Li, "Growth-associated gene expression after stroke: evidence for a growth-promoting region in peri-infarct cortex," *Experimental Neurology*, vol. 193, no. 2, pp. 291–311, 2005.

[43] R. P. Stroemer, T. A. Kent, and C. E. Hulsebosch, "Enhanced neocortical neural sprouting, synaptogenesis, and behavioral recovery with D-amphetamine therapy after neocortical infarction in rats," *Stroke*, vol. 29, no. 11, pp. 2381–2395, 1998.

[44] E. MacDonald, H. van der Lee, D. Pocock et al., "A novel phosphodiesterase type 4 inhibitor, HT-0712, enhances rehabilitation-dependent motor recovery and cortical reorganization after focal cortical ischemia," *Neurorehabilitation and Neural Repair*, vol. 21, no. 6, pp. 486–496, 2007.

[45] A. N. Clarkson and S. T. Carmichael, "Cortical excitability and post-stroke recovery," *Biochemical Society Transactions*, vol. 37, no. 6, pp. 1412–1414, 2009.

[46] S. Schmidt, C. Bruehl, C. Frahm, C. Redecker, and O. W. Witte, "Age dependence of excitatory-inhibitorybalance following stroke," *Neurobiology of Aging*. In press.

[47] S. Schmidt, C. Redecker, C. Bruehl, and O. W. Witte, "Age-related decline of functional inhibition in rat cortex," *Neurobiology of Aging*, vol. 31, no. 3, pp. 504–511, 2010.

[48] N. Jaenisch, O. W. Witte, and C. Frahm, "Downregulation of potassium chloride cotransporter KCC2 after transient focal cerebral ischemia," *Stroke*, vol. 41, no. 3, pp. e151–e159, 2010.

[49] S. T. Carmichael, "Targets for neural repair therapies after stroke," *Stroke*, vol. 41, no. 10, supplement, pp. S124–S126, 2010.

[50] S. T. Carmichael, "Themes and strategies for studying the biology of stroke recovery in the poststroke epoch," *Stroke*, vol. 39, no. 4, pp. 1380–1388, 2008.

[51] J. J. Ohab, S. Fleming, A. Blesch, and S. T. Carmichael, "A neurovascular niche for neurogenesis after stroke," *Journal of Neuroscience*, vol. 26, no. 50, pp. 13007–13016, 2006.

[52] Z. G. Zhang and M. Chopp, "Neurorestorative therapies for stroke: underlying mechanisms and translation to the clinic," *The Lancet Neurology*, vol. 8, no. 5, pp. 491–500, 2009.

[53] J. Liauw, S. Hoang, M. Choi et al., "Thrombospondins 1 and 2 are necessary for synaptic plasticity and functional recovery after stroke," *Journal of Cerebral Blood Flow and Metabolism*, vol. 28, no. 10, pp. 1722–1732, 2008.

[54] C. E. Brown, K. Aminoltejari, H. Erb, I. R. Winship, and T. H. Murphy, "In vivo voltage-sensitive dye imaging in adult mice reveals that somatosensory maps lost to stroke are replaced over weeks by new structural and functional circuits with prolonged modes of activation within both the peri-infarct zone and distant sites," *Journal of Neuroscience*, vol. 29, no. 6, pp. 1719–1734, 2009.

[55] C. Calautti and J. C. Baron, "Functional neuroimaging studies of motor recovery after stroke in adults: a review," *Stroke*, vol. 34, no. 6, pp. 1553–1566, 2003.

[56] R. M. Dijkhuizen, A. B. Singhal, J. B. Mandeville et al., "Correlation between brain reorganization, ischemic damage, and neurologic status after transient focal cerebral ischemia in rats: a functional magnetic resonance imaging study," *Journal of Neuroscience*, vol. 23, no. 2, pp. 510–517, 2003.

[57] P. Lipton, "Ischemic cell death in brain neurons," *Physiological Reviews*, vol. 79, no. 4, pp. 1431–1568, 1999.

[58] P. Nicotera and S. A. Lipton, "Excitotoxins in neuronal apoptosis and necrosis," *Journal of Cerebral Blood Flow and Metabolism*, vol. 19, no. 6, pp. 583–591, 1999.

[59] R. D. Schwartz, X. Yu, M. R. Katzman, D. M. Hayden-Hixson, and J. M. Perry, "Diazepam, given postischemia, protects selectively vulnerable neurons in the rat hippocampus and striatum," *Journal of Neuroscience*, vol. 15, no. 1, pp. 529–539, 1995.

[60] A. R. Green, A. H. Hainsworth, and D. M. Jackson, "GABA potentiation: a logical pharmacological approach for the treatment of acute ischaemic stroke," *Neuropharmacology*, vol. 39, no. 9, pp. 1483–1494, 2000.

[61] R. D. Schwartz-Bloom and R. Sah, "γ-aminobutyric acid A neurotransmission and cerebral ischemia," *Journal of Neurochemistry*, vol. 77, no. 2, pp. 353–371, 2001.

[62] R. D. Schwartz-Bloom, K. A. Miller, D. A. Evenson, B. J. Crain, and J. V. Nadler, "Benzodiazepines protect hippocampal neurons from degeneration after transient cerebral ischemia: an ultrastructural study," *Neuroscience*, vol. 98, no. 3, pp. 471–484, 2000.

[63] B. Alicke and R. D. Schwartz-Bloom, "Rapid down-regulation of GABA(A) receptors in the gerbil hippocampus following transient cerebral ischemia," *Journal of Neurochemistry*, vol. 65, no. 6, pp. 2808–2811, 1995.

[64] A. N. Clarkson, J. Clarkson, D. M. Jackson, and I. A. Sammut, "Mitochondrial involvement in transhemispheric diaschisis following hypoxia-ischemia: clomethiazole-mediated amelioration," *Neuroscience*, vol. 144, no. 2, pp. 547–561, 2007.

[65] A. N. Clarkson, H. Liu, R. Rahman, D. M. Jackson, I. Appleton, and D. S. Kerr, "Clomethiazole: mechanisms underlying lasting neuroprotection following hypoxia-ischemia," *FASEB Journal*, vol. 19, no. 8, pp. 1036–1038, 2005.

[66] M. D. Ginsberg, "Neuroprotection for ischemic stroke: past, present and future," *Neuropharmacology*, vol. 55, no. 3, pp. 363–389, 2008.

[67] P. Lyden, A. Shuaib, K. Ng et al., "Clomethiazole acute stroke study in ischemic stroke (CLASS-I): final results," *Stroke*, vol. 33, no. 1, pp. 122–128, 2002.

[68] L. Cohen, B. Chaaban, and M. O. Habert, "Transient Improvement of aphasia with zolpidem," *New England Journal of Medicine*, vol. 350, no. 9, pp. 949–950, 2004.

[69] J. R. Inglefield, J. M. Perry, and R. D. Schwartz, "Postischemic inhibition of GABA reuptake by tiagabine slows neuronal death in the gerbil hippocampus," *Hippocampus*, vol. 5, no. 5, pp. 460–468, 1995.

[70] D. J. Cash and K. Subbarao, "Two desensitization processes of GABA receptor from rat brain. Rapid measurements of chloride ion flux using quench-flow techniques," *FEBS Letters*, vol. 217, no. 1, pp. 129–133, 1987.

[71] J. R. Huguenard and B. E. Alger, "Whole-cell voltage-clamp study of the fading of GABA-activated currents in acutely dissociated hippocampal neurons," *Journal of Neurophysiology*, vol. 56, no. 1, pp. 1–18, 1986.

[72] M. H. J. Tehrani and E. M. Barnes Jr., "Agonist-dependent internalization of γ-aminobutyric acid(A)/benzodiazepine receptors in chick cortical neurons," *Journal of Neurochemistry*, vol. 57, no. 4, pp. 1307–1312, 1991.

[73] Y. Ben-Ari, R. Khazipov, X. Leinekugel, O. Caillard, and J. L. Gaiarsa, "GABA(A), NMDA and AMPA receptors: a developmentally regulated "menage a trois"," *Trends in Neurosciences*, vol. 20, no. 11, pp. 523–529, 1997.

[74] M. M. McCarthy, A. P. Auger, and T. S. Perrot-Sinal, "Getting excited about GABA and sex differences in the brain," *Trends in Neurosciences*, vol. 25, no. 6, pp. 307–312, 2002.

[75] C. Redecker, H. J. Luhmann, G. Hagemann, J. M. Fritschy, and O. W. Witte, "Differential downregulation of GABA(A) receptor subunits in widespread brain regions in the freeze-lesion model of focal cortical malformations," *Journal of Neuroscience*, vol. 20, no. 13, pp. 5045–5053, 2000.

[76] C. Redecker, W. Wang, J. M. Fritschy, and O. W. Witte, "Widespread and long-lasting alterations in GABAA-receptor subtypes after focal cortical infarcts in rats: mediation by NMDA-dependent processes," *Journal of Cerebral Blood Flow and Metabolism*, vol. 22, no. 12, pp. 1463–1475, 2002.

[77] M. Que, K. Schiene, O. W. Witte, and K. Zilles, "Widespread up-regulation of N-methyl-D-aspartate receptors after focal photothrombotic lesion in rat brain," *Neuroscience Letters*, vol. 273, no. 2, pp. 77–80, 1999.

[78] A. Scimemi, A. Semyanov, G. Sperk, D. M. Kullmann, and M. C. Walker, "Multiple and plastic receptors mediate tonic GABAA receptor currents in the hippocampus," *Journal of Neuroscience*, vol. 25, no. 43, pp. 10016–10024, 2005.

[79] S. J. Mitchell and R. A. Silver, "Shunting inhibition modulates neuronal gain during synaptic excitation," *Neuron*, vol. 38, no. 3, pp. 433–445, 2003.

[80] R. M. McKernan and P. J. Whiting, "Which GABAA-receptor subtypes really occur in the brain?" *Trends in Neurosciences*, vol. 19, no. 4, pp. 139–143, 1996.

[81] M. Farrant and Z. Nusser, "Variations on an inhibitory theme: phasic and tonic activation of $GABA_A$ receptors," *Nature Reviews Neuroscience*, vol. 6, no. 3, pp. 215–229, 2005.

[82] N. C. Saxena and R. L. Macdonald, "Assembly of GABA(A) receptor subunits: role of the δ subunit," *Journal of Neuroscience*, vol. 14, no. 11, pp. 7077–7086, 1994.

[83] M. T. Bianchi and R. L. Macdonald, "Neurosteroids shift partial agonist activation of GABAA receptor channels from low- to high-efficacy gating patterns," *Journal of Neuroscience*, vol. 23, no. 34, pp. 10934–10943, 2003.

[84] S. Mertens, D. Benke, and H. Mohler, "GABAA receptor populations with novel subunit combinations and drug binding profiles identified in brain by α5- and δ-subunit-specific immunopurification," *Journal of Biological Chemistry*, vol. 268, no. 8, pp. 5965–5973, 1993.

[85] A. Baude, C. Bleasdale, Y. Dalezios, P. Somogyi, and T. Klausberger, "Immunoreactivity for the GABAA receptor α1 subunit, somatostatin and connexin36 distinguishes axoaxonic, basket, and bistratified interneurons of the rat hippocampus," *Cerebral Cortex*, vol. 17, no. 9, pp. 2094–2107, 2007.

[86] C. Sun, W. Sieghart, and J. Kapur, "Distribution of α1, α4, γ2, and δ subunits of GABAA receptors in hippocampal granule cells," *Brain Research*, vol. 1029, no. 2, pp. 207–216, 2004.

[87] D. W. Cope, P. Wulff, A. Oberto et al., "Abolition of zolpidem sensitivity in mice with a point mutation in the GABAA receptor γ2 subunit," *Neuropharmacology*, vol. 47, no. 1, pp. 17–34, 2004.

[88] J. Liepert, "Motor cortex excitability in stroke before and after constraint-induced movement therapy," *Cognitive and Behavioral Neurology*, vol. 19, no. 1, pp. 41–47, 2006.

[89] A. Floyer-Lea, M. Wylezinska, T. Kincses, and P. M. Matthews, "Rapid modulation of GABA concentration in human sensorimotor cortex during motor learning," *Journal of Neurophysiology*, vol. 95, no. 3, pp. 1639–1644, 2006.

[90] R. M. Lazar, B. F. Fitzsimmons, R. S. Marshall et al., "Reemergence of stroke deficits with midazolam challenge," *Stroke*, vol. 33, no. 1, pp. 283–285, 2002.

[91] J. P. van der Zijden, P. van Eijsden, R. A. De Graaf, and R. M. Dijkhuizen, "1H/13C MR spectroscopic imaging of regionally specific metabolic alterations after experimental stroke," *Brain*, vol. 131, no. 8, pp. 2209–2219, 2008.

[92] C. M. Stinear, J. P. Coxon, and W. D. Byblow, "Primary motor cortex and movement prevention: where Stop meets Go," *Neuroscience and Biobehavioral Reviews*, vol. 33, no. 5, pp. 662–673, 2009.

[93] J. W. Stinear and W. D. Byblow, "Disinhibition in the human motor cortex is enhanced by synchronous upper limb movements," *Journal of Physiology*, vol. 543, no. 1, pp. 307–316, 2002.

27

Mechanisms Underlying Tolerance after Long-Term Benzodiazepine Use: A Future for Subtype-Selective GABA$_A$ Receptor Modulators?

Christiaan H. Vinkers[1,2] and Berend Olivier[1,3]

[1] Division of Pharmacology, Utrecht Institute for Pharmaceutical Sciences and Rudolf Magnus Institute of Neuroscience, Utrecht University, Universiteitsweg 99, 3584CG Utrecht, The Netherlands
[2] Department of Psychiatry, Rudolf Magnus Institute of Neuroscience, University Medical Center Utrecht, Utrecht, The Netherlands
[3] Department of Psychiatry, Yale University School of Medicine, New Haven, CT, USA

Correspondence should be addressed to Christiaan H. Vinkers, c.h.vinkers@uu.nl

Academic Editor: John Atack

Despite decades of basic and clinical research, our understanding of how benzodiazepines tend to lose their efficacy over time (tolerance) is at least incomplete. In appears that tolerance develops relatively quickly for the sedative and anticonvulsant actions of benzodiazepines, whereas tolerance to anxiolytic and amnesic effects probably does not develop at all. In light of this evidence, we review the current evidence for the neuroadaptive mechanisms underlying benzodiazepine tolerance, including changes of (i) the GABA$_A$ receptor (subunit expression and receptor coupling), (ii) intracellular changes stemming from transcriptional and neurotrophic factors, (iii) ionotropic glutamate receptors, (iv) other neurotransmitters (serotonin, dopamine, and acetylcholine systems), and (v) the neurosteroid system. From the large variance in the studies, it appears that either different (simultaneous) tolerance mechanisms occur depending on the benzodiazepine effect, or that the tolerance-inducing mechanism depends on the activated GABA$_A$ receptor subtypes. Importantly, there is no convincing evidence that tolerance occurs with α subunit subtype-selective compounds acting at the benzodiazepine site.

1. Introduction

Shortly after their development in the 1960s, benzodiazepines became very popular as they exerted many desirable effects such as reduction of anxiety, anticonvulsant properties, and myorelaxation combined with a rather low toxicity [1]. However, their use is associated with many side effects precluding their long-term use, including sedation, amnesia, cognitive impairment, and ataxia. Even though guidelines generally recommend limiting benzodiazepines to short-term use, long-term use still often occurs. Chronic benzodiazepine treatment can result in the development of benzodiazepine dependence [2]. DSM-IV criteria for benzodiazepine dependence consist of various psychological (behavioral) and physical symptoms, including tolerance, withdrawal symptoms when drug intake is stopped and

dose escalation [3]. Indeed, chronically treated patients become less sensitive to some effects of benzodiazepines (tolerance) which may include anticonvulsant, sedative, hypnotic, and myorelaxant effects of benzodiazepines. Also, benzodiazepine discontinuation may result in the appearance of a characteristic withdrawal syndrome with heightened anxiety, insomnia, and sensory disturbances [4]. In fact, tolerance and withdrawal could be two manifestations of the same compensatory mechanism, with withdrawal occurring when the counterbalancing benzodiazepine effect is absent [5]. This is supported by the fact that acutely induced benzodiazepine effects are opposite to the withdrawal symptoms, and that changes in glucose use in the Papez circuit (including the cingulate cortex and mammillary body) were also observed on withdrawal, implying a common circuitry in the withdrawal process [6]. However, physical dependence (usually defined by withdrawal symptoms) does not require the presence of tolerance, and tolerance may develop without any signs of physical dependence [7].

Presently, despite decades of basic and clinical research, our understanding how benzodiazepines tend to lose their efficacy over time (i.e., tolerance) is at least incomplete. Here we review the current knowledge on the neuroadaptive mechanisms underlying benzodiazepine tolerance. This paper does not specifically address the addictive properties of benzodiazepines and their effects on the dopamine system or their abuse liability potential (including their nonmedical use in popular culture), which are described in detail elsewhere [8–10].

Benzodiazepine tolerance is considered to constitute an adaptive mechanism following chronic treatment, and it may thus be regarded as an example of neuronal plasticity. Efforts have been made to explain tolerance at the molecular or functional level of the GABA$_A$ receptor because classical (nonselective) benzodiazepines modulate inhibitory GABA$_A$ receptors possessing α_1, α_2, α_3, or α_5 subunits. On the other hand, the excitatory glutamate system has also been implicated to play a role in the development of benzodiazepine tolerance [5]. Enhanced understanding of the dynamic process leading to reduced benzodiazepine efficacy following chronic treatment could accelerate the development of compounds that would maintain efficacy during chronic treatment [11]. Indeed, increasing knowledge on the specific functions of different GABA$_A$ receptor subunits has led to a breakthrough of novel and more selective drugs acting at the benzodiazepine site of the GABA$_A$ receptor. It is interesting but beyond the scope of the review to draw a comparison between benzodiazepine tolerance and alcohol tolerance as alcohol (albeit with low potency) acts at the GABA$_A$ receptor [12].

Firstly, we will discuss the molecular basis of the GABA$_A$ receptor system before taking a closer look at the clinical aspects of the development of benzodiazepine tolerance. Then, the putative molecular mechanisms underlying benzodiazepine tolerance will be extensively discussed, followed by a section specifically addressing the issue of tolerance development with novel and more selective benzodiazepines in the light of the putative tolerance mechanisms associated with classical benzodiazepines. From a clinical perspective, the understanding of tolerance is important because long-term benzodiazepine treatment with continuing efficacy—using either existing or novel and more selective drugs—could offer potential benefits to several groups of patients.

2. Benzodiazepines and the GABA$_A$ System

2.1. GABA$_A$ Receptors. GABA$_A$ receptors constitute the major fast inhibitory neurotransmitter system in the brain. They are composed of five transmembrane-spanning subunits that assemble to form a ligand-gated chloride channel with various possible subunits (α_{1-6}, β_{1-3}, γ_{1-3}, δ, ε, θ, and π) resulting in GABA$_A$ receptor heterogeneity [13]. Binding of GABA to the GABA$_A$ receptor increases the influx of negatively charged chloride ions, resulting in an inhibitory postsynaptic signal (IPSP). Although in theory a vast number of subunits combinations could be expected,

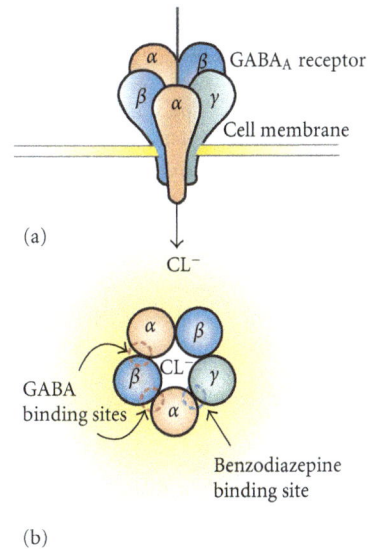

(a)

(b)

FIGURE 1: Representation of the GABA$_A$ receptor structure. The inhibitory GABA$_A$ receptor consists of five subunits that together form a ligand-gated chloride (Cl) channel (a). When GABA binds (between the α and the β subunit of the GABA$_A$ receptor), chloride ions flow into the neuron, resulting in a hyperpolarization of the cell membrane (a). Classical nonselective benzodiazepines allosterically enhance the inhibitory actions of GABA by binding between the α_1, α_2, α_3, or α_5 subunit and the γ subunit (b). Although the GABA$_A$ receptor displays a large molecular heterogeneity depending on the subunit composition, the most common subtype is a pentamer with 2α, 2β, and 1γ subunit.

GABA$_A$ receptors are found in typical subunit compositions with the most common receptor subtype being composed of two α, two β, and one γ subunit [14] (Figure 1). In situ hybridization and immunohistochemical studies have shown that GABA$_A$ receptor subunits display a distinct CNS distribution with a differential cellular localization pattern, suggesting that GABA$_A$ receptor subunits have a specialized function (Table 1) [14]. Overall, a high expression of GABAergic subunits is present in the cortex, hippocampus, and basal ganglia [15]. Of the GABAergic subunits, α_1, β_1, β_2, β_3, and γ_2 subunits are found throughout the brain. In contrast, the α_2, α_3, α_4, α_5, α_6, γ_1, and δ subunits have a specific regional expression pattern. The α_1 subunit is highly coassembled with β_2 and γ_2 subunits and is synaptically located on neuronal cell bodies. GABA$_A$ receptors that contain an α_2 or α_3 subunit are less abundant and are codistributed with the β_3 and γ_2 subunits. The α_2 subunit is present in the cortex, hippocampus, amygdale, and hypothalamus, and often its expression is negatively correlated with the expression of α_1 subunits. The expression of the α_3 subunit is highest in the cortex, hippocampus,

TABLE 1: Localization of common GABA$_A$ receptor subtypes in the brain (adapted from [19]).

Subtype	Frequency	Localization
$\alpha_1\beta_2\gamma_2$	Major (60%) synaptic	Cerebral cortex (layer I–VI), hippocampus, striatum, cerebellum, amygdala, brainstem.
$\alpha_2\beta_n\gamma_2$	Minor (15–20%) synaptic	Cerebral cortex (layers I–IV), hippocampus, striatum, hypothalamus, amygdala.
$\alpha_3\beta_n\gamma_2$	Minor (10–15%) synaptic	Cerebral cortex (layers V–VI), hippocampus, cerebellum, amygdala, brainstem (including raphe nuclei and locus coeruleus), spinal cord.
$\alpha_4\beta_n\delta/\gamma$	Minor (<10%) extrasynaptic	Hippocampus (dentate gyrus), thalamus, cortex.
$\alpha_5\beta_n\gamma_2$	Minor (<5%) extrasynaptic	Cerebral cortex, hippocampus, amygdala, hypothalamus, spinal cord.
$\alpha_6\beta_n\gamma_2/\delta$	Minor (<5%)(extra) synaptic	Cerebellum.

amygdala, thalamus, and brainstem, although it is also expressed in monoaminergic neurons (e.g., the raphe nuclei and the locus coeruleus in the brainstem) and cholinergic neurons in the forebrain. α_5 subunits are predominantly expressed in the hippocampus where they comprise 15–20% of the diazepam-sensitive GABA$_A$ receptors [16]. Regarding cellular localization, cortical and hippocampal pyramidal cells receive input from morphologically distinct GABAergic interneurons that innervate different pyramidal cell parts depending on the type of interneuron (e.g., chandelier and basket cells) with a specialized postsynaptic expression of α subunits [17, 18].

Thus, GABA$_A$ receptor subtypes probably possess diverging functional properties dependent on the subunit composition, contributing to the GABA signaling complexity [13]. Additionally, GABA$_A$ receptors are found synaptically as well as extrasynaptically. Synaptic receptors usually contain γ subunits and mediate fast phasic inhibition accompanied by transient high GABA concentrations [16]. By contrast, GABA has higher potency (at μM concentrations) at extrasynaptic GABA$_A$ receptors that usually contain a δ subunit, preferentially assemble with α_6 or α_4 subunits and have slow desensitization kinetics [20]. Also, α_5 subunits may be localized extrasynaptically [21]. Extrasynaptic tonic inhibition—which is not modified by benzodiazepines—is suggested to modulate excitability of neuronal networks throughout the brain.

2.2. Benzodiazepines from a Nonspecific towards a Subunit-Specific Pharmacology. Classical benzodiazepines allosterically modulate GABA-induced IPSPs by binding to the benzodiazepine site of GABA$_A$ receptors that contain an α_1, α_2, α_3, or α_5 subunit in combination with a β and a γ_2 subunit (Figure 1). The exact binding site of benzodiazepines

at the GABA$_A$ receptor is located between the α and γ subunit. In contrast, benzodiazepines do not interact with GABA$_A$ receptors that contain an α_4- or α_6-subunit. In addition to benzodiazepines, other drug classes can bind to the GABA$_A$ receptor complex, including several anticonvulsants, ethanol, barbiturates, neurosteroids, and some anesthetics [15]. The fact that classical benzodiazepines nonselectively bind to different α subunits led to the hypothesis that the pharmacological profile with anxiolytic, sedative, anticonvulsive and myorelaxant properties may be further dissected. Both genetic and pharmacological approaches explored the hypothesis that α subunits differentially contribute to the different effects of classical benzodiazepines The genetic approach consisted of point mutations into specific α subunits (α_1(H101R), α_2(H101R), α_3(H126R), and α_5(H105R)), turning them functionally insensitive to benzodiazepines without altering their GABA sensitivity [22]. Pharmacological research on the GABA$_A$ receptor has focused on the development of compounds that show differential efficacy across the various α subunits [13]. Such drugs generally bind with equal affinity to all α subunits (i.e., α_1, α_2, α_3, and α_5 subunits), but selectively alter the capacity to increase GABA binding to one or more of them. Using this strategy, various efficacy-selective (and some affinity-selective) compounds have been developed with preferential agonistic activity at the α_1 (zolpidem and zaleplon), $\alpha_{2/3}$ (TPA023, L838, 417, and SL651498), or inverse agonist activity the α_5 subunit (α5IA, L-655,708, and MRK-016) (see also Table 2).

In line with a specific central localization and distribution of GABAergic subunits, these genetic and pharmacological approaches have demonstrated that different α subunits of the GABA$_A$ receptor mediate the distinct effects of benzodiazepines. Specifically, α_1-containing GABA$_A$ receptors probably mediate the sedative, amnesic, and anticonvulsant actions of classical benzodiazepines [13, 23]. In contrast, muscle relaxation and anxiety reduction after benzodiazepine administration was primarily ascribed to α_2 (and possibly α_3) subunit activation [24], whereas α_5 subunit-containing GABA$_A$ receptors appear to be involved in learning and memory [25, 26].

In light of the topic of this review, studies investigating the contribution of GABAergic subunits in benzodiazepine abuse liability, drug reinforcement, and tolerance development are of particular interest. Unfortunately, studies applying genetic and subtype-selective methodologies to examine the development of tolerance are scarce. One study using α subunit point mutation mice implicated a critical role for α_5 subunits together with α_1 subunits in the decreasing sedative efficacy of the classical benzodiazepine diazepam after chronic treatment [27]. We will discuss this finding in detail later in this paper. Studies on the background of physical dependence and abuse liability using subtype-selective GABA$_A$R modulators are more abundant. Using self-administration studies, it was shown that efficacy at α_1-containing GABA$_A$ subtypes significantly contributed to the reinforcing effects and withdrawal symptoms of benzodiazepines [8, 28, 29]. Specifically, TPA123, which still possesses 23% intrinsic activity at α_1 subunits still led

TABLE 2: Summary of novel GABA$_A$ receptor subtype selective compounds.

Target	Name	Efficacy (compared to a classical benzodiazepine)	Affinity/Remarks	Ref
α_1	Zolpidem	Comparable at $\alpha_1/\alpha_2/\alpha_3/\alpha_5$	5-10-fold higher affinity for α_1 versus $\alpha_{2/3}$ > 1000 fold higher affinity for α_1 versus α_5	[15]
$\alpha_{2/3}$	TPA023	α_1 (0%), α_2 (11%), α_3 (21%), α_5 (5%)	Equivalent affinity	[8]
$\alpha_{2/3}$	TPA123	α_1 (23%), α_2 (35%), α_3 (43%), α_5 (19%)	Equivalent affinity. Reinforcing efficacy and physiological dependence remained present	[8]
$\alpha_{2/3}$	L838,417	α_1 (1.5%), α_2 (43%), α_3 (43%), α_5 (39%)	Equivalent affinity	[23]
$\alpha_{2/3}$	SL651498	α_1 (45%), α_2 (115%), α_3 (83%), α_5 (50%) Compared to zolpidem for α_1 efficacy	5–10-fold increased affinity for $\alpha_{2/3}$, 10–20 fold lower affinity for α_5	[31]

to benzodiazepine-like drug reinforcement and withdrawal symptoms, whereas TPA023 with 0% α_1 intrinsic activity did not, even at full GABA$_A$ receptor-binding capacity [8]. However, there is still the possibility that the lower α_2 and α_3 efficacy of TPA023 may have contributed to the absence of drug reinforcement and withdrawal. In support, L-838,417 also led to continued self-administration, even though it lacks efficacy for the α_1 subtype [30]. In any case, the α_5 subunit may not be directly involved in the abuse potential of classical benzodiazepines as the α_1-preferring hypnotic zolpidem with no affinity for the α_5 subunit still led to self-administration in primates [30]. This finding is surprising as it suggests that the α_5 subunit may be involved in tolerance development but not in drug reinforcement. Consequently, these processes could be independently mediated, even though they are both incorporated in the definition of benzodiazepine dependence.

2.3. GABA Metabolism. As benzodiazepines enhance the inhibitory effects of GABA and shift the GABA concentration-response curve to the left, the synaptic GABA concentration affects benzodiazepine efficacy. GABA is converted from glutamate by the enzyme glutamic acid decarboxylase (GAD) that maintains intracellular levels of GABA and exists in two independent isoforms (GAD$_{65}$ and GAD$_{67}$). In contrast to the localization of GAD$_{67}$ in the neuronal body, GAD$_{65}$ is primarily expressed in axon terminals, suggesting a role for GAD$_{65}$ in synaptic neurotransmission and a more general role for GAD$_{67}$ in regulating GABA synthesis [32]. Synaptic GABA is removed from the cleft into the presynaptic axon terminals by GABA transporters (GATs). So far, four GAT subtypes have been identified, with the highly expressed GAT$_1$ and GAT$_4$ being the most widely distributed [33].

3. The Development of Benzodiazepine Tolerance

Before examining the possible mechanisms underlying the development of benzodiazepine tolerance after long-term exposure, it is important to review its evidence and determine whether it is clinically relevant. Overall, there is

little doubt that benzodiazepines are acutely effective in reducing anxiety, sleep latency and preventing convulsions. The tolerance that is eventually thought to develop appears to occur at different rates and to a different degree for each of the benzodiazepine effects [34]. Preclinical studies have shown that tolerance to the sedative and hypnotic effects occurs rather rapidly, followed by tolerance to the anticonvulsant effects, whereas tolerance to the anxiolytic effects of benzodiazepines are absent or partially develop after long-term treatment (for reviews, see [34–36]). As these preclinical studies have already been extensively reviewed, and novel preclinical studies on benzodiazepine tolerance have been limited in the last years to our knowledge, it is beyond this paper to reproduce all preclinical data on tolerance development. In general, preclinical studies are in agreement with the clinical divergent picture, even though in most preclinical studies, tolerance is not directly related to the applied dose, dosing interval, or the drug's plasma levels or half-life. Here, we will focus on the clinical evidence for (the rate of) tolerance development for each benzodiazepine action, even though we will also include preclinical studies when clinical studies are lacking or inconclusive.

3.1. Clinical Studies on Sedative and Hypnotic Tolerance. A study in low-dose benzodiazepine-dependent subjects showed a complete loss of hypnotic activity independent of the half-life of the prescribed benzodiazepine, even though a substantial suppression of REM sleep still occurred [37]. Also, other studies have shown that chronic users displayed no increase in sedation or motor impairment after the acute application of a benzodiazepine [38–40]. Moreover, tolerance to benzodiazepine-induced decreased reaction speed was shown after 10 days of alprazolam treatment [41]. Oral administration of triazolam, a short acting benzodiazepine, initially improved both sleep induction and maintenance, but latency to sleep and the number of awakenings were back to baseline values after two weeks of triazolam use [42]. Importantly, early-morning insomnia associated with short-acting benzodiazepines triazolam and midazolam markedly worsened after 7 days of treatment [43]. However, conflicting studies with triazolam exist that did not show any tolerance development [44, 45]. Another study applying the longer-acting benzodiazepine temazepam (15 or 30 mg) for either 26 or 54 nights in 7-8 subjects with chronic insomnia found no development of drug tolerance due to long-term temazepam administration [46]. Flurazepam, which has a relatively long elimination half-life, was shown to be effective for initiating and maintaining sleep with intermediate and long-term use (over 4 weeks), even though daytime sedation diminished during prolonged use [47]. Thus, even though tolerance to the sedative effects quickly emerges in most studies, these effects seem to be most prominent with benzodiazepines with a short half-life. Tolerance could thus depend on the half life of the applied benzodiazepine. However, this may be an overgeneralization, as a review showed that tolerance in human subjects only marginally emerged after chronic treatment with the short-acting drugs midazolam and zolpidem, even though the short-acting drug triazolam was associated with tolerance [48]. A limitation of most studies is their relatively short duration of exposure. Another issue is that convincing evidence for improved sleep after long-term use is lacking [49], yet this may not be the sole result of tolerance but could also be attributable to a generalized lack of efficacy. In support, in human subjects, discontinuation of benzodiazepines did not decrease sleep quality compared to a group that stayed on benzodiazepines up to 52 weeks after cessation [50], or even increased sleep quality and slow wave sleep after discontinuation in insomnia patients [51].

3.2. Clinical Studies on Anticonvulsant Tolerance. The use of benzodiazepines over a longer period of time in epilepsy is limited due to the development of tolerance [52]. In line with preclinical studies [53–55], tolerance develops during the first several months in 30–50% of epilepsy patients treated with either clobazam or clonazepam [56]. Thus, benzodiazepines are only prescribed in acute epileptic seizures or in a status epilepticus. However, in certain cases, intermittent use may be indicated, which may reduce the likelihood of tolerance [57]. Chronic treatment in rodents with the α_1-preferential compound CL218, 572 resulted in loss of picrotoxin-induced seizures [58]. In contrast to classical benzodiazepines, partial GABA$_A$ receptor PAMs including bretazenil did not result in anticonvulsant tolerance in several preclinical studies [54, 59, 60]. However, to our knowledge, these drugs have not been tested for (continuing) anticonvulsant activity in humans, precluding firm conclusions on their tolerance-inducing effects in epilepsy patients.

3.3. Clinical Studies on Amnesic Tolerance. Most studies have found continued short-term memory impairment after acute administration of benzodiazepines in chronically treated subjects [38, 39, 61]. Also, no tolerance for memory-impairing effects of alprazolam was found during a 10-day acute treatment [41]. However, another study reported tolerance to the acute amnesic effects of alprazolam after chronic use [40]. A major concern is that loss of memory associated with benzodiazepine use may be lasting, even after treatment discontinuation [62, 63], although other studies reported improved cognitive functioning after discontinuation with increased speed and accuracy of information processing,

improved reaction time and working memory [50, 64–66]. Collectively, clinical data do not support the existence of tolerance to benzodiazepine-induced cognitive impairments.

3.4. Clinical Studies on Anxiolytic Tolerance. If developing al all, tolerance to the anxiolytic effects seems to develop more slowly compared to tolerance to the hypnotic effects. In patients with panic disorder, neither anxiolytic tolerance nor daily dose increase was observed after 8 weeks of alprazolam treatment with continued efficacy [67]. This was confirmed by another study in panic disorder patients who already chronically took alprazolam. Here, no differences were found in cortisol responsivity or anxiolytic efficacy compared to alprazolam-naïve patients, independent of disease severity [40]. Another double-blind study allocated 180 chronically anxious outpatients to diazepam (15 to 40 mg/day) and found that prolonged diazepam treatment (6–22 weeks) did not result in tolerance to the anxiolytic effects of diazepam [68]. Furthermore, additional studies all show a continuing anxiolytic effect, at least for panic disorder [69–72], generalized anxiety disorder [73], and social phobia [74–76]. Although a declining anxiolytic efficacy after long-term use of benzodiazepines cannot be clearly established, it is important to remember that other disadvantages prevent benzodiazepines to chronically treat anxiety symptoms, such as continued memory impairment, accident risk, hip fractures, and withdrawal symptoms [7, 77]. In conclusion, there is no solid evidence from the existing literature that anxiolytic efficacy declines following chronic benzodiazepine use in humans.

3.5. Clinical Studies on Drug Reinforcement Tolerance. The relevant topic of benzodiazepine tolerance to the reinforcing effects of benzodiazepines was already discussed by Licata and Rowlett [9]. They concluded that tolerance to reinforcing effects of benzodiazepines appears unlikely, supported by studies in nonhuman primates in which midazolam and zolpidem maintained stable self-injection and physical dependence under conditions of chronic continuous availability [78, 79]. Also, in humans, tolerance to drug reinforcement could lead to dose escalation that would maintain the vicious cycle of tolerance and dependence. In clinical practice, the majority of patients do not escalate their dose, suggesting that drug reinforcement tolerance may not emerge [80].

3.6. Conclusion. In conclusion, tolerance develops relatively quickly for the sedative, hypnotic, and anticonvulsant actions of benzodiazepines. Tolerance to anxiolytic and amnesic effects most probably does not appear at all. The fact that benzodiazepine dosage may be hard to reduce after chronic use can be ascribed to physical dependence to avoid withdrawal symptoms rather than the development of tolerance.

With diverging rates and varying completeness of tolerance development, it may be speculated that either (i) different tolerance mechanisms exist depending on the benzodiazepine effect, or that (ii) a uniform mechanism accounts for tolerance but revolves around the subunit composition of the targeted GABA$_A$ receptor subtype and the brain region involved. However, from the presented evidence it is difficult to conclude that benzodiazepines indeed produce a robust and reproducible tolerance for all (side) effects. It is clear however, that benzodiazepine tolerance is not a uniform process for all clinical effects and does not apply to all available benzodiazepines. However, it is not known which factors predict whether a certain benzodiazepine possesses the potential to produce tolerance. Unfortunately, many studies address the physical dependence of benzodiazepines and their abuse potential, but do not specifically investigate tolerance.

4. Mechanisms Underlying Tolerance

4.1. General. Decades of research into the molecular effects of long-term benzodiazepine treatment have already importantly advanced our understanding of tolerance and several excellent reviews on this topic have already been published [5, 11, 34, 77]. The general assumption is that chronic benzodiazepine use leads to compensating changes in the central nervous system. This way, the GABAA receptor may become less responsive to the continuing acute effects of benzodiazepines, either as a result of adaptations in the GABAA receptor itself, intracellular mechanisms, or changes in other neurotransmitter systems, such as the glutamatergic system. Although adaptive processes probably play an important role, it is important to realize that the development of tolerance is not uniform for all its actions, and differences between preclinical and clinical tolerance development may exist. Therefore, the possibility that not one but multiple adaptive mechanisms simultaneously coexist complicates research into benzodiazepine tolerance. Moreover, these adaptive changes could be limited to one or more specific brain areas. This makes it very challenging to single out one a priori unifying mechanism underlying tolerance. In support, a study in rats using 2-deoxyglucose quantitative autoradiography showed that during chronic diazepam treatment, heterogeneous tolerance to the diazepam-induced reduction of glucose utilization occurred in the brain, depending on treatment duration and brain region [6]. Whereas acute diazepam administration resulted in reductions in glucose utilization throughout the brain, 3 days of diazepam treatment led to tolerance in brain structures associated with sensory processing (parietal cortex, auditory cortex, cochlear nucleus) which was interpreted to correlate with reduced sedation. After 28-day diazepam treatment, tolerance to the depressant effect of diazepam on cerebral glucose occurred in the mamillary body, subiculum, and caudate nucleus, whereas changes in the frontal cortex approached significance. Of particular interest is the finding that none of the amygdaloid nuclei showed any blunting over time, in line with persistent anxiolytic effects of benzodiazepines.

Before taking a closer look at specific mechanisms that have been proposed to underlie benzodiazepine tolerance, it is important to note that pharmacokinetic factors probably do not play a major role in the development of tolerance [81]. In support, plasma levels after acute diazepam administration did not differ between chronically alprazolam-treated

and untreated panic disorder patients, even though sedative and amnesic tolerance was observed [40]. The most obvious candidate to mediate the adaptive changes in cellular and synaptic function after chronic benzodiazepine treatment is the GABAA receptor. Therefore, we will first discuss the evidence supporting changes in the GABA system (including GABAA receptor coupling and GABA receptor expression) after chronic benzodiazepine exposure.

4.2. GABAA System Hypotheses

4.2.1. Mechanism 1: GABAA Receptor Uncoupling. One explanation for a loss of benzodiazepine function is a loss in GABAA receptor allosteric coupling. The GABAA receptor contains two GABA-binding sites and one benzodiazepine-binding site that are allosterically coupled, that is, binding to the benzodiazepine-binding site potentiates binding of GABA to the GABA-binding site (Figure 1). Benzodiazepines are generally referred to as positive allosteric modulators (PAMs) because their binding alters the GABAA receptor conformation with an increased capacity to bind GABA, leading to increased channel opening frequency, increased chloride influx, and, consequently, to hyperpolarization. GABAA receptor uncoupling is defined as a decreased ability of benzodiazepines to enhance GABA-induced IPSPs at the GABAA receptor. In terms of tolerance development, it has been hypothesized that chronic treatment affects the benzodiazepines' capacity to pharmacologically enhance the GABA response (i.e., tolerance leads to uncoupling). A decreased coupling may develop as a result of changed GABAA receptor subunit composition, alterations to the GABAA receptor itself (including phosphorylation) or its second messenger ligands, or any process affecting the conformational state of the GABAA receptor. The receptor uncoupling hypothesis is attractive as it does not assume any changes in subunit expression and ligand binding yet uses the knowledge on the specialized functions of the GABAA receptor and the different subunits. However, the uncoupling process is an aspecific process as it can be induced by exposure to different classes of GABAA receptor modulators acting at different modulatory sites, such as neurosteroids and barbiturates [82].

Already in 1984, an electrophysiological study indicated that allosteric coupling may play a role by showing a 50% decrease in the GABA enhancement of benzodiazepine-binding without significant changes in benzodiazepine-binding site density or affinity [83]. Also, more recent indications for reduced allosteric coupling were found after chronic treatment using transfected cell lines that express GABAA receptors or in neurons [84–94]. The mechanisms underlying possible differences in coupling remain poorly understood. If the GABAA receptor assembly process is modified, GABA receptor composition can be modified due to subunit replacements or altered expression in the receptor. This way, GABAA receptors with a different functionality could potentially possess reduced benzodiazepine sensitivity due to reduced GABAA receptor coupling. To our knowledge, no studies exist which have directly investigated GABAA receptor subunit composition after chronic exposure. Another mechanism to affect receptor coupling is GABA$_A$ receptor phosphorylation. GABA$_A$ receptors are phosphorylated by various protein kinases and dephosphorylated by phosphatases [95]. Dynamic functional alterations in GABA$_A$ receptor phosphorylation status may directly affect the inhibitory synaptic strength, with changes in channel openings (or indirectly influence receptor trafficking). However, the precise effects of phosphorylation on neuronal GABA$_A$ receptor function are complex, even though key residues within the intracellular loop of the GABA$_A$ receptor seem of particular importance. Using whole-cell patch-clamp recordings of GABA$_A$ receptor IPSCs in hippocampal neurons, brain-region-dependent effects of activation of cAMP-dependent protein kinase A (PKA) or Ca^{2+}/phospholipid-dependent protein kinase C (PKC) were shown [96]. Also, PKA activity was found to be directly involved in changed GABA$_A$ receptor functioning in hippocampal pyramidal cells following chronic flurazepam treatment [97]. Probably, phosphorylation patterns rather than individual sites are of importance, supported by the finding that mutation to one PKA phosphorylation site is not involved in tolerance [90]. Using a point mutation genetic approach, transcriptional reduction was found in calcium-/calmodulin-dependent kinase IIα and MAP kinase phosphatase-1in control mice but not in α1(H101R) after acute administration of diazepam [98]. Unfortunately, no chronic treatment was included in these studies.

It remains to be seen whether changes in allosteric coupling are relevant to the development of tolerance *in vivo*. Because benzodiazepine tolerance gradually develops over days to weeks, this would suggest that structural changes take place, whereas posttranslational compensation would be expected to be directly manifest. In support, uncoupling seems to develop rapidly, with the classical benzodiazepine chlordiazepoxide (applied together with GABA) stimulating the rate and extent of desensitization produced in a single neuron within several seconds [99]. Also, the observed uncoupling after chronic benzodiazepine treatment is rapidly reversed by a brief exposure *in vivo* to the benzodiazepine antagonist flumazenil [83, 86].

4.2.2. Mechanism 2: Alterations in GABA$_A$ Receptor Subunit Expression. The most straightforward hypothesis to explain impaired sensitivity after chronic benzodiazepine exposure would be a general downregulation of GABA$_A$ receptors throughout the brain. Indeed, the process of tolerance requires GABA$_A$ receptors at least to some extent, as cell lines expressing one specific type of the GABA$_A$R are susceptible to tolerance [86, 87, 90]. Because classical (nonselective) benzodiazepines bind to GABA$_A$ receptors that contain an α_1, α_2, α_3, or α_5 subunit, it could be expected that expression of receptors containing these α subunits (plus a γ_2 subunit) is changed. Of course, this would depend on the cellular and anatomical distribution of GABA$_A$ receptors. Already earlier in Section 2.1, the differentiated and unique distribution of GABAergic subunits in the CNS was discussed. With regard to the benzodiazepine-sensitive α subunits, the α_1 subunit is ubiquitously expressed in the entire brain, whereas the other α subunits (α_2, α_3 and α_5) display a more restricted

pattern of expression (see Table 1). If receptor internalization simply downregulates GABA$_A$ receptor density, then a priori regional differentiation would be expected based on receptor distribution.

The processes that control the assembly, membrane trafficking, and synaptic accumulation of GABA$_A$ receptors are complex (for review, see [100]). In short, GABA$_A$ receptors are assembled from individual subunits out of the endoplasmic reticulum within minutes after their translation, with amino acid sequences in the N-terminus influencing the GABA$_A$ receptor subtype (Figure 2). Then, receptor trafficking to the plasma membrane takes place, facilitated by diverse helper GABA$_A$ receptor-associated proteins (among that GABARAP, BIG2, PRIP, gephyrin, and radixin). Ultimately, (clathrin-dependent) endocytosis occurs after receptor dephosphorylation, after which degradation or recycling may ensue (Figure 2). If prolonged activation of the GABA system leads to receptor downregulation, then this could be established by interfering at multiple steps of the dynamic GABA$_A$ receptor life cycle. These include decreased subunit mRNA transcription, subunit degradation in the endoplasmic reticulum (e.g., by ubiquitylation), decreased expression of GABA$_A$ receptor-associated helper proteins, and alterations in the endocytosis of specific GABA$_A$ receptor subtypes. The finding that the protein synthesis inhibitor cycloheximide and the RNA synthesis inhibitor actinomycin D blocked the effects of chronic diazepam exposure in recombinant cells expressing GABA$_A$ receptors indicates that GABA$_A$ receptor synthesis is of at least some importance [87].

Up to now, a plethora of studies have tried to address whether chronic benzodiazepine treatment indeed affects GABA$_A$ receptor expression (and thus benzodiazepine binding sites) using compounds with different subtype selectivity profiles at different doses and varying treatment duration. A recent excellent review summarized all data on the regulation of GABA$_A$ receptor subunit after chronic benzodiazepine treatment that was mostly studied in rats [102]. It is beyond the scope of this review to repeat the meticulous work laid down in this paper. Of all subunits, α, β, and γ subunits have been mostly examined. This paper confirms that both for mRNA and protein subunit levels, the available evidence leads to a divergent and sometimes conflicting picture, although the majority of the studies essentially do not show any significant difference in subunit expression [102]. Furthermore, a lack of consistency appears for subunit changes in different specific brain areas. Moreover, the length and method of chronic treatment seem relevant since differences in GABA$_A$ receptor subunit mRNA levels after chronic diazepam treatment in rats can depend on whether diazepam is administered as daily systemic injections or via osmotic minipumps [103]. Binding studies also generally report no changes in benzodiazepine binding after chronic treatment [92, 93, 104]. Together, GABA$_A$ receptor expression (both mRNA and protein levels) is not consistently and robustly altered after various long-term treatment regimens. Thus, a general central downregulation or even consistent region-specific changes in GABA$_A$ receptor expression after chronic benzodiazepine use are not supported by the literature. Even though methodological differences (e.g., treatment regimen,

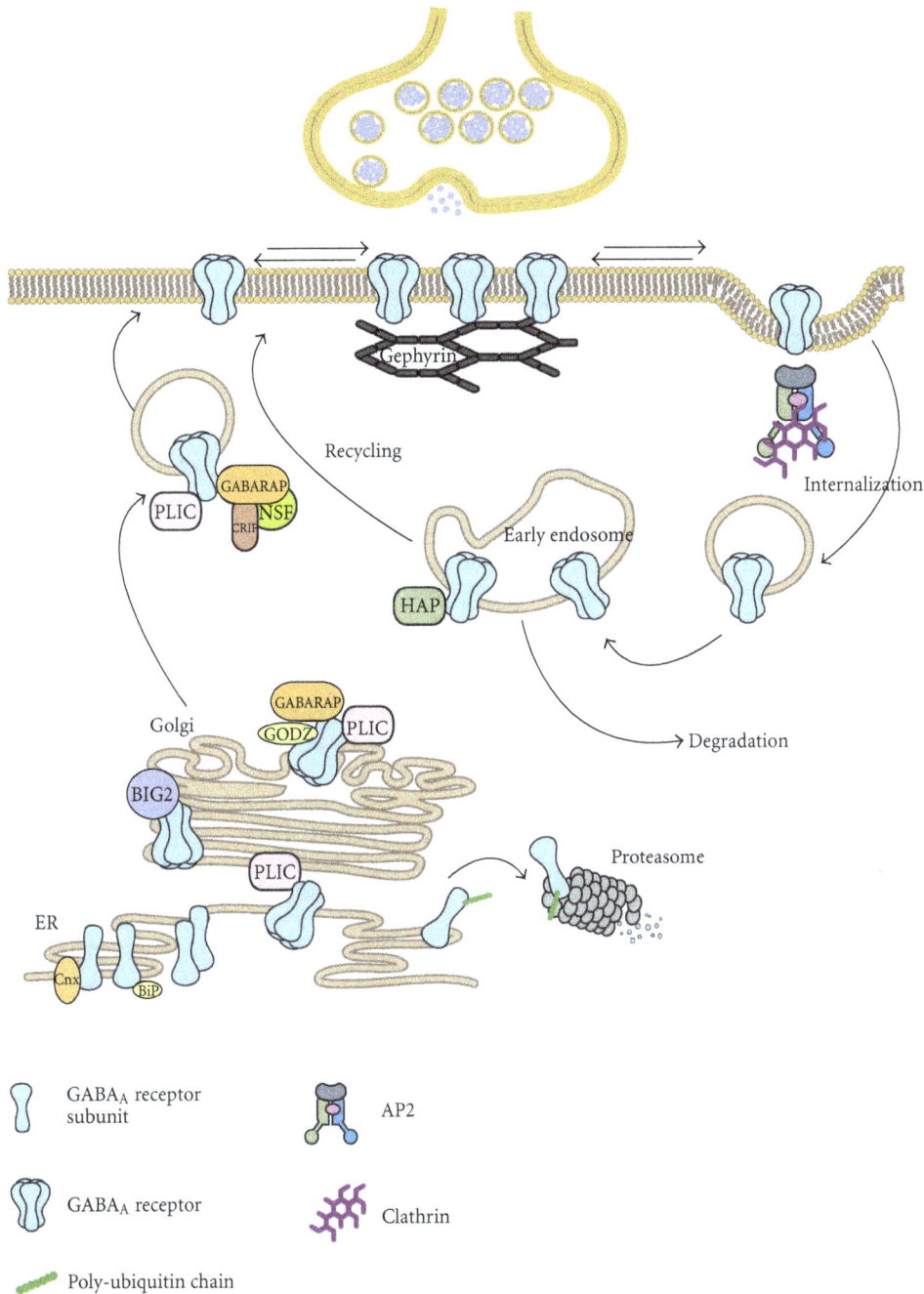

FIGURE 2: GABA$_A$ receptor trafficking and associated proteins. GABA$_A$ receptors are assembled from individual subunits in the endoplasmatic reticulum (ER) where the chaperones BiP and Calnexin assist in quality control. Unassembled GABA$_A$ receptor subunits that are to be targeted for ER-associated degradation are ubiquitinated and degraded in the proteasome. The ubiquitin-like protein PLIC can interact with GABA$_A$ receptors thereby inhibiting their targeting for proteasomal degradation. Assembled pentameric GABA$_A$ receptors exit the ER and bind the guanidine exchange factor brefeldin-A-inhibited GDP/GTP exchange factor 2 (BIG2) in the Golgi. Here they also interact with the palmitoylase transferase GODZ and Gamma-aminobutyric acid receptor-associated protein (GABARAP). GABARAP interacts with the NEM sensitive fusion (NSF) protein, as does the GABA$_A$ receptor β subunit, and this association may facilitate transport of the receptor complexes to the cell surface. GABA$_A$ receptors are inserted at extrasynaptic sites and can diffuse along the plasma membrane in and out of synaptic domains. At synapses they are stabilized by an interaction with the scaffolding protein Gephyrin. The interaction of the GABA$_A$ receptor intracellular loops with the $\mu 2$ subunit of the adaptin complex AP2 is important for GABA$_A$ receptor internalization. GABA$_A$ receptors are delivered by a clathrin-mediated pathway to early endosomes where they can be targeted for degradation in the lysosome or for recycling upon binding of Huntington-associated protein (HAP1). Reprinted by permission from Elsevier, reprinted from [101].

species, route of administration, and applied drug) may account for some conflicting findings, the results seem overall inconsistent. Moreover, molecular results are often not combined with behavioral tests, preventing a direct correlation between behavioral tolerance and molecular changes. Clinical studies applying *in vivo* binding or postmortem GABA$_A$ receptor expression after chronic benzodiazepine treatment are to the knowledge of the authors lacking.

Changes in rates of GABA$_A$ receptor endocytosis, receptor membrane insertion, intracellular trafficking, and association with helper GABA$_A$ receptor-associated proteins could still play a role, leading to a reduction in membrane surface receptors without affecting overall subunit protein expression (e.g., see [105]). Another interesting suggestion is that a possible loss of synaptic function after chronic exposure could be due to a shift to a perisynaptic or even an extrasynaptic localization of GABA$_A$ receptors, away from clustering of GABA$_A$ receptors at synapses (Figure 2) [106]. At least in alcohol research, such dynamic changes in plasticity at inhibitory synapses have been shown [107]. Moreover, it cannot be excluded that particular subunits play a role in the development of tolerance after chronic treatment in the absence a direct up- or downregulation. Using the previously mentioned α subunit point mutation mice, acutely administered diazepam still reduced locomotor activity in $\alpha5$ (H105R) mice even after chronic 8-day diazepam treatment at a combined daily dose of 15 mg/kg [27]. This suggests that the α_1 subunit that mediates the sedative effects remains responsive, indicating that simultaneous activation of the α_1 and α_5 subunit may be necessary for tolerance to the locomotor-reducing effects of classical benzodiazepines. Specifically, it was hypothesized that increased phasic signaling would alter extrasynaptic tonic inhibition mediated by α_5-containing GABA$_A$ receptors, whereas a decrease in hippocampal α_5-specific binding was reported in diazepam-tolerant mice. Also, in contrast to α_1-, α_2-, and α_3-containing receptors, α_5-containing GABA$_A$ receptors are located extrasynaptically at the base of dendritic spines where they can modulate excitatory glutamatergic input. However, $\alpha1$(H101R) mice are not sensitive to the acute sedative benzodiazepine effects, making a comparison to isolated α_1 subunit activation not possible. Moreover, only tolerance to the sedative effects of diazepam was reported. Thus, it may still be possible that tolerance to other benzodiazepine effects is mediated by other subunits.

4.3. Glutamate System Hypotheses

4.3.1. General.
From the previous sections, we conclude that compensatory changes solely arising from the GABA system may at most partially explain the tolerance arising following chronic treatment with benzodiazepines. Glutamate is an excitatory neurotransmitter acting on glutamate receptors. Together with the GABA system, they constitute the two fast-acting and opposing neurotransmitter systems that can modulate synaptic plasticity. In support, close neuroanatomical connections exist between GABAergic and glutamatergic neurons [108, 109]. With a presence in at least 30–50% of all synapses in the CNS, inhibitory GABA

and excitatory glutamate together coordinate the balance in the brain's excitability. Therefore, it is not surprising that as these two opposing and fast-acting neurotransmitter systems form a delicate balance, chronic (increased) activation of the GABAergic system during benzodiazepine treatment may pertubate glutamatergic transmission. The basis of benzodiazepine tolerance could then lie in sensitization of the glutamatergic system—a putative process that could account for the withdrawal symptoms after chronic benzodiazepine discontinuation [5, 110]. Such sensitization is reminiscent to adaptive glutamatergic processes as seen in kindling experiments, although it should be noted that kindling only occurs with intermittent and not after continuous treatment [111]. Glutamatergic sensitization could thus play a role in the development of tolerance as well as withdrawal symptoms upon cessation of treatment. Glutamatergic changes after benzodiazepine withdrawal will not be discussed here, but there are indications that the glutamatergic system plays a role in withdrawal states with accompanying increases in anxiety and seizure activity (for review see [5]). However, glutamate receptor mRNA and protein changes may be dynamic during withdrawal, with unchanged levels during the early phase of withdrawal but changes occurring several days later [112]. This consequently complicates the interpretation of withdrawal studies and their significance for our understanding of benzodiazepine tolerance.

Similar to the GABAergic system, the glutamate system is diverse and complex, generally being divided into ionotropic and metabotropic receptor types. Ionotropic glutamate receptors form a class of heteromeric ligand-gated cation channels that potentiate the influx of K$^+$, Na$^+$, or Ca^{2+} ions following glutamate binding. Three classes of the ionotropic glutamate receptor occur in het central nervous system: the NMDA receptor (N-methyl-D-aspartate), the AMPA receptor (alpha-amino-3-hydroxy-5-methyl-4-isoxazole-4-propionic acid), and the kainate receptor (for a recent review see [113]). Functional NMDA receptors contain two obligatory GluN$_1$ and two regulatory GluN$_{2/3}$ subunits and are vital for synaptic plasticity (for review, see [114]). Each GluN subunit contains extracellular loops where coagonists glycine or D-serine (GluN$_1$ and GluN$_3$ subunits) and glutamate (GluN$_2$ subunits) can bind [115]. Although the channel is blocked by Mg^{2+} ions, changes in membrane potential can make the channel permeable to Na$^+$, Ca^{2+}, and K$^+$ ions. The central distribution of GluN$_2$ subunits eventually ensures heterogeneity in the NMDA receptor system. AMPA receptors are widespread heterotetrameric ligand-gated ion channels composed of four types of subunits (GluR$_{1-4}$), and are crucial to long-term synaptic plasticity such as long-term potentiation (for review see [116]). Although glutamate possesses lower affinity for the AMPA receptor compared to NMDA receptors, faster excitation-inducing kinetics are present at the AMPA receptor. Relevant to this review, a study showed that AMPA receptor desensitization was caused by a rupture of a domain interface which allowed the ion channel to close, providing a simple yet elegant explanation [117]. Kainate receptors are made up of four subunits, GluR$_5$, GluR$_6$, GluR$_7$, KA$_1$, and KA$_2$, which are similar to AMPA and NMDA receptor subunits and can be arranged in different ways to form a functional tetramer (for review, see [118]). Compared to NMDA and AMPA receptors, synaptic kainate receptors exhibit slow rise and decay properties.

4.3.2. Mechanism 3: Role of Ionotropic Glutamatergic Receptors.
Several studies have addressed the compensatory glutamate sensitization hypothesis during chronic benzodiazepine exposure to account for the development of tolerance (as reviewed by [5, 110]).

In rodents, the development of tolerance to the sedative effects of the classical benzodiazepines diazepam and chlordiazepoxide was prevented by coadministration of the NMDA receptor antagonists CPP, dizocilpine, MK-801, and ketamine [119–121]. Also, lorazepam-induced tolerance to its acute anticonvulsant effects was partially prevented with simultaneous CPP treatment [122]. In contrast, the development of tolerance to the anxiolytic effects of diazepam in a social interaction test was not blocked by concomitant administration of dizocilpine [123]. This suggests that the mechanism underlying tolerance to the anxiolytic effects of diazepam is different from that underlying tolerance to the sedative effects. Increases in cortical mRNA of NMDA NR_1 and NR_{2B} subunits have been reported in rats tolerant to diazepam [124, 125], which were prevented by concomitant treatment with the NMDA receptor antagonist MK-801 [126]. However, another study showed decreases in hippocampal NR_{2B} subunits after chronic flurazepam treatment, even though the total amount of NMDA receptors was unchanged [127].

In support, after long-term (but not acute) lorazepam treatment, no differences were found in the affinity or density of NMDA receptors, even though increased *in vitro* glutamate release and NMDA-induced cGMP efflux in the hippocampus was reported [128]. Together, these data suggest that NMDA-dependent mechanisms contribute to the development of benzodiazepine tolerance. However, as anxiolytic tolerance was not blocked by NMDA receptor antagonism, the NMDA system could also play a differential role in tolerance depending on the specific behavioral effects [123]. Moreover, a straightforward glutamate sensitization may be an oversimplification, as tolerance to the sedative effects of lorazepam after 21-day treatment correlated with a decreased rather than an increased sensitivity for glutamate (using$^{[(3)H]}$ glutamate binding) [129].

Even though the AMPA receptor antagonist GYKI 52466 did not affect the development of tolerance to the sedative effects of diazepam [121], changes in AMPA receptor subunits have been reported to be altered after long-term benzodiazepine exposure [130]. Specifically, significant reductions of mGLuR1 (cortex and amygdala) and mGluR2 mRNA (amygdala) were reported in rats treated chronically with diazepam, even though the effects were complex and dependent on treatment route (subcutaneous or intraperitoneal injections). Adding to the complexity of the published data, another study did not show changes in hippocampal GluR1-3 subunit proteins following chronic flurazepam treatment, even though mEPSCs were found and nonspecific binding was increased using the AMPA receptor

antagonist$^{[(3)H]}$ Ro48-8587 [131]. A genetic approach with GluR$_1$ knockout mice showed that after subchronic flurazepam treatment, these mice developed a reduced and incomplete tolerance to the muscle relaxation and sedative effects of flurazepam, even though acute flurazepam effects were comparable between knockout and wild-type mice [132].

With regard to glutamatergic kainate receptors, we found no pharmacological or genetic studies investigating the development of tolerance.

Together, the evidence does not support a universal and replicable glutamatergic component, even though there are indications that NMDA receptor blockade can prevent tolerance to at least some behavioral benzodiazepine effects. However, molecular data are diverse and sometimes inconsistent, which are reminiscent of the molecular changes in the GABA system after chronic benzodiazepine treatment (see Section 4.2.2).

4.4. Other Mechanisms

4.4.1. Mechanism 4: Transcriptional and Neurotrophic Factors.
Although the hypothesis that downstream signaling events adjust in response to chronic exposure to benzodiazepines seems plausible, a surprising paucity of data exist in this field. It is tempting to speculate on the expression of diverse helper GABA$_A$ receptor-associated proteins (including GABARAP, BIG2, PRIP, gephyrin, and radixin) after long-term benzodiazepine use (Figure 2). In addition, changes in intracellularly located cAMP-response-element-binding protein (CREB) or calcium, vital in various second messenger systems, could be altered, and prolonged GABA concentrations in a neuronal culture have been shown to affect voltage-gated calcium channels [133]. However, until further studies provide additional proof for chronic benzodiazepine-induced downstream intracellular changes, the evidence that this process plays a role is inconclusive.

Neurotrophic proteins support neuronal survival, synaptic growth, and differentiation throughout the brain via tyrosine kinase receptors (Trk) and, with lower affinity, via p75 receptors (p75NTRs) [134]. Neurotrophic factors that have discovered so far include brain-derived neurotrophic factor (BDNF), neurotrophin-3 (NT-3) and neurotrophin-4 (NT-4), and nerve growth factor (NGF). Since they act as potent factors in regulating fast synaptic inhibition, adaptations leading to tolerance following chronic benzodiazepine treatment could in part be mediated via these neurotrophic factors. In support, BDNF (and NT-4) was found to acutely reduce postsynaptic GABA$_A$ receptor immunoreactivity via activation of TrkB receptors [135–139], even though one study reported an increase [140], and another study reports that chronic BDNF treatment potentiates GABAergic inhibition [141]. This reduced immunoreactivity was hypothesized to be caused by a reduction in GABA$_A$ receptor surface expression and was accompanied by reduced postsynaptic responses with the direct GABA$_A$ receptor agonist muscimol [142]. Mechanistically, BDNF-induced suppression of GABAergic signaling was hypothesized to stem from altered GABA$_A$ receptor composition, increased GABA$_A$ receptor

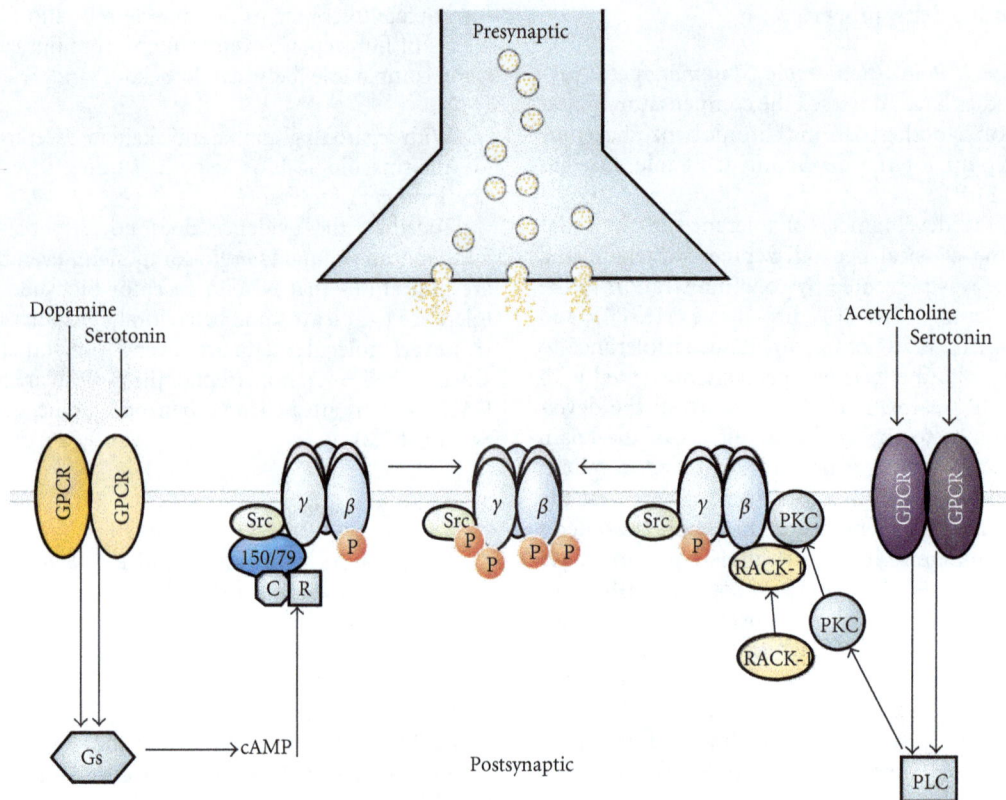

FIGURE 3: Functional crosstalk between G-protein coupled receptors (GPCRs) (which are present in the serotonin, dopamine, acetylcholine system) and $GABA_A$ receptors is facilitated through multiple protein kinases and scaffold proteins. $GABA_A$ receptor β and $\gamma2$ subunits are phosphorylated (P) by PKA and PKC upon the activation of individual GPCRs for dopamine and serotonin. PKA phosphorylation of $GABA_A$ receptor $\beta1$ and $\beta3$ subunits is dependent upon AKAP150/79, which directly interacts with these receptor subunits. AKAP150/79 also binds inactive PKA composed of regulatory (R) and catalytic (C) subunits. In addition, PKC phosphorylates the receptor $\beta1$–3 and $\gamma2$ subunits. Upon the activation of the appropriate GPCR, PKC-mediated phosphorylation is facilitated by the direct (but independent) interaction of the receptor for activated C kinase (RACK-1) and the β isoform of PKC with the $GABA_A$ receptor $\beta1$–3 subunits. RACK-1 facilitates functional regulation of $GABA_A$ receptors by controlling the activity of PKC associated with these proteins. The $GABA_A$ receptor $\gamma2$ subunit is also phosphorylated by Src, and this kinase is capable of binding to receptor β and $\gamma2$ subunits. Finally, the functional effects of phosphorylation are diverse and range from inhibitions to enhancements of $GABA_A$ receptor activity, dependent upon the receptor subunit composition. Reprinted by permission from Elsevier, reprinted from [95].

phosphorylation, decreased subunit synthesis, or increased postsynaptic receptor internalization or diffusion [139]. Interestingly, all these proposed mechanisms were already discussed in this paper. Thus, neurotrophin-induced changes may not be an independent mechanism, but be a player in a causal chain of events. Again, to our knowledge, no studies exist on the effects of chronic benzodiazepine treatment on neurotrophic expression and functionality.

4.4.2. Mechanism 5: Serotonin, Dopamine, Acetylcholine Systems. There is ample evidence that the serotonin, dopamine, and acetylcholine receptor systems can modulate the $GABA_A$ receptor functionality [143–146] (Figure 3). For example,

the receptor for activated C kinase (RACK-1) potentiated PKC-dependent phosphorylation of $GABA_A$ receptors mediated by the activation of muscarinic acetylcholine receptors [145], and serotonergic neurotransmission inhibited GABAergic signaling via $GABA_A$ receptor PKC-dependent phosphorylation, again with involvement of RACK-1 [144]. Altogether, these neurotransmitter systems act via G-protein-coupled receptors to activate protein kinases (PKA and PKC) and scaffold proteins that may subsequently modulate $GABA_A$ receptor β and $\gamma2$ subunit phosphorylation (Figure 3) [95].

However, studies investigating the role of the serotonin, dopamine, and acetylcholine system in response to chronic benzodiazepine treatment are scarce. Three weeks of diazepam treatment (25 mg/day) in healthy male volunteers resulted in tolerance to the prolactin and growth hormone response induced by the 5-HT precursor L-tryptophan, even though sedative effects of L-tryptophan remained present [147]. Another study showed that chronic diazepam treatment resulted not only in diazepam tolerance but also in a very modest reduced efficacy of the 5-HT$_{1A}$ receptor agonist 8-OH-DPAT to induce flat body posture and forepaw treading [148]. In contrast, only acute but not chronic diazepam treatment decreased basal extracellular dopamine levels in rats, even though both acute and chronic treatment regimens could reverse the stress-induced rise of cortical dopamine levels [149].

4.4.3. Mechanism 6: Neurosteroids. There is ample and convincing evidence that neurosteroids are endogenous allosteric regulators that interact with GABA$_A$ receptors to modulate both tonic (extrasynaptic) and phasic (synaptic) inhibition (for reviews, see [150, 151]). Also, acute or chronic neurosteroid treatment may change GABA$_A$ receptor subunit expression, especially extrasynaptic α_4 and δ subunits [151]. In light of the plasticity-inducing actions of neurosteroids on inhibitory signaling, long-term enhancement of the GABA system with benzodiazepines may in turn evoke changes in the neurosteroids system such as changes in neurosteroid synthesis and metabolism, although classical benzodiazepines may differ in their potency to cause such changes [152]. In support, ovariectomy attenuated the development of tolerance to the anticonvulsant actions of diazepam [153]. Moreover, co-administration of the neurosteroids allopregnanolone or pregnenolone (but not dehydroepiandrosterone) prevented the development of tolerance after chronic treatment with either triazolam and diazepam [154]. Adding to the complexity of the putative involvement of neurosteroids in benzodiazepine tolerance, factors such as GABA$_A$ receptor subunit composition, phosphorylation mechanisms, and ((extra)synaptic) localization—which are all factors that were already found to be involved in tolerance development—influence the specific dynamics of neurosteroid activity.

4.4.4. Conclusion. From our review of the literature on the various mechanisms that may underlie benzodiazepine tolerance, it occurs that there is a considerable variance in the published data. The heterogeneity of the data lies in the application of different methodologies, species, treatment regimens, and benzodiazepines. Specifically, we have considered classical benzodiazepines as a homogenous drug class since they all lead to a nonspecific enhancement of GABA$_A$ receptors that contain an α_1, α_2, α_3, or α_5 subunit. However, *in vivo* pharmacodynamic potency and pharmacokinetic half-life differences could greatly impact on tolerance processes [7]. In support, subchronic treatment with different classical benzodiazepines lead to differential propensity for FG7142-induced seizures in mice, with triazolam, clonazepam, and diazepam producing around seizures in around 80% of the mice, whereas alprazolam and midazolam did so in 60% of the animals and lorazepam

in 40% of the animals [155]. Surprisingly, chlordiazepoxide did not lead to any precipitated seizures, even though a comparable GABA$_A$ receptor occupancy was obtained. Therefore, the assumption that classical benzodiazepines act as a homogeneous class probably complicates the interpretation of the current literature.

Altogether, it appears that none of the proposed putative mechanisms can sufficiently explain tolerance development. Thus, multiple mechanisms may (synergistically) coexist, or an additional yet undiscovered mechanism may be present. However, the complex and adaptive nature of the GABA system and the existing heterogeneous literature on benzodiazepine tolerance suggest that one unifying tolerance mechanism may be a vast oversimplification. In any case, the proposed tolerance mechanisms are not completely independent, exemplified by the fact that neurotrophic factors and neurosteroids are influenced by GABA$_A$ receptor composition and phosphorylation status, which are themselves proposed to be involved in benzodiazepine tolerance. Unfortunately, the present literature does not consistently support a clear recommendation in terms of a pharmacological GABA$_A$ receptor profile (e.g., subunit preference) to aid in the development of novel and more selective benzodiazepines that lack tolerance development and are suitable for long-term treatment.

5. Tolerance to Novel Subtype-Selective Benzodiazepines

Here, we will review the evidence for tolerance development with novel GABA$_A$ receptor subtype selective compounds that provide the direct opportunity to evaluate their roles in tolerance. With the development of subunit-selective benzodiazepines, it has become possible to dissect the different effects of classical benzodiazepines (see Section 2.2 and Table 2). However, declining efficacy over time is a complex process which may not be easily attributed to one specific α subunit. Still, if novel drugs possess reduced propensity to lead to tolerance development, this will be greatly welcomed from a clinical perspective. Continuing efficacy with these drugs would advance the clinical use of drugs acting at the GABA$_A$ receptor benzodiazepine site. Unfortunately, not many studies have directly addressed tolerance development using these novel compounds. Recent data from our laboratory suggest that no tolerance develops to the acute hypothermic, anxiolytic, or sedative effect of diazepam in mice treated for 28 days with the GABA$_A$-α_2/α_3 selective compound TPA023 (Table 2) [156], indicating that chronic activation of GABA$_A$-α_2/α_3 receptors does not lead to anxiolytic tolerance after acute diazepam challenge (unpublished data). Also, in contrast to morphine, no analgesic tolerance occurred in rats after a 9-day treatment with the $\alpha_{2/3}$ subtype GABA$_A$ receptor positive allosteric modulator L838,417 using a model of neuropathic pain [157]. From these data, it seems that tolerance development after chronic administration of GABA$_A$-α_2/α_3 subtype selective drugs may not develop, or, alternatively, that tolerance to diazepam's sedative actions needs concomitant activation of GABA$_A$-α_1/GABA$_A$-α_5 receptors. In support of the latter hypothesis, ligands that do not bind to the α_5 subunit such as zolpidem have a reduced tendency to engender tolerance [158, 159], supported by studies in which chronic treatment with zolpidem (but not midazolam) did not produce any tolerance to sedative and anticonvulsant effects in mice and rats [160–162].

In addition to studies directly assessing tolerance, several studies have investigated the precipitated withdrawal after (sub) chronic treatment with subtype-selective compounds. Compounds with selective efficacy at α_2, α_3, and α_5 GABA$_A$ receptor subtypes were shown to lead to differential seizures susceptibility in mice in response to the inverse agonist FG-7142 [155]. Chronic treatment with zolpidem, as well as the selective compounds L-838,417 (partial agonist at $\alpha2$ GABA$_A$, $\alpha3$GABA$_A$, and $\alpha5$GABA$_A$ receptors) and SL651498 (full agonist at $\alpha2$GABA$_A$ and $\alpha3$GABA$_A$ receptors, partial agonist at $\alpha1$GABA$_A$ and $\alpha5$GABA$_A$ receptors), did not result in seizures following FG-7142 administration [31, 155] (Table 2). Similarly, chronic treatment with TPA023 (partial agonist at $\alpha2$GABA$_A$, $\alpha3$GABA$_A$, and $\alpha5$GABA$_A$ receptors) also did not result in FG-7142-induced seizures in mice [156]. However, because these studies do not specifically address tolerance development, the rather general conclusion from these studies is that partial or selective modulation of the GABA$_A$ receptor results in a reduced liability for physical dependence. Thus, it is important to note that, even though zolpidem does not seem to engender any obvious tolerance development, zolpidem can lead to withdrawal symptoms that are comparable to those seen after chronic classical benzodiazepine treatment [29, 77]. Thus, tolerance and withdrawal symptoms may constitute separate entities in benzodiazepine dependence. In support, one study demonstrated that marked withdrawal symptoms appeared upon abrupt discontinuation of chronic clorazepate treatment in dogs, even though tolerance was present to a rather limited extent [163].

Together, it can be concluded that so far, α_2/α_3 subtype selective compounds have neither been found to lead to tolerance nor withdrawal symptoms. This would constitute a significant improvement over currently used benzodiazepines, even though the anxiolytic profile of these compounds remains to be determined [164], and abuse liability may still be present [8]. However, interpretations should be made with caution since chronic treatment with nonselective partial positive allosteric modulators such as bretazenil did neither result in anticonvulsant tolerance [54, 59, 60] nor in FG-7142-precipitated seizures [155]. These studies implicate that the potency of classical and subtype-selective compounds, in addition to or despite subtype selectivity, may also be of importance in the development of tolerance. It could be also hypothesized that low efficacy at the α_1 subunit, rather than selectivity or reduced efficacy at α_2/α_3 subtypes, may be the causal mechanism preventing tolerance development. Also, the clinical anxiolytic efficacy of α_2/α_3 subtype selective compounds has not yet been established. In addition to a specific efficacy profile, tolerance development may also depend on a compound's *affinity* at certain GABA$_A$ receptor subtypes. This way, tolerance processes may be different with affinity-selective compounds

such as zolpidem compared to efficacy-selective compounds such as TPA023. Circumstantial evidence stems from the fact that α_1-preferential affinity-selective compounds such as zolpidem produce physical dependence [165], even though the compound TPA123 that possesses 23% efficacy at the α_1 subunit (but is not affinity selective) did also result in physical dependence [8]. However, based on the currently available evidence, no definite conclusions can be drawn regarding the subtype involved in tolerance. Also, it is not possible to distinguish tolerance processes in selective binding (affinity) and selective activation (efficacy).

6. Conclusion

In the present paper, we summarized the rather inconsistent data regarding changes in several neurotransmitter systems to explain the development of tolerance. Specifically, we addressed possible changes at the level of (i) the GABA$_A$ receptor (subunit expression and receptor coupling), (ii) intracellular changes stemming from transcriptional and neurotrophic factors, (iii) ionotropic glutamate receptors, (iv) other neurotransmitters (serotonin, dopamine, and acetylcholine systems), and (v) the neurosteroid system. From the large variance in the studies, it appears that either different (simultaneous) tolerance mechanisms occur depending on the benzodiazepine effect, or that one tolerance-inducing mechanism depends on the activated GABA$_A$ receptor subtypes. This is not unlikely, given that tolerance is a heterogeneous process that occurs at different rates for the various effects and also depends on the profile of the (subtype selective) benzodiazepine. Adaptations could then occur on different time scales depending on the receptor subtype and brain region involved. In line with this hypothesis, tolerance develops relatively quickly for the sedative and anticonvulsant actions of benzodiazepines, whereas tolerance to anxiolytic and amnesic effects most probably do not develop at all. It is intriguing that anxiolytic effects of classical benzodiazepines may not decline during prolonged treatment. In addition to subtype selectivity, additional factors may be important for a (subtype-selective) benzodiazepine to cause tolerance, including GABA$_A$ receptor potency (efficacy) and *in vivo* receptor occupancy over time. The finding that partial agonists with an overall but comparable lower efficacy at all α subunits of the GABA$_A$ receptor such as bretazenil did not result in anticonvulsant tolerance raises the possibility that chronic clinical use of these compounds is associated with a lower tolerance.

An important question is how the development of tolerance of benzodiazepines could be reduced. One interesting suggestion could be—rather than intermittent use that can be defined by an individual—to develop benzodiazepine dosing schedules with varying daily doses including placebos. This could result in continued clinical efficacy (obviously depending on the indication) and utilize the placebo effect. The other possibility to reduce tolerance is the currently developing and promising body of literature on subtype-selective GABA$_A$ receptor PAMs. From the literature we reviewed, it appears that α_2/α_3 subtype selective compounds do not lead to tolerance or withdrawal symptoms. However, the underlying mechanism (reduced α_1 efficacy or a generally reduced efficacy profile) is unknown. Also, it is presently unclear whether this lack of tolerance also applies to α_1- and α_5-selective GABAergic positive allosteric modulators, although a broad and unspecific tolerance resulting from selective (and often low potency) compounds seems unlikely.

In conclusion, the development of tolerance following chronic benzodiazepine treatment is a complex process in which multiple processes may simultaneously act to cause varying rates of tolerance depending on the studied effect and the administered drug. There is no convincing evidence that subtype-selective compounds acting at the benzodiazepine site lead to tolerance at a level comparable to classical benzodiazepines. If this is indeed the case, one consequence may be that such subtype-selective compounds are unlikely to engender clinical tolerance, which would be a clinically significant improvement over classical benzodiazepines.

References

[1] M. Lader, "History of benzodiazepine dependence," *Journal of Substance Abuse Treatment*, vol. 8, no. 1-2, pp. 53–59, 1991.

[2] R. T. Owen and P. Tyrer, "Benzodiazepine dependence. A review of the evidence," *Drugs*, vol. 25, no. 4, pp. 385–398, 1983.

[3] American Psychiatric Association, *Diagnostic and Statistical Manual of Mental Disorders: DSM-IV-TR*, 2000.

[4] H. Petursson, "The benzodiazepine withdrawal syndrome," *Addiction*, vol. 89, no. 11, pp. 1455–1459, 1994.

[5] C. Allison and J. A. Pratt, "Neuroadaptive processes in GABAergic and glutamatergic systems in benzodiazepine dependence," *Pharmacology and Therapeutics*, vol. 98, no. 2, pp. 171–195, 2003.

[6] J. A. Pratt, R. R. Brett, and D. J. Laurie, "Benzodiazepine dependence: from neural circuits to gene expression," *Pharmacology Biochemistry and Behavior*, vol. 59, no. 4, pp. 925–934, 1998.

[7] J. H. Woods, J. L. Katz, and G. Winger, "Benzodiazepines: use, abuse, and consequences," *Pharmacological Reviews*, vol. 44, no. 2, pp. 151–347, 1992.

[8] N. A. Ator, J. R. Atack, R. J. Hargreaves, H. D. Burns, and G. R. Dawson, "Reducing abuse liability of GABAA/benzodiazepine ligands via selective partial agonist efficacy at α_1 and $\alpha_{2/3}$ subtypes," *Journal of Pharmacology and Experimental Therapeutics*, vol. 332, no. 1, pp. 4–16, 2010.

[9] S. C. Licata and J. K. Rowlett, "Abuse and dependence liability of benzodiazepine-type drugs: GABAA receptor modulation and beyond," *Pharmacology Biochemistry and Behavior*, vol. 90, no. 1, pp. 74–89, 2008.

[10] K. R. Tan, M. Brown, G. Labouébe et al., "Neural bases for addictive properties of benzodiazepines," *Nature*, vol. 463, no. 7282, pp. 769–774, 2010.

[11] K. A. Wafford, "GABAA receptor subtypes: any clues to the mechanism of benzodiazepine dependence?" *Current Opinion in Pharmacology*, vol. 5, no. 1, pp. 47–52, 2005.

[12] J. H. Krystal, J. Staley, G. Mason et al., "γ-aminobutyric acid type A receptors and alcoholism: intoxication, dependence, vulnerability, and treatment," *Archives of General Psychiatry*, vol. 63, no. 9, pp. 957–968, 2006.

[13] U. Rudolph and H. Mohler, "GABA-based therapeutic approaches: GABAA receptor subtype functions," *Current Opinion in Pharmacology*, vol. 6, no. 1, pp. 18–23, 2006.

[14] R. M. McKernan and P. J. Whiting, "Which GABAA-receptor subtypes really occur in the brain?" *Trends in Neurosciences*, vol. 19, no. 4, pp. 139–143, 1996.

[15] W. Sieghart, "Structure and pharmacology of γ-aminobutyric acidA receptor subtypes," *Pharmacological Reviews*, vol. 47, no. 2, pp. 181–234, 1995.

[16] W. Sieghart and G. Sperk, "Subunit composition, distribution and function of GABAA receptor subtypes," *Current Topics in Medicinal Chemistry*, vol. 2, no. 8, pp. 795–816, 2002.

[17] S. R. Cobb, E. H. Buhl, K. Halasy, O. Paulsen, and P. Somogyl, "Synchronization of neuronal activity in hippocampus by individual GABAergic interneurons," *Nature*, vol. 378, no. 6552, pp. 75–78, 1995.

[18] D. A. Lewis, R. Y. Cho, C. S. Carter et al., "Subunit-selective modulation of GABA type A receptor neurotransmission and cognition in schizophrenia," *American Journal of Psychiatry*, vol. 165, no. 12, pp. 1585–1593, 2008.

[19] H. Mohler, J. M. Fritschy, and U. Rudolph, "A new benzodiazepine pharmacology," *Journal of Pharmacology and Experimental Therapeutics*, vol. 300, no. 1, pp. 2–8, 2002.

[20] D. Belelli, N. L. Harrison, J. Maguire, R. L. Macdonald, M. C. Walker, and D. W. Cope, "Extrasynaptic GABAA receptors: form, pharmacology, and function," *Journal of Neuroscience*, vol. 29, no. 41, pp. 12757–12763, 2009.

[21] D. R. Serwanski, C. P. Miralles, S. B. Christie, A. K. Mehta, X. Li, and A. L. De Blas, "Synaptic and nonsynaptic localization of GABAA receptors containing the $\alpha5$ subunit in the rat brain," *Journal of Comparative Neurology*, vol. 499, no. 3, pp. 458–470, 2006.

[22] U. Rudolph, F. Crestani, D. Benke et al., "Benzodiazepine actions mediated by specific γ-aminobutyric acidA receptor subtypes," *Nature*, vol. 401, no. 6755, pp. 796–800, 1999.

[23] R. M. McKernan, T. W. Rosahl, D. S. Reynolds et al., "Sedative but not anxiolytic properties of benzodiazepines are mediated by the GABAA receptor $\alpha1$ subtype," *Nature Neuroscience*, vol. 3, no. 6, pp. 587–592, 2000.

[24] J. R. Atack, "GABAA receptor subtype-selective modulators. I. alpha2/alpha3-selective agonists as non-sedating anxiolytics," *Current Topics in Medicinal Chemistry*, vol. 2, pp. 331–360, 2010.

[25] N. Collinson, F. M. Kuenzi, W. Jarolimek et al., "Enhanced learning and memory and altered GABAergic synaptic transmission in mice lacking the $\alpha5$ subunit of the GABAA receptor," *Journal of Neuroscience*, vol. 22, no. 13, pp. 5572–5580, 2002.

[26] G. R. Dawson, K. A. Maubach, N. Collinson et al., "An inverse agonist selective for $\alpha5$ subunit-containing GABAA receptors enhances cognition," *Journal of Pharmacology and Experimental Therapeutics*, vol. 316, no. 3, pp. 1335–1345, 2006.

[27] C. van Rijnsoever, M. Täuber, M. K. Choulli et al., "Requirement of $\alpha5$-GABAA receptors for the development of tolerance to the sedative action of diazepam in mice," *Journal of Neuroscience*, vol. 24, no. 30, pp. 6785–6790, 2004.

[28] N. A. Ator, "Contributions of GABAA receptor subtype selectivity to abuse liability and dependence potential of pharmacological treatments for anxiety and sleep disorders," *CNS Spectrums*, vol. 10, no. 1, pp. 31–39, 2005.

[29] R. R. Griffiths, C. A. Sannerud, N. A. Ator, and J. V. Brady, "Zolpidem behavioral pharmacology in baboons: self-injection, discrimination, tolerance and withdrawal," *Journal of Pharmacology and Experimental Therapeutics*, vol. 260, no. 3, pp. 1199–1208, 1992.

[30] J. K. Rowlett, D. M. Platt, S. Lelas, J. R. Atack, and G. R. Dawson, "Different GABA$_A$ receptor subtypes mediate the anxiolytic, abuse-related, and motor effects of benzodiazepine-like drugs in primates," *Proceedings of the National Academy of Sciences of the United States of America*, vol. 102, no. 3, pp. 915–920, 2005.

[31] G. Griebel, G. Perrault, J. Simiand et al., "SL651498: an anxioselective compound with functional selectivity for alpha2- and alpha3-containing gamma-aminobutyric acid$_A$ GABA$_A$ receptors," *Journal of Pharmacology and Experimental Therapeutics*, vol. 298, no. 2, pp. 753–768, 2001.

[32] F. M. Benes, M. S. Todtenkopf, P. Logiotatos, and M. Williams, "Glutamate decarboxylase(65)-immunoreactive terminals in cingulate and prefrontal cortices of schizophrenic and bipolar brain," *Journal of Chemical Neuroanatomy*, vol. 20, no. 3-4, pp. 259–269, 2000.

[33] A. Schousboe, A. Sarup, O. M. Larsson, and H. S. White, "GABA transporters as drug targets for modulation of GABAergic activity," *Biochemical Pharmacology*, vol. 68, no. 8, pp. 1557–1563, 2004.

[34] A. N. Bateson, "Basic pharmacologic mechanisms involved in benzodiazepine tolerance and withdrawal," *Current Pharmaceutical Design*, vol. 8, no. 1, pp. 5–21, 2002.

[35] S. E. File, "Tolerance to the behavioral actions of benzodiazepines," *Neuroscience and Biobehavioral Reviews*, vol. 9, no. 1, pp. 113–121, 1985.

[36] S. E. File, "The history of benzodiazepine dependence: a review of animal studies," *Neuroscience and Biobehavioral Reviews*, vol. 14, no. 2, pp. 135–146, 1990.

[37] D. Schneider-Helmert, "Why low-dose benzodiazepine-dependent insomniacs can't escape their sleeping pills," *Acta Psychiatrica Scandinavica*, vol. 78, no. 6, pp. 706–711, 1988.

[38] I. Lucki and K. Rickels, "The behavioral effects of benzodiazepines following long-term use," *Psychopharmacology Bulletin*, vol. 22, no. 2, pp. 424–433, 1986.

[39] I. Lucki, K. Rickels, and A. M. Geller, "Chronic use of benzodiazepines and psychomotor and cognitive test performance," *Psychopharmacology*, vol. 88, no. 4, pp. 426–433, 1986.

[40] D. S. Cowley, P. P. Roy-Byrne, A. Radant et al., "Benzodiazepine sensitivity in panic disorder: effects of chronic alprazolam treatment," *Neuropsychopharmacology*, vol. 12, no. 2, pp. 147–157, 1995.

[41] D. Allen, H. V. Curran, and M. Lader, "The effects of repeated doses of clomipramine and alprazolam on physiological, psychomotor and cognitive functions in normal subjects," *European Journal of Clinical Pharmacology*, vol. 40, no. 4, pp. 355–362, 1991.

[42] A. Kales, M. B. Scharf, and J. D. Kales, "Rebound insomnia: a new clinical syndrome," *Science*, vol. 201, no. 4360, pp. 1039–1041, 1978.

[43] A. Kales, C. R. Soldatos, E. O. Bixler, and J. D. Kales, "Early morning insomnia with rapidly eliminated benzodiazepines," *Science*, vol. 220, no. 4592, pp. 95–97, 1983.

[44] V. Pegram, P. Hyde, and P. Linton, "Chronic use of triazolam: the effects on the sleep patterns of insomniacs," *Journal of International Medical Research*, vol. 8, no. 3, pp. 224–231, 1980.

[45] T. Roth, M. Kramer, and T. Lutz, "Intermediate use of triazolam: a sleep laboratory study," *Journal of International Medical Research*, vol. 4, no. 1, pp. 59–63, 1976.

[46] M. M. Mitler, M. A. Carskadon, R. L. Phillips et al., "Hypnotic efficacy of temazepam: a long-term sleep laboratory evaluation," *British Journal of Clinical Pharmacology*, vol. 8, no. 1, pp. 63S–68S, 1979.

[47] A. Kales and J. D. Kales, "Sleep laboratory studies of hypnotic drugs: efficacy and withdrawal effects," *Journal of Clinical Psychopharmacology*, vol. 3, no. 2, pp. 140–150, 1983.

[48] C. R. Soldatos, D. G. Dikeos, and A. Whitehead, "Tolerance and rebound insomnia with rapidly eliminated hypnotics: a meta-analysis of sleep laboratory studies," *International Clinical Psychopharmacology*, vol. 14, no. 5, pp. 287–303, 1999.

[49] M. Monane, R. J. Glynn, and J. Avorn, "The impact of sedative-hypnotic use on sleep symptoms in elderly nursing home residents," *Clinical Pharmacology and Therapeutics*, vol. 59, no. 1, pp. 83–92, 1996.

[50] H. V. Curran, R. Collins, S. Fletcher, S. C. Y. Kee, B. Woods, and S. Iliffe, "Older adults and withdrawal from benzodiazepine hypnotics in general practice: effects on cognitive function, sleep, mood and quality of life," *Psychological Medicine*, vol. 33, no. 7, pp. 1223–1237, 2003.

[51] D. Poyares, C. Guilleminault, M. M. Ohayon, and S. Tufik, "Chronic benzodiazepine usage and withdrawal in insomnia patients," *Journal of Psychiatric Research*, vol. 38, no. 3, pp. 327–334, 2004.

[52] T. R. Browne and J. K. Penry, "Benzodiazepines in the treatment of epilepsy: a review," *Epilepsia*, vol. 14, no. 3, pp. 277–310, 1973.

[53] W. Loscher, C. Rundfeldt, D. Honack, and U. Ebert, "Long-term studies on anticonvulsant tolerance and withdrawal characteristics of benzodiazepine receptor ligands in different seizure models in mice. I. Comparison of diazepam, clonazepam, clobazam and abecarnil," *Journal of Pharmacology and Experimental Therapeutics*, vol. 279, no. 2, pp. 561–572, 1996.

[54] C. Rundfeldt, P. Wlaz, D. Honack, and W. Loscher, "Anticonvulsant tolerance and withdrawal characteristics of benzodiazepine receptor ligands in different seizure models in mice. Comparison of diazepam, Bretazenil and Abecarnil," *Journal of Pharmacology and Experimental Therapeutics*, vol. 275, no. 2, pp. 693–702, 1995.

[55] S. F. Gonsalves and D. W. Gallager, "Time course for development of anticonvulsant tolerance and GABAergic subsensitivity after chronic diazepam," *Brain Research*, vol. 405, no. 1, pp. 94–99, 1987.

[56] D. Ko, J. M. Rho, C. M. DeGiorgio, and S. Sato, "Benzodiazpines," in *Epilepsy: A Comprehensive Textbook*, J. J. Engel and T. A. Pedley, Eds., pp. 1475–1489, Lippincott-Raven, Philadelphia, Pa, USA, 1997.

[57] M. J. Brodie, "Established anticonvulsants and treatment of refractory epilepsy," *The Lancet*, vol. 336, no. 8711, pp. 350–354, 1990.

[58] S. E. File and L. Wilks, "Effects of acute and chronic treatment on the pro- and anti-convulsant actions of CL 218, 872, PK 8165 and PK 9084, putative ligands for the benzodiazepine receptor," *Journal of Pharmacy and Pharmacology*, vol. 37, no. 4, pp. 252–256, 1985.

[59] M. Feely, P. Boyland, A. Picardo, A. Cox, and J. P. Gent, "Lack of anticonvulsant tolerance with RU 32698 and Ro 17-1812," *European Journal of Pharmacology*, vol. 164, no. 2, pp. 377–380, 1989.

[60] W. Loscher, C. Rundfeldt, D. Honack, and U. Ebert, "Long-term studies on anticonvulsant tolerance and withdrawal characteristics of benzodiazepine receptor ligands in different seizure models in mice. II. The novel imidazoquinazolines NNC 14-0185 and NNC 14-0189," *Journal of Pharmacology*

and Experimental Therapeutics, vol. 279, no. 2, pp. 573–581, 1996.

[61] H. V. Curran, A. Bond, G. O'Sullivan et al., "Memory functions, alprazolam and exposure therapy: a controlled longitudinal study of agoraphobia with panic disorder," *Psychological Medicine*, vol. 24, no. 4, pp. 969–976, 1994.

[62] P. R. Tata, J. Rollings, M. Collins, A. Pickering, and R. R. Jacobson, "Lack of cognitive recovery following withdrawal from long-term benzodiazepine use," *Psychological Medicine*, vol. 24, no. 1, pp. 203–213, 1994.

[63] M. J. Barker, K. M. Greenwood, M. Jackson, and S. F. Crowe, "Persistence of cognitive effects after withdrawal from long-term benzodiazepine use: a meta-analysis," *Archives of Clinical Neuropsychology*, vol. 19, no. 3, pp. 437–454, 2004.

[64] K. Tsunoda, H. Uchida, T. Suzuki, K. Watanabe, T. Yamashima, and H. Kashima, "Effects of discontinuing benzodiazepine-derivative hypnotics on postural sway and cognitive functions in the elderly," *International Journal of Geriatric Psychiatry*, vol. 25, no. 12, pp. 1259–1265, 2010.

[65] U. Tonne, A. J. Hiltunen, B. Vikander et al., "Neuropsychological changes during steady-state drug use, withdrawal and abstinence in primary benzodiazepine-dependent patients," *Acta Psychiatrica Scandinavica*, vol. 91, no. 5, pp. 299–304, 1995.

[66] K. Rickels, I. Lucki, E. Schweizer, F. García-España, and W. G. Case, "Psychomotor performance of long-term benzodiazepine users before, during, and after benzodiazepine discontinuation," *Journal of Clinical Psychopharmacology*, vol. 19, no. 2, pp. 107–113, 1999.

[67] E. Schweizer, K. Rickels, S. Weiss, and S. Zavodnick, "Maintenance drug treatment of panic disorder: I. Results of a prospective, placebo-controlled comparison of alprazolam and imipramine," *Archives of General Psychiatry*, vol. 50, no. 1, pp. 51–60, 1993.

[68] K. Rickels, G. Case, R. W. Downing, and A. Winokur, "Long-term diazepam therapy and clinical outcome," *The Journal of the American Medical Association*, vol. 250, no. 6, pp. 767–771, 1983.

[69] D. S. Charney and S. W. Woods, "Benzodiazepine treatment of panic disorder: a comparison of alprazolam and lorazepam," *Journal of Clinical Psychiatry*, vol. 50, no. 11, pp. 418–423, 1989.

[70] J. C. Ballenger, "Long-term pharmacologic treatment of panic disorder," *Journal of Clinical Psychiatry*, vol. 52, no. 2, supplement, pp. 18–23, 1991.

[71] G. D. Burrows, F. K. Judd, and T. R. Norman, "Long-term drug treatment of panic disorder," *Journal of Psychiatric Research*, vol. 27, supplement 1, pp. 111–125, 1993.

[72] M. H. Pollack, G. E. Tesar, J. F. Rosenbaum, and S. A. Spier, "Clonazepam in the treatment of panic disorder and agoraphobia: a one-year follow-up," *Journal of Clinical Psychopharmacology*, vol. 6, no. 5, pp. 302–304, 1986.

[73] J. B. Cohn and C. S. Wilcox, "Long-term comparison of alprazolam, lorazepam and placebo in patients with an anxiety disorder," *Pharmacotherapy*, vol. 4, no. 2, pp. 93–98, 1984.

[74] S. M. Sutherland, L. A. Tupler, J. T. Colket, and J. R. T. Davidson, "A 2-year follow-up of social phobia: status after a brief medication trial," *Journal of Nervous and Mental Disease*, vol. 184, no. 12, pp. 731–738, 1996.

[75] J. R. T. Davidson, S. M. Ford, R. D. Smith, and N. L. S. Potts, "Long-term treatment of social phobia with clonazepam," *Journal of Clinical Psychiatry*, vol. 52, no. 11, supplement, pp. 16–20, 1991.

[76] M. W. Otto, M. H. Pollack, R. A. Gould et al., "A comparison of the efficacy of clonazepam and cognitive-behavioral group therapy for the treatment of social phobia," *Journal of Anxiety Disorders*, vol. 14, no. 4, pp. 345–358, 2000.

[77] R. R. Griffiths and E. M. Weerts, "Benzodiazepine self-administration in humans and laboratory animals—implications for problems of long-term use and abuse," *Psychopharmacology*, vol. 134, no. 1, pp. 1–37, 1997.

[78] E. M. Weerts and R. R. Griffiths, "Zolpidem self-injection with concurrent physical dependence under conditions of long-term continuous availability in baboons," *Behavioural Pharmacology*, vol. 9, no. 3, pp. 285–297, 1998.

[79] E. M. Weerts, B. J. Kaminski, and R. R. Griffiths, "Stable low-rate midazolam self-injection with concurrent physical dependence under conditions of long-term continuous availability in baboons," *Psychopharmacology*, vol. 135, no. 1, pp. 70–81, 1998.

[80] S. B. Soumerai, L. Simoni-Wastila, C. Singer et al., "Lack of relationship between long-term use of benzodiazepines and escalation to high dosages," *Psychiatric Services*, vol. 54, no. 7, pp. 1006–1011, 2003.

[81] C. Fernandes, S. E. File, and D. Berry, "Evidence against oppositional and pharmacokinetic mechanisms of tolerance to diazepam's sedative effects," *Brain Research*, vol. 734, no. 1-2, pp. 236–242, 1996.

[82] L. K. Friedman, T. T. Gibbs, and D. H. Farb, "γ-aminobutyric acid$_A$ receptor regulation: heterologous uncoupling of modulatory site interactions induced by chronic steroid, barbiturate, benzodiazepine, or GABA treatment in culture," *Brain Research*, vol. 707, no. 1, pp. 100–109, 1996.

[83] D. W. Gallager, J. M. Lakoski, and S. F. S. L. Gonsalves Rauch, "Chronic benzodiazepine treatment decreases postsynaptic GABA sensitivity," *Nature*, vol. 308, no. 5954, pp. 74–77, 1984.

[84] G. Wong, T. Lyon, and P. Skolnick, "Chronic exposure to benzodiazepine receptor ligands uncouples the γ—aminobutyric acid type A receptor in WSS-1 cells," *Molecular Pharmacology*, vol. 46, no. 6, pp. 1056–1062, 1994.

[85] E. I. Tietz, T. H. Chiu, and H. C. Rosenberg, "Regional GABA/benzodiazepine receptor/chloride channel coupling after acute and chronic benzodiazepine treatment," *European Journal of Pharmacology*, vol. 167, no. 1, pp. 57–65, 1989.

[86] R. J. Primus, J. Yu, J. Xu et al., "Allosteric uncoupling after chronic benzodiazepine exposure of recombinant γ-aminobutyric acid$_A$ receptors expressed in Sf9 cells: ligand efficacy and subtype selectivity," *Journal of Pharmacology and Experimental Therapeutics*, vol. 276, no. 3, pp. 882–890, 1996.

[87] D. Pericic, D. S. Strac, M. J. Jembrek, and J. Vlainic, "Allosteric uncoupling and up-regulation of benzodiazepine and GABA recognition sites following chronic diazepam treatment of HEK 293 cells stably transfected with $\alpha 1\beta 2\gamma 2S$ subunits of GABA$_A$ receptors," *Naunyn-Schmiedeberg's Archives of Pharmacology*, vol. 375, no. 3, pp. 177–187, 2007.

[88] R. L. Klein and R. A. Harris, "Regulation of GABA$_A$ receptor structure and function by chronic drug treatments in vivo and with stably transfected cells," *Japanese Journal of Pharmacology*, vol. 70, no. 1, pp. 1–15, 1996.

[89] R. L. Klein, M. P. Mascia, P. C. Harkness, K. L. Hadingham, P. J. Whiting, and R. A. Harris, "Regulation of allosteric coupling and function of stably expressed γ-aminobutyric acid GABA$_A$ receptors by chronic treatment with GABA$_A$ and benzodiazepine agonists," *Journal of Pharmacology and Experimental Therapeutics*, vol. 274, no. 3, pp. 1484–1492, 1995.

[90] N. J. Ali and R. W. Olsen, "Chronic benzodiazepine treatment of cells expressing recombinant GABA$_A$ receptors uncouples allosteric binding: studies on possible mechanisms," *Journal of Neurochemistry*, vol. 79, no. 5, pp. 1100–1108, 2001.

[91] V. Itier, P. Granger, G. Perrault, H. Depoortere, B. Scatton, and P. Avenet, "Protracted treatment with diazepam reduces benzodiazepine1 receptor-mediated potentiation of gamma-aminobutyric acid-induced currents in dissociated rat hippocampal neurons," *Journal of Pharmacology and Experimental Therapeutics*, vol. 279, no. 3, pp. 1092–1099, 1996.

[92] C. Heninger and D. W. Gallager, "Altered γ-aminobutyric acid/benzodiazepine interaction after chronic diazepam exposure," *Neuropharmacology*, vol. 27, no. 10, pp. 1073–1076, 1988.

[93] R. R. Brett and J. A. Pratt, "Changes in benzodiazepine-GABA receptor coupling in an accumbens-habenula circuit after chronic diazepam treatment," *British Journal of Pharmacology*, vol. 116, no. 5, pp. 2375–2384, 1995.

[94] D. J. Roca, I. Rozenberg, M. Farrant, and D. H. Farb, "Chronic agonist exposure induces down-regulation and allosteric uncoupling of the γ-aminobutyric acid/benzodiazepine receptor complex," *Molecular Pharmacology*, vol. 37, no. 1, pp. 37–43, 1990.

[95] J. T. Kittler and S. J. Moss, "Modulation of GABA$_A$ receptor activity by phosphorylation and receptor trafficking: implications for the efficacy of synaptic inhibition," *Current Opinion in Neurobiology*, vol. 13, no. 3, pp. 341–347, 2003.

[96] P. Poisbeau, M. C. Cheney, M. D. Browning, and I. Mody, "Modulation of synaptic GABA$_A$ receptor function by PKA and PKC in adult hippocampal neurons," *Journal of Neuroscience*, vol. 19, no. 2, pp. 674–683, 1999.

[97] S. M. Lilly, X. J. Zeng, and E. I. Tietz, "Role of protein kinase A in GABA$_A$ receptor dysfunction in CA1 pyramidal cells following chronic benzodiazepine treatment," *Journal of Neurochemistry*, vol. 85, no. 4, pp. 988–998, 2003.

[98] L. Huopaniemi,, R. Keist, A. Randolph, U. Certa, and U. Rudolph, "Diazepam-induced adaptive plasticity revealed by alpha1 GABA$_A$ receptor-specific expression profiling," *Journal of Neurochemistry*, vol. 88, no. 5, pp. 1059–1067, 2004.

[99] D. Mierlak and D. H. Farb, "Modulation of neurotransmitter receptor desensitization chlordiazepoxide stimulates fading of the GABA response," *Journal of Neuroscience*, vol. 8, no. 3, pp. 814–820, 1988.

[100] T. C. Jacob, S. J. Moss, and R. Jurd, "GABA$_A$ receptor trafficking and its role in the dynamic modulation of neuronal inhibition," *Nature Reviews Neuroscience*, vol. 9, no. 5, pp. 331–343, 2008.

[101] I. L. Arancibia-Cárcamo and J. T. Kittler, "Regulation of GABA$_A$ receptor membrane trafficking and synaptic localization," *Pharmacology and Therapeutics*, vol. 123, no. 1, pp. 17–31, 2009.

[102] M. Uusi-Oukari and E. R. Korpi, "Regulation of GABA$_A$ receptor subunit expression by pharmacological agents," *Pharmacological Reviews*, vol. 62, no. 1, pp. 97–135, 2010.

[103] M. I. Arnot, M. Davies, I. L. Martin, and A. N. Bateson, "GABA$_A$ receptor gene expression in rat cortex: differential effects of two chronic diazepam treatment regimes," *Journal of Neuroscience Research*, vol. 64, no. 6, pp. 617–625, 2001.

[104] H. J. Little, D. J. Nutt, and S. C. Taylor, "Bidirectional effects of chronic treatment with agonists and inverse agonists at the benzodiazepine receptor," *Brain Research Bulletin*, vol. 19, no. 3, pp. 371–378, 1987.

[105] M. H. Tehrani and E. M. Barnes Jr., "Sequestration of gamma-aminobutyric acid$_A$ receptors on clathrin-coated vesicles during chronic benzodiazepine administration *in vivo*," *Journal of Pharmacology and Experimental Therapeutics*, vol. 283, no. 1, pp. 384–390, 1997.

[106] E. M. Barnes Jr., "Intracellular trafficking of GABA$_A$ receptors," *Life Sciences*, vol. 66, no. 12, pp. 1063–1070, 2000.

[107] J. Liang, N. Zhang, E. Cagetti, C. R. Houser, R. W. Olsen, and I. Spigelman, "Chronic intermittent ethanol-induced switch of ethanol actions from extrasynaptic to synaptic hippocampal GABA$_A$ receptors," *Journal of Neuroscience*, vol. 26, no. 6, pp. 1749–1758, 2006.

[108] J. P. Herman, N. K. Mueller, and H. Figueiredo, "Role of GABA and glutamate circuitry in hypothalamo-pituitary-adrenocortical stress integration," *Annals of the New York Academy of Sciences*, vol. 1018, pp. 35–45, 2004.

[109] H. Homayoun and B. Moghaddam, "NMDA receptor hypofunction produces opposite effects on prefrontal cortex interneurons and pyramidal neurons," *Journal of Neuroscience*, vol. 27, no. 43, pp. 11496–11500, 2007.

[110] D. N. Stephens, "A glutamatergic hypothesis of drug dependence: extrapolations from benzodiazepine receptor ligands," *Behavioural Pharmacology*, vol. 6, no. 5-6, pp. 425–446, 1995.

[111] R. J. Marley, C. Heninger, T. D. Hernandez, and D. W. Gallager, "Chronic administration of β-carboline-3-carboxylic acid methylamide by continuous intraventricular infusion increases GABAergic function," *Neuropharmacology*, vol. 30, no. 3, pp. 245–251, 1991.

[112] E. Izzo, J. Auta, F. Impagnatiello, C. Pesold, A. Guidotti, and E. Costa, "Glutamic acid decarboxylase and glutamate receptor changes during tolerance and dependence to benzodiazepines," *Proceedings of the National Academy of Sciences of the United States of America*, vol. 98, no. 6, pp. 3483–3488, 2001.

[113] S. F. Traynelis, L. P. Wollmuth, C. J. McBain et al., "Glutamate receptor ion channels: structure, regulation, and function," *Pharmacological Reviews*, vol. 62, no. 3, pp. 405–496, 2010.

[114] L. Bard and L. Groc, "Glutamate receptor dynamics and protein interaction: lessons from the NMDA receptor," *Molecular and Cellular Neuroscience*, vol. 48, no. 4, pp. 298–307, 2011.

[115] P. Paoletti and J. Neyton, "NMDA receptor subunits: function and pharmacology," *Current Opinion in Pharmacology*, vol. 7, no. 1, pp. 39–47, 2007.

[116] T. Nakagawa, "The biochemistry, ultrastructure, and subunit assembly mechanism of AMPA receptors," *Molecular Neurobiology*, vol. 42, no. 3, pp. 161–184, 2010.

[117] N. Armstrong, J. Jasti, M. Beich-Frandsen, and E. Gouaux, "Measurement of conformational changes accompanying desensitization in an Ionotropic glutamate receptor," *Cell*, vol. 127, no. 1, pp. 85–97, 2006.

[118] J. Lerma, "Kainate receptor physiology," *Current Opinion in Pharmacology*, vol. 6, no. 1, pp. 89–97, 2006.

[119] J. M. Khanna, A. Chau, and G. Shah, "Effect of NMDA antagonists on rapid tolerance to benzodiazepines," *Brain Research Bulletin*, vol. 42, no. 2, pp. 99–103, 1997.

[120] S. E. File and C. Fernandes, "Dizocilpine prevents the development of tolerance to the sedative effects of diazepam in rats," *Pharmacology Biochemistry and Behavior*, vol. 47, no. 4, pp. 823–826, 1994.

[121] K. G. Steppuhn and L. Turski, "Diazepam dependence prevented by glutamate antagonists," *Proceedings of the National Academy of Sciences of the United States of America*, vol. 90, no. 14, pp. 6889–6893, 1993.

[122] J. M. Koff, G. A. Pritchard, D. J. Greenblatt, and L. G. Miller, "The NMDA receptor competitive antagonist CPP modulates benzodiazepine tolerance and discontinuation," *Pharmacology*, vol. 55, no. 5, pp. 217–227, 1997.

[123] C. Fernandes and S. E. File, "Dizocilpine does not prevent the development of tolerance to the anxiolytic effects of diazepam in rats," *Brain Research*, vol. 815, no. 2, pp. 431–434, 1999.

[124] M. Tsuda, H. Shimizu, Y. Yajima, T. Suzuki, and M. Misawa, "Hypersusceptibility to DMCM-induced seizures during diazepam withdrawal in mice: evidence for upregulation of NMDA receptors," *Naunyn-Schmiedeberg's Archives of Pharmacology*, vol. 357, no. 3, pp. 309–315, 1998.

[125] M. F. Perez, R. Salmiron, and O. A. Ramirez, "NMDA-NR1 and -NR2B subunits mRNA expression in the hippocampus of rats tolerant to diazepam," *Behavioural Brain Research*, vol. 144, no. 1-2, pp. 119–124, 2003.

[126] R. S. Almiron, M. F. Perez, and O. A. Ramirez, "MK-801 prevents the increased NMDA-NR1 and NR2B subunits mRNA expression observed in the hippocampus of rats tolerant to diazepam," *Brain Research*, vol. 1008, no. 1, pp. 54–60, 2004.

[127] B. J. Van Sickle, A. S. Cox, K. Schak, L. J. Greenfield, and E. I. Tietz, "Chronic benzodiazepine administration alters hippocampal CA1 neuron excitability: NMDA receptor function and expression," *Neuropharmacology*, vol. 43, no. 4, pp. 595–606, 2002.

[128] C. Bonavita, A. Ferrero, M. Cereseto, M. Velardez, M. Rubio, and S. Wikinski, "Adaptive changes in the rat hippocampal glutamatergic neurotransmission are observed during long-term treatment with lorazepam," *Psychopharmacology*, vol. 166, no. 2, pp. 163–167, 2003.

[129] C. D. Bonavita, V. Bisagno, C. G. Bonelli, G. B. Acosta, M. C. Rubio, and S. I. Wikinski, "Tolerance to the sedative effect of lorazepam correlates with a diminution in cortical release and affinity for glutamate," *Neuropharmacology*, vol. 42, no. 5, pp. 619–625, 2002.

[130] C. Allison and J. A. Pratt, "Differential effects of two chronic diazepam treatment regimes on withdrawal anxiety and AMPA receptor characteristics," *Neuropsychopharmacology*, vol. 31, no. 3, pp. 602–619, 2006.

[131] B. J. Van Sickle and E. I. Tietz, "Selective enhancement of AMPA receptor-mediated function in hippocampal CA1 neurons from chronic benzodiazepine-treated rats," *Neuropharmacology*, vol. 43, no. 1, pp. 11–27, 2002.

[132] T. Aitta-aho, O. Y. Vekovischeva, P. J. Neuvonen, and E. R. Korpi, "Reduced benzodiazepine tolerance, but increased flumazenil-precipitated withdrawal in AMPA-receptor GluR-A subunit-deficient mice," *Pharmacology Biochemistry and Behavior*, vol. 92, no. 2, pp. 283–290, 2009.

[133] H. R. Lyons, M. B. Land, T. T. Gibbs, and D. H. Farb, "Distinct signal transduction pathways for GABA-induced GABAA receptor down-regulation and uncoupling in neuronal culture: a role for voltage-gated calcium channels," *Journal of Neurochemistry*, vol. 78, no. 5, pp. 1114–1125, 2001.

[134] B. Lu, P. T. Pang, and N. H. Woo, "The yin and yang of neurotrophin action," *Nature Reviews Neuroscience*, vol. 6, no. 8, pp. 603–614, 2005.

[135] I. Brunig, S. Penschuck, B. Berninger, J. Benson, and J. M. Fritschy, "BDNF reduces miniature inhibitory postsynaptic currents by rapid downregulation of GABA_A receptor surface expression," *European Journal of Neuroscience*, vol. 13, no. 7, pp. 1320–1328, 2001.

[136] J. N. Jovanovic, P. Thomas, J. T. Kittler, T. G. Smart, and S. J. Moss, "Brain-derived neurotrophic factor modulates fast synaptic inhibition by regulating GABA_A receptor phosphorylation, activity, and cell-surface stability," *Journal of Neuroscience*, vol. 24, no. 2, pp. 522–530, 2004.

[137] T. Tanaka, H. Saito, and N. Matsuki, "Inhibition of GABA_A synaptic responses by brain-derived neurotrophic factor (BDNF) in rat hippocampus," *Journal of Neuroscience*, vol. 17, no. 9, pp. 2959–2966, 1997.

[138] Q. Cheng and H. H. Yeh, "Brain-derived neurotrophic factor attenuates mouse cerebellar granule cell GABA_A receptor-mediated responses via postsynaptic mechanisms," *Journal of Physiology*, vol. 548, no. 3, pp. 711–721, 2003.

[139] C. Henneberger, R. Jüttner, T. Rothe, and R. Grantyn, "Postsynaptic action of BDNF on GABAergic synaptic transmission in the superficial layers of the mouse superior colliculus," *Journal of Neurophysiology*, vol. 88, no. 2, pp. 595–603, 2002.

[140] Y. Mizoguchi, T. Kanematsu, M. Hirata, and J. Nabekura, "A rapid increase in the total number of cell surface functional GABA_A receptors induced by brain-derived neurotrophic factor in rat visual cortex," *Journal of Biological Chemistry*, vol. 278, no. 45, pp. 44097–44102, 2003.

[141] M. M. Bolton, A. J. Pittman, D. C. Lo, and Lo, "Brain-derived neurotrophic factor differentially regulates excitatory and inhibitory synaptic transmission in hippocampal cultures," *Journal of Neuroscience*, vol. 20, no. 9, pp. 3221–3232, 2000.

[142] S. A. Hewitt and J. S. Bains, "Brain-derived neurotrophic factor silences GABA synapses onto hypothalamic neuroendocrine cells through a postsynaptic dynamin-mediated mechanism," *Journal of Neurophysiology*, vol. 95, no. 4, pp. 2193–2198, 2006.

[143] Z. Yan, "Regulation of GABAergic inhibition by serotonin signaling in prefrontal cortex: molecular mechanisms and functional implications," *Molecular Neurobiology*, vol. 26, no. 2-3, pp. 203–216, 2002.

[144] J. Feng, X. Cai, J. Zhao, and Z. Yan, "Serotonin receptors modulate GABA_A receptor channels through activation of anchored protein kinase C in prefrontal cortical neurons," *Journal of Neuroscience*, vol. 21, no. 17, pp. 6502–6511, 2001.

[145] N. J. Brandon, J. N. Jovanovic, T. G. Smart, and S. J. Moss, "Receptor for activated C kinase-1 facilitates protein kinase C-dependent phosphorylation and functional modulation of GABA_A receptors with the activation of G-protein-coupled receptors," *Journal of Neuroscience*, vol. 22, no. 15, pp. 6353–6361, 2002.

[146] X. Wang, P. Zhong, and Z. Yan, "Dopamine D4 receptors modulate GABAergic signaling in pyramidal neurons of prefrontal cortex," *Journal of Neuroscience*, vol. 22, no. 21, pp. 9185–9193, 2002.

[147] D. J. Nutt, P. J. Cowen, and M. Franklin, "The effect of diazepam on indices of 5-HT function in man," *Pharmacology Biochemistry and Behavior*, vol. 24, no. 5, pp. 1491–1495, 1986.

[148] A. Khan and D. J. Haleem, "Tolerance in the anxiolytic profile following repeated administration of diazepam but not buspirone is associated with a decrease in the responsiveness of postsynaptic 5-HT-1A receptors," *Acta Biologica Hungarica*, vol. 58, no. 4, pp. 345–357, 2007.

[149] A. A. Hegarty and W. H. Vogel, "The effect of acute and chronic diazepam treatment on stress-induced changes in cortical dopamine in the rat," *Pharmacology Biochemistry and Behavior*, vol. 52, no. 4, pp. 771–778, 1995.

[150] J. J. Lambert, M. A. Cooper, R. D. J. Simmons, C. J. Weir, and D. Belelli, "Neurosteroids: endogenous allosteric modulators of GABA$_A$ receptors," *Psychoneuroendocrinology*, vol. 34, supplement 1, pp. S48–S58, 2009.

[151] M. B. Herd, D. Belelli, and J. J. Lambert, "Neurosteroid modulation of synaptic and extrasynaptic GABA$_A$ receptors," *Pharmacology and Therapeutics*, vol. 116, no. 1, pp. 20–34, 2007.

[152] N. Usami, T. Yamamoto, S. Shintani et al., "Substrate specificity of human 3(20)α-hydroxysteroid dehydrogenase for neurosteroids and its inhibition by benzodiazepines," *Biological and Pharmaceutical Bulletin*, vol. 25, no. 4, pp. 441–445, 2002.

[153] M. A. Wilson and R. Biscardi, "Effects of gender and gonadectomy on responses to chronic benzodiazepine receptor agonist exposure in rats," *European Journal of Pharmacology*, vol. 215, no. 1, pp. 99–107, 1992.

[154] D. S. Reddy and S. K. Kulkarni, "Neurosteroid coadministration prevents development of tolerance and augments recovery from benzodiazepine withdrawal anxiety and hyperactivity in mice," *Methods and Findings in Experimental and Clinical Pharmacology*, vol. 19, no. 6, pp. 395–405, 1997.

[155] N. R. Mirza and E. O. Nielsen, "Do subtype-selective gamma-aminobutyric acid A receptor modulators have a reduced propensity to induce physical dependence in mice?" *Journal of Pharmacology and Experimental Therapeutics*, vol. 316, no. 3, pp. 1378–1385, 2006.

[156] J. R. Atack, K. A. Wafford, S. J. Tye et al., "TPA023 [7-(1, 1-dimethylethyl)-6-(2-ethyl-2H-1, 2, 4-triazol-3-ylmethoxy)-3-(2-fluor ophenyl)-1, 2, 4-triazolo[4, 3-b]pyridazine], an agonist selective for alpha2- and alpha3-containing GABA$_A$ receptors, is a nonsedating anxiolytic in rodents and primates," *Journal of Pharmacology and Experimental Therapeutics*, vol. 316, no. 1, pp. 410–422, 2006.

[157] J. Knabl, R. Witschi, K. Hosl et al., "Reversal of pathological pain through specific spinal GABA$_A$ receptor subtypes," *Nature*, vol. 451, no. 7176, pp. 330–334, 2008.

[158] G. Zammit, "Comparative tolerability of newer agents for insomnia," *Drug Safety*, vol. 32, no. 9, pp. 735–748, 2009.

[159] A. Ravishankar and T. Carnwath, "Zolpidem tolerance and dependence—two case reports," *Journal of Psychopharmacology*, vol. 12, no. 1, pp. 103–104, 1998.

[160] D. J. Sanger and B. Zivkovic, "Differential development of tolerance to the depressant effects of benzodiazepine and non-benzodiazepine agonists at the omega (BZ) modulatory sites of GABA$_A$ receptors," *Neuropharmacology*, vol. 31, no. 7, pp. 693–700, 1992.

[161] D. J. Sanger and B. Zivkovic, "Investigation of the development of tolerance to the actions of zolpidem and midazolam," *Neuropharmacology*, vol. 26, no. 10, pp. 1513–1518, 1987.

[162] G. Perrault, E. Morel, D. J. Sanger, and B. Zivkovic, "Lack of tolerance and physical dependence upon repeated treatment with the novel hypnotic zolpidem," *Journal of Pharmacology and Experimental Therapeutics*, vol. 263, no. 1, pp. 298–303, 1992.

[163] R. Scherkl, D. Kurudi, and H. H. Frey, "Clorazepate in dogs: tolerance to the anticonvulsant effect and signs of physical dependence," *Epilepsy Research*, vol. 3, no. 2, pp. 144–150, 1989.

[164] J. R. Atack, "Subtype-selective GABA$_A$ receptor modulation yields a novel pharmacological profile: the design and development of TPA023," *Advances in Pharmacology*, vol. 57, pp. 137–185, 2009.

[165] N. A. Ator, "Zaleplon and triazolam: drug discrimination, plasma levels, and self-administration in baboons," *Drug and Alcohol Dependence*, vol. 61, no. 1, pp. 55–68, 2000.

28

Effect of Coenzyme-Q10 on Doxorubicin-Induced Nephrotoxicity in Rats

Azza A. K. El-Sheikh,[1] Mohamed A. Morsy,[1] Marwa M. Mahmoud,[1] Rehab A. Rifaai,[2] and Aly M. Abdelrahman[1]

[1] Department of Pharmacology, Faculty of Medicine, Minia University, 61511 El-Minia, Egypt
[2] Department of Histology, Faculty of Medicine, Minia University, 61511 El-Minia, Egypt

Correspondence should be addressed to Mohamed A. Morsy, mamm222@hotmail.com

Academic Editor: Ismail Laher

Nephrotoxicity is one of the limiting factors for using doxorubicin (Dox) as an anticancer chemotherapeutic. Here, we investigated possible protective effect of coenzyme-Q10 (CoQ10) on Dox-induced nephrotoxicity and the mechanisms involved. Two doses (10 and 100 mg/kg) of CoQ10 were administered orally to rats for 8 days, in the presence or absence of nephrotoxicity induced by a single intraperitoneal injection of Dox (15 mg/kg) at day 4 of the experiment. Our results showed that the low dose of CoQ10 succeeded in reversing Dox-induced nephrotoxicity to control levels (e.g., levels of blood urea nitrogen and serum creatinine, concentrations of renal reduced glutathione (GSH) and malondialdehyde, catalase activity and caspase 3 expression, and renal histopathology). Alternatively, the high dose of CoQ10 showed no superior nephroprotection over the low dose, as there were no significant improvements in renal histopathology, catalase activity, or caspase 3 expression compared to the Dox-treated group. Interestingly, the high dose of CoQ10 alone significantly decreased renal GSH level as well as catalase activity and caused a mild induction of caspase 3 expression compared to control, probably due to a prooxidant effect at this dose of CoQ10. We conclude that CoQ10 protects from Dox-induced nephrotoxicity with a precaution to dosage adjustment.

1. Introduction

Doxorubicin (Dox), also known as adriamycin, is a broad spectrum anticancer anthracycline antibiotic that has been successfully used in treatment of a variety of hematological malignancies and solid tumors. Unfortunately, the use of Dox has been limited by the occurrence of dose-dependent toxicities to vital organs, as the heart, the kidney, and the liver [1]. The exact mechanism of Dox-induced nephrotoxicity is not yet completely understood. Renal Dox-induced toxicity may be part of a multiorgan damage mediated mainly through free radical formation eventually leading to membrane lipid peroxidation [2]. Induction of apoptosis and modulation of nitric oxide (NO) [3] are other mechanisms that may be involved in toxic adverse effects associated with Dox therapy. In addition, Dox may induce nephrotoxicity through its direct renal damaging effect, as it accumulates preferentially in the kidney [4]. Dox toxic effects to other organs as the heart and the liver may modulate blood supply to the kidney and alter xenobiotic detoxification processes, respectively, thus indirectly contributing to Dox-induced nephropathy.

A number of antioxidant compounds have been proposed as chemopreventive therapy for Dox-induced toxicity [5]. Of these compounds, the antioxidant coenzyme-Q10 (CoQ10) has been tried to minimize cardiotoxicity related to Dox therapy [6], but its effect on Dox-induced nephrotoxicity has not yet been elucidated. CoQ10, also known as ubiquinone, is the only naturally-occurring lipid soluble antioxidant that is endogenously synthesized [7]. Meat, fish, nuts, and certain oils are some of the richest nutritional sources of CoQ10, while much lower levels can be found in most dairy products, vegetables, fruits, and cereals [8]. It is used as a dietary supplementation

and as a cotherapy in conjunction with medication in a number of conditions, including cardiovascular diseases, cancer, muscular neurodegenerative disorders, and diabetes [9].

The nephroprotective effect of CoQ10 is still controversial. On one hand, CoQ10 showed nephroprotective effects in some animal models [10, 11]. On the other hand, no renal protection has been reported in another animal study [12]. Furthermore, a study conducted on renal transplant recipient patients showed that despite the evident antioxidant effect of CoQ10, the kidney function reflected by creatinine level was not improved [13]. In the present work, an attempt was made to investigate the effect of CoQ10 on renal damage induced by Dox therapy.

2. Materials and Methods

2.1. Chemicals. CoQ10 powder was a generous gift from Mepaco (Egypt). Dox hydrochloride 10 mg vial (Pharmacia Italia, SPA, Italy), polyclonal rabbit/antirat caspase 3 antibody (1 mg/mL; Lab Vision, USA), biotinylated goat antirabbit secondary antibody (Transduction Laboratories, USA), kits for total protein concentration (Diamond diagnostics, Egypt), blood urea nitrogen (BUN), creatinine, reduced glutathione (GSH), and catalase (Biodiagnostic, Egypt) were purchased.

2.2. Animals and Experimental Design. Adult male Wistar rats weighing 185–250 g were obtained from the National Research Centre, Giza, Egypt. Animals were kept in standard housing conditions (12 h lighting cycle and 24 ± 2°C temperature), three or four rats/cage, and were left to acclimatize for one week. Rats were supplied with laboratory chow and tap water ad libitum. This work was ethically approved by the members of the board of the Faculty of Medicine, Minia University, Egypt (7/2010) in accordance with the EEC Directive of 1986 (86/609/EEC). Animals were randomly assigned to different experimental groups with no statistically significant difference in weight between groups. Animal groups were control-untreated group ($n = 7$), CoQ10L group ($n = 7$) treated with low (L) dose of CoQ10 of 10 mg/kg orally [10], CoQ10H group ($n = 7$) treated with high (H) dose of CoQ10 of 100 mg/kg orally [14], Dox-treated group ($n = 15$) receiving a single ip injection of Dox in a dose of 15 mg/kg (the dose was selected based on our preliminary experiments and a previous study by Ajith et al. [15] as renal toxicity was not seen at lower doses) given 5 days before animal sacrifice, Dox/CoQ10L and Dox/CoQ10H groups ($n = 12$ each) receiving similar Dox treatment, together with similar low or high doses of CoQ10, respectively, for 8 consecutive days, starting 3 days prior to Dox injection. Larger numbers of animals were assigned for groups receiving Dox, as higher rate of mortality was anticipated based on our preliminary experiments. CoQ10 powder, prepared in 1% carboxymethylcellulose, was administered by stomach tube. Animal not receiving CoQ10 received the same volume of 1% carboxymethylcellulose.

Similarly, animals not receiving Dox were injected with the same volume of distilled water ip (Dox vehicle).

2.3. Evaluation of Renal Function. After 5 days of Dox injection, each rat was weighed then sacrificed by cervical dislocation. Venous blood samples were collected from the jugular vein, centrifuged at 5000 rpm for 15 min (Janetzki T30 centrifuge). As a marker of renal function and nephrotoxicity, BUN and serum creatinine were determined using colorimetric diagnostic kits according to the manufacturer's instructions.

2.4. Renal Homogenate Preparation and Determination of Protein Concentration. After sacrifice, both kidneys were rapidly excised and weighed. A longitudinal section of the left kidney was fixed in 10% formalin then embedded in paraffin for histopathological and immunohistochemical examinations. The rest of the kidneys were snap frozen in liquid nitrogen and kept at −80°C. For preparing renal tissue homogenate for biochemical analysis, kidney was homogenized (Glas-Col homogenizer), and a 20% w/v homogenate was prepared in ice-cold phosphate buffer (0.01 M, pH 7.4). The homogenate was centrifuged at 3000 rpm for 20 min, and the supernatant was kept at −80°C till used. Protein concentration was determined in the supernatant by total protein kit using spectrophotometer (Beckman DU-64 UV/VIS).

2.5. Evaluation of Renal GSH and Catalase Levels. Evaluation of renal antioxidant defense mechanisms was done by assessment of renal tissue GSH and catalase enzyme levels. For GSH, a spectrophotometric kit was used. Briefly, the method is based on that the sulfhydryl group of GSH reacts with 5,5′-dithio-*bis*-2-nitrobenzoic acid (Ellman's reagent) and produces a yellow colored 5-thio-2-nitrobenzoic acid which was measured colorimetrically at 405 nm using Beckman DU-64 UV/VIS spectrophotometer. Results were expressed as μmol/g renal protein. Assessment of renal homogenate catalase antioxidant enzyme activity was determined from the rate of decomposition of H_2O_2 at 510 nm after the addition of tissue homogenate as described by colorimetric kit. The results were expressed as unit/g renal protein.

2.6. Assessment of Renal Lipid Peroxides and NO Levels. Renal lipid peroxidation was determined as thiobarbituric acid reacting substance and is expressed as equivalents of malondialdehyde (MDA), using 1,1,3,3-tetramethoxypropane as standard [16]. Results were expressed as nmol/g renal protein. The assessment of stable oxidation end products of NO, nitrite, and nitrate served as an index of NO production. This method was based on Griess reaction [17] that depends on the spectrophotometric measurement of total nitrites at 540 nm after the conversion of nitrate to nitrite by copperized cadmium granules. Results were expressed as nmol/100 mg renal protein.

2.7. Histopathological and Immunohistochemical Examination. Renal tissue that fixed in 10% formalin and embedded

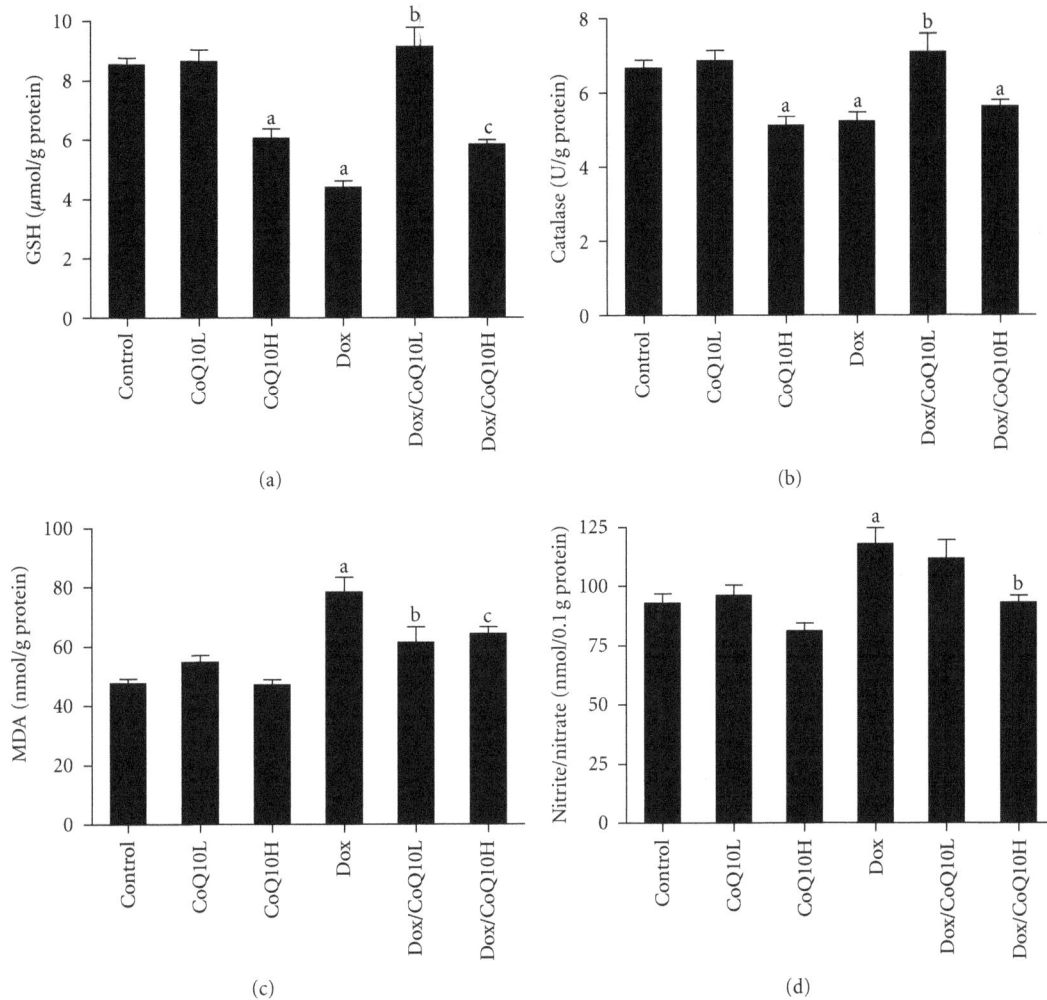

(a)

(b)

(c)

(d)

FIGURE 1: Effect of low and high doses of coenzyme Q10 (CoQ10) on renal (a) reduced glutathione (GSH), (b) catalase, (c) malondialdehyde (MDA), and (d) nitric oxide (nitrite/nitrate) levels in rats exposed to doxorubicin- (Dox-) induced nephrotoxicity. Animal groups tested are control-untreated group, animals treated with low or high dose CoQ10 alone (CoQ10L or CoQ10H, resp.), and animals treated with Dox or with Dox together with low or high CoQ10 dose (Dox/CoQ10L or Dox/CoQ10H, resp.). Values are represented as means ± SE of 6–11 observations. [a]Significant difference compared to control, [b]significant difference compared to Dox, without significant difference from control, and [c]significant difference compared to Dox, with significant difference from control. Significant difference is reported when $P < 0.05$.

in paraffin were sectioned by a microtome at 5 μm thickness and stained with hematoxylin and eosin for routine histopathological assessment. Three slides from each animal group, each with three sections, were subjected to semiquantitative microscopical analysis using light microscopy (Olympus CX41). Renal changes were graded as mild, moderate, or severe. Scores +, ++, and +++ are mild, moderate, and severe levels, revealing less than 25, 50, and 75% histopathological alterations of total fields examined, respectively.

Immunohistochemical staining was performed for caspase 3 using polyclonal rabbit/antirat caspase 3 antibody. Briefly, sections were deparaffinized, hydrated then washed in 0.1 M phosphate buffer. Sections were then treated with 0.01% trypsin for 10 min at 37°C then washed with phosphate buffer for 5 min. Endogenous peroxidases were

quenched by treatment with 0.5% H_2O_2 in methanol, and nonspecific binding was blocked by normal goat serum diluted 1 : 50 in 0.1 M phosphate buffer. Tissues were incubated in the primary antibody (caspase 3; 1 : 1000) overnight at 4°C. Afterwards, tissues were washed and incubated in biotinylated goat antirabbit secondary antibody (1 : 2000) for 30 min. Following further 30 min incubation in vectastain ABC reagent, the substrate diaminobenzidine was added for 6 min, which gives brown color at the immunoreactive sites.

2.8. Statistical Analysis. Data was analyzed by one way ANOVA followed by Dunnett Multiple Comparison Test. The values are represented as means ± SEM. Chi-square test was used to analyze the significance of animal mortality results. All statistical analysis was done using GraphPad

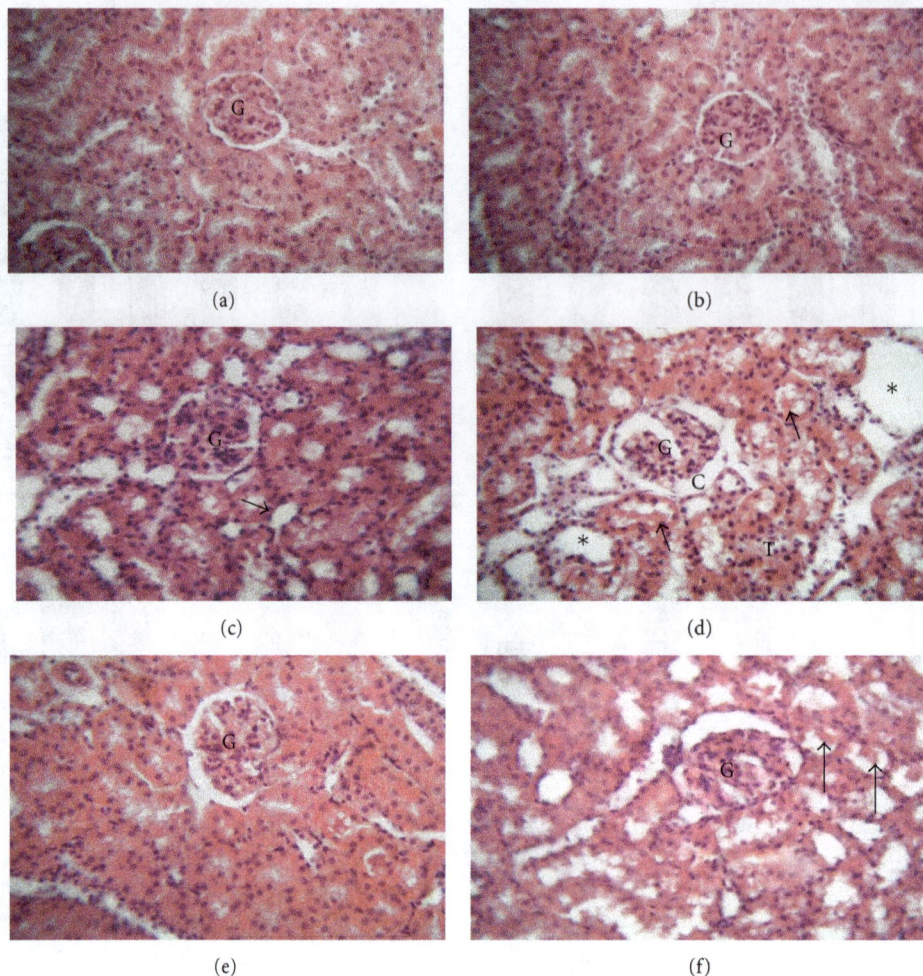

FIGURE 2: Effect of coenzyme Q10 (CoQ10) on kidney histopathological picture of doxorubicin- (Dox-) treated and untreated rats. A photomicrograph of a section in rat kidney (H and E ×400) of ((a) and (b)) untreated control and low dose CoQ10 treated (CoQ10L) groups, respectively, with normal structure of renal glomeruli (G) and cortical tubules; (c) high dose CoQ10 treated (CoQ10H) group with normal renal glomeruli (G), but mild degeneration of the epithelial lining of some tubules (arrow); (d) Dox-treated group with dilated Bowman's space (c), severe degenerative changes observed in the renal tubules with exfoliated cells (T). Some tubules are filled with protein casts (arrows) and some showing cystic dilatation (stars); (e) Dox/CoQ10L group with regeneration of renal tubular epithelial cells and normal morphology of renal cortex and glomeruli (G); (f) Dox/CoQ10H group with marked degeneration of renal tubules with exfoliated epithelial cells and casts (arrows).

Prism software (version 5). The differences were considered significant when the calculated P value is less than 0.05.

3. Results

3.1. Effect of CoQ10 on Mortality and Kidney/Body Weight Ratio in Dox-Treated Rats. At sacrifice time, no mortality was observed in animals of control, CoQ10L, and CoQ10H groups (Table 1). On the other hand, Dox treatment significantly increased animal mortality. Coadministration of CoQ10 in both Dox/CoQ10L and Dox/CoQ10H groups did not result in statistically significant improvement in mortality. Kidney/body weight ratio was not affected by sole administration of CoQ10 in low or high dose. Treatment with Dox significantly increased the kidney/body weight

ratio, which was not changed by administration of either doses of CoQ10.

3.2. Effect of CoQ10 on BUN and Creatinine in Dox-Treated Rats. Results of BUN and creatinine are summarized in Table 1. Rats receiving a single dose of Dox (15 mg/kg, ip) showed significant increase in BUN and creatinine levels compared to control group. Concomitant CoQ10 in low dose with Dox resulted in significant reduction of BUN and creatinine to levels comparable to normal controls. On the other hand, the high dose of CoQ10 resulted in less improvement of BUN and creatinine levels that were significant from Dox-treated group, but were still significantly higher from control. Neither the low nor the high CoQ10 alone, without Dox treatment, had any effect on these two markers of renal function compared to control.

TABLE 1: Effect of coenzyme Q10 (CoQ10) on percent of animal mortality, kidney/body weight ratio, blood urea nitrogen (BUN), and creatinine in doxorubicin- (Dox-) induced nephrotoxicity in rats.

Groups	Mortality %	Kd/Wt	BUN (mg/dL)	Creatinine (mg/dL)
Control	0	5.9 ± 0.8	8 ± 1	0.95 ± 0.04
CoQ10L	0	5.9 ± 0.6	8 ± 2	0.9 ± 0.1
CoQ10H	0	6.4 ± 0.7	10 ± 1	0.9 ± 0.1
Dox	40[a]	7.2 ± 0.6[a]	358 ± 97[a]	2.6 ± 0.3[a]
Dox/CoQ10L	25	6.7 ± 0.8	31 ± 7[b]	1.7 ± 0.1[b]
Dox/CoQ10H	8	6.8 ± 1.1	98 ± 31[c]	1.9 ± 0.2[c]

CoQ10L and CoQ10H are rats treated with low and high doses of CoQ10, respectively; Kd/Wt is kidney/body weight * 1000 ratio. Values are representation of 6–11 observations as means ± SEM, except survival which is represented as a percentage. [a]Significant difference compared to control, [b]significant difference compared to Dox group, with no statistically significant difference compared to control, and [c]significant difference compared to Dox group, but with also significant difference compared to control group. Results are considered significantly different when $P < 0.05$.

TABLE 2: Effect of coenzyme Q10 (CoQ10) on severity of histopathological lesions in doxorubicin- (Dox-) induced nephrotoxicity in rats.

Groups	Tubular degeneration	Tubular dilatation	Dilated Bowman's space	Protein casts
Control	0	0	0	0
CoQ10L	0	0	0	0
CoQ10H	++	+	0	0
Dox	+++	++	+	++
Dox/CoQ10L	+	0	0	+
Dox/CoQ10H	+++	++	+	+

CoQ10L and CoQ10H are rat groups treated with low (L) or high (H) dose CoQ10, respectively. Score level 0 was considered normal. Scores +, ++, and +++ are mild, moderate, and severe levels, revealing less than 25, 50, and 75% histopathological alterations of total fields examined, respectively. Score represents values obtained from tissue sections of 3 animals of each group, 5 fields/section (×400).

3.3. Effect of CoQ10 on Renal GSH, Catalase, Lipid Peroxidation, and NO Levels in Dox-Induced Nephrotoxicity.

Treatment with Dox caused significant decrease in renal GSH and catalase levels compared with untreated control (Figures 1(a) and 1(b), resp.). Concomitant treatment of Dox with the low dose of CoQ10 restored renal GSH and catalase values to levels statistically comparable to control. On the other hand, concomitant treatment of Dox with the high dose of CoQ10 had no effect on renal catalase level, with less improvement on renal GSH that was significantly higher than Dox group but still significantly lower than control. The high dose of CoQ10, without Dox treatment, showed significant decrease of renal GSH and catalase compared to control.

Renal MDA was evaluated as an indicator of kidney lipid peroxidation (Figure 1(c)) and nitrite/nitrate ratio as an indicator of renal NO levels (Figure 1(d)). Dox significantly increased renal MDA and nitrite/nitrate ratio compared to control. Administrating CoQ10 in the low dose to Dox-treated animals retrieved MDA to levels statistically insignificant from control but had no effect on nitrite/nitrate ratio. On the other hand, giving CoQ10 in the high dose to Dox-treated animals improved MDA compared to Dox group but was still statistically significant from control and restored nitrite/nitrate ratio to levels comparable to that of control. CoQ10 alone in the low or the high dose had no significant effect on either renal MDA or NO levels.

3.4. Effect of CoQ10 on Renal Histopathology in Dox-Treated Rats.

Histopathological examination revealed that control and CoQ10L groups had normal structure of renal glomeruli and cortical tubules (Figures 2(a) and 2(b); Table 2). On the other hand, Dox-treated group presented with dilated Bowman's space and marked degeneration of renal tubules that showed exfoliated cells, protein casts, and cystic dilatation (Figure 2(d)). Concomitant administration of CoQ10 in the low dose with Dox resulted in reversal of histopathological damage induced by Dox, with regeneration of renal epithelial cells lining of cortical tubules and restoration of normal morphology to renal cortex (Figure 2(e)). The high dose of CoQ10 given with Dox, however, did not reverse morphological changes seen in Dox group, but showed marked degeneration of renal tubules with exfoliated epithelial cells and casts comparable to Dox group (Figure 2(f)). Furthermore, the high dose without Dox treatment in CoQ10H group showed degeneration of the epithelial lining of some tubules (Figure 2(c)).

3.5. Effect of CoQ10 on Renal Apoptosis in Dox-Induced Nephrotoxicity.

As a marker of apoptosis, induction of caspase 3 was evaluated by immunohistochemical staining (Figure 3). Semiquantitative analysis was further performed to calculate the degree of significance (Figure 4). Immunohistochemical staining of rat kidney showed that administration of Dox caused significant increase in the immunoreactivity of caspase 3 compared to control, which was highly expressed in renal glomeruli and tubules both cytoplasmically and in some nuclei (Figure 3(d)). Concomitant administration of CoQ10 in the low dose with Dox significantly decreased caspase 3 expression to levels significant from Dox alone (Figure 3(e)). On the other hand, the high dose of CoQ10 with Dox failed to produce a similar effect, as it showed high caspase 3 expression in the glomeruli and renal tubules (Figure 3(f)). Interestingly, administration of the high dose of CoQ10, but not low dose, without Dox caused significant expression of caspase 3 compared to control (Figure 3(c)).

4. Discussion

Despite the extensive clinical utilization of Dox in the treatment of cancer patients, the mechanism by which it produces its nephrotoxic adverse effect is still under intense debate. One of the mechanisms suggested is free radical formation and oxidative stress [1]. The level of the endogenous antioxidant CoQ10 seems to increase in

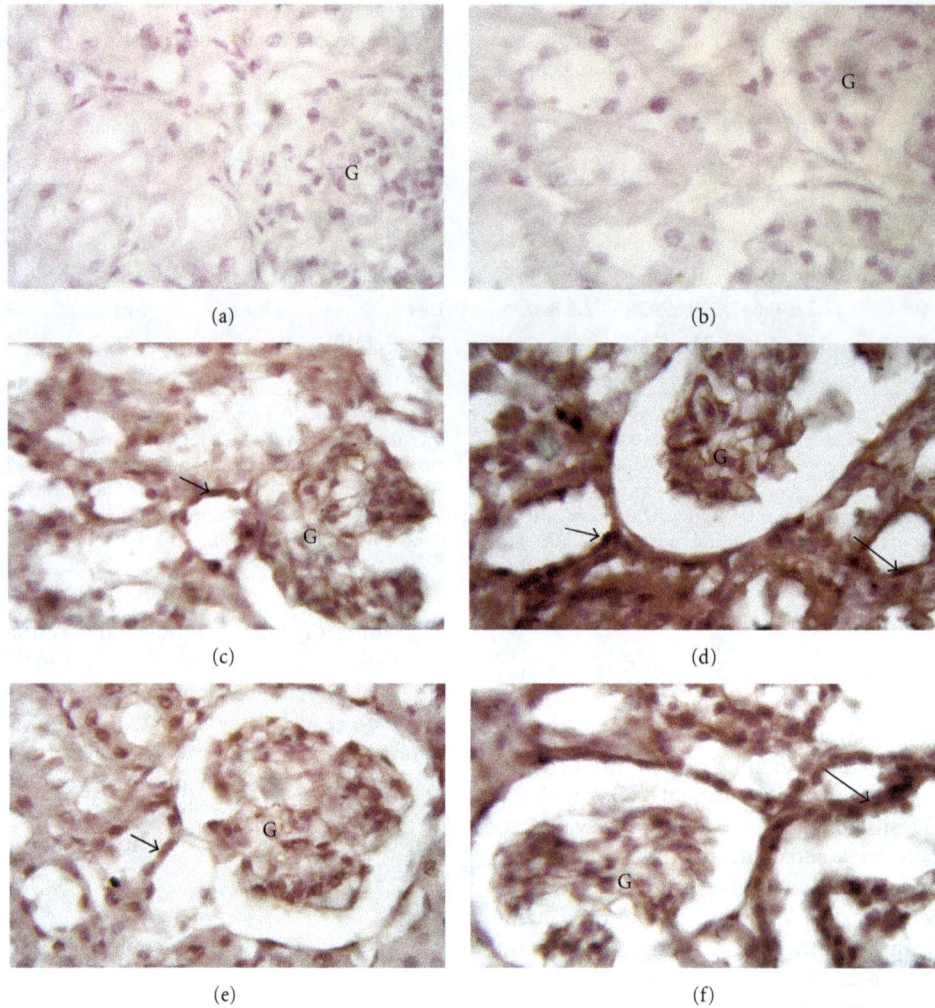

FIGURE 3: Effect of coenzyme Q10 (CoQ10) on caspase 3 immunohistochemical staining of doxorubicin- (Dox-) treated and untreated rat kidney. Localization of caspase 3 immunoreactivity in the kidney cortex ($\times$1000) of ((a) and (b)) untreated control and low dose CoQ10 treated (CoQ10L) groups, respectively, showing negative immunoreactivity; (c) high dose CoQ10 treated group (CoQ10H) showing faint expression within the glomeruli (G) and the renal tubules (arrow); (d) Dox-treated group showing high expression in the renal glomeruli (G) and renal tubules. The expression is mainly cytoplasmic, but with some nuclei showing positive expression (arrows); (e) Dox/CoQ10L group showing faint expression within the glomeruli (G) and the renal tubules (arrow); (f) Dox/CoQ10H group showing high expression in the glomeruli (G) and the renal tubules (arrow).

human plasma after Dox therapy [18]. This is probably through upregulation of CoQ10 gene expression as a cellular defense mechanism against chemotherapy to promote cell survival [19]. This directed our attention to investigate the role of CoQ10 as a possible nephroprotective agent against Dox-induced renal damage, especially after its success in protecting from Dox-induced cardiotoxicity [6].

The dose of Dox used in this study corresponds to the dose that is currently being used in clinical practice [20]. In the present study, this dose produced acute renal function deterioration in the animal group receiving it. Such alteration in renal function was completely restored to levels statistically insignificant from control by prophylactic coadministration of CoQ10 in a low dose. The high dose of CoQ10 also improved Dox-induced renal function deterioration, but still significantly higher than control levels. This

indicates that increasing CoQ10 dose does not confer more nephroprotection against Dox-induced renal damage.

Improvement of Dox-induced nephrotoxicity was previously tried by compounds that partially succeeded in preserving normal renal function and structure probably through their antioxidant effects, as caffeic acid phenethyl ester [21], Zingiber officinale Roscoe [15], and Solanum torvum [22]. Here, a prophylactic low dose of CoQ10, 3 days before and extending 5 days concurrently with Dox treatment, restored most of kidney antioxidant parameters and apoptotic signs to control levels. The enhanced renal antioxidant status resulting from low dose CoQ10 prophylactic treatment could explain its nephroprotective effect. Such nephroprotective effect is probably not accompanied by any alteration in Dox disposition, including metabolism, biliary excretion, and clearance [23], nor with deterioration in Dox

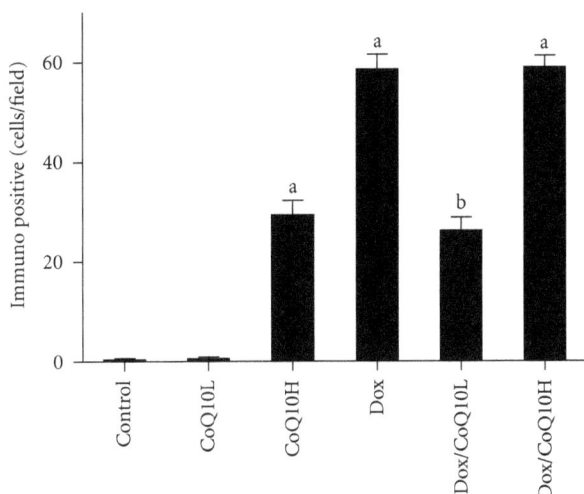

FIGURE 4: Effect of two doses of coenzyme Q10 (CoQ10) on renal caspase 3 immunohistochemical semiquantitative analysis in rats exposed to doxorubicin- (Dox-) induced nephrotoxicity. Kidneys were isolated from control untreated group, animals treated with low or high dose CoQ10 (CoQ10L or CoQ10H, resp.), and animals treated with Dox, or with Dox together with CoQ10L or CoQ10H, respectively. Values are represented as means ± SE of number of immuno-positive cells for caspase 3 in sections of 3 animals of each group, 5 fields/section. [a]Significant difference compared with control and [b]significant difference compared to Dox, with significant difference from control. Significant difference is reported when $P < 0.05$.

antineoplastic properties as reported in breast cancer cell cultures [24].

Increasing the dose of CoQ10 given with Dox therapy did not show any improvement in renal function or histopathological structure over low CoQ10 dose. Furthermore, cotherapy of Dox with the higher CoQ10 dose resulted in disappointing effects concerning renal antioxidant status and apoptosis. These results imply a prooxidant effect of CoQ10 in the high dose. Indeed, some antioxidants were reported to possess prooxidant effects at higher doses, as the flavonoids: quercetin, myricetin, kaempferol [25], and curcumin [26] that were found to mediate induction of reactive oxygen species at high concentration. Some studies suggested a similar prooxidant effect for CoQ10 in vitro [27–29]. This was further supported by the prooxidant effects reported for the CoQ10 analog, known as mitochondrial-targeted coenzyme Q mitoQ [30]. A study conducted on renal hemodialysis patients showed that CoQ10 suppressed the oxidative stress and still, unexpectedly, decreased oxygen radical absorbing capacity [31]. In these patients suffering from diminished renal function, concentration of CoQ10 may be higher than normal, which probably resulted in the appearance of such prooxidant effect. Here, we provide for the first time a mechanistic proof of prooxidant mechanisms of high dose CoQ10 in vivo, which, when given alone, resulted in oxidative stress evident by decreased renal GSH and catalase levels and induced mild renal apoptosis implicated by renal caspase 3 expression.

In conclusion, at a dose of 10 mg/kg, CoQ10 protects against Dox-induced nephrotoxicity in rats. However, increasing the dose of CoQ10 concomitantly given with Dox to 100 mg/kg is not more nephroprotective. This is probably due to a prooxidant effect of CoQ10 manifested at the high dose and seen even when it is given alone without Dox.

Conflict of Interests

The authors reported no conflict of interests.

References

[1] C. Carvalho, R. X. Santos, S. Cardoso et al., "Doxorubicin: the good, the bad and the ugly effect," Current Medicinal Chemistry, vol. 16, no. 25, pp. 3267–3285, 2009.

[2] S. Ghibu, S. Delemasure, C. Richard et al., "General oxidative stress during doxorubicin-induced cardiotoxicity in rats: absence of cardioprotection and low antioxidant efficiency of alpha-lipoic acid," Biochimie, vol. 94, no. 4, pp. 932–939, 2011.

[3] H. Mizutani, S. Tada-Oikawa, Y. Hiraku, M. Kojima, and S. Kawanishi, "Mechanism of apoptosis induced by doxorubicin through the generation of hydrogen peroxide," Life Sciences, vol. 76, no. 13, pp. 1439–1453, 2005.

[4] V. W. Lee and D. C. Harris, "Adriamycin nephropathy: a model of focal segmental glomerulosclerosis," Nephrology, vol. 16, no. 1, pp. 30–38, 2011.

[5] S. Granados-Principal, J. L. Quiles, C. L. Ramirez-Tortosa, P. Sanchez-Rovira, and M. Ramirez-Tortosa, "New advances in molecular mechanisms and the prevention of adriamycin toxicity by antioxidant nutrients," Food and Chemical Toxicology, vol. 48, no. 6, pp. 1425–1438, 2010.

[6] K. A. Conklin, "Coenzyme Q10 for prevention of anthracycline-induced cardiotoxicity," Integrative Cancer Therapies, vol. 4, no. 2, pp. 110–130, 2005.

[7] G. P. Littarru and L. Tiano, "Bioenergetic and antioxidant properties of coenzyme Q10: recent developments," Molecular Biotechnology, vol. 37, no. 1, pp. 31–37, 2007.

[8] I. Pravst, K. Žmitek, and J. Žmitek, "Coenzyme Q10 contents in foods and fortification strategies," Critical Reviews in Food Science and Nutrition, vol. 50, no. 4, pp. 269–280, 2010.

[9] J. M. Villalba, C. Parrado, M. Santos-Gonzalez, and F. J. Alcain, "Therapeutic use of coenzyme Q10 and coenzyme Q10-related compounds and formulations," Expert Opinion on Investigational Drugs, vol. 19, no. 4, pp. 535–554, 2010.

[10] A. A. Fouad, A. I. Al-Sultan, S. M. Refaie, and M. T. Yacoubi, "Coenzyme Q10 treatment ameliorates acute cisplatin nephrotoxicity in mice," Toxicology, vol. 274, no. 1–3, pp. 49–56, 2010.

[11] M. F. Persson, S. Franzen, S. B. Catrina et al., "Coenzyme Q10 prevents GDP-sensitive mitochondrial uncoupling, glomerular hyperfiltration and proteinuria in kidneys from db/db mice as a model of type 2 diabetes," Diabetologia, vol. 55, no. 5, pp. 1535–1543, 2012.

[12] E. Sutken, E. Aral, F. Ozdemir, S. Uslu, O. Alatas, and O. Colak, "Protective role of melatonin and coenzyme Q10 in ochratoxin A toxicity in rat liver and kidney," International Journal of Toxicology, vol. 26, no. 1, pp. 81–87, 2007.

[13] A. Długosz, J. Kuźniar, E. Sawicka et al., "Oxidative stress and coenzyme Q10 supplementation in renal transplant recipients," International Urology and Nephrology, vol. 36, no. 2, pp. 253–258, 2004.

[14] H. S. El-Abhar, "Coenzyme Q10: a novel gastroprotective effect via modulation of vascular permeability, prostaglandin E2, nitric oxide and redox status in indomethacin-induced gastric ulcer model," *European Journal of Pharmacology*, vol. 649, no. 1–3, pp. 314–319, 2010.

[15] T. A. Ajith, M. S. Aswathy, and U. Hema, "Protective effect of Zingiber officinale roscoe against anticancer drug doxorubicin-induced acute nephrotoxicity," *Food and Chemical Toxicology*, vol. 46, no. 9, pp. 3178–3181, 2008.

[16] J. A. Buege and S. D. Aust, "Microsomal lipid peroxidation," *Methods in Enzymology*, vol. 52, pp. 302–310, 1978.

[17] K. V. H. Sastry, R. P. Moudgal, J. Mohan, J. S. Tyagi, and G. S. Rao, "Spectrophotometric determination of serum nitrite and nitrate by copper-cadmium alloy," *Analytical Biochemistry*, vol. 306, no. 1, pp. 79–82, 2002.

[18] S. Eaton, R. Skinner, J. P. Hale et al., "Plasma coenzyme Q10 in children and adolescents undergoing doxorubicin therapy," *Clinica Chimica Acta*, vol. 302, no. 1-2, pp. 1–9, 2000.

[19] G. Brea-Calvo, A. Rodríguez-Hernández, D. J. Fernández-Ayala, P. Navas, and J. A. Sánchez-Alcázar, "Chemotherapy induces an increase in coenzyme Q10 levels in cancer cell lines," *Free Radical Biology & Medicine*, vol. 40, no. 8, pp. 1293–1302, 2006.

[20] B. A. Chabner, D. P. Ryan, L. Paz-Ares, R. Garcia-Carbonevo, and P. Calabresi, "Antineoplastic agents," in *Goodman and Gilman's the Pharmacological Basis of Therapeutics*, J. G. Hardman, L. E. Limbird, and A. G. Gilman, Eds., pp. 1389–1459, McGraw-Hill, New York, NY, USA, 2001.

[21] M. Yagmurca, H. Erdogan, M. Iraz, A. Songur, M. Ucar, and E. Fadillioglu, "Caffeic acid phenethyl ester as a protective agent against doxorubicin nephrotoxicity in rats," *Clinica Chimica Acta*, vol. 348, no. 1-2, pp. 27–34, 2004.

[22] M. Mohan, S. Kamble, P. Gadhi, and S. Kasture, "Protective effect of Solanum torvum on doxorubicin-induced nephrotoxicity in rats," *Food and Chemical Toxicology*, vol. 48, no. 1, pp. 436–440, 2010.

[23] Q. Zhou and B. Chowbay, "Effect of coenzyme Q10 on the disposition of doxorubicin in rats," *European Journal of Drug Metabolism and Pharmacokinetics*, vol. 27, no. 3, pp. 185–192, 2002.

[24] H. Greenlee, J. Shaw, Y. K. Lau, A. Naini, and M. Maurer, "Lack of effect of coenzyme q10 on doxorubicin cytotoxicity in breast cancer cell cultures," *Integrative Cancer Therapies*, vol. 11, no. 3, pp. 243–250, 2012.

[25] S. C. Sahu and G. C. Gray, "Pro-oxidant activity of flavanoids: effects on glutathione and glutathione S-transferase in isolated rat liver nuclei," *Cancer Letters*, vol. 104, no. 2, pp. 193–196, 1996.

[26] V. Tanwar, J. Sachdeva, M. Golechha, S. Kumari, and D. S. Arya, "Curcumin protects rat myocardium against isoproterenol-induced ischemic injury: attenuation of ventricular dysfunction through increased expression of hsp27 alongwith strengthening antioxidant defense system," *Journal of Cardiovascular Pharmacology*, vol. 55, no. 4, pp. 377–384, 2010.

[27] R. E. Beyer, "The participation of coenzyme Q in free radical production and antioxidation," *Free Radical Biology and Medicine*, vol. 8, no. 6, pp. 545–565, 1990.

[28] R. E. Beyer, "An analysis of the role of coenzyme Q in free radical generation and as an antioxidant," *Biochemistry and Cell Biology*, vol. 70, no. 6, pp. 390–403, 1992.

[29] A. W. Linnane, M. Kios, and L. Vitetta, "Coenzyme Q10—Its role as a prooxidant in the formation of superoxide anion/hydrogen peroxide and the regulation of the metabolome," *Mitochondrion*, vol. 7, pp. S51–S61, 2007.

[30] L. Plecitá-Hlavatá, J. Ježek, and P. Ježek, "Pro-oxidant mitochondrial matrix-targeted ubiquinone MitoQ10 acts as antioxidant at retarded electron transport or proton pumping within Complex I," *International Journal of Biochemistry and Cell Biology*, vol. 41, no. 8-9, pp. 1697–1707, 2009.

[31] T. Sakata, R. Furuya, T. Shimazu, M. Odamaki, S. Ohkawa, and H. Kumagai, "Coenzyme Q10 administration suppresses both oxidative and antioxidative markers in hemodialysis patients," *Blood Purification*, vol. 26, no. 4, pp. 371–378, 2008.

Permissions

All chapters in this book were first published in APS, by Hindawi Publishing Corporation; hereby published with permission under the Creative Commons Attribution License or equivalent. Every chapter published in this book has been scrutinized by our experts. Their significance has been extensively debated. The topics covered herein carry significant findings which will fuel the growth of the discipline. They may even be implemented as practical applications or may be referred to as a beginning point for another development.

The contributors of this book come from diverse backgrounds, making this book a truly international effort. This book will bring forth new frontiers with its revolutionizing research information and detailed analysis of the nascent developments around the world.

We would like to thank all the contributing authors for lending their expertise to make the book truly unique. They have played a crucial role in the development of this book. Without their invaluable contributions this book wouldn't have been possible. They have made vital efforts to compile up to date information on the varied aspects of this subject to make this book a valuable addition to the collection of many professionals and students.

This book was conceptualized with the vision of imparting up-to-date information and advanced data in this field. To ensure the same, a matchless editorial board was set up. Every individual on the board went through rigorous rounds of assessment to prove their worth. After which they invested a large part of their time researching and compiling the most relevant data for our readers.

The editorial board has been involved in producing this book since its inception. They have spent rigorous hours researching and exploring the diverse topics which have resulted in the successful publishing of this book. They have passed on their knowledge of decades through this book. To expedite this challenging task, the publisher supported the team at every step. A small team of assistant editors was also appointed to further simplify the editing procedure and attain best results for the readers.

Apart from the editorial board, the designing team has also invested a significant amount of their time in understanding the subject and creating the most relevant covers. They scrutinized every image to scout for the most suitable representation of the subject and create an appropriate cover for the book.

The publishing team has been an ardent support to the editorial, designing and production team. Their endless efforts to recruit the best for this project, has resulted in the accomplishment of this book. They are a veteran in the field of academics and their pool of knowledge is as vast as their experience in printing. Their expertise and guidance has proved useful at every step. Their uncompromising quality standards have made this book an exceptional effort. Their encouragement from time to time has been an inspiration for everyone.

The publisher and the editorial board hope that this book will prove to be a valuable piece of knowledge for researchers, students, practitioners and scholars across the globe.

List of Contributors

Xia Chen
Phase I Unit of Clinical Pharmacological Research Center, Peking Union Medical College Hospital, 100032 Beijing, China

Sanne de Haas, Marieke de Kam and Joop van Gerven
Centre for Human Drug Research, 2333 CL Leiden, The Netherlands

Dhirender Kaushik, Ajay Kumar and Pawan Kaushik
Institute of Pharmaceutical Sciences, Kurukshetra University, Kurukshetra 136 119, India

A. C. Rana
Rayat College of Pharmacy, Ropar, Punjab 144 533, India

Alex Brenchat, Maria Rocasalbas, Daniel Zamanillo, JoséMiguel Vela and Luz Romero
Department of Pharmacology, Drug Discovery and Preclinical Development, ESTEVE, Avenida Mare de Déu de Montserrat 221, 08041 Barcelona, Spain

Michel Hamon
UMR 894 INSERM-CPN/UPMC, Faculté de Médecine Pierre et Marie Curie, Site Pitié-Salpêtriére, 91 boulevard de l'Hôpital, 75634 Paris Cedex 13, France

Naila Rasheed
Department of Medical Biochemistry, College of Medicine, Qassim University, P.O. BOX 6655, Buraidah 51452, Saudi Arabia

Abdullah Alghasham
Department of Pharmacology and Therapeutics, College of Medicine, Qassim University, P.O. BOX 6655, Buraidah 51452, Saudi Arabia

Kanaiya Panchal and Snehal Patel
Department of Pharmacology, Nirma University, Ahmedabad, Gujarat 382 481, India

Parloop Bhatt
Department of Pharmacology, L. M. College of Pharmacy, Ahmedabad, Gujarat 380009, India

J. A. Shilpi
Pharmacy Discipline, Khulna University, Khulna 9208, Bangladesh

M. E. Islam, M. Billah and K. M. D. Islam
Biotechnology and Genetics Discipline, Khulna University, Khulna 9208, Bangladesh

F. Sabrin
Department of Biotechnology and Genetic Engineering, Mawlana Bhashani Science and Technology University, Santosh, Tangail 1902, Bangladesh

S. J. Uddin
School of Pharmacy, Griffith University, QLD 4222, Australia

L. Nahar
Leicester School of Pharmacy, De Montfort University, The Gateway, Leicester LE1 9BH, UK

S. D. Sarker
Department of Pharmacy, School of Applied Sciences, University of Wolverhampton, MA Building, Wulfruna Street, Wolverhampton WV1 1LY, UK

Muhammad Bilal Azmi
Department of Biochemistry, University of Karachi, Karachi 75270, Pakistan
Quality Enhancement Cell, Dow University of Health Sciences, Karachi 74200, Pakistan

Shamim A. Qureshi
Department of Biochemistry, University of Karachi, Karachi 75270, Pakistan

Dinesh Dhingra and Varun Kumar
Department of Pharmaceutical Sciences, Guru Jambheshwar University of Science and Technology, Haryana, Hisar 125001, India

M. E.Nadia, A. S.Nazrun, M. Norazlina, N. M. Isa, M. Norliza and S. ImaNirwana
Department of Pharmacology, Faculty of Medicine, The National University of Malaysia, Kuala Lumpur campus, 50300 Kuala Lumpur, Malaysia

Takuhiro Uto, OsamuMorinaga and Yukihiro Shoyama
Department of Pharmacognosy, Faculty of Pharmaceutical Sciences, Nagasaki International University, 2825-7 Huis Ten Bosch, Sasebo, Nagasaki 859-3298, Japan

De-Xing Hou
Course of Biological Science and Technology, United Graduate School of Agricultural Sciences, Kagoshima University, Korimoto 1-21-24, Kagoshima 890-0065, Japan

S. Abakuks and A. M. Deters
Institute for Pharmaceutical Biology and Phytochemistry, Westphalian Wilhelms University of Münster, Hittorfstra Be 56, 48149 Münster, Germany

Harquin Simplice Foyet and Armand Abdou Bouba
Department of Agriculture, Livestock and By-Products, The Higher Institute of the Sahel, University of Maroua, P.O. Box 46, Maroua, Cameroon

David Emery Tsala
Department of Life and Earth Sciences, Higher Teachers' Training College, University of Maroua, P.O. Box 55, Maroua, Cameroon

Lucian Hritcu
Department of Biology, Alexandru Ioan Cuza University, Bou/evard Carol I 11, 700506 Iasi, Romania

Sudeep Karve
College of Pharmacy, The Ohio State University, Columbus, OH 43210, USA
RTI Health Solutions, Research Triangle Park, Durham, NC 27709, USA

Deborah Levine
Department of Internal Medicine, College of Medicine, The Ohio State University, Columbus, OH, USA
Division of Health Services Management and Policy, College of Public Health, The Ohio State University, Columbus, OH 43210, USA
Ann Arbor VA Healthcare System and Departments of Medicine and Neurology, The University of Michigan, Ann Arbor, MI 48109, USA

Eric Seiber
Health Services Management and Policy, The Ohio State University, Columbus, OH 43210, USA

MilapNahata
College of Pharmacy, The Ohio State University, Columbus, OH 43210, USA

RajeshBalkrishnan
Department of Clinical, Social and Administrative Sciences, University of Michigan, Ann Arbor, MI 48109, USA
Clinical, Social and Administrative Sciences, College of Pharmacy, University of Michigan, 428 Church Street, Ann Arbor, MI 48109, USA

Reza Shafiee-Nick and Hassan Rakhshandeh
Pharmacological Research Center of Medicinal Plants, School of Medicine, Mashhad University of Medical Sciences, Mashhad 9177948564, Iran
Department of Pharmacology, School of Medicine, Mashhad University of Medical Sciences, Mashhad 9177948564, Iran

Ahmad Ghorbani and Farzaneh Vafaee Bagheri
Pharmacological Research Center of Medicinal Plants, School of Medicine, Mashhad University of Medical Sciences, Mashhad 9177948564, Iran

George J. Amabeoku and Joseph Kabatende
Discipline of Pharmacology, School of Pharmacy, University of the Western Cape, Private Bag X17, Bellville 7535, South Africa

A. S. Nazrun, M. Norazlina, M. Norliza and S. Ima Nirwana
Department of Pharmacology, Faculty of Medicine, The National University of Malaysia, 50300 Kuala Lumpur, Malaysia

Brett Froeliger and Rachel Victoria Kozink
Department of Psychiatry and Behavioral Sciences, Duke University Medical Center, Durham, NC 27708, USA

Jean Crowell Beckham
Department of Psychiatry and Behavioral Sciences, Duke University Medical Center, Durham, NC 27708, USA
Durham Veterans Affairs Medical Center, Durham, NC 27708, USA
VISN 6, Mental Illness Research, Education, and Clinical Center (MIRECC), Durham, NC 27708, USA

Michelle Feldman Dennis
Department of Psychiatry and Behavioral Sciences, Duke University Medical Center, Durham, NC 27708, USA
Durham Veterans Affairs Medical Center, Durham, NC 27708, USA

Francis JosephMcClernon
Department of Psychiatry and Behavioral Sciences, Duke University Medical Center, Durham, NC 27708, USA
Durham Veterans Affairs Medical Center, Durham, NC 27708, USA

Matthew L. Banks and S. Stevens Negus
Department of Pharmacology and Toxicology, Virginia Commonwealth University, P.O. Box 980613, Richmond, VA 23298, USA

EtienneMokondjimobe, Jean Akiana, Ulrich Oswald Ndalla, Regis Dossou-Yovo, Joseph Mboussa and Henri-Joseph Parra
Faculty of Health Sciences, Anti-Tuberculosis Centre, National Laboratory of Public Health, Marien Ngouabi University, Brazzaville, Democratic Republic of Congo

Benjamin Longo-Mbenza
Faculty of Health Sciences, Walter Sisulu University, Private Bag X1, Eastern Cape, Mthatha 5117, South Africa

Rachad Alnamer and Abdelaziz Benjouad
Laboratory of Genetic Immunology and Biochemistry, Department of Biology, Faculty of Science, Mohammed V Agdal University, BP 6203, Rabat Instituts, Agdal, Rabat, Morocco

KatimAlaoui and Yahia Cherrah
Laboratory of Pharmacology and Toxicology, Department of Drugs Sciences, Faculty of Medicine and Pharmacy, Mohammed V Souissi University, ERTP, BP 6203, Rabat Instituts, Agdal, Rabat, Morocco

El Houcine Bouidida
National Laboratory of Drugs Controlled, BP 6203, Rabat Instituts, Agdal, Rabat, Morocco

Rehab AlJamal-Naylor
Avipero Ltd., 5th Floor, 125 Princes Street, Edinburgh EH2 4AD, UK

Linda Wilson
School of Biomedical Sciences, The University of Edinburgh, Hugh Robson Building, George Square, Edinburgh EH8 9XD, UK

SusanMcIntyre, Beth Harrison and David J. Harrison
Division of Pathology, Institute of Genetics and Molecular Medicine, The University of Edinburgh, Western General Hospital, Edinburgh EH4 2XU, UK

Fiona Rossi and Mark Marsden
MRC Centre for Inflammation Research, The Queen's Medical Research Institute, The University of Edinburgh, 47 Little France Crescent, Edinburgh EH16 4TJ, UK

Tamotsu Imanishi
Department of Veterinary Medicine, Faculty of Agriculture, Iwate University, Ueda, Morioka 020-8550, Japan
Department of Food Safety, Pharmaceutical and Medical Safety Bureau, Ministry of Health, Labour and Welfare, Kasumigaseki, Chiyoda, Tokyo 100-8916, Japan

Muhammad Mubarak Hossain
Department of Veterinary Medicine, Faculty of Agriculture, Iwate University, Ueda, Morioka 020-8550, Japan
Department of Environmental and Occupational Medicine, Robert Wood Johnson Medical School, University of Medicine and Dentistry of New Jersey, 170 Frelinghuysen Road, Piscataway, NJ 08854, USA

Ping Xu
Department of Veterinary Medicine, Faculty of Agriculture, Iwate University, Ueda, Morioka 020-8550, Japan

Itaru Sato and Tadahiko Suzuki
Department of Veterinary Medicine, Faculty of Agriculture, Iwate University, Ueda, Morioka 020-8550, Japan

Haruo Kobayashi
Department of Veterinary Medicine, Faculty of Agriculture, Iwate University, Ueda, Morioka 020-8550, Japan
7-272 Aza-Mukaishinden, Ukai, Takizawa-mura, Iwate-gun, Iwate Prefecture 020-0172, Japan

SadollahMohammadi
Department of Pharmacology and Toxicology, School of Pharmacy, Tabriz University of Medical Sciences, Tabriz 5165665931, Iran
Division of Molecular Toxicology, Institute of Environmental Medicine, Karolinska Institutet (KI), Box 210, 17177 Stockholm, Sweden
Department of Pharmacology and Physiology, School of Medicine, Ardabil University of Medical Sciences, Ardabil 56135665, Iran

Moslem Najaf
Department of Pharmacology and Toxicology, School of Pharmacy, Tabriz University of Medical Sciences, Tabriz 5165665931, Iran

Hossein Hamzeiy
Department of Pharmacology and Toxicology, School of Pharmacy, Tabriz University of Medical Sciences, Tabriz 5165665931, Iran
Research Center for Pharmaceutical Nanotechnology (RCPN), Tabriz University of Medical Sciences, Tabriz 5165691749, Iran

Nasrin Maleki-Dizaji
Department of Pharmacology and Toxicology, School of Pharmacy, Tabriz University of Medical Sciences, Tabriz 5165665931, Iran
Drug Applied Research Center (DARC), Tabriz University of Medical Sciences, Tabriz 5165665811, Iran

Masoud Pezeshkian
Department of Cardiac Surgery and Cardiovascular Research Center, School of Medicine, Tabriz University of Medical Sciences, Tabriz 5166615573, Iran

Homayon Sadeghi-Bazargani
Department of Statistics and Epidemiology, School of Health and Nutrition, Tabriz University of Medical Sciences, Tabriz 5166614711, Iran

Masoud Darabi
Department of Biochemistry and Clinical Laboratories, School of Medicine, Tabriz University of Medical Sciences, Tabriz 5166615731, Iran

Sara Mostafalou
Department of Toxicology, Pharmaceutical Sciences Research Center (PSRC) and School of Pharmacy, Tehran University of Medical Sciences, Tehran 141556451, Iran

Shahab Bohlooli
Department of Pharmacology and Physiology, School of Medicine, Ardabil University of Medical Sciences, Ardabil 56135665, Iran

Alireza Garjani
Department of Pharmacology and Toxicology, School of Pharmacy, Tabriz University of Medical Sciences, Tabriz 5165665931, Iran
Research Center for Pharmaceutical Nanotechnology (RCPN), Tabriz University of Medical Sciences, Tabriz 5165691749, Iran
Drug Applied Research Center (DARC), Tabriz University of Medical Sciences, Tabriz 5165665811, Iran

SayedeMaryam Naghibi, Mahmoud Hosseini, Fatemeh Khani, Motahare Rahimi and Farzaneh Vafaee
Neuroscience Research Center and Department of Physiology, School of Medicine, Mashhad University of Medical Sciences, Mashhad, Iran

Hassan Rakhshandeh and Azita Aghaie
Pharmacological Research Center of Medicinal Plants
and Department of Pharmacology, School of Medicine,
Mashhad University of Medical Sciences, Mashhad
9177948564, Iran

**Vaishali D. Shewale,Tushar A. Deshmukh and Vijay
R. Patil**
Tapi Valley Education Society, Hon'ble, Loksevak
Madhukarrao Chaudhari College of Pharmacy, Faizpur
425 503, India
Department of Pharmacognosy, Hon'ble, Loksevak
Madhukarrao Chaudhari College of Pharmacy, Faizpur
425 503, Maharashtra, India

Liladhar S. Patil
Tapi Valley Education Society, Hon'ble, Loksevak
Madhukarrao Chaudhari College of Pharmacy, Faizpur
425 503, India
Department of Biotechnology, Hon'ble, Loksevak
Madhukarrao Chaudhari College of Pharmacy, Faizpur
425 503, Maharashtra, India

Andrew N. Clarkson
Departments of Anatomy and Psychology, University of
Otago, P.O. Box 913, Dunedin 9013, New Zealand

Christiaan H. Vinkers
Division of Pharmacology, Utrecht Institute for
Pharmaceutical Sciences and Rudolf Magnus Institute of
Neuroscience, Utrecht University, Universiteitsweg 99,
3584CG Utrecht, The Netherlands
Department of Psychiatry, Rudolf Magnus Institute
of Neuroscience, University Medical Center Utrecht,
Utrecht, The Netherlands

Berend Olivier
Division of Pharmacology, Utrecht Institute for
Pharmaceutical Sciences and Rudolf Magnus Institute of
Neuroscience, Utrecht University, Universiteitsweg 99,
3584CG Utrecht, The Netherlands
Department of Psychiatry, Yale University School of
Medicine, New Haven, CT, USA

**Azza A. K. El-Sheikh, Mohamed A.Morsy, Marwa
M.Mahmoud and Aly M. Abdelrahman**
Department of Pharmacology, Faculty of Medicine, Minia
University, 61511 El-Minia, Egypt

Rehab A. Rifaai
Department of Histology, Faculty of Medicine, Minia
University, 61511 El-Minia, Egypt